Community Health in
the 21st Century

Second Edition

Related Benjamin Cummings Health Titles

Anspaugh/Ezell, *Teaching Today's Health,* Sixth Edition (2001)

Barr, *Introduction to U.S. Health Policy* (2002)

Buckingham, *A Primer on International Health* (2001)

Cottrell/Girvan/McKenzie, *Principles & Foundations of Health Promotion and Education,* Second Edition (2002)

Donatelle, *Access to Health,* Seventh Edition (2002)

Donatelle, *Health: The Basics,* Fourth Edition (2001)

Donnelly, Eburne, Kittleson, *Mental Health: Dimensions of Self-Esteem and Emotional Well-Being* (2001)

Girdano/Dusek/Everly, *Controlling Stress and Tension,* Sixth Edition (2001)

Karren/Hafen/Smith/Frandsen, *Mind/Body Health,* Second Edition (2002)

McKenzie/Smeltzer, *Planning, Implementing, and Evaluating Health Promotion Programs: A Primer,* Third Edition (2001)

Neutens/Rubinson, *Research Techniques for the Health Sciences,* Third Edition (2002)

Seaward, *Health of the Human Spirit: Spiritual Dimensions for Personal Health and Well-Being* (2001)

Skinner, *Promoting Health through Organizational Change* (2002)

Check out these and other Benjamin Cummings health titles at: www.aw.com/bc.

Community Health in the 21st Century

Second Edition

Patricia A. Reagan
University of Utah

Jodi Brookins-Fisher
Central Michigan University

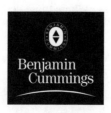

Benjamin
Cummings

San Francisco   Boston   New York
Cape Town   Hong Kong   London   Madris   Mexico City
Montreal   Munich   Paris   Singapore   Sydney   Tokyo   Toronto

Publisher: Daryl Fox
Acquisitions Editor: Deirdre McGill
Project Editor: Susan Teahan
Publishing Assistant: Michelle Cadden
Managing Editor, Production: Wendy Earl
Production Editor: Leslie Austin
Text and Cover Design: Brad Greene
Copy Editor and Proofreader: Martha Ghent
Compositors: Cecelia Morales and Brad Greene
Illustrations: Karl Miyajima
Indexer: Sylvia Coates
Manufacturing Buyer: Stacey Weinberger
Marketing Manager: Sandra Lindelof
Cover Photograph: David Bradford

Photo Credits
p. 39, Corbis; p. 47, Joe Imel/AP/Wide World Photos; p. 55, F. Hoffmann/The Image-
Works; p. 57, Robert Harbison; p. 84, Robert Harbison; p. 91, Reuters/Corbis/Bettmann;
p. 109, AP/Wide World; p. 258, Ruth Fremson/AP/Wide World Photos; p. 277, Robert
Harbison; p. 312, Robert Harbison; p. 338, Robert Harbison; p. 439, Robert Harbison;
p. 478, Will Faller; All other photos supplied by the authors.

Library of Congress Cataloging-in-Publication Data

Reagan, Patricia A.
  Community health in the 21st Century / Patricia A. Reagan, Jodi Brookins-Fisher.--
2nd ed.
    p. cm.
  Includes bibliographical references and index.
  ISBN 0-205-34281-7 (pbk. : alk. paper)
  1. World health. 2. Public health. I. Title: Community health in the twenty-first
century. II. Brookins-Fisher, Jodi. III. Title.

RA441 .R43 2002
362.1'09'05--dc21

                            2001047344

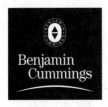

ISBN 0-205-34281-7

13 14 15 16 17 — HPC — 12 11 10 09

www.aw.com/bc

CONTENTS

Continued

v

Continued

Continued

PREFACE

This text is designed to introduce students to the broad, challenging, controversial, academic discipline and profession of community health education. While previous community health education textbooks have done a good job of introducing students to the facts and realities of the health problems associated with communities, they have generally failed to address the social/political reasons why many community health problems continue to exist.

Community Health in the 21st Century goes beyond the data accumulated from many government, volunteer, and academic sources. It dares to ask students to think critically about the difficult decisions faced by those who finance health care services, education, and legislation and to look at the implications of those decisions.

This textbook also looks at communities and their health status in the United States as part of a global community. In the twenty-first century, epidemics, environmental threats, political upheaval, and the status of women and other minorities will not be provincial issues. An epidemic in Zaire becomes a potential epidemic in Washington, D.C. as tourists, governmental officials, business representatives, and immigrants easily and quickly travel beyond borders. When people with HIV are discriminated against in China or Russia, the impact is felt right here at home, where many people living with HIV/AIDS are still active participants in international travel and work. Oil spills, radioactive waste accidents, civil war, famine, epidemics, and discrimination on the basis of race, class, gender, sexual orientation, physical and mental abilities, and health status all magnify beyond their origin and affect all of us. This textbook asks the reader to think in global terms as one looks into her or his own community and identifies the potential health concerns that exist there.

Community health in the twenty-first century must include advocacy, compassion, and open-mindedness toward social issues and culturally unique issues, once thought to be the purview of other disciplines such as sociology, criminology, social work, and law. One cannot look forward without looking back, critiquing past interventions and programs and determining what has worked and what has failed. This text strives to provide the insight and perspectives of a variety of social and political ideologies.

Special Features

Throughout this text, the authors have included short quotes from community health educators from all parts of the country who are actually putting knowledge into practice. The individual reflections about the twenty-first century introduce the reader to the different professions of people working in the field, and the many academic degrees that make up the community health profession. In addition, the following special features reflect the authors' desire to incorporate a realistic view of community health today and in the future and to provide useful learning aids that will assist in the comprehension of material.

- People are recognized as the most important part of community health issues. Special populations are incorporated throughout the text to provide a global and holistic perspective.

- Valuable tools, such as Internet information and addresses, prevention ideas, and related organizations, provide excellent resources for students.

- Chapter Objectives, Summaries, Cybersites with World Wide Web addresses, questions, exercises, and notes in every chapter help students understand and apply the chapter content.

- Informational boxes in every chapter present interesting and current data.

- In-chapter discussion questions and politically and socially conscious exercises in each chapter allow for critical thinking and provide discussion about one's own community issues.

- Special emphasis on environmental health issues illustrates the relationship between humans and their environment and prepares community health educators to be observant and knowledgeable (Chapters 18–21).

In the twenty-first century the community health educator will rely heavily on data that are accessible through Internet sources. Most assessment, demographic, morbidity, mortality, and vital statistics data that will be used may be found on web sites managed by government agencies, private health organizations, and volunteer agencies. Many of these sites will have search engines that have the capability to search out the most recent data and present it in the form of tables and charts. Many sites will also have the most recent documentation of surveys with results and analysis available for use in program planning, grant writing, and evaluation endeavors.

Each chapter in this text provides a hands-on experience for the student to learn how to use the Internet data search engines currently available. The exercise will give an example of how to use the site, direct URL addresses, and give an experience that will walk the student through a simple analysis of a question related to the chapter just studied.

The authors encourage students to go beyond assigned exercises and dig deeply into the myriad of resources available through each web site. The more familiar the community health educator is with services available through the Internet, the more efficient and successful will be the work in one's community.

Acknowledgments

The authors would like to thank the following reviewers for their input: Sheila Parker, University of Arizona; Linda Jackson, University of Maryland; Hollis Matsen, San Francisco State University; Silvea Thomas, Kingsborough Community College; Carol Mikanowicz, Youngstown State University; Eva Allen, University of Southern California at Sumter; and Kerry Redican, Virginia Polytechnical University.

Section I

A Framework for Community Health

Chapters 1 through 5 look at the history, administration, global demographics, and the science of community health. They provide the framework upon which the prevention of health risks and the promotion of healthy living is made in the United States. At the end of each chapter throughout this text, the reader will find some Internet sites that may enhance and update the information in the chapter.

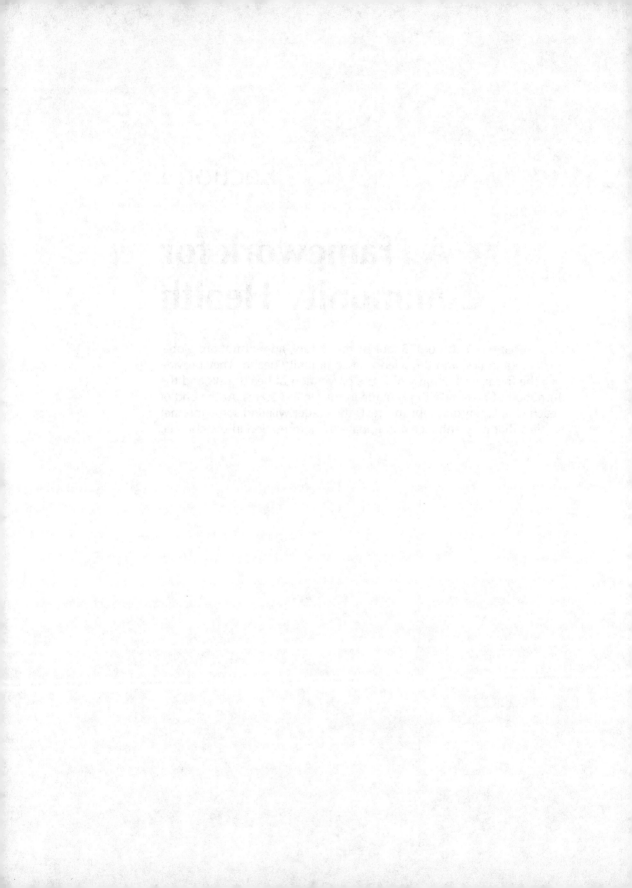

CHAPTER 1

An Introduction to Community Health

Community Health in the 21st Century
Early in the 21st century the major challenge will be in using the present
and future technology to health educate the public. Advances in technology
will allow opportunities for individualized educational programming as
well as educating the population at large. It will be very important that
community health educators be grounded in the art of the electronic com-
munication and methodology.

—Loren Bensley, Ed.D.
Health Promotion and Rehabilitation

Chapter Objectives

The student will:

1. understand that he or she are part of a global community and the health of one nation or people affects the planet as a whole.

2. recognize that community health is dynamic, political, and controversial. To face community health issues one must define a community as diverse, with many views, beliefs, values and concerns.

3. realize that community health issues change as problems are solved and new issues arise. Just because an issue appears to be solved, it may reemerge tomorrow.

4. be able to identify the priority areas for the Healthy People 2010 objectives, their modifiable risk factors and trends from 1990 to 2010.

5. list the educational skills, roles, responsibilities, and credentialing criteria of community health educators.

6. identify the political and ethical responsibilities of community health educators.

The Global Nature of Community Health

It is not news that most Americans are at risk for one of the major killers: cardiovascular disease, cancer, stroke, or accidents. What is becoming more apparent and equally distressing is that communities and the environment are also at risk for major chronic, acute, disabling, and terminal illnesses such as

HIV/AIDS, loss of the ozone layer, water pollution, and homelessness. Community health has always included the goal of making communities, as entities, healthier. Unlike the community health problems of the past, however, which were often managed by individual towns or geographical communities, the cost of community health is now a *global* responsibility. Efforts at solving problems require the multidisciplinary approach of theorists and clinicians, administrators and legislators, academics and bureaucrats. No longer can problem solving be focused on one issue at a time or approached through one solution. The complexity of health problems requires looking at the interaction of a variety of systems that overlap and are dependent upon each other. When change occurs in one context, a myriad of effects within other systems must be adjusted or accommodated. The health of people and the environment has become a very sophisticated, complex discipline. Most important to remember is that where we live, who we are, how we live, what we believe, our social and political environment, and our personal and professional interactions influence personal and community health. Lifestyle is the number one contributor to our health (50 percent), followed by our genetic inheritance (20 percent), the environment (20 percent) and finally medical interventions (10 percent). (Figure 1.1)

Throughout this text, the environment will be woven into many aspects of community health. It is the authors' belief that global/environmental concerns cannot be separated from human health concerns. They are interconnected. We, as humans, cannot forget our place on this planet Earth, nor how our own actions affect the planet, which in turn, affects our health. Schaffer and Anundsen (1993) sum up these beliefs succinctly: "Just as we need to reconnect in new ways with family, neighbors, co-workers, and those different from us if we are to survive as a species, we also need to develop a new relationship with the earth and its diverse species if we are to survive as a planetary community."[1] Each community health issue ties into a larger community health issue, which to some degree ties into a planetary community health issue.

What Is Community Health?

In its simplest form, community health involves identifying and finding solutions to health problems of a specific "community." More profoundly, community health is a field of practice encompassing and coordinating at the local level the overlapping aspects of school health, public health, employee health, maternal and child health, environmental health protection, and the personal health practices of individuals and families.[2] Community is a key concept because a health concern involves a specific group of people within certain parameters.

A community may be the city of Des Moines, Iowa; it may be a small ethnic neighborhood within Boston; it may be all fifty-year-old, male Native Americans living on a Navajo reservation in New Mexico; or it may be a group of people with a similar agenda who call themselves a community. As you can see, a community becomes special given how it defines itself or is defined. Its unique quality may be that of race, ethnicity, age, orientation, beliefs, occupation, political agenda, economic status, religion, rural or urban housing, com-

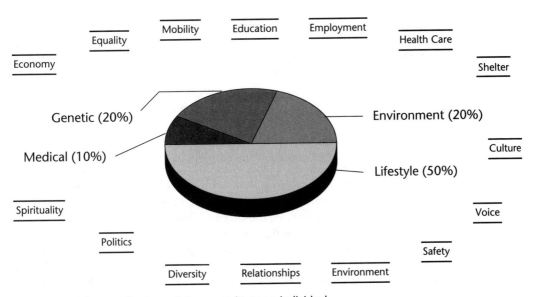

Figure 1.1 The contributions of a community to an individual.

mon language, physical ability, or some other quality that draws any group of people into a common bond. It is the common bond of a community, regardless of size or number of people, that at some particular moment in time becomes defined as a "community" whose unique health issue becomes the focus of the field of practice called community health.

Another interesting description of community defines it as a "dynamic whole that emerges when a group of people participate in common practices, depend on one another, make decisions together, identify themselves as part of something larger than the sum of their individual relationships, and commit themselves for the long term to their own, one another's, and the group's well-being."[3] As further stated, the chief characteristic of a community is commitment; and true commitment requires trust, honesty, compassion, and respect of all the members. Certainly, the more we understand the community in which we are working, the more effective we will be in dealing with community health issues.

Community or Public Health?

In the nineteenth century, the United States, even the world, was a society of "island communities" with considerable economic and political autonomy.[4] This is no longer the case. We are all part of the whole. This text will use the term public health as often as community health because the public is the product of many communities of diverse people whose interests and needs usually overlap when we look at issues of health. Within our public are religious, political, sexual orientations; genderized, geographical, and socioeconomically dispersed persons; and socially differentiated communities. Each has its own unique health risks and needs. However, each is part of public concern and welfare.

Commonly, public health is thought of as the sum of all official (governmental) agencies and efforts to promote, protect, and preserve the health of people whom these agencies serve. Public health is most often defined as such because of the governmental and tax implications associated with promoting and protecting health, while community health is much broader, including volunteer agencies, private programs, and individual citizens. Truly, community health requires the cooperation and integration of the public and the private sectors. Therefore, it is often difficult to distinguish the health efforts of protection and promotion as being exclusively public health or community health.

The public nature of the global community includes all species, all subgroups, and all institutions. There are few problems found to be so isolated and so private as to be contained within any defined community, not crossing outside community parameters. Public or community awareness, attention, and intervention are usually better than isolated attempts at health promotion. Public and community health means working together to help people help themselves, not to merely survive, but to achieve their maximum potential. It requires the integrated knowledge, dedication, and skills of nursing, medicine, social work, nutrition, and engineering professionals, and also professional health educators, environmentalists, feminists, educators, consumers, and other interested community members.

Community and public health's approach to addressing health problems in a community has been described as a five-step process:

1. Define the health problem.
2. Identify the risk factors associated with the problem.
3. Develop and test community-level interventions to control or prevent the cause of the problem.
4. Implement interventions to improve the health of the population.
5. Monitor those interventions to assess their effectiveness.

Essentially, the main task of community and public health is prevention of health problems through interventions, and the mobilization of a community to minimize or treat an immediate health problem. The ten great pubic health achievements of the twentieth century are found in Box 1.1.

What Are the Latest Community Health Issues?

This is a noble question of an inquisitive community health professional-to-be, but one that is difficult to answer. Remember, each community has its own unique health concerns. Also, many of these local problems are becoming national, and even worldwide concerns (again the link to public health). Professionals in the field would probably differ over the ranking of important community health issues today, depending on where and with whom they work. Many, however, would probably agree that virtually all health issues must receive attention from a variety of professionals and disciplines within the community if we want to adequately address quality of life through a healthy environment.

BOX 1.1 Ten Great Public Health Achievements—United States, 1900–1999, as Determined by the CDC

- Vaccination
- Motor-vehicle safety
- Safer workplaces
- Control of infectious diseases
- Decline in deaths from coronary heart disease and stroke

- Safer and healthier foods
- Healthier mothers and babies
- Family planning
- Fluoridation of drinking water
- Recognition of tobacco use as a health hazard

Two community health issues to highlight are HIV disease and violence. Both are having tremendous detrimental impact on communities, and both have received nationwide attention, no matter where you might reside. Some no longer view HIV disease as an epidemic.[5] That does not mean it is no longer a health issue; quite the contrary. HIV disease is now endemic (common) in every community in the United States and on the planet. Each community must have its own action plan to prevent this disease from infecting and affecting more people. Even within a geographical community there will need to be different action plans for groups of people within that larger community. For example, the injection drug using population needs different prevention programs than the adolescent high school population, although both are at risk for HIV infection.

Violence is another national concern which with specific community implications. First of all, violence needs to be defined by each community. Is it gangs we are concerned with or domestic violence? Child abuse or gay bashing? Once we understand which type of violence is permeating our community (or which one we will deal with first), we need to design a prevention/intervention plan. A gang prevention program for Saginaw, Michigan, will not necessarily be effective in Omaha, Nebraska. As an aspiring community health professional, you see the point. It all comes back to our definition of a particular community. What we do for prevention of health problems will depend on the community structure.

In January 2000 an immediate national community health concern was the flu epidemic. This health crisis was preceded the previous year by the devastating hurricanes in the southeastern part of the United States. Often, ongoing community health efforts associated with chronic health issues must be set aside to address very immediate health problems: outbreaks of food poisoning, contaminated water, natural disasters, severe accidents, infectious disease outbreaks in schools. There is seldom a time when one can adequately state with confidence what the most immediate and most important community health issues are or will be. Every day brings new challenges and new threats to the health of a community.

The year 2000 has brought a renewed appreciation for community health. While the political climate and lobbying efforts of big business, the military, or private organizations often affect the financial and community commitment to prevention and surveillance of health hazards, the end of the 1990s began to address the very significant importance of clean water, air, and food products. There was a renewed emphasis on violence as a result of school tragedies, prevention of youth smoking, protection from sexually transmitted diseases, and greater concern on preventable infectious disease. The twenty-first century appears to hold a similar commitment to health promotion through community, public and personal health initiatives. Perhaps the current understanding of the importance of prevention and risk reduction can be summed up with this play on a popular bumper sticker: "If you think prevention is expensive, wait until you see disease."

A Focus on Prevention

There has been a movement in community health, as well as health care in general, toward prevention. This involves developing programs, curricula, campaigns, and activities to prevent a community health problem from developing in the first place. Prevention is a healthier, cheaper way to address any health issue than intervention or treatment. Throughout the text, prevention programs across the United States will be highlighted in individual chapters. Prevention has been a goal at the national level as well. One such national effort to establish prevention guidelines has been through the Healthy People 2000 objectives for the nation.

Healthy People 2010

In the 1970s the United States Public Health Service laid the foundations for a national health campaign called **Healthy People 2000**, with the first Surgeon General's *Report On Health Promotion And Disease Prevention* (Box 1.2). The 1980

BOX 1.2 *Healthy People 2000 Primary Objectives by Age Group*

1. Improve infant health, and by 1990, reduce infant mortality by at least 35 percent to fewer than 9 per 1,000. Special focus is on low birth weight and birth defects.

2. Improve child health, and by 1990, reduce death among those 1 to 14 years by at least 20 percent to fewer than 34 per 100,000. Special focus is on growth, development, and injuries.

3. Improve health and habits of adolescent aged 15 to 24 to reduce death by at least 20 percent to fewer than 93 per

100,000. Special focus is on motor vehicle accidents, alcohol, and drugs.

4. Improve health of adults between 15 and 64 years by at least 25 percent to fewer than 400 per 100,000. Special focus is on heart attacks, strokes, and cancer.

5. Improve health and quality of life for older adults to reduce the average annual number of days of restricted activity due to acute and chronic conditions by 20 percent to fewer than 30 days per year for people over 65 years. Special focus is on functional independence, influenza, and pneumonia.[6]

Table 1.1   Modifiable risk factors for leading causes of death.

Cause of Death	Modifiable Risk Factors
Heart disease	Smoking, high blood-pressure, high blood cholesterol, physical inactivity, diabetes, overweight, stress
Cancer	Smoking, diets high in fats, diets low in fruits/vegetables and grains, worksite carcinogens, environmental carcinogens, alcohol
Stroke	High blood pressure, smoking, high blood-cholesterol, stress
Motor-vehicle injuries	Alcohol, no seat belts, speed, roadway design
Other accidents	Alcohol, drug abuse, smoking (fires), product design, handgun availability
Chronic lung disease	Smoking, worksite exposures
Homicide	Handgun availability, alcohol, drug abuse, stress
Suicide	Stress, alcohol, drug abuse
Cirrhosis of liver	Alcohol, possible nutrient deficiencies
Influenza/pneumonia	Smoking
Diabetes	Obesity

(*Source:* McGinnis, J. M. et. al (1991). In *Oxford textbook of public health,* Vol. 2, p. 127. Used by permission of Oxford University Press)

publication *Promoting Health/Preventing Disease: Objectives for the Nation* committed the United States to disease prevention and health promotion strategies for substantially changing the patterns of death, disease, and disability in the population by the year 1990. Table 1.1 describes the modifiable risk factors thought to contribute to virtually every one of the ten leading causes of death and disability.[7] It will not come as a surprise that stopping smoking and reducing alcohol use would decrease almost every cause of death. The process of setting objectives was based on these risk factors and created the three broad working categories for 1990: (1) preventive health services for individuals, (2) health protection for population groups, and (3) health promotion for population groups.

Twenty-two priority areas, as listed in Table 1.2, were also identified and grouped into four categories: (1) health promotion, (2) health protection, (3) preventive services, and (4) surveillance and data systems.

Given the many goals and objectives of this important plan, it was clear from the outset that achieving the original 1990 targets would require a national, integrated effort of health care delivery systems, health organizations, academics, insurers, employers, and consumer groups as well as federal, state, and local governments. Such cooperation was not always found in the 1980s, however; in 1980, 226 specific and measurable disease prevention objectives for the nation, to be achieved by 1990, were published in a landmark document, *Promoting Health/Preventing Disease: Objectives for the Nation.*[8] McGinnis (1991) stated that attaining the 1990 objectives depended upon successful implementation at the state and local level.

By 1987, a Public Health Foundation study of health departments in all fifty states, the District of Columbia, and the four U.S. territories found that 84

Table 1.2   Healthy People 2000 priority areas.

Health Promotion	Preventive Services
1. Physical activity and fitness	14. Maternal and infant health
2. Nutrition	15. Heart disease and stroke
3. Tobacco	16. Cancer
4. Alcohol and other drugs	17. Diabetes and chronic disabling conditions
5. Family planning	18. HIV infection
6. Mental health and mental disorders	19. Sexually transmitted diseases
7. Violent and abusive behavior	20. Immunization and infectious diseases
8. Educational and community-based programs	21. Clinical preventive services
Health Protection	**Surveillance and Data Systems**
9. Unintentional injuries	22. Surveillance and data systems
10. Occupational safety and health	**Age-Related Objectives**
11. Environmental health	Children
12. Food and drug safety	Adolescents and young adults
13. Oral health	Adults
	Older adults

(*Source:* U.S. Dept. of HHS. PHS, *Healthy People 2000: National Health Promotion and Disease Prevention Objectives,* Full Report. DHHS Pub. No. 91-5212. Washington, DC: USGPO, 1991)

percent surveyed had established health objectives. Further, forty states had established centralized units within the state to promote and coordinate disease prevention/health promotion activities. Legislation to implement such activities had been introduced in about two-thirds of the states by 1985.

A 1985 mid-course review (Figure 1.2) revealed that the United States had made substantial progress toward the original four age group specific mortality goals established in 1979. Approximately half of the 226 specific objectives had either been achieved at midpoint or were on course. By 1985, 13 percent of the 1990 objectives had already been accomplished. Just over 26 percent were unlikely to be achieved, and data were lacking on the remaining 26 percent of the objectives. Trends were in the wrong direction for less than 4 percent of the objectives.[9]

As 1990 came and went, it became necessary to set new goals and objectives for the year 2000. In the 1990s, Healthy People 2000 defined three broad goals: to increase the span of healthy life; to reduce health disparities; and to achieve access to preventive services for all U.S. citizens. The objectives are organized into twenty-two priority areas with about 300 unduplicated main objectives. Subobjectives for minorities and other special populations were also established to meet unique needs and health problems. These populations include low income people, members of some racial and ethnic minority groups, and people

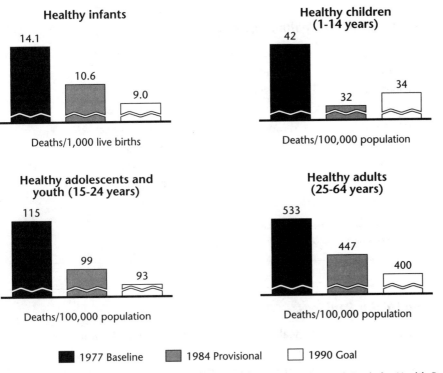

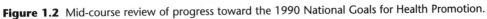

Figure 1.2 Mid-course review of progress toward the 1990 National Goals for Health Promotion.

with disabilities. It is of some concern to community health that sexual orientation has yet to be included among the target population objectives.

> *Discussion:* As you continue through this book, you may want to compare the national objectives with goals and objectives that have been set by your state health departments. Your state health department will send you its Healthy People 2010 objectives by request. Start that comparison by reading Box 1.3 and Box 1.4 and see if your state is ranked healthy or unhealthy.

The beginning of the twenty-first century introduced the nation to the proposed Healthy People 2010: National Health Promotion and Disease Prevention Objectives (Figure 1.3). Healthy People 2010 has been revised through the input and interaction of many national forums. The new plan will include greater emphasis on public and professional participation, an increase in priority areas, concern for special populations, and the increased use of statistical models to assist in establishing meaningful numerical targets.[10] The 2010 plan also looks at projections in the coming years that include an increase in population size, an increase in median age and older Americans as a cohort, changes

BOX 1.3 State Health Rankings, 2000

Healthiest States	Most Improved	Worst Health
New Hampshire	Arkansas	Mississippi
Minnesota	Delaware	Louisiana
Hawaii	Hawaii	South Carolina
Utah	Montana	West Virginia
Massachusetts	South Dakota	Nevada
Vermont		Arkansas
Colorado		Alabama
Wisconsin		Florida

(*Source:* Adapted from Health Care State Rankings, 2000
www.unitedhealthgroup.com/sr2000/overallrank.html)

BOX 1.4 State Health Rankings, 2000

Health Component	Most Healthy	Least Healthy
Prevalence of smoking	Utah/Hawaii	Kentucky/Nevada
Motor vehicle deaths	Massachusetts/Connecticut	Alabama/Mississippi
Violent crime	North Dakota/Vermont	Florida/New Mexico
Heart disease	Utah/Hawaii	Mississippi/West Virginia
Unemployment	Iowa/New Hampshire	West Virginia/Alaska
Prenatal care	Rhode Island/New Hampshire	New Mexico/Utah
Primary care	Hawaii	Mississippi
Occupational safety	Massachusetts/Arizona	Montana/Wyoming
Infant mortality	Minnesota/New Hampshire	Mississippi/Alabama
Lack health insurance	Nebraska/Iowa	Texas/Arizona
Total mortality	Hawaii/North Dakota	West Virginia/Kentucky

(*Source:* Adapted from Health Care State Rankings, 2000
www.unitedhealthgroup.com/sr2000/components/mortality/total.html)

in racial and ethnic compositions with increases in Hispanic, African American, Asian, and Pacific Islander populations, and a decrease in the white population. There is concern that communicable diseases may increase as pathogens become antibiotic resistant, and new issues such as road rage, and even computer rage, may pose new challenges to community health.

Healthy People 2010 Framework

Vision of 2010:
Healthy People in Healthy Communities

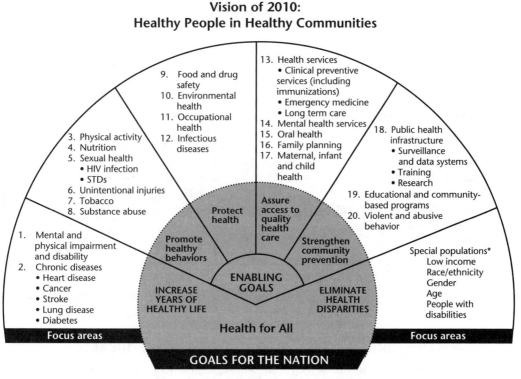

* Special population groups need to be considered as objectives are developed in all focus areas.

Figure 1.3 Healthy People 2010: Goals for the Nation.
(*Source:* U.S. Department of Human Services (1997), *Developing Objectives for Healthy People 2000*)

The 2010 plan has a "broadened prevention science base; improved surveillance and data systems; a heightened awareness and demand for preventive health services and quality health care; and changes in demographics, science, technology, and disease spread."[11] The proposed goals for 2010 are to (1) increase quality and years of life; and (2) eliminate health disparities by race, education, disability, geography, or sexual orientation. The goals will be monitored through 467 objectives and the twenty-eight focus areas given in Box 1.5.

The objectives of Healthy People 2010 are classified according to health status, risk reduction, public awareness, professional education and awareness, and service and protection. While significant improvements have been made in the nation's health over the past decade, gains have not been universal. Therefore, many of the year 2010 objectives focus upon specific populations that have a higher risk of disease or disability compared to the total population.

BOX 1.5 Health People 2010 Focus Areas

 1. Access to Quality Health Services
 2. Arthritis, Osteoporosis, Chronic Back
    Conditions
 3. Cancer
 4. Chronic Kidney Disease
 5. Diabetes
 6. Disability and Secondary Conditions
 7. Educational and Community-Based
    Programs
 8. Environmental Health
 9. Family Planning
10. Food Safety
11. Health Communication
12. Heart Disease and Stroke
13. HIV

14. Immunization and Infectious Diseases
15. Injury and Violence Prevention
16. Maternal, Infant, and Child Health
17. Medical Product Safety
18. Mental Health and Mental Disorders
19. Nutrition and Overweight
20. Occupational Safety and Health
21. Oral Health
22. Physical Activity and Fitness
23. Public Health Infrastructure
24. Respiratory Diseases
25. Sexually Transmitted Diseases
26. Substance Abuse
27. Tobacco Use
28. Vision and Hearing

Throughout this text the **Healthy People 2000** or **2010 Objectives** will appear in boxes in each chapter.

The Roles of the Community Health Educator

While the school health educator addresses the health problems associated with individuals and groups within school systems, the community health educator is primarily concerned with the health of a community and the groups within that community. His or her role is to "elicit, facilitate, and maintain positive health practices by assuring that people have the skills and support needed for their voluntary adoption of activities conducive to their health."[12]

The community health educator is a generalist; an applied scientist and educator who uses the knowledge and skills of the natural, behavioral, health, and environmental sciences to prevent disease and injury and to promote human well-being in the context of the global environmental community.[13] This community health practitioner basically combines the tasks of many professionals employed in communities and adds the broader skills and interests of an educator. Depending upon the agency in which one works, the responsibilities of a community health educator are diverse. Community health educators start at their desk, planning, but they spend a great deal of time talking with groups, visiting organizations, conducting workshops, evaluating programs, lobbying legislatures, interviewing with media, counseling clients, or attending conferences and workshops. Depending on how public and community health tasks are delineated in any state, the tasks and roles of the community health educator may be:

- Making inspections of restaurants, nursing homes, playgrounds
- Conducting special studies of at-risk populations
- Sampling air, water, and food
- Reviewing plans for health curriculum and promotion projects
- Acting as an educator and public relations officer
- Community organizing for volunteer agencies
- Planning programs for youth, older Americans, special interest groups
- Acting as a consultant to civic groups, business, industry, and individuals
- Enforcing environmental and public health laws
- Conducting evaluations of program outcomes
- Advocating for target populations with which he or she works

Among the areas he or she may be involved in are:

- Personal health assessment
- Accident prevention
- Air pollution control
- Communicable disease prevention/control
- Environmental emergencies
- Food processing and food handling
- Outbreaks of foodborne and waterborne infections
- Hazardous substances control
- Housing
- Indoor environment standards
- Vector control
- Minority population advocacy
- School health issues
- Migrant labor camp inspections and education
- Noise control and abatement
- Home health care
- Occupational health and safety
- Consumer product safety
- Radiation control
- Public nursing clinics
- Public and private sewage
- Chronic disease prevention/control
- Health education and health promotion
- Water pollution control

- Promotion of risk reduction behaviors
- Assessment of health status

General competencies and academic preparation of this new twenty-first century community health educator are:

- Computer competency
- Ability to surf the net and use databases
- Chemistry
- Biology
- Microbiology
- Math
- Physics
- Marketing
- Foreign language
- Epidemiology
- Risk assessment
- Communication techniques
- Facilitating groups
- Program planning and evaluation
- Educational methods
- Presentation skills
- Knowledge of public health laws and regulations
- Relationships with local, state, and federal agencies
- Relationships with health departments, business, industry, voluntary agencies, and public agencies
- Cultural awareness/sensitivity
- Health education

Professional attitudes are also important in the community health educator. He or she should be:

- People oriented
- Politically active
- Dedicated to the environment
- A promoter of diversity and equity
- A promoter of individual and public welfare
- Aware of his or her own "isms"
- Ethical

Sadly, it has taken decades to raise the consciousness of a nation about the health risks of unhealthy lifestyle behaviors. Now, community health education becomes even more complex as we must also take on the health risks of neglect, racism, sexism, ageism, classism, heterosexism, and homophobia. Community health practitioners should also be advocates for the environment and work by all means possible to prevent the exacerbation of risks that threaten our planet.

Who Are Community Health Educators?

Community health educators are as diverse as the discipline itself. Although one may obtain a degree in community health or related disciplines such as public health, health education, health science, or health promotion; many working in the field come from different professions. For example, nurses are often community health educators. In hospitals, clinics, schools, or homes they often give information to help their clients obtain or maintain healthier lifestyles. Physicians and physician assistants may also educate in many of the same ways. Those working in environmental fields educate by instructing the public in areas ranging from how to prevent lead poisoning to information on the damaging effects of automobile emissions. Community health educators may be as formal as an instructor in a classroom or as informal as a marcher in a parade on women's reproductive health concerns. However, since our nation is not the healthiest, it requires those specifically trained to lead the way toward optimal health. In academic programs specifically targeted at graduating community health professionals, many of the skills previously listed should be taught.

Community Health Education Specialist (C.H.E.S)

With the demand for personal and community healthful living, the need for professionals skilled in the knowledge of health information, program planning, program implementation, marketing, evaluation, statistical analysis, and health teaching has grown proportionately. Today, professional, personal, and community health educators are one of the important links from the medical community to the lay community, from the classroom to the boardroom, from the city to the country. The new focus on prevention has been promoted by insurance companies, businesses, the medical profession, and the Commission On Health Care Reform. Such a commitment to health promotion formalizes and encourages the role of health educators in seeking the goal of improving the health of the nation and reducing health care costs. It has been a major shift for health education to move from a focus on shaping individual behavior to a community-focused effort supporting changes in policies and legislation.[14]

The Joint Committee on Health Education Terminology defines **health education** as the "continuum of learning which enables people, as individuals and as members of social structures, to voluntarily make decisions, modify behaviors and change social conditions in ways which are health enhancing."[15]

Health educators have taken to the front lines of local, state, and private agencies; public schools and universities; legislative committees; conservative and liberal health-related organizations. They have demonstrated measurable leadership in the promotion of personal, community, and environmental health.

Many people in the past have been informal health educators although their titles may not have reflected this unique professional role. Medical professionals such as physicians, nurses, and dentists have always promoted healthful behavior on the parts of their clients and patients. Legislatures have enacted health education programs and health and safety laws that protect specific populations. Municipal leaders have passed laws that promote the health and welfare of their unique communities. City and state workers have encouraged community and environmental health promotion by establishing standards of health and safety regulations and programs to assist in the implementation of health programs. Parents, school, and religious teachers are health educators in their everyday teaching of children in matters of personal hygiene, safety, respect for the environment, and self-esteem. The formal role of health education is, however, a specialized discipline that requires the training, practice, and status comparable to other health professions.

The professional health educator receives at least an undergraduate degree with specialized training. The science of assessing health needs, reducing risky behavior, promoting healthful behaviors, administering health promotion programs, evaluating such programs, and serving as a community resource for a myriad of personal and community health issues has become a rigorous curriculum with practical as well as theoretical training. In 1978, the Role Delineation Project created a standardized body of knowledge, skills, and competencies required by all entry level health educators. Universities and colleges that award an undergraduate degree in Health Education now may prepare students with a curriculum that covers the necessary competencies required for entry-level health educators who may or may not then certify through national testing as a **Certified Health Education Specialist (C.H.E.S).**

The National Commission for Health Educators Credentialing is an independent, nonprofit national agency established to set guidelines and a framework for development of competency-based curriculum. The commission describes the benefits of being certified within the profession as:

1. Attests to the individual knowledge and skills essential to the field of practice
2. Assists employers to identify qualified practitioners
3. Helps assure consumers of validity of services offered
4. Enhances the profession
5. Recognizes a commitment to professional standards
6. Delineates the scope of the practice
7. Provides recognition to individual health education specialists

In 1985, The National Task Force on the Preparation and Practice of Health Educators delineated seven areas of responsibility as minimal for competency as a health educator:

1. Assessing individual and community needs for health education
2. Planning effective health education programs

3. Implementing health education programs

4. Evaluating the effectiveness of health education programs

5. Coordinating provision of health education services

6. Acting as a resource person in health education

7. Communicating health and health education needs, concerns and resources[16]

Today, public, private, and volunteer agencies acknowledge, recruit, and hire those health educators who have earned credentials through the national process of certification of health educators. The national certification process is based upon the standardization of health education competencies that were developed through collaboration of health education programs and community health educators throughout the country. Annual examinations, much like those given to nurses and social workers, are now conducted for health education specialists from a variety of disciplines. The individual certification and the added awareness of the strengths of certified health education specialists by state and local health education programs should provide a greater incentive to hire and promote health educators who have a broad, comprehensive, nationally recognized curricular background. Uniformity of skills and knowledge will ultimately promote leadership and continued professional recognition within the growing health education field.

Is Community Health Political?

Public and community health education is not without controversy and criticism. Despite positive contributions to the planet, the actual ability to protect all people is at times quite equivocal. From a political point of view, liberals have historically portrayed public health heroically as government intervention to protect the working classes from the worst excesses of industrialization and urbanization. A more radical view of public health is that the unionized working classes, in their confrontation with the business and management classes over many health related issues, often lose maximum protection through industry resistance and government acquiescence to economic concerns.[17] All citizens are right to stress the unbelievable economic cost of escalating health care and tending to the planet. Conservatives often view public and environmental health efforts as extremist, and in fact, contrary to the economic survival of our nation. The conservative voice is one of understandable caution. How can all political positions realize their concerns without compromising our existence? Perhaps the answer is left to new scholars reading this text.

For example, even in the early 1800s, the debate between opposing political positions raged over the need to quarantine ships to protect port cities from disease, which interfered with shipping and the economic interest of trade and growth. Opponents of quarantine argued that disease was internally generated by the filthy conditions of the docks, streets, and alleys that provided an ideal environment for "putrefactive fermentation." Little justification for disrupting commerce seemed legitimate given the lack of knowledge about the etiology of disease, and contradictory evidence suggested no clear victor between opposing viewpoints of how to solve health problems. Health regulations were written and revised more in response to political pressures than to shifts in medical thinking. Quarantine regulations were alternately relaxed in response to pressure from merchants and strengthened under the immediate threat of epidemics.[18]

Can you see the similarity of quarantining debates to current community health issues? AIDS is a present example. Many "experts" debate cause, effect, and solution. Ultimately politicians and those in power determine regulations, such as mandatory testing or quarantine legislation, that are revised or rescinded due to grassroots or professional activism. The question of whether to allow those infected with HIV into the country, despite any medical reason not to, illustrates one of the many issues that impact health.

This text does not claim to be unbiased in how it perceives the state of the planet's health and those who should be improving community health. The authors believe that the planet is in dire need of health improvement and that we all must be involved in addressing the issues that exist. While most problems have no immediate or simple solution, there are some proactive suggestions made. Another important theme in this text is that community health problems have multiple causes. Multifactors cannot easily be simplified into the traditional, balanced paradigm of host, agent, and environment. Underlying many health problems are also the "isms"—racism, ageism, sexism, heterosexism, classism, homophobia. These should not be ignored when searching for cause, effect, or solution.

Many of the historical leaders in the public health movement were social reformers and activists as well as statespeople acting in the public interest. Foremost were Edwin Chadwick, Lemuel Shattuck, Florence Nightingale, Dorthea Dix, Maggie Kuhn, and Margaret Sanger. Today, leadership is also in the hands of untiring reformers: Byllye Avery, Founder of the National Black Women's Health Project; C. Everett Koop, former Surgeon General of the United States; Marian Wright Edelman, Founder and President of the Children's Defense Fund; Mathilde Krim, Founder and Chairperson of the American Foundation for AIDS Research; Larry Kramer, founder of ACT-UP (AIDS Coalition to Unleash Power). Look around your own community. Who are the movers and shakers identified with community health issues? Are they well-paid professionals or grassroots community volunteers? Are they associated with big business or social services? Are you among them? Until the planet and its occupants are healthy, there is room for more leadership at the top. There is room for community health educators and other health professionals to get personally, professionally, and politically involved in reform. Like the above predecessors, community health educators may be the social reformers and activists of the future. In public health, like feminism, "the personal is political."

In the twenty-first century, issues of domestic economy will be addressed side by side with the issues of health and the environment. The year 2000 and forthcoming century provide an amazing opportunity for school health educa-

Community health educators are
usually seen at health fairs promoting
programs to reduce health risks.

tors, environmental health educators, community health educators, and public health educators to make a major contribution to the planet and to society. Jobs in the health arena should increase with an emphasis on health care reform that promotes prevention. Environmental technology should proliferate. The new bioethical and fundamental issues of how to best work with and in our environment add a greater intellectual depth to curriculum and program planning. These are exciting times. This is a teachable moment in our history. It is a time for community health educators to be on the front line of creating situations in which people can become empowered to participate in their own reconceptualization of power, hierarchy, and health as a right, not a privilege.

Public Health Ethics

Like the medical profession, which has a Hippocratic oath to guide it, the public and community health professions have tried to establish a universally accepted set of standards and ethics. The objectives of public health services and of public health information systems are utilitarian. Their overall aim is to attain the maximum good for the maximum number within current resource constraints. This approach departs fundamentally from the ethics of clinical practice where a clinician is expected to act on behalf of her or his patient. It also conflicts with the basic principles of social justice where, in stark and very explicit contrast, one person's life and one person's rights must not be differentiated from another.[19] Unfortunately, in looking at the health of a community, there are often conflicting interests as well as the need to curtail some people's behaviors to protect the greater number. For instance, while the ideal is a home with plumbing and electricity, an individual or family has the right to live in a dwelling without such amenities if other healthful accommodations are made, unless germs may be spread to neighbors, children playing nearby, or even the occupants themselves. For example, the Amish live in such a nontraditional environment. Another departure from public health norms is allowing a child to attend school unimmunized when his or her family's religion—for example, Christian Scientists—does not believe in immunization. Sometimes the threat to other children and school staff must be weighed against the cultural and religious beliefs of citizens. You can see where ethical dilemmas can easily occur and must be settled through compromise, negotiation, and alternative practices.

Obviously, where individual rights and community health are in contrast, conflict can and does occur. The continued battle for abortion rights versus fetal rights, the controversy over mandatory vaccination of school age children versus the religious beliefs of parents, or the right of Parkinson's disease patients to be treated with fetal tissue make public health decisions difficult, challenging, and provocative for those of us who work in the field. As biotechnology expands, ethics for public health grows proportionately. Professional organizations and professional ethicists must begin to anticipate and grapple with the complexities of public health, biomedical advances, and individual rights and responsibilities.

Community health educators have the responsibility to maintain professional demeanor and interaction with those to whom they report and to those whom they serve. Among those qualities considered professional and ethical are confidentiality, dissemination of current data and information, personal and direct interaction with stakeholders, informed consent of subjects who are part of research projects, and one's best attempt to balance privacy with the need to know.

In 1976, the Society for Public Health Education (SOPHE) developed a formalized standard code of ethics to serve as a guide for all health educators:

1. I will accurately represent my capability, education, training, and experience.

2. I will maintain my competence at the highest level through continuing study, training, and research.

3. I will report research findings and practice activities honestly and without distortion.

4. I will not discriminate because of race, color, national origin, religion, age, sex, or socioeconomic status in rendering service, employing, training, or promoting others.

5. I value privacy, dignity, and worth of the individual, and will use skills consistent with these values.

6. I will observe the principle of informed consent with respect to individuals and groups served.

7. I will support change by choice, not by coercion.

8. I will foster an educational environment that nurtures individual growth and development.

9. If I become aware of unethical practices, I am accountable for taking appropriate action concerning these practices.[20]

In 1991, the Association for the Advancement of Health Education (AAHE) Ethics Committee refined and revised the ethical code for those involved with community health education. Among the principles of the Code of Ethics are:

1. The health educator's ultimate responsibility is to educate the general public about health. When there is a conflict of interest among stakeholders, health

educators must consider all issues and give priority to those whose goals are closest to the principles of self-determination and freedom of choice.

2. Health educators are responsible for the reputation of their discipline and should uphold high professional standards.

3. Health educators should consult with colleagues in order to avoid unethical conduct.

4. Health educators should seek to promote integrity in the delivery of health education by adapting strategies and methods to the needs of different populations.

5. Health educator preparation should include personal and professional honesty, integrity, and knowledge.

6. Health educators will recognize the boundaries of their professional competence and provide only those services and programs for which they are qualified.

7. Health educators will plan and conduct research in accordance with federal and state laws and professional standards.[21]

Community health educators must personally prepare to deal with two ethical dilemmas. First, who should decide whether to introduce change and the consequence of change into a person's or a family's life? For example, at what point does the community health educator intervene to require or encourage HIV testing? How and when is the best way to teach pregnant women to improve nutrition? Second, what right does a health educator have to impose his or her ideas and standards of behavior upon others? For example, should the community health educator articulate his or her views on abortion? Should the community health educator encourage birth control to teenage audiences?

For community health education, values and ethical behavior should be founded upon (1) respect for human life in all its social manifestations, (2) respect for the dignity and beliefs of others, and (3) respect for the highest professional competence at all levels of preparation and practice. Community health educators should practice nondiscrimination against race, religion, age, gender, sexual orientation, cultural background, or social class. They should involve those to be affected by change in the planning and implementation of that change. They should avoid manipulative methods to ensure free and open choice among all options. Some in the field would argue that our established codes of ethics are too general to accomplish these tasks.

It is not enough to promote health and prevent illness. Both must be accomplished through professional, ethical, and sensitive techniques and procedures throughout all levels of community health, whether it be the local health department or the Public Health Service.

Summary

As community health students, we are part of a long history of caring and tending to the peoples of the planet. We may actually be one of the oldest professions and we will certainly be a profession that does not become obsolete from lack of opportunity. Early on, many community health efforts were based on those of ancient nations. Later, with the discovery of pathogens to many diseases, community health focused on prevention. There has also been somewhat of a broadening of community health's scope to include issues of chronic, as well as communicable, disease prevention. Truly, if any time in history should practice community health promotion, it would be the present. Professionals must now look at the many dimensions of community health problems, while incorporating the vast knowledge learned from our history.

Community health education can no longer think of itself as a small part of a big system, tackling overwhelming problems in a global community. Community health education's time has come. The priorities of creating a healthy people for the twenty-first century require the vigilant efforts of health promotion programs worldwide. We no longer can think provincially as members of a local community. Everything we do contributes to our global community, either positively or negatively.

CYBERSITES RELATED TO CHAPTER 1

American Public Health Association
   www.apha.org

American Alliance for Health, Physical Education, Recreation, and Dance
   www.aapherd.org

Healthy People 2010
   www.health.gov/healthypeople

QUESTIONS

1. How do you define community health?
2. What are the community health issues of your college/university "community"?
3. What would our society be like if there were no "isms"?
4. Why is the health of the planet so important at this time?
5. What are the consequences to developed countries if they ignore developing countries?
6. What is the value of becoming a Certified Community Health Specialist?

EXERCISES

1. Expand your horizons. Imagine yourself able to serve somewhere in the world in a public health capacity. There are no financial or personal limitations. Where would you go? Why would you go? What would be your mission when you got there? How would you prepare? What would you expect to bring home?

2. Visit your state and local health departments. What are the state and local health departments doing for the Healthy People 2010 objectives and goals? How are they being implemented? What is the role of your state legislature, universities, private businesses, and consumer groups in meeting these objectives?

INTERNET INTERACTIVE ACTIVITY

Working with the National Objectives of Healthy People 2010

Healthy People 2010 is a national health promotion and disease prevention initiative that brings together national, state, and local government agencies; nonprofit, voluntary, and professional organizations; businesses; communities; and individuals to improve the health of all Americans, eliminate disparities in health, and improve years and quality of healthy life. The priority focus of all state and most local health departments will for the next ten years be directed toward meeting the objectives set forth in Healthy People 2010.

As a community health educator, being familiar with the Healthy People 2010 objectives is a major responsibility in terms of program planning, evaluation, grant writing, and community interaction with target populations. You can find complete documents by starting at the homepage for Healthy People 2010:

www.health.gov/healthypeople/document/eight/focus

Exercise

There are twenty-eight focus areas in Healthy People 2010. They can be found by clicking **Proceed to the Table of Contents** on the homepage.

1. Go through each of the focus areas by clicking on the HTML link for objectives for improving health.

2. From the objectives given for each area, select two that you think your community should address, given your current knowledge of your community.

3. Give an example of a risk reduction or prevention program idea that your community might consider for each of the twenty-eight objectives.

REFERENCES

1. Shaffer, Carolyn and Anundsen, Kristen (1993). *Creating community anywhere: finding support and connection in a fragmented world.* New York: Putnam.

2. Green, Lawrence (1990). *Community health.* St. Louis: Times Mirror/Mosby.

3. Shaffer & Anundsen, op. cit.

4. Fee, Elizabeth (1991). The origins and development of public health in the U.S. In *Oxford textbook of public health,* Vol. 1, p. 3.

5. Rothenberger, John (1994). Presentation to College Health 2000. July 30, Scottsdale, Arizona.

6. Basch, Paul (1990). *Textbook of international health.* New York: Oxford University Press.

7. Ibid.

8. U.S. Dept. of HHS, Office of Disease Prevention and Health Promotion (1997). *Developing Objectives for Healthy People 2000.* Washington, DC.

9. McGinnis, J. M., Harrell, J. A., & Artz, L. M. (1991). Objectives-based strategies for disease prevention. In *International textbook of public health,* Vol. 2, Oxford Press, pp. 127–144.

10. U.S. Dept. of HHS, Office of Disease Prevention and Health Promotion (1997). *Developing Objectives for Healthy People 2000.* Washington, DC.

11. Ibid.

12. Green, op. cit.

13. Koren, Herman (1991). *Handbook of environmental health and safety,* Vol. I. Chelsea, MI: Lewis Publishing.

14. Breckon, Donald J. (1998). *Community health education: Settings, roles and skills.* Gaithersberg, MD: Aspen Publications.

15. Ibid.

16. Ibid.

17. Basch, op. cit.

18. Ibid.

19. Ibid.

20. Ibid.

21. Greenberg, J., & Gold, R. (1992). *The health education ethics book.* Dubuque, IA: Wm. C. Brown.

CHAPTER 2

The History, Administration, and Organization of Community Health

Community Health in the 21st Century
There will be more for-profit health education programs taking the place
of programs that are funded today by grants and foundations. Computers
and technology will increase. Prevention will be more popular.

—Lisa Appelhans, B.S. Health Education;
Health Promotion Coordinator

Chapter Objectives

The student will:

1. describe the primary role of the federal, state, and local governments in providing health services.

2. give examples of health problems addressed by private, philanthropic, and volunteer organizations.

3. compare fee for service health care with socialized health care.

4. historically outline the progression of community and public health education

The Origins and History of Public and Community Health

Today's immediate health problems and the related conditions of the planet's air, soil, and water have historical roots. One hundred years ago trash was tossed in wooden barrels in front of buildings and city air was filled with the particulate matter of smoke stacks, chimneys, and burning trash. Toilet waste was often thrown directly into the water running down street gutters, and horse manure produced tons of waste on city streets. Public health in the 1700s and 1800s included regulation of graveyards, fat rendering factories, sugar boilers, dryers, glue boilers, and slaughterhouses. As colonial towns began to reek with the smell of waste, religious leaders or town physicians were called upon to "exorcize" the evil smells. New regulations were imposed that demanded clean privies and alleys and the removal of dead animals and decaying foods.

Sometimes prayer was called upon as a public health mechanism and many clergy took credit for saving the health of communities as well as souls.[1]

In England, Edwin Chadwick gradually recognized the importance of sanitation in the maintenance of public health and prepared the 1842 *Report ... on an Inquiry into the Sanitary Condition of the Labouring Population of Great Britain*, upon which American public health was born. Although from 1832 the recurring threat of cholera pandemics was a major impetus to create boards of health, little else was officially targeted by communities. Public health was primarily a police function of quarantine because epidemics galvanized the public into restrictive enforcement. **Endemic** (common) diseases such as measles, diphtheria, influenza, and malaria brought only stoic indifference. The 1842 report gave boards of health a basis upon which to develop and establish their legitimacy.

Using the Chadwick report as a model, in 1848 John Griscom in New York and Lemuel Shattuck in Boston wrote *Reports on the Sanitary Conditions of their States*. Upon these documents the modern state and local health departments were built. Today, thirty-six of Shattuck's fifty recommendations are accepted as standard practice.

Among the fifty Shattuck recommendations still practiced in the 1990s are:

1. Establish state and local boards of health.
2. Collect and analyze vital statistics.
3. Exchange health information.
4. Initiate sanitation programs for towns and buildings.
5. Maintain a system of sanitary inspections.
6. Study the health of school children.
7. Control food adulteration.
8. Control smoke nuisances.
9. Preach health from the pulpit.
10. Teach the science of sanitation in medical schools.

Ancient and Premodern History

When the United States finally began to conscientiously address the health hazards of its towns and cities, public health established programs built upon thousands of years of historical knowledge. Ancient Egyptians worshiped the scarabaeus or dung beetle because of its scavenging powers and its symbolic contributions to cleanliness of the environment. People were admonished to keep their houses clean, to bathe frequently, and keep drinking water pure. Excavated tombs have revealed water closets, medicinal plants, and signs of public health engineering.

Over 36,000 mummies found in Egypt, China, and elsewhere have been rich sources of medical information and have shown that schistosomiasis, arteriosclerosis, emphysema, silicosis and anthracosis, dental caries, osteomyelitis, gout, and tuberculosis among many others are long-standing maladies for humans.[2] Evidence of treatment modalities exist in ancient manuscripts and excavated artifacts. Interestingly, not one of 25,000 Egyptian mummies shows any evidence of syphilis, a disease often blamed on ancient peoples.

The Hebrews of the Old Testament may have actually taken many of their proscriptions for health from even more ancient cultures. The hygienic codes (Mosaic law) of early Jews kept them free from contagious disease, poor sanitation, parasites, sexually transmitted diseases, and unwanted maternity. Circumcision was probably adopted from the Egyptians who practiced circumcision in 2000 BC.

Europe and the United States have recently discovered the secrets of the Chinese barefoot doctors. Chinese medicine dates back to about 3322 BC to Fu Hsi, who taught his people about the treatment of diseases. As early as 2700 BC, Shen-Nung published a book listing 365 kinds of medicines: 46 from minerals, 67 from animals, and 252 from plants. Acupuncture is now used as an alternative to Western medicinal ways of treating pain and illness in non-Chinese cultures. New research agendas are being prepared to test the flora and herbs of past and less developed populations to determine the efficacy to healing modern maladies.

Born to the Greek god Asklepios were two daughters, Hygeia (whose name gave us hygiene) and Panakeia (panacea). Hygeia taught the people how to stay well and Panakeia healed the sick with her medicines. As intertwined as the gods and the Greek people often were, Greek citizens clearly recognized the social and temporal nature of disease. Theano, presumably the wife of Pythagoras, was devoted to medicine, hygiene, physics, and ethics.

Greek tradition did not spring fully formed from the pen of Hippocrates. From the Minoans came ideas of hygiene, healing temples, and the caduceus, the symbol of medicine. Egypt contributed its pharmaceutical lore and surgical techniques. Mesopotamia added different drugs and basic organization of medical practice. Add to these diverse cultural contributions myth, magic, folklore, and the legacy of spiritual healing and Greek tradition is born.[3]

The Romans brought to civilization the use of aqueducts, baths, maintenance of streets, wholesomeness of food, hospitals, and public toilets. Despite their interest in public health, they had little understanding of anatomy and physiology keeping medicine quite primitive. They also had no idea of the hazard of lead to humans. The Romans adopted lead for water pipes that apparently disabled many unwitting Roman citizens. The word "plumbing" is, in fact, derived from the Latin name for lead, plumbum.[4]

Much of the knowledge produced by these sophisticated civilizations was unheeded or lost during the middle ages when an estimated 4 million "healers" were burned as witches because of their ability to heal. Ascetic monks equated cleanliness and knowledge with sin.[5] The result was that crowded cities and misinformation reduced the health standards of water, sanitation, and personal hygiene, and increased epidemic disease such as the bubonic plague or **Black Death.** A classic description of the horror of this bacterial pandemic spread by the bite of a flea carried on a rat is described in *The Plague* by Camus.[6] The first

pandemic (worldwide outbreak), was an outbreak of bubonic plague also known as the Plague of Justinian, which struck in 542 AD and decimated the known world from Asia to Ireland. However, the great Black Death of the fourteenth century is the most destructive epidemic in known history. Europe alone lost perhaps 25 million people, half its total population by 1500, and throughout the Middle East, India, and China similar devastation resulted in the additional deaths of tens of millions. The black plague killed 90 percent of the population of Florence, Italy, and 50 percent of the citizens of Paris, France.[7]

Less devastating, but equally horrifying were epidemics of smallpox, diphtheria, measles, influenza, tuberculosis, scabies, anthrax, and trachoma. A belief in **miasma,** the theory that disease spreads vis-à-vis noxious air or vapor contaminated by the putrefaction of refuge and sewage, preceded germ theory and left Europe and the United States without the scientific theoretical base to prevent these serious, population-decimating illnesses.

Smallpox has been the greatest killer of humankind over all recorded time. Ramses V (1157 BC) of Egypt appears to have had smallpox. It killed three and one-half million Aztecs and 90 percent of the Native Americans living near the American colonies in 1617. Smallpox has often been spread by religious missionaries. As Islam spread in 570 AD, so did smallpox. The Crusades spread smallpox in the 1100s, and the Puritans deliberately passed smallpox to the Native Americans in the 1700s as a form of germ warfare. The Hudson Bay Company was asked by the United States government to distribute smallpox-contaminated blankets to natives who were on land that the government wanted to acquire.

The Middle Ages and Precolonization

During the Middle Ages in Europe, classical medical knowledge was retained by the Arabs, who established settlements in Spain, Portugal, and Sicily. Much of European medieval thought was expended on the rivalry with Islam, and although the Crusades generally failed, contacts with the Muslim world opened new vistas to Europeans. About 1500 AD, concepts of cleanliness and sanitation began to reemerge in European cities.

Trade, exploration, war, and world discovery spread disease all over the world in the sixteenth and seventeenth centuries as sick sailors infected native populations with the scourges of sexually transmitted disease, measles, cholera, yellow fever, typhoid, and other contagious diseases. Certainly one of the greatest social diseases to plague the world was the enslavement of an estimated 11 million north and west Africans. In addition to the inhumanity of slavery, transported Africans brought their indigenous pathogens to countries that had no natural immunity to new pathogens. Imported were amoebic and bacillary dysentery, helminth parasites such as the hookworm, schistosomiasis, and the filarial worm, which caused elephantiasis.

On the American continents, Native Americans were using laxatives, diuretics, emetics, and antipyretic drugs. In South America, natives used cocaine, quinine, curare, and ipecac and did sophisticated skull surgery called "trepanation." Much of what was known then is still used today by native peoples and modern medicine.

Change in science comes slowly, and the change from miasma to germ theory in Europe was evidence of this pace. The period from 1750 to the beginning of the twentieth century, known as the Industrial Revolution, reintroduced good public health methods to developing countries, including our own. Unfortunately, the massive development of power-driven factories also increased public health problems associated with industrialization. In France, scientist Louis Pasteur had the greatest impact on medicine and public health by establishing empirically that fermentation in wine, beer, and milk was due to microorganisms, not vapors. His work influenced British surgeon Joseph Lister who introduced the practice of antisepsis to the operating theaters in 1865. Despite obvious success with theory and practice, there were critics, such as Dr. Hughes Bennett, Professor of Medicine at Edinburgh University in England:

> *Where are the germs? Show them to us and we will believe. Has anyone seen these germs? The dust has been ransacked for these organic germs—collected and carefully examined with a microscope, near the soil and on the summits of the highest buildings ... yet all without results ...*"[8]

Early Health Care in the United States

In 1798, the United States federal government established a public health service known as the Marine Hospital Service. This agency was created by President John Adams to care for sick and disabled merchant seamen and to prevent the spread of epidemic diseases. The merchant marines were the link to economic development, transportation, and defense and thus was one of the first priorities of a new nation.

During the 1800s millions of European immigrants came to the United States, settling in major seaports on the east coast. Crowding exacerbated the already existing problems of sanitation, housing, pests, and vermin (rodents), drainage, and solid waste disposal. The poor sanitary conditions led to outbreaks of communicable diseases and ultimately to establishment of public health departments and the implementation of the recommendations of Lemuel Shattuck.

The colonists came to the Americas for freedom, but by the mid-1800s they found themselves at war over the freedom of other unwilling immigrants, African slaves, who had been shipped here in the 1700s and 1800s. In the South, slave owners established their own public health regulations by controlling the lives, housing, food, clothing, sanitation, discipline, and reproduction of their slaves. Outbreaks of communicable diseases were seasonally epidemic, and serious musculoskeletal deformities caused by floggings (beatings) were common.[9]

The Civil War of 1865, to free the slaves from their inhuman treatment, demonstrated the dramatic health effects and costs of war. Over two-thirds of the 360,000 Union soldiers were killed by infectious diseases rather than enemy bullets. It is estimated that at least three-fourths of the Confederate soldiers' deaths were due to disease. The ravages of dysentery, spread by inadequate sanitation, were appalling. It was the nurse and activist Florence Nightingale who promoted health through camp inspections, distribution of educational materials, and providing nursing care.[10]

The post–Civil War era brought a time of healing for a divided nation, social reform, and the beginning of comprehensive sanitation and public health services in industrial cities. Middle- and upper-class women were prime movers of these reforms. They demanded improved housing, child labor laws, temperance (movement to control alcohol), and reduction in maternal and child deaths. Their movement was called by some "municipal housekeeping."[11] This was a time of increased awareness about community health; recent discoveries were leading to prevention efforts.

Other issues began to crop up as related to disease, one being poverty. The 1920s saw an expansion of urban communities that increased disease. There was also the concern about the inequality of the distribution of wealth. This movement continues today as we search for factors associated with our current leading killers in America: chronic diseases.

Today the practice of public health overlaps several other disciplines in medicine and the social sciences, and requires the collaboration of a myriad of organizations and agencies of the public and private sectors. The sum total of this massive task of saving the planet and its inhabitants is called **Community Health Promotion (CHP)**. CHP is any combination of educational, social, and environmental actions conducive to the health of a population in a geographically defined area.[12] The issues, while still the same as in times past, also now include lifestyle changes, sexual freedom, mobility, violence, biomedical technology, issues of longevity, as well as the survival and long-term effects of premature infants. Another major modern concern is mental health, which includes alcoholism and drug abuse, relationship dependency, genetic abnormalities, lead poisoning, abuse of pharmaceuticals, and learning disabilities. The discipline is now broad, complex, high-tech, and challenging.

Health Care Delivery

Providing health care has been a priority of all peoples, whether it is done within the nuclear family or as a community responsibility. The concept of an organized health care delivery system in the United States, what we call "traditional medicine," is built on a fee for service system, and is a manifestation of this century. Such a system has not been particularly cost effective, efficient, or equitable, and attempts to change the system have been proposed for decades. Often economically disadvantaged citizens have trouble accessing a private, fee for service system, and become part of a community's backup resources. Changes in the 1990s appeared to be heading toward a more socialized system, with a single payer (the government), primarily encouraging health maintenance group practices. The delivery of health care will probably not change dramatically for those who have the ability to pay for private, individualized care, but to meet the demands of such an economically diverse nation, many will see new health care delivery practices in their lifetime.

In terms of community health that encompasses personal and public health—unlike Europe, which has a smaller, more homogeneous population and a national health scheme—the United States has a very complex health care system that is epitomized by a "pluralistic" arrangement of public and private partnerships that collaborate to provide the financing and delivery of health care services for individuals and communities. The framework is largely local and decentralized with much of the work being done by voluntary, private, or nongovernmental bodies. The basic ideology and structure is a continually changing blend of private free-market dynamics and organized programs of financing, delivery, and regulation of services. Ideally, the provision of health services is within a free market of consumers and providers who, in theory, are expected to be regulated by competition. Unfortunately, the theory has not worked well in practice as evinced by skyrocketing costs, inequitable access to care, 43 million uninsured Americans, and bake sales that are held for kidney patients or bone marrow transplants.

In 1993 Hillary Rodham Clinton was appointed to head a commission on health care reform in an attempt to "heal the system" and reform the current health care system. Preliminary reports from the Commission on Health Care Reform suggested a move away from a free-market system of health care to a more socialized or federally administered system. Such a change would be a radical departure in the United States but would resemble both the Canadian and British health care systems of providing care to all their citizens.

Although responsibility for health care in the United States is, in unique fashion, both a public and private affair, in recent years, government—especially the federal government—has emerged as perhaps the single most important force shaping our health care system, albeit piecemeal. The role of state and local government, however, cannot be underestimated. President Reagan's New Federalism gave more responsibility to state and local governments through block grants. At the same time however, economic retrenchment such as Proposition 13 in California and similar cutbacks in the northwestern and northeastern states made it overwhelmingly difficult for state and local government to manage adequate public health.

As seen within the overall health care system, two themes seem to emerge when public and community health education are reviewed: (1) steady fragmentation of health services and (2) the expanding role of the federal government. Fragmentation has occurred as select agencies, both public and private, have assumed responsibility or have been required, by evidence of neglect for a particular health area, to take responsibility for services that are not adequately served by state health departments.[13] The result is a good portion of our population who are medically underserved (Table 2.1). A coordinated community health education system that meets the numerous needs of a variety of populations seldom exists outside small communities.

Table 2.1   Medically underserved by state.

State	%	Rank	State	%	Rank
Alabama	27.6	4	Montana	17.0	19
Alaska	0	51	Nebraska	2.9	50
Arizona	17.5	18	Nevada	10.0	41
Arkansas	27.6	4	New Hampshire	7.6	46
California	21.5	9	New Jersey	11.1	37
Colorado	14.9	25	New Mexico	22.9	8
Connecticut	4.4	49	New York	20.8	11
Delaware	13.7	28	North Carolina	15.7	22
District of Columbia	25.4	6	North Dakota	6.2	47
Florida	18.7	16	Ohio	14.4	26
Georgia	20.2	12	Oklahoma	23.6	7
Hawaii	8.3	45	Oregon	11.2	35
Idaho	17.6	17	Pennsylvania	11.3	34
Illinois	19.8	13	Rhode Island	11.2	35
Indiana	12.1	31	South Carolina	19.3	14
Iowa	10.4	38	South Dakota	10.3	39
Kansas	11.8	32	Tennessee	18.9	15
Kentucky	16.4	20	Texas	21.3	10
Louisiana	31.8	2	Utah	11.4	33
Maine	8.6	44	Vermont	5.3	48
Maryland	15.0	24	Virginia	10.2	40
Massachusetts	12.9	29	Washington	15.9	21
Michigan	15.2	23	West Virginia	29.7	3
Minnesota	9.9	42	Wisconsin	12.7	30
Mississippi	33.3	1	Wyoming	8.9	43
Missouri	14.2	27			

Discussion: What does it mean to be medically underserved?

When describing responsibility for health care, most textbooks show a hierarchical system that on paper appears to work smoothly and resourcefully to meet public health needs. The diagrammed systems shown in Figures 2.1, 2.2, and 2.3 illustrate the organizational hierarchy of the health organizations at the federal, state, and local levels. In theory, these levels of health administration are financed by public tax monies to oversee national health concerns and emergencies along with state and local needs and interest in efficient, coordi-

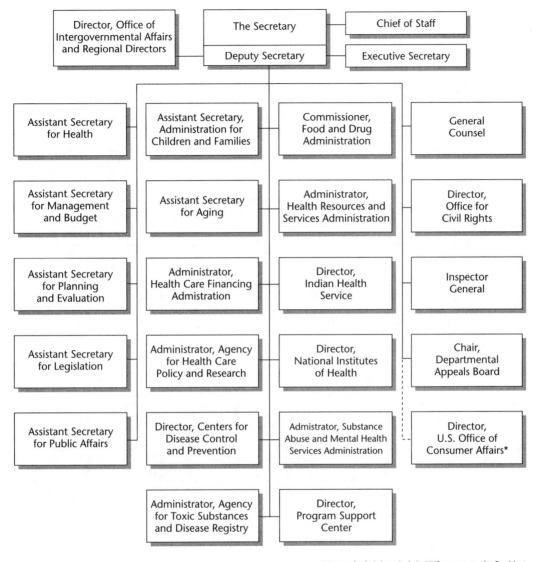

Figure 2.1 The U.S. Department of Health and Human Services.

* Located administratively in HHS; reports to the President.

nated, and cooperative ways. In actuality, duplication of services, neglect of some constituents, competition for funding, moral agendas of lobby groups, "isms" and phobias, and political agendas often create a system that is very fractured, resulting in many target persons and groups falling between the cracks of the health care system.

An attempt to solve these problems was made with the 1974 National Health Planning and Resource Development Act. This Act was designed to

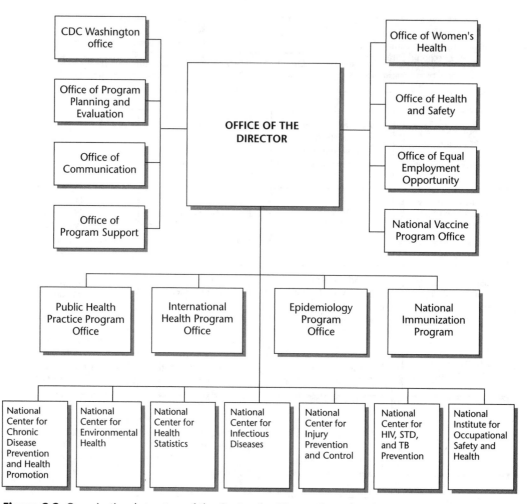

Figure 2.2 Organizational structure of the Centers for Disease Control and Prevention (1998).

establish a nationwide network of health planning agencies, administered by the Public Health Service.[14]

Administrative problems of health officials at all levels have been compounded by the reemergence of old health problems such as measles, tuberculosis, sexually transmitted diseases, mental illnesses, and emergence of new problems like AIDS, those without health insurance, immigration, hazardous waste, and environmental health issues. Without financial and personal resources from the federal government, states and local municipalities find themselves unable to address these and other problems, and must rely on community-based groups such as local health foundations to address massive problems. There is little wonder why there is anger, suspicion, and often no coordination among agencies and organizations when everyone feels at risk.

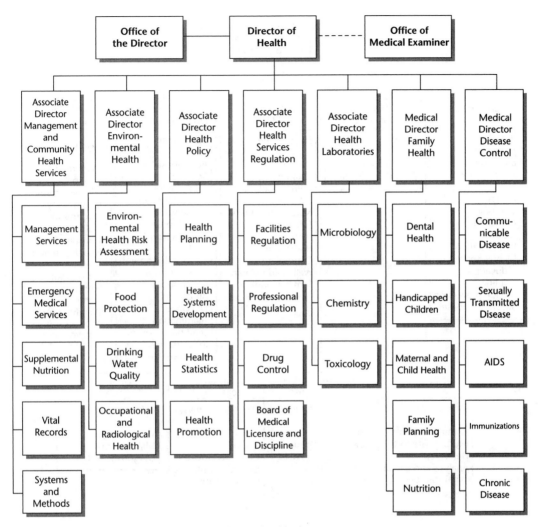

Figure 2.3 Organization chart for a typical state health department.

The Role of Federal Government

There is no constitutionally defined role for the federal government in health; however, over the years, the federal role has come to include (1) responsibility for certain populations such as merchant seamen, members of the armed services, veterans, and Native Americans; (2) the regulation of interstate commerce of drugs and food; (3) grants in aid to states and institutions; and (4) the administration of the Medicare insurance program for older Americans and Medicaid for selected population groups.

Today there are over fifty departments, agencies, and bureaus within the federal government that deal with health. The most specific government agency

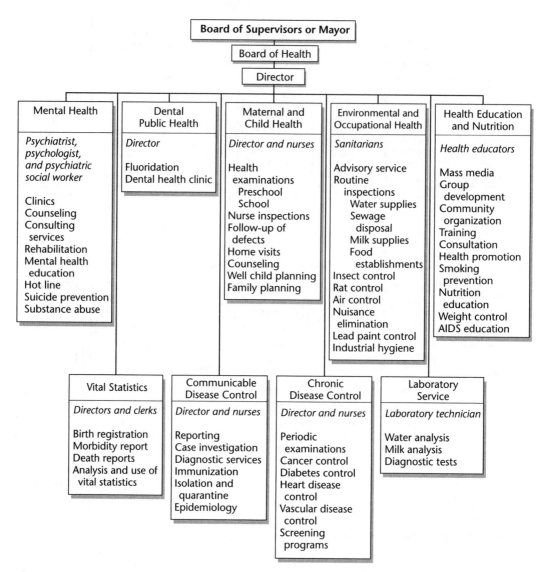

Figure 2.4 Organization chart for a typical city or county health department (many variations may be found).

associated with health is the **Department of Health and Human Services (HHS),** known until 1980 as the Department of Health, Education, and Welfare. This branch of the federal government is responsible for the administration of nationwide programs such as Medicare and related programs.

Health and Human Services currently consists of twelve operating divisions whose heads report independently and directly to the Secretary of HHS. Eight of the twelve divisions of HHS are now specifically part of the Public Health Service whose administrative officer is the Assistant Secretary for Health.

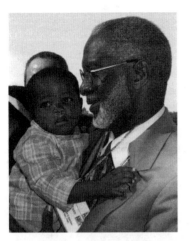

Surgeon General, David Satcher, MD, holding a 7-month old baby girl with AIDS whose mother recently passed away from complications of AIDS.

Agencies Outside of the Public Health Service

1. **The Administration on Aging** administers the Older Americans Act of 1965, tracking characteristics and needs of older people.

2. **The Administration for Children and Families** was established in 1991 and was formerly known as the Family Services Administration. This branch oversees assistance and service programs to those families and children in need.

3. **The Agency for Health Policy and Research** is the only agency charged with producing and disseminating scientific and policy relevant information and data about the cost of health care.

4. **The Agency for Toxic Substances and Disease Registry** oversees the SuperFund legislation passed in 1980 and discussed in a later chapter. The mission of this agency is "to prevent exposure and adverse human health effects ..." associated with hazardous substances.

Agencies within the Public Health Service:

1. **The Centers for Disease Control and Prevention (CDC)** provide leadership and consultation to state and local health departments and agencies, and is the primary federal governmental agency responsible for the implementation of Healthy People 2010 at the state and local levels. The CDC is comprised of six centers, one institute, and six program offices that serve the nation as a means of gathering and disseminating health information as well as investigating disease conditions, especially epidemics.

   The centers include the:

   - National Center for Chronic Disease Prevention and Health Promotion (NCCDPHP)
   - National Center for HIV, STD, and TB Diseases (NCHSTP)
   - National Center for Injury Prevention and Control (NCIPC)

BOX 2.1 The CDC Headquarters

Did you ever wonder why the CDC is located in Atlanta, Georgia, when most other federal government agencies are centered around Washington, D.C.? The CDC was started as an agency to pursue malaria control; the Office of Malaria Control in War Areas. Most of the malaria epidemic existed in Central America. Since Florida was highly underde- veloped at its inception in 1942, Atlanta was chosen as the next logical location for head- quarters. Today, the CDC is a highly organ- ized network of buildings. Since there is little room to expand, there is a unique system of operations underground, allowing the CDC to grow as needed.[15]

BOX 2.2 How the CDC Can Help

The CDC is very user-friendly, even to those community health professionals working at the local level. The Centers are also a source of many publications, brochures, and resources that are free to the public in specific quantities. In a time of limited resources for all types of community health programs, one should be aware of how the CDC can help. Call the public information line at (404) 639- 3534; or 1-800-458-5231 for an HIV/AIDS publications catalog.

- National Center for Infectious Diseases (NCID)
- National Center for Environmental Health (NCEH)
- National Center for Injury Prevention and Control (NCIPC)

  The six program offices include the:

- Epidemiology Program Office (EPO)
- International Health Program Office (IHOP)
- National Immunization Program (NIP)
- Public Health Practice Program Office (PHPPO)
- Office of Minority Health (OMH)
- Office of Women's Health (OWH)

  The Institutes housed in the Public Health Service are the:

- National Institute for Occupational Safety and Health (NIOSH)
- National Center for Health Statistics
- National Center for Infectious Diseases
- National Center for Prevention Services
- National Institute for Occupational Safety and Health

  The CDC also has three Program offices:

- Epidemiology Program Office

- International Health Program Office
- Public Health Practice Program Office[16]

The CDC publishes the *Morbidity and Mortality Weekly Report* (*MMWR*) which reports the most current incidence and prevalence statistics for forty-nine reportable diseases from around the country. The *MMWR* also provides a means of disseminating and describing new regulatory changes or health information pertinent to public health and safety for local communities.

2. **The Food and Drug Administration (FDA)** monitors the safety of consumed products, resulting from the 1906 Pure Food and Drug Act. The FDA's main concern is that our food, medicine, cosmetics, and so on, are effective and safe for human consumption. The products they cover range from food additives to food labeling; from radiation levels to the nation's blood supply. The FDA also monitors the safety of new medical products and licenses new products. The agency does not monitor the safety of meat or milk, which is regulated by the Department of Agriculture.

3. **The Health Care Financing Administration (HCFA)** manages our **Medicare** and **Medicaid** programs, which have been in existence since the mid-1960s. (Both programs are detailed in Chapter 3.) Briefly, Medicare provides health insurance to older Americans and those with disabilities who receive social security or railroad retirement benefits. Medicaid provides some health insurance coverage to economically disadvantaged Americans. Medicaid also sets standards of health care and ensures that all federally-funded health care programs are safe to participating Americans.

4. **The Health Resources and Services Administration** is concerned with programs that increase accessibility of resources to at-risk populations. Essentially this agency serves the poor, uninsured, and geographically isolated populations who are severely underserved by private health care systems.

5. **The Indian Health Service** provides health care services to tribal Indians and improves their health status.

6. **National Institutes of Health (NIH)** conduct health-related research and work closely with university research projects. NIH have actually been around since 1887 when they began as a research laboratory. Their epicenter is Bethesda, Maryland, outside of Washington, D.C. There are thirteen research institutes, a hospital, a library, and an international center in the NIH. The Institutes conduct research in many areas including heart disease, cancer, and HIV/AIDS. Many of their monies support research programs at the university, hospital, and nonprofit levels; in fact, 40 percent of all biomedical research done in the United States is supported by the NIH.[17] The thirteen institutes within the NIH are:

- National Cancer Institute
- National Heart, Lung, and Blood Institute
- National Institute of Diabetes and Digestive and Kidney Diseases
- National Institute of Arthritis, Musculoskeletal, and Skin Diseases

- National Institute of Allergy and Infectious Diseases
- National Institute of Child Health and Human Development
- National Institute of Aging
- National Institute of Dental Research
- National Institute of Environmental Health Sciences
- National Institute of General Medical Sciences
- National Institute of Neurological Disorders and Stroke
- National Eye Institute
- National Center for Research Resources

7. **Substance Abuse and Mental Health Services Administration** conducts research and supports programs regarding mental illness, substance abuse, and addictive disorders.

8. **The Program Support Center** was created in 1995 to provide cost-effective, efficient, and responsive administrative support services to all components of the HHS. The services provided include human resources, financial management, administrative, operations, and information technology.

The Public Health Service also has the lead federal government role in ensuring the health needs of a nation after a disaster. The Federal Response Plan, which becomes effective upon a Presidential Declaration of a Federal Disaster, initiates a plan of action directed by the PHS. The Emergency Support Functions (ESF) include:

- Assessment of health and medical needs
- Health surveillance
- Medical care personnel
- Health and medical equipment and supplies
- Patient evacuation
- In-hospital care
- Food, drug, and medical device safety
- Work health and safety
- Radiological hazards
- Chemical hazards
- Biological hazards
- Mental health
- Public health information
- Vector control
- Potable water, waste water, and solid waste disposal
- Victim identification and mortuary services[18]

Within the federal government, virtually all cabinet departments contribute in some way to health service, delivery, or prevention. For example, besides the Department of Health and Human Services, the **Department of Agriculture** is probably one of the most important to community health, as it is responsible for the inspection of meat, poultry, eggs, and milk. It administers the food stamp program and the program for Women, Infants, and Children (WIC). The 1993 outbreak and subsequent mortality by E. coli bacterial infection in fast food meat in the northwest emphasized the critical need for more and better food inspection.

The **Department of Labor** oversees the Occupational Safety and Health Administration (OSHA), which is responsible for industrial health and safety. They regulate mine safety, children's labor safety, and migrant labor laws. The department collects data related to industrial health injuries and assesses need for further regulation.

The **Department of Commerce** conducts the census by which health care trends can be determined and program planning can be implemented. The department also has the unusual responsibility of Merchant Marine health programs.

The **Department of Defense** conducts research into many personal, environmental, and public health issues. Much of the technology that comes from defense research filters into the public medical system through cooperation and resources.

The **Department of Interior** is responsible for mine safety through the Bureau of Mines and for fish and wildlife environmental safety through the United States Fish and Wildlife Service. The Department of the Interior, through the National Park Service, is responsible for national park concessions and park and camping sanitation.

The **Department of Energy** helps set regulations for the safe and efficient use of energy resources.

The **Environmental Protection Agency** (EPA) is not a cabinet office, however, it controls billions of dollars designated for cleanup of hazardous waste sites, and cleaning up air and water pollution through control of toxic agents in the environment.

The **Department of Veterans Affairs** oversees veterans' benefits, services, and job opportunities.

The Role of State Health Departments

Ironically, despite the increasing activity of the federal government in health matters, public health is still largely in the hands of state and local authorities. The principal role of the federal government is to set minimum standards of public health and encourage states and communities to meet or exceed these standards, to assist in training personnel, to gather statistics, to aid with emergency problems, and provide advice. States then develop rules and regulations to protect its individuals. The chief means by which the federal government promotes its health policies is through a system of federal funding to states in various block grants or delegated grants, usually requiring matching funds. The initial purpose of block grants was to provide more authority to states and local agencies about health programs, since these agencies work directly with the people served. There are over 3,000 state and local health departments in the United States. All fifty states have a state health department, although they all operate somewhat differently from each other. In 2000, one out of every three United States citizens received direct services from these state and local health departments. State and local health departments are also the greatest source of employment for community and public health educators. State health department budgets are often the largest of all state expenses primarily due to Medicaid. State health departments are under the auspices of the governor, who hires or appoints a Director or Commissioner for Health. At the state level the director is traditionally a physician, although this isn't always the case. Local health directors may also be nonmedically trained administrators.

With funding through state tax revenues, fees and licensing permits, laboratory fees, clinical service fees, and federal block grants, state agencies provide services in four broad budget areas: (1) personal health, (2) environmental health, (3) health resources, and (4) public health laboratories.

Personal health services focus on special populations including programs for children with disabilities, maternal and child health care, chronic disease control and prevention, dental health, inpatient mental health, communicable disease control and prevention, STD prevention, public health nursing, nutrition, health education, and screening services. More than half of the federal dollars received by state health departments goes to the Women, Infants and Children program (WIC), which provides nutritional food supplements to a family's diet through special coupons.

In many states, environmental health is actually a primary responsibility of a state's environmental protection agency. These agencies are responsible for environmental quality (air, noise, radiation, and pesticide), waste management, water resources, coastal resources, fish and game, parks and forestry. State EPAs also develop standards, conduct inspections, regulate licensure, and enforce sanitary codes and public health laws. They may also monitor the health and safety regulations in mobile home parks, migrant camps, recreational areas, and youth camps. They are particularly concerned with the food safety and water sanitation.[19] However, similar activities occur at state health departments.

Under health resources, the state health department regulates emergency medical services and the collection of vital statistics, which are discussed in Chapter 5. Briefly, the state health departments collect and monitor statistics from local health departments and other agencies. Data are collected regarding many subjects, such as marriages, births, deaths, and disease trends.

State laboratories test human and animal specimens and environmental samples. Public health laboratories are essential to the microbiotic analysis of health issues. Most states have their own laboratories, but some localities contract their lab work with private labs. Lab work includes testing blood and tissue for communicable diseases, testing for hereditary and metabolic diseases, sanitation and environmental testing, and testing for sexually transmitted diseases, including HIV.

State health departments also participate in the Healthy People 2010 initiative. If Healthy People 2010 is truly going to be accomplished, state and local health departments will need to work with other community agencies to achieve the goals and objectives set.

The Role of Local Health Departments

There are approximately 3,000 local health departments that serve over 95.4 percent of the population. Most local health departments are actually county-wide or combinations of a few cities and counties. The local health departments have at least one full-time public health professional and may provide local services in nursing, public health education, environmental sanitation, chronic disease control, communicable disease control, health statistics and records, school health services, maternal, and child health programs and home health care. Many larger local health departments also provide dental health, emergency services, animal control, alcohol and drug abuse prevention, laboratory services, and mental health. Local health departments are also a primary source of health education activity. In general, local health departments are required by law to provide personal health services and sanitation services. They often work with other community agencies in providing these needed services.

Often the local health department is the first source of health care for the poor, transient, or underserved populations. They may provide necessary outreach to homeless shelters, prostitutes, travelers' aid groups, and migrants. Local health departments usually operate on a free or nominal fee basis. Sometimes the vastness of the geographical dimensions of a local community and the lack of economic resources (taxes) make the provision of health care for all its citizens impossible. Community health promotion services are often the first to be eliminated in local health cutbacks. Only programs required by legislation are often retained during financial austerity. As they struggle onward, local health departments may also be involved in Healthy People 2010.

Philanthropic Organizations

Philanthropic organizations include many foundations that are established by a single donor or family, and they aid a wide variety of activities through the allocation of grant monies. Well-known philanthropic organizations include the W. K. Kellogg Foundation of Battle Creek, Michigan, and the Robert Woods Johnson Foundation of New Jersey, that work in developing and expanding educations program in health and agriculture. The Milbank Memorial Fund of New York is interested in the application of social and behavioral sciences to public health and preventive medicine and has supported work in demography, vital statistics, population, and general health problems. The Ford Foundation of New York has concentrated its work in less developed countries (LDC) in education, economic development and planning, food production, and child survival.

The Rockefeller Foundation is probably the best known for its historical beginnings and significant contributions to public health. During the building of the Panama Canal, the Panama Canal Commission waged a successful campaign against mosquitoes and their diseases, malaria and yellow fever. United States industrialists brought some of the lessons of Panama home to the southern United States. John D. Rockefeller convinced the General Education Board to support "the general organization of rural communities for economic, social, and educational purposes." The soon to become Rockefeller Foundation played a major part in ridding the southern United States of hookworm and malaria in the early part of the 1900s by allocating one million dollars to the Eradication of Hookworm Disease program. The yellow fever vaccine was developed in Rockefeller Foundation laboratories in 1936. Rockefeller Foundation money eradicated the *Anopheles gambiae* (malaria-carrying mosquito) in Brazil in 1938. Although Rockefeller was not 100 percent successful in eradicating hookworm, he was a major force behind expanding the role of public health agencies in the United States and abroad.

Volunteer Organizations

Volunteer organizations often emerge as the result of a need not being met by government agencies. They tend to organize around a cause such as AIDS, drunk driving, a chronic illness support group, or an emergency situation. The leadership may receive a salary, however, almost all community health education is centered around a volunteer staff of lay people who are trained to address a health issue and then implement a particular program. These organizations may disappear as need is reduced or interest wanes.

Most often voluntary agencies raise money for immediate health needs within their "community" and for ongoing research; and they provide education to professionals and families associated with the health concern addressed.

Quasi-Governmental Health Organizations

The American Red Cross—first known as the National Relief Organization—was established by Clara Barton (1821–1912) and her army of women volunteers, who went to the Civil War battlefront to administer to wounded soldiers. The United States Congress responded to Barton's plea to set up relief agencies much like those that were found in Europe. In July 1882, the United States then approved the treaty covering the Red Cross and its place in the international Geneva Convention Treaty. The International Red Cross emphasis is on helping the survivors of natural disasters. It has served in all wars since its beginning, and it has been a recognized part of the international philanthropic community: "There is no doubt that the day is not far distant—if it has not already come—when the American people will recognize the Red Cross as one of the wisest and best systems of philanthropic work in modern times" (editorial in the Chicago Inter Ocean, 1884).[20] Over one hundred years later, the Red Cross has lived up to this prediction, serving a worldwide population in many capacities.

Although the American Red Cross is a volunteer organization, it has been given, over time, some official responsibilities. Essentially, the American Red

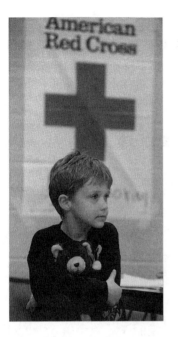

The American Red Cross is often the first volunteer agency on the scene of a disaster in urban or rural America, often providing shelter for those who lose their homes.

Cross oversees much of the collection of blood in the United States. Further, the American Red Cross is often an official disaster emissary of the United States government.

Professional Organizations

Most professionals in the health care field are able to affiliate with associations promoting advancement in their fields, providing accreditation and certification, and updating membership on important developments within the field through professional journals. Common to most professional organizations are forums to exchange and discuss current research, opportunities for continuing education, and establishment of professional ethics and national leadership. In 1988 there were more than 17,000 members combined in eight health education units of seven national organizations that comprised the Coalition of National Health Education Organizations.[21]

Well known among the myriad of professional medical organizations are **The American Medical Association (AMA),** the **American Nurses Association,** and the **American Dental Association.** Community Health Educators are primarily affiliated most often with the **American Public Health Association (APHA),** the **American Alliance for Health, Physical Education, Recreation and Dance (AAHPERD),** the **Society for Public Health Education (SOPHE),** the **American College Health Association (ACHA),** and the **American School Health Association (ASHA).** Most states have their own public health, medical, and health education associations as well.

BOX 2.3 Addresses of Professional Health Organizations

1. American College Health Association
   2807 Central Street, Evanston, Illinois
   60201

2. American Public Health Association
   800 I Street N.W. Washington, DC
   20001-3710

3. Association for the Advancement of
   Health Education
   1900 Association Drive, Reston,
   Virginia 22091

4. Society for Public Health Education
   2001 Addison Street, Suite 220, Berkeley, California 94704

5. American Alliance for Health, Physical
   Education, Recreation and Dance
   1900 Association Drive, Reston, Virginia
   22091

BOX 2.4 Global Health Targets

1. Health equity: childhood stunting
2. Survival: MMR, CMR, life expectancy
3. Reverse global trends of five major
   pandemics
4. Eradicate and eliminate certain
   diseases
5. Improve access to water, sanitation,
   food, and shelter

6. Measures to promote health
7. Develop, implement, and monitor
   national HFA policies
8. Improve access to comprehensive
   essential, quality health care
9. Implement global and national health
   information and surveillance systems
10. Support research for health

International Organizations

The most widely known and admired of international health agencies is probably the **World Health Organization (WHO).** The WHO, located in Geneva,
Switzerland, is the guiding and lead agency for most worldwide or global health
initiatives that cross global borders. It was the WHO that was the lead agency
for the eradication of smallpox on the planet in 1977.

Approximately 189 nations hold membership in the WHO at any time.
Each nation pays dues in proportion to its ability to pay, and participates in the
planning and policy decisions through the World Health Assembly that is comprised of delegates from member nations.

The purpose of WHO is to (1) provide funds to improve health and control
pacific diseases, and (2) provide central technical services, advisors, and personnel. Much like Healthy People 2010, the WHO has created a collaborative
program with the United Nations Children's Fund called **Health for All in the
21st Century.** The modification of goals for this program for the next millennium are in process. Global health targets are given in Box 2.4.

Summary

Given the current fiscal and political environment, any major expansion of the state and local role in health would be very surprising. Yet, the numbers of people needing health assistance, and the number of new health problems that are emerging in the environment, require some sort of vigilance and increased attention. Many state fiscal conditions have seriously deteriorated since mid 1982. The widening gap between needs and resources available to meet them are making policy decisions and resource allocation decisions very complex and painful. The solution probably lies in a reorganization of the United States health care system; one that is broad, fair, streamlined, and not based solely on making money. In other words, "health care for people, not profit." Much like former Vice President Gore's attempt to "reinvent government," health care must also be reinvented. It will also require rethinking the national agenda. Answers should be sought as to what programs in and out of health care have become relatively obsolete, which tasks can be given to the private sector, which need to be reclaimed with vigor, and how equal access to health care can be obtained.

CYBERSITES RELATED TO CHAPTER 2

Centers for Disease Control
   www.cdc.gov

National Institutes of Health Directory
   www.med.nyu.edu/keyword.html

U.S. Department of Health & Human Services
   www.dhhs.gov

QUESTIONS

1. Does personal medical care or public health have the greater effect on health itself? How and why?

2. How do the primary responsibilities of the local health departments differ from those of the state health departments? Why are these differences necessary?

3. What are the advantages to a community health educator in belonging to a professional organization?

4. Describe similarities and differences in the health problems of the 1800s and the 1900s. What will be the health problems of the new millennium?

5. What were some of the key breakthroughs in early research that helped pave the way toward prevention?

6. How is "community health" history interwoven into "public health" history?

EXERCISES

1. Put yourself in the position of a person in need of public assistance. Go to your local social service agency and apply for Medicaid, Food Stamps, or WIC supplemental food program. How can we make public assistance a more dignified experience for those who need this service?

2. Imagine yourself on a national health planning committee. What are five suggestions you would contribute for reorganizing health care in the United States? What would be your priority health issues? What changes would you make in the health organization for your local community?

INTERNET INTERACTIVE ACTIVITY

The Wonder of Wonder: Using the Internet to Update Mortality and Morbidity Data

Throughout this text students will be able to find specific mortality and morbidity data for their communities, state, or regions by using programs available through the Internet. For community health professions, the CDC Wonder program is a fast and efficient means of finding data by demographic characteristics. For instance, what if you wanted to know the mortality incidence and rate for men and women of all races for the author's city, Salt Lake City, Utah? Follow the steps below to determine these data.

1. Using your Internet browser, go to the following web address:

   www.cdc.gov/nchs/datawh/cdcwond.htm

2. You will get to the next page:

   wonder.cdc.gov/

   On this page you will click on **Searches and Queries** which will take you to instructions for using the data base.

   wonder.cdc.gov/rchtml/Convert/data/AdHoc.html

3. On this page you will log on as an **Anonymous user,** which should take you to

   wonder.cdc.gov/

4. You are now ready to search for the answer to the question, What were the number and rate of deaths in Salt Lake City, Utah, in the most recent year for men and women of all races and ages? So click on **Get Data,** which takes you to

   wonder.cdc.gov/SearchesQueriesSelect.shtml

5. Among the data sets you see **Mortality,** which you click and which takes you to

   wonder.cdc.gov/mortJ.shtml

6. Now you tell Wonder what data you want

Utah

Salt Lake County

All races

All genders

All ages

For the most recent year available

no age adjusted rates

no specific mortality codes

displayed by gender

7.   **Send,** which takes you to

wonder.cdc.gov/wonder/usr/anonymous/ANONDE816F542D/
WQ0NE5PH.PCW.00.html

This page reports

Gender	Death Count	Population	Death Rate
Male	4,906	830,562	590.68
Female	4,688	837,252	559.92

You now know that among all men of all races and all ages, there were 4,906 deaths between 1996–1997, which was a rate of 590.68 per 100,000. Among all women of all races and all ages there were 4,688 deaths with a rate of 559.92 per 100,000.

Using Wonder, follow the directions above and find the mortality rate for your city. You may change the variables as your curiosity moves you.

REFERENCES

1. Fee, Elizabeth (1991). The origins and development of public health in the U.S. In *Oxford textbook of public health*. Vol. 1, p. 3.

2. Basch, Paul (1990). *Textbook of international health*. New York: Oxford University Press.

3. Ibid.

4. Kime, Robert E. (1992). *Environment and health*. Guilford, CT: Dushkin Publishing.

5. Klein, Richard J., & Freedman, Mary Ann (1993). *Revisions to Healthy People 2000 baselines*. Statistical Notes, U.S. Dept. of HHS, CDC. Number 5, July.

6. Camus, Albert (1948). *The plague*. London: Hamish Hamilton.

7. Basch, op. cit.

8. Bryan, Jenny (1988). *Health and science*. New York: Hampstead Press.

9. Fee, op. cit.

10. Ibid.

11. Ibid.

12. Green, Lawrence W. (1990). *Community health.* St. Louis: Times Mirror/Mosby.

13. Schneider, Mary Jane (2000). *Introduction to public health.* Gaithersburg, MD: Aspen Publishers.

14. McKenzie, James (1999). *Introduction to community health.* Sudbury, MA: Jones and Bartlett.

15. Etheridge, Elizabeth W. (1992). *Sentinel for health.* Berkeley: University of California Press.

16. Centers for Disease Control and Prevention: *CDC Fact Book, FY 1992,* U.S. Department of Health and Human Services.

17. Schneider, op. cit.

18. Ginzburg, Harold, & Jevec, Robert J. (1993). The Public Health Service's response to Hurricane Andrew. *Public Health Reports 108*(2), March/April, p. 241.

19. Miller, Dean (1992). *Dimensions of community health.* New York: Wm. C. Brown.

20. Schneider, op. cit.

21. Directory of the Coalition of National Health Education Organizations, 1988–1989. New York: National Center for Health Education, 1988, pp. 1–8.

CHAPTER 3

Financing and Providing
Health Care

Chapter Objectives

The student will:

1. compare fee for service health care with socialized health care.

2. explain how Americans are insured and how uninsured citizens finance their health care.

3. outline the basic services of Medicaid.

4. outline the basic services of Medicare.

5. name the four health block grants and describe what is covered under each grant.

The Economics of Health Care

Health care is a service that may be purchased by individuals in the United States through private health care plans, employer-based insurance or deduction payments, or government entitlement plans such as Medicaid. The economics of health care differ from other industries. Traditionally, health care has suffered from little competition, little consumer input, consumer ignorance, barriers to entry, and little government regulation. It is no wonder that in the twenty-first century paying for health care is a complex and controversial priority for the American public.

After defense costs, the cost of health care is the most overwhelming of all economic responsibilities for Americans. In 1999, health care spending in the United States was $4,000 per person. In 1999 total health care expenditures were more than a trillion dollars in the United States.[1] This is an enormous amount when compared to other developed countries where the average per capita annual cost for health services is about $475, and less than $25 in developing countries. A comparison of the percent of gross domestic health expenditures among developed countries is given in Table 3.1. This disparity is painfully real and perhaps quite questionable when it comes to the problem of providing for a healthy society.[2]

Discussion: Is the expenditure on military as compared to health excessive or necessary in the twenty-first century?

Table 3.1   Health expenditures as percent of
gross domestic product (1998).

Country	Health Expenditure
United States	13.9
Australia	8.4
Canada	7.6
Denmark	8.0
Italy	7.7
Japan	7.2
Mexico	4.7
United Kingdom	6.8

(*Sources:* Centers for Disease Control. National Center for Health Statistics)

The burgeoning cost of providing health care to 273 million people is "breaking the bank" of our federal government and private industry, impoverishing many Americans who suffer catastrophic illnesses, and results in a system that does not provide comprehensive and equitable health care. While changing the health care system is a national priority, the economic realities of the twenty-first century made such reform seem only an illusion.

The 1992 Congress had before it thirty-two health care bills that had been introduced as an attempt to save a failing health care system and provide health care coverage or increase access. Proposed health policy in the 1990s was a hybrid of free-market forces and government regulation. Naturally, the role of the federal government in our health care is controversial. Liberals tend to see the government's role as necessary, while conservatives see it as intrusive. In general, however, most citizens hoped that no matter what national plan was approved, or for whom you work or what kind of health care provider you pick, you would be guaranteed a package of benefits likely to cover doctors' and hospital bills, prescription drugs and preventive care, as well as some benefits that many current health insurance plans do not now cover, such as outpatient mental health care or home health care.

The cost of a new, national health care plan would not be less than health care now costs us, at least in the beginning. In fact, there will probably be new taxes to pay the estimated $100 billion a year cost. The payoff would be that all Americans (or at least a good percentage) would have coverage, not only those who do not live in poverty, are not unemployed, or work for employers who do not provide minimum health care plans. The health care plans were ambitious but vital to the welfare of a country that now makes over 90 million Americans dependents of government entitlements.

The diversity of health plans really boiled down to managed competition; employers, and other consumers forming large purchasing networks. Insurance companies, **health maintenance organizations (HMOs)** (prepaid health plans that provide a range of services in return for a fixed monthly premium), or other health plans bid for their business, offering attractive core-benefits packages. In theory, the tremendous buying power of the networks create competition among health plans and ensure quality and low prices.

The care provided is essentially defined as **managed care**, an organized network of doctors and hospitals much like existing HMOs. Managed care was not nationalized during the revisioning of health care in the United States, but it did emerge as the primary tool for changing the traditional fee for service system that still prevails for people with adequate, private, health insurance.

The Result

As a result of tremendous lobbying efforts by all who would be affected by a change the health care system, the non-action by Congress, and initiatives of the private sector to implement change, in the year 2000 the United States, in general, did participate in what is nationally called managed care. However, despite some non-legislated changes, there has not been a decrease in the number of uninsured and underserved Americans. The percent of uninsured by state is given in Table 3.2. The cost of providing health care has not decreased, and some health services have actually become more difficult to access than before "reform." Managed care today describes strategies that health care organizations use to control the cost, quantity, and quality of medical services. In some organizations, it is defined as a style of practice.

While all managed care organizations insure plan members and furnish the care they receive, they carry out these functions in diverse ways. Managed care organizations can be for-profit or not-for-profit, local or part of a national chain, tightly managed staff modes or looser organizations that contract with independent providers, group practices, or networks. In 2000, 81 million Americans were enrolled in health maintenance organizations (HMOs) and as many as 130 million were insured in one or another form of managed care. Nationally, more than 25 percent of Medicaid recipients and 10 percent of Medicare beneficiaries are enrolled in managed care organizations. The most rapid rate of growth has been in for-profit managed care organizations.[3]

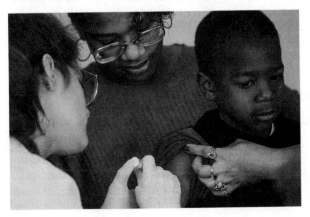

Managed care encourages early prevention.

Table 3.2   Percent uninsured, by state (1999).

State	Percent Uninsured	State	Percent Uninsured	State	Percent Uninsured
Alabama	14.3	Kentucky	14.5	North Dakota	11.8
Alaska	19.1	Louisiana	22.5	Ohio	11.0
Arizona	21.2	Maine	11.9	Oklahoma	17.5
Arkansas	14.7	Maryland	11.8	Oregon	14.6
California	20.3	Massachusetts	10.5	Pennsylvania	9.4
Colorado	16.8	Michigan	11.2	Rhode Island	6.9
Connecticut	9.8	Minnesota	8.0	South Carolina	17.6
Delaware	11.4	Mississippi	16.6	South Dakota	11.8
District of Columbia	15.4	Missouri	8.6	Tennessee	11.5
Florida	19.2	Montana	18.6	Texas	23.2
Georgia	16.1	Nebraska	10.8	Utah	14.2
Hawaii	11.1	Nevada	20.7	Vermont	12.3
Idaho	19.1	New Hampshire	10.2	Virginia	14.1
Illinois	14.1	New Jersey	13.4	Washington	15.8
Indiana	10.8	New Mexico	25.8	West Virginia	17.1
Iowa	8.3	New York	16.4	Wisconsin	11.0
Kansas	12.1	North Carolina	15.4	Wyoming	16.1

(*Source:* U.S. Census Bureau)

Some would say that managed care has been relatively successful since there has been a slowing of medical inflation.[4] It has also emphasized prevention and health education in an attempt to keep enrollees healthy. However, there are many criticisms. HMOs have dropped Medicare patients in some communities, many patients have been denied treatment that was previously covered, financial incentives to physicians translate into less care for patients, and choice is very limited.[5] In terms of community health, the primary problem with managed care has been the continuing dilemma of 40+ million uninsured Americans who delay routine preventive measures, delay early interventions and often put others at risk. Additionally, under managed care public hospitals in inner cites bear the brunt of caring for the sickest uninsured patients, and many are at risk of closing for lack of funding.[6]

Why Is There Inadequate Health Care for All Americans?

Ironically, despite an entire decade of "health care reform" no other industrialized country in the world has the large numbers of uninsured citizens that the United States does, spends more per capita, or devotes a greater percentage of their economies to health care.[7] To understand the cost of the health care

---

BOX 3.1 *What Drives Health Care Costs?*

1. The aging of the population.
2. Advances in medical technology.
3. The expectations of the American public as to the kind of health care it deserves.
4. Third party payers (users feel little pain).

5. The tax system that allows an employee to receive health benefits tax free and thus reduces economic incentives for health care.
6. Medical malpractice insurance premiums.
7. The refusal to recognize that infinite needs have run into finite resources.

(*Source:* Black, Douglas (1991). Inequalities in health. *Public Health*, Vol. 105: 23–27)

---

dilemma, one must begin to understand some of the variables that contribute to poor health care: poverty, unemployment, homelessness, single parents, hunger, inefficiency, and the insurance system.

Poverty

The 1980s took a terrible toll on the health of the nation. Despite the longest economic recovery in U.S. history, the number of poor grew significantly, while the number of uninsured increased by nearly 20 percent between 1980 and 1987[8] to a total of 43 million in 2000. Persons living below poverty in 1999 are given in Figure 3.1.

There is probably no simple, single explanation for the association between low income and poor health. To determine which variable is the leading one and which is the dependent one, we need to recognize that in differing circumstances each is capable of playing the leading role. The onset of illness in the family breadwinner is very likely to cause descent in the social scale and loss of access to health care. If the illness is severe enough it may lead to unemployment, which

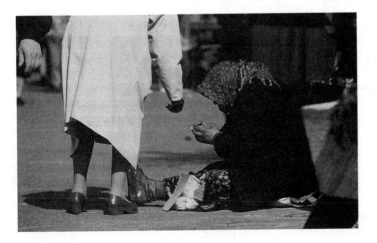

It is hard to believe that in a country that has so much, poverty still overwhelms many cities and contributes to many health problems.

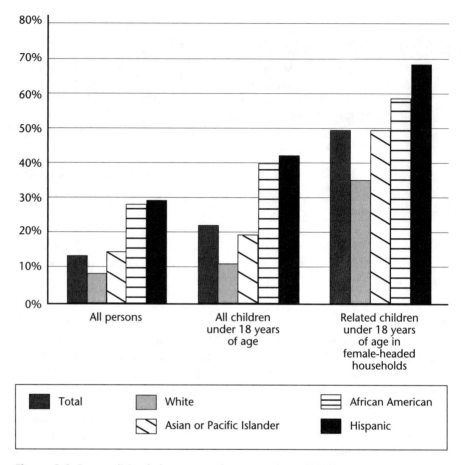

Figure 3.1 Persons living below poverty by race and age (1999).
(*Sources:* Centers for Disease Control. National Center for Health Statistics. National Health Interview Survey)

initiates a series of losses associated with poor health. Poverty and other forms of social deprivation bring with them a constellation of disadvantages, some of which are recognized as risks to health—loss of purchasing power, poor housing, overcrowding, greater liability to accidents in cramped homes and in the street, violence, and diet that even if adequate in quantity may be deficient in quality and lacking in expensive "protective" foods such as fruit and vegetables.

Other variables include difficulty in accessing health care, inadequate use of preventive measures, the specific risks of certain occupations, some of which are also ill paid, and the greater prevalence among manual workers of behaviors that are harmful to health, of which smoking is by far the worst. All of these are aggravated by poor coping skills, poor decision making, and lack of resiliency. This is called blaming the victim by some, but it may be challenged on the pragmatic ground that failure to cope is as independent as diagnosis and treatment, and can lead to no practical action.[9]

Table 3.3   Poverty in the United States (1998).

Characteristic	Number (in millions)	Percent	Characteristic	Number (in millions)	Percent
Total People	34,476	12.7	**Residence**		
Family Status			Inside metropolitan areas	26,997	12.3
In families	25,370	11.2	Inside central cities	14,921	18.5
Householder	7,186	10.0	Outside central cities	12,076	8.7
Related children under 18	12,845	18.3	Outside metrolpolitan areas	7,479	14.4
Related children under 6	4,775	20.6	**Total Families**	7,186	10.0
			White, total	4,829	8.0
In unrelated subfamilies	628	48.8	White, non-Hispanic	3,264	6.1
Reference person	247	47.4	Black, total	1,981	23.4
Children under 18	361	50.5	Asian and Pacific Islander, total	270	11.0
Unrelated individual	8,478	19.9			
Male	3,465	17.0	Hispanic origin, all races	1,648	22.7
Female	5,013	22.6	**Type of Family**		
Race and Hispanic Origin			Married couple	2,879	5.3
			White	2,400	5.0
White, total	23,454	10.5	White, non-Hispanic	1,639	3.8
White, non-Hispanic	15,799	8.2	Black	290	7.3
Black, total	9,091	26.1	Hispanic origin, all races	775	15.7
Asian and Pacific Islander, total	1,360	12.5	Female householder, no husband present	3,831	29.9
Hispanic origin, all races	8,070	25.6	White	2,123	24.9
Age			White, non-Hispanic	1,428	20.7
Under 18 years	13,467	18.9	Black	1,557	40.8
18 to 64 years	17,623	10.5	Hispanic origin, all races	756	43.7
18 to 24 years	4,312	16.6			
25 to 34 years	4,582	11.9			
35 to 44 years	4,082	9.1			
45 to 54 years	2,444	6.9			
55 to 59 years	1,165	9.2			
60 to 64 years	1,039	10.1			
65 years and over	3,386	10.5			

(*Source:* U.S. Census Bureau)

Poverty does not cause a specific illness. However, the environment of poverty does lead to morbidity (illness) and mortality (death). Those social and economic institutions that distribute income, employment, housing, child care, health care, and education are not accessible and forthcoming for all. As a result, during periods of economic prosperity the poor are not given the opportunity to participate, and during recessionary times they are vulnerable to a greater depth of poverty.

Table 3.3 gives a picture of the 34,476 million people living in poverty in the United States in 1998. The U.S. 1998 federal poverty level for one person

Table 3.4   Income poverty by region of the world (1987–1998).

Region	Population covered by at least one (percent)	People living on less than $1 a day (millions)				
		1987	1990	1993	1996	1998
East Asia and the Pacific	90.8	417.5	452.4	431.9	265.1	278.3
(excluding China)	71.1	114.1	92.0	83.5	55.1	65.1
Europe and Central Asia	81.7	1.1	7.1	18.3	23.8	24.0
Latin America and the Caribbean	88.0	63.7	73.8	70.8	76.0	78.2
Middle East and North Africa	52.5	9.3	5.7	5.0	5.0	5.5
South Asia	97.9	474.4	495.1	505.1	531.7	522.0
Sub-Saharan Africa	72.9	217.2	242.3	273.3	289.0	290.9
Total	88.1	1,183.2	1,276.4	1,304.3	1,190.6	1,198.9
(excluding China)	84.2	879.8	915.9	955.9	980.5	985.7

(*Source:* The World Bank Group. PovertyNet. www.worldbank.org/data/trends/income.htm)

was $9,500, $11,000 for a couple, and $16,036 for a family of four. The median household income was $37,005 in 1998.

The 1990 census indicated that 37.7 million residents in the United States live below the poverty level and 20 percent, or 5.7 million, older people were poor or nearly poor. The majority of poor are black females, followed by Hispanic females. Children represent nearly 40 percent of all the nation's poor,[10] and in 1998, one-fourth of children younger than age 6 lived in households with incomes below the national poverty line of $16,036 for a family of four. Poor older citizens spend more than 45 percent of their income on housing. They may spend nearly 20 percent of their limited incomes on out-of-pocket health care expenses.

> *Discussion:* Should people in poverty be getting more or less of the tax supported health services than those who pay into the tax base?

This trend is worldwide. In 1990 the poorest fifth of the world population had less than 3 percent of the economic product while the richest fifth had 74 percent of it. One-fifth of the world lives in absolute poverty. Table 3.4 shows the disparity of poverty in some countries of the world. Those who live in absolute poverty are 25 percent of Asians, 62 percent of sub-Saharan Africans, 35 percent of Latin Americans, and 28 percent of North Africans and Mideastern peoples. Given the relationship between economic status and health, it is not unusual to see morbidity and mortality increasing among the poor of the planet. In many nations, per capita income is continuing to decline with total global poverty having risen in the 1980s. In many places the total average annual health expenditure per person is less than $4.00 in United States currency. In the thirty-seven poorest countries of the world, health expenditures for children decreased by 50 percent from 1989 to 1995.[11]

In relationship to physical health, a study noted that low-income persons had higher rates of premature death, tended to die younger, were frequently ill, had less time disability free, and were less happy. Living in poverty means enduring inadequate housing, clothing and food, workplaces that are frequently hazardous; limited recreational opportunities; and a sometimes inaccessible health care system that responds in a reactive rather than a preventive manner.

Living in poverty also negatively affects coping abilities and strains both formal and informal social support.[12] The interaction of the above factors, which hinder or damage health for those living in poverty, are especially hard on individuals and families.

Ultimately, those living in poverty depend upon the resources of those who are not for survival and health care. Medicaid, financing of health care for low income persons, is a major budget expense for every state in the United States and thus for every taxpayer.

Poverty among children is a significant category that greatly increases morbidity and mortality and has long-term consequences. The emphasis on improving the circumstances of children trapped in poverty goes to the heart of the problem for the future. Children First, a non-profit advocacy group, proposes several steps to reducing childhood poverty. These solutions include increasing the minimum wage, expanding job training, reducing budget cuts in human services, expanding health and child care benefits, improving child support collections, and conducting adult literacy and English classes. These solutions are rooted in social changes that require public commitment.

Poverty also contributes to malnutrition, which increases the infant and childhood mortality rates. Studies are now indicating that malnutrition and infectious diseases are related in their ill effects. Malnutrition clearly makes many infectious diseases such as measles more severe. The diarrhea and dysentery associated with many diseases impacts calorie intake, thus increasing mortality.

Unemployment

Gorlick[13] asks the question, does unemployment kill? While the relationship between unemployment and mortality is controversial, the link between unemployment and morbidity appears to be more direct, especially psychiatric morbidity. Increased psychological disturbance in men has been linked to being unemployed, poor, divorced, of lower socioeconomic status, having a stressful marital relationship, and personal or spousal ill health. Many appropriately use the words "intense pain" and "traumatic" to describe long-term unemployment and confirm a statistical association between unemployment and death within one year. In urban areas where unemployment runs up to 75 percent, death rates are disproportionately high. Such areas are called "death zones."[14]

In the United States, being insured is almost always correlated with employment. The high cost of health care makes out-of-pocket health care expenses or insurance premiums almost prohibitive to the average person. Most families depend upon employer-subsidized health care insurance. The result of high unemployment or employment that does not include health insurance are the 43 million uninsured in 2000 (16.2% of the population). Because health insurance is tied to employment, it is also difficult for people to change jobs without putting their insurance eligibility at risk. Universal health insurance would reduce the stress of unemployment, would give people more flexibility in job choices and produce a blanket of security for those who work full- or part-time without health insurance.

A 1996 law was designed to protect health coverage for workers who quit work or switch jobs. It would allow one to transfer health insurance to a new job. This law was opposed by insurers. A 1998 report by the General Accounting Office found some companies charging $15,000 a year for new insurance policies.[15]

Homelessness

There are varying degrees of homelessness ranging from people living in insecure, unsafe, or unaffordable housing who are at risk of homelessness to people living on the street, in parks, or squats who are in a state of outright homelessness. "Homelessness may represent a single acute episode in a person's life, or a condition into which individuals enter and exit repeatedly over the course of their lives."[16]

During the 1980s there were significant increases in the numbers of homeless people that continued into the 1990s. Despite former President Ronald Reagan's pronouncement that "the homeless ... are homeless, you might say, by choice,"[17] the majority of homeless seek the alternative of a safe, private, livable home. It is estimated that 700,000 people are homeless and as many as 3 million are without shelter each night in the United States. Up to 2 million people experience homelessness in any year.[18]

In 1998 among those who were homeless, 36 percent were families with children, 25 percent children, 47 percent single men, and 14 percent single women.[19] The last government census of homeless was taken in 1996. Figure 3.2 gives the number of homeless in February in 1996 in selected cities. The census found that 46 percent suffered with alcohol problems, 38 percent had drug problems, and 45 percent suffered mental health problems.[20]

Studies show that most homeless are not deinstitutionalized mental patients as is frequently thought; one in four homeless citizens have jobs and more than one-third are in families with children. Nearly half of all poor households in the nation pay at least 70 percent of their income for housing.[21] Small children have become the fastest growing sector of the homeless—the average homeless family includes a parent with two or three children. The average child is six years old, the average parent twenty-seven.[22]

More important than physical and psychological disability may be decreases in low-income housing units (since 1980, 2.5 million low-income housing units have been torn down and have not been replaced). The shortage of affordable

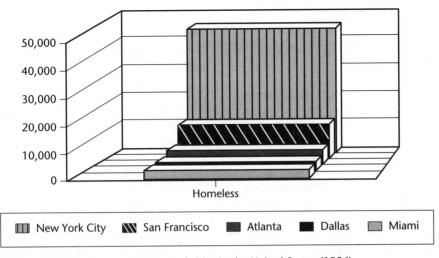

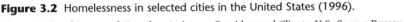

Figure 3.2 Homelessness in selected cities in the United States (1996).

(*Source:* National Survey of Homeless Assistance Providers and Clients. U.S. Census Bureau, 1996)

housing is at crisis proportions. Almost 50 percent of single room occupancy (SRO) housing has been demolished. Federal funds for the creation and maintenance of subsidized housing was reduced from $32 billion in 1981 to $8 billion in 1985. Poor families face three to ten years on public waiting lists for low income housing. On the average, people outnumber available housing five to one.[23]

In one study of U.S. homeless, 45 percent of the respondents said their health worsened since they were without a place to live. Respiratory infections and hypertension are the most prevalent health problems of the homeless, with the exception of alcohol and drug abuse. A study by the Massachusetts Medical Society noted that the most frequent illnesses among a sample of the homeless were trauma (31 percent), upper respiratory disorders (28 percent), limb disorders (19 percent), mental illness (16 percent), skin diseases (15 percent), hypertension (14 percent), and neurological illnesses (12 percent).[24]

Inadequate housing contributes to other long-term health problems as well. Quality and density of childhood housing are predictive of somatic and psychiatric hospitalization as well as conviction for criminal offenses in adulthood. A person without an address cannot realistically apply for a job, and without a job, poverty is inevitable. Providing health care to the millions of homeless in our communities is falling more often on community health education efforts. Community outreach programs are being called upon to provide personal hygiene necessities, encourage medical professional volunteer services, and do health risk prevention in shelters and on the street.

Low-Income Single Parents

Besides possible homelessness, low-income single parents, especially single mothers, experience significantly greater health problems than mothers in dual parenting situations. There is an increase in severe psychiatric disturbance, more frequent and severe headaches, and high rates of tranquilizer and analgesic use.

The primary barrier to adequate health care for the single-parent family is the cost of health care, dental care, and routine visits. Additional barriers to health care include time constraints, inadequate health care information, and work or educational commitments. Again, the state is the primary recipient of low-income health care costs through Medicaid or subsidizing nonpayment through increased costs to those with insurance or resources.

Insurance

In 2001, the primary means of paying for health care in the United States was "third party payment," or insurance. On any given day, approximately 2 percent of the working population of the United States are disabled by illness. At least 20 percent of the population are sufficiently sick each year to require the services of a physician. The cost of hospitalization has skyrocketed. Medical care is the fastest rising item in the consumer price index, with hospital costs accounting for the largest proportion of this increase. While third-party payments cover most of the expense, in some cases it may cover as little as a quarter of the total cost of an illness.[25]

Commercial medical insurance plans were first offered in the United States in the middle of the nineteenth century. Most plans are now designed to cover hospital costs with the exception of a co-payment or a deductible payment. Coverage for out-patient care is usually much more limited or requires additional insurance coverage.

The alternative to private insurance for many is a pre-paid fixed payment membership in a Health Maintenance Organization (HMO) such as Kaiser-Permanente or Family Health Practice, or a membership in a Preferred Provider Organization (PPO).

Health Maintenance Organizations (HMOs)   The Nixon administration expanded the options available for health insurance by enacting legislation for Health Maintenance Organizations (HMOs). With HMOs, payment is made in advance for services based on a fixed contract fee by a certain population. Usually, it is a group plan, provided by an employer as an option to private insurance.

HMOs strive to provide adequate health care emphasizing prevention. The result is standard health care, which costs 28 percent less than traditional fee-for-service systems. Usually, there is 100 percent coverage of services.

Although good health care is administered in a cost-containing manner, HMOs are not without their problems. High start-up costs are a concern, although they are increasing in popularity. There is also a concern with quality of health care since a patient is not guaranteed to see the same health care provider at every visit. HMOs employ physician assistants and nurse practitioners, whom although adequately trained, may not be perceived as qualified as a medical doctor to some patients. Members want to have a say in who provides their care, and they may not have that option. Also, with an emphasis on prevention one may not be able to come in for a visit without first trying home remedies. For example, for a common cold, a provider may offer advice about some over-the-counter medications for a few days, and then if symptoms persist, schedule an appointment. Some persons may not like the fact they cannot come in based on their perceived need, and cannot necessarily choose his or her specialist of choice, or choose when to visit. HMOs usually require an office visit first, and then they may approve certain specialists with whom they are associated.

Preferred Provider Organizations   This system, also developed in the 1970s, provides the consumer with a combination between traditional fee-for-service and HMOs. PPO's negotiate a lower fee-for-service with selected hospitals and health care providers in the area. Employees pay into the system, and 100 percent coverage is usually provided. There may be minimal copayments for visits. Instead of going to a central location for most services, like an HMO, consumers may go to a variety of providers, including specialists, of their choice. However, if they are not part of the system, the consumer must pay traditional fees.

> ***Discussion:*** What might account for the high and low rates of uninsured in the various U.S. states?

George Lundberg of the American Medical Association says "it is not a coincidence that the United States of America and the Republic of South Africa are the only two developed, industrialized countries that do not have a national health policy. Both have substantial numbers of underserved people who are different ethnically from the controlling group." Do you feel Dr. Lundberg's statement to be true?

The Health Care System

Growing inequalities in United States health care delivery services are creating the emergence of a two-tiered system. A 1986 study found 89 percent of black or Hispanic and 81 percent of unemployed patients were transferred to public hospitals because they did not have medical insurance. These transfers occurred even though many patients were in unstable or intensive care conditions.

The study also found that there were dramatic ethnic, racial, and age inequalities for health insurance coverage. Hispanics, blacks, and young urban city dwellers were more likely to spend at least a month without health insurance during the more than two years studied by the government. The American Medical Association refers to this as a "de facto" state of affairs, not as deliberate racism. While 82 percent of whites have health insurance only 58 percent of blacks, 54 percent of Mexican Americans, 51 percent of Puerto Ricans, and 69 percent of Cuban Americans are insured.

Whites, the middle aged, and suburbanites were more likely to be covered. Over 37 million older Americans, thanks to federal Medicare coverage, had the most extensive coverage of any group.[26] About 40 million economically disad-

Table 3.5   Medicaid recipients, 1998 (in millions).

Basis of Eligibility	Number of Recipients
All recipients	**40.6**
Aged (65 and over)	3.9
Blind and disabled	6.6
Adults with dependents	8.0
Children under 2 years	18.3
Other Title XIX	4.4

(*Source:* Statistical Abstracts of the U.S. 2000 Census)

Table 3.6   Medicaid and Medicare: percent of coverage.

Characteristic	Medicaid	Medicare	Characteristic	Medicaid	Medicare
Total	2.5	6.7	**Hispanic origin and race**		
Total, age adjusted	7.8	20.7	All Hispanic	27.6	34.9
Total, crude	7.9	20.8	White, non-Hispanic	5.4	18.3
Age			Black, non-Hispanic	19.0	34.0
65–74 years	7.5	20.3	**Percent of poverty level**		
75 years and over	8.4	21.5	Below 100 percent	41.0	26.9
75–84 years	7.9	20.5	100–149 percent	14.5	28.6
85 years and over	10.2	25.2	150–199 percent	5.1	23.1
Sex			200 percent or more	2.5	15.0
Male	5.2	19.6	**Geographic region**		
Female	9.7	21.5	Northeast	6.4	19.5
Race			Midwest	5.0	15.2
White	6.4	19.2	South	9.7	21.3
Black	19.3	33.9	West	9.9	28.5

(*Source:* Health Care Financing Administration)

vantaged were covered by Medicaid in 1998[27] (Table 3.5). Characteristics of these recipients are shown in Table 3.6.

Traditional Financing of Health Care

In 1998, among the more than 182 million Americans who lived in a household with at least one employed adult, 15.7 percent were uninsured. Nearly one in five children was completely uninsured even though United States health expenditure exceeds 11 percent of the United States Gross National Product (GNP), and the per capita health expenditures in the United States exceed those of virtually every other industrialized nation. Health care costs for the average family were approximately $9,000 in the year 2000. Where this money was spent is shown in Figure 3.3. There is no question that there is a tremendous inequity in health care in the United States. Part of the problem may be the federal government's reluctance to assure access to personal health care to all its citizens.

In 1998, a three-year federal program finally went into effect that would insure 2.4 million low-income children. Thirty-eight state plans for providing this insurance had been approved with others pending. The $24 billion program helps states provide health insurance for children in working families that earn too much for Medicaid, but not enough to afford private health insurance. Early results show a decrease in preventable childhood illnesses and a reduction in child mortality.

With the exception of Medicare, which insures those over sixty-five years old, Medicaid programs that assist eligible low-income people and some with disabilities, and a small number of programs for the uninsured and undeserved, federal laws pertaining to the provision of personal health services are generally intended to foster voluntary, privately negotiated coverage.[28] The result has been a fragmented, disjointed, selective, private health care system.

In 1987, 86 percent of the privately insured obtained their health care coverage through a private employer-based system. However, a move away from unionized jobs in manufacturing and a push toward non-unionized service sector jobs, which carry few fringe benefits and are usually at the lowest end of the pay scale, leave one-fourth of working people with no benefits. For more than

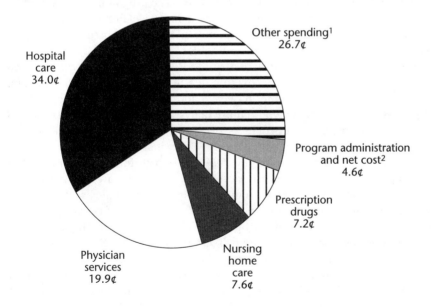

[1] Includes dentist services, other professional services, home health care, durable medical products, over-the-counter medicines and sundries, public health, and research and construction.

[2] For private health insurance.

Figure 3.3 One dollar spent on health care (1997).

(*Source:* Health Care Financing Administration, Office of the Actuary, National Health Statistics Group)

three decades, Congress has introduced national health insurance packages, but even in 1992 plans that would essentially socialize and universalize health care, or require employers to provide benefits, could not get past administrations that want less government involvement and less intrusion into business. Admittedly, it appears obvious that the cost of change to taxpayers will be significant.

Not only is business adamantly opposed to providing health insurance, but insurance companies, afraid of the burden of insuring millions of mostly low-income families, oppose similar legislation. What both are unwilling to consider is the probable savings to the federal government (taxpayers) resulting from reduced reliance by low-income working families on public programs for the uninsured.[29]

Medicare

When President Lyndon B. Johnson signed Medicare into law in 1965, he said, "No longer will older Americans be denied the healing miracle of modern medicine. No longer will illness crush and destroy the savings that they have so carefully put away over a lifetime."[30] Although that optimism fell short of reality in 2000, Medicare is still the most important source of health care financing for about 95 percent of people over the age of 65 and workers with disabilities (40.6 million persons in 1998).[31] The Medicare program was enacted on July 30, 1965 as Title XVIII of the Social Security Act. The program, administered by the Health Care Financing Administration, makes available two separate but complementary health insurance programs. In 1998, combined Medicaid and Medicare costs represented $412 billion dollars.

Part A, the **Basic Hospital Insurance Benefits Plan,** provides limited payment for hospital insurance, covering nearly all persons aged 65 years and over, disabled beneficiaries under 65 years, and workers and their dependents with end-stage renal disease who require dialysis or kidney transplant. Patients must first meet a $676 deductible as of 1994.[32] Part A services are limited within time periods called "benefit periods." There is an extra sixty days of inpatient hospital care called "reserve days." Medicare pays for about 40 percent of the medical care costs of older Americans. The poorer you are, the greater the percentage of income you spend on medical care. Older people are now spending 18.5 percent of their income on health care, more than they were spending before the passage of the Medicare bill.[33] It is also believed that Medicare is one of the most efficient systems for the delivery of health care. Ninety-eight cents of every dollar spent by Medicare is for benefit payments, compared to only sixty cents of every dollar spent by private insurance.[34] Part A is financed for the most part by the 1.45 percent payroll tax paid by employees and matched by employers. In 1998, 39 million people over 65 and 6 million disabled people were enrolled with an average expenditure of $5,300 a year.[35]

Not covered by Part A are private rooms in a hospital or nursing home, private nursing, routine physical exams, eyeglasses, hearing aids, most immunizing vaccines, ordinary dental care, dentures, orthopedic shoes, services required as a result of war, and drugs and medicines with or without a prescription.

Changes in Medicare in 1997 have added two important services to Part A. The HCFA has adopted the Healthy People 2010 goal of achieving at least a 60 percent influenza immunization rate among older Americans. Further, HCFA adopted the Healthy People 2010 goal of achieving a mammography screening rate of at least 60 percent for Medicare beneficiaries.

Part B, the **Supplementary Medical Insurance Plan,** is voluntary and assists in outpatient costs.[36] Part B provides limited payment for some doctors' services, outpatient hospital services, certain ambulance services, and some other medical services and supplies. If you choose Part B, you pay a monthly premium deducted from your Social Security benefits that in 2001 was $50.00 per month.[37] After patients meet a $100 deductible, Medicare covers 80 percent of certain physician and non-hospital costs. As of December 1998, Medicare Part B covered 36.8 million people.

In 1984, Congress approved the most fundamental change in the Medicare law since its enactment in 1964. Medicare's traditional method of payment to

---

BOX 3.2 *Title XVIII Health Insurance for the Aged and Disabled (Medicare)*

Part A. Hospital Insurance

Benefits include
1. Hospital inpatient services
   a. up to 90 days during any illness
   b. deductible coinsurance after the 60th hospital day
   c. lifetime limit for inpatient psychiatric care—190 days
2. Post-hospital extended care service
   a. up to 100 days in skilled nursing facility
   b. three-day hospital admission required
3. Post-hospital home health services
   a. approved skilled nursing care or physical or speech therapy
4. Exclusions
   a. excluded are private duty nurses and the cost of the first three pints of blood
5. Financing
   a. Part A is financed by an additional social security tax on employees, employers, and self-employed persons

Part B. Supplemental Medical Insurance

1. Physicians's services
   a. private and hospital-based medical doctors and specialists
   b. limited service by dentists, podiatrists, optometrists, and chiropractors
2. Hospital outpatient services
   a. diagnostic procedures
   b. home health services
   c. renal dialysis
   d. limited supplies, equipment, etc.
3. Exclusions
   a. glasses, dentures, hearing aids, drugs, dental care, physical examinations
4. Financing
   a. Part B is financed by a monthly premium plus government matching

hospitals, patterned after private insurance repayment models, was replaced by 467 **diagnosis-related groups (DRGs).** The DRG reimbursement provides a fixed payment for each DRG (i.e., appendicitis, pneumonia, hysterectomy, and others) that is adjusted according to whether hospitals are located in urban or rural areas. In theory, this payment plan is an attempt to keep health care costs down by providing incentives for hospitals to increase profitability by providing less care after the patient has been admitted. This should lead to a reduction in ancillary services and length of stay. In reality, DRGs have been very controversial. Not only has this program literally put some hospitals out of business because they cannot adequately recoup for long-term care that is often necessary, but many patients are released prematurely, in an effort to save money, only to have long-term effects.

The retrenchment of federal government in the 1980s created dramatic reductions in program coverage that added to its single greatest void, the failure to cover long-term care services for the chronically ill, elderly, and disabled persons.

Five of six major items of the Medicare legislation enacted under the Reagan administration and continued under former President Bush were designed to reduce program costs. The changes reduced Medicare expenditures by more than $17 billion; however, the reductions were not evenly spread out through the health care industry. Both administrations claimed that providers, not beneficiaries, would absorb the impact of the cuts. While physicians' income from Medicare continued to grow at the same rate as during the prior decade, hospital revenues from Medicare shrank and out-of-pocket costs to those who utilized Medicare increased.[38]

Medicaid

One of the most troublesome issues in health during the 1980s and 1990s was the political machinations of Medicaid. Medicaid, enacted in 1965, is the largest federal public assistance program for the poor. The program is funded by federal and state governments and is administered by states, if they choose to participate, covering 28 million people as of 1998. States are given considerable discretion in establishing eligibility, defining benefits, and establishing reimbursement. States are allowed to include not only the financially needy, but also the medically needy, the aged, blind, and disabled poor as well as their dependent children and families. The result is a massive, fractured program that does not even serve many of those who need this assistance.

Most hard hit as a result of early efforts to reduce social welfare spending were pregnant women and children and certain low-income working families that were often headed by single mothers. Major reductions in federal Medicaid funding occurred when U.S. poverty levels were climbing, thus increasing the need for Medicaid. Structural changes in Aid to Families with Dependent Children (AFDC) (cash welfare programs) eliminated more than 500,000 families with children from eligibility. Fifty percent of all families with children who were eliminated from the program were left completely uninsured. In 1986,

---

BOX 3.3 *Title XIX Grants to States for Medical Assistance Programs (Medicaid)*

Federal matching grants are made available, at the option of the states, for medical assistance programs for:

1. Recipients of federally aided public assistance
2. Recipients of Supplemental Security Income benefits (SSI)
3. Medically indigent and the aged, blind, and disabled
4. Other needy children

Programs for AFDC and SSI recipients are to include some of five basic services:

1. In-hospital service
2. Outpatient hospital services
3. Laboratory and x-ray services
4. Skilled nursing home services
5. Physicians' services

Also to be included:

1. Screening of eligible children for defects and chronic conditions
2. Family planning services

Financing

1. Federal matching is 50 to 83 percent of costs according to state's per capita income.

All states except Arizona have established Medicaid programs.

Congress passed legislation extending Medicaid coverage to children under five years old and pregnant women with incomes below the poverty level.[39]

A "mid-course correction" by the Reagan administration led to some reforms for a threatened Medicaid program. In the face of massive unemployment, the loss of private health insurance, and the resulting millions of people without access to health care, modest expansions of Medicaid benefits to cover pregnant women, infants, and young children of the working poor were passed in 1984. Ironically, this first major reform in Medicaid since 1965 came from an unlikely coalition of liberal Democrats and conservative Republicans in Congress. From their unique prospective, all were essentially concerned about the health of children and their understanding of the inherent cost effectiveness of preventive investment in child health. It is a shame that the long-term cost effectiveness of preventive education and resources for other health risks has not received the same bipartisan cooperation.

Changes in the "welfare system" of the United States in the 1990s gave new attention to the needs of children and their health. By 2002 all poor children under 19 years will be covered by Medicaid.[40] In 1998, $142 billion was spent in Medicaid for 40.6 million recipients. Medicaid recipients by race are given in Table 3.7.

Eligible health care services in the year 2000 included:

- inpatient and outpatient hospital services
- pre-natal care
- vaccines
- nursing facilities
- rural health

Table 3.7   Medicaid recipients by race (1994–1998).

	Recipients (millions)			
	1994	**1995**	**1996**	**1998**
Total	35.1	36.3	36.1	40.6
White	16.0	16.5	16.2	16.7
Black	8.7	9.0	8.6	9.8
Native American or Alaskan Native	0.3	0.3	0.3	0.3
Asian	0.8	0.8	0.8	1.0
Hispanic	5.9	6.3	6.3	6.4
Unknown	3.3	3.5	3.9	6.3

(*Source:* Statistical Abstracts of the United States, 2000)

- family planning
- nurse-midwives
- screening of children under 2 years
- laboratory and x-ray services
- physicians' services, plus other forms of health care covered at the option of the individual states[41]

Decentralization of Health Care

The concept of **decentralization,** having maximum participation in the assessment, planning, and implementation of health programs at its most immediate level is the ideal goal of health promotion in communities. Unfortunately, the magnitude of the diverse social, health, economic, cultural, and personal beliefs and issues at any level, and the lack of adequate economic resources available, have made complete decentralization an unrealistic means of providing good health care. Issues of community health have required leadership and financial support from the highest levels of government. These issues have not always received such support, and the result has been discouragement and disagreement at the local levels which have made decentralization difficult to realize.

Block Grants

The Reagan administration's program of decentralization specifically emphasized reducing the overall growth in federal spending. These programs were designed to decrease the rate of domestic spending, reduce federal support for state and local governments, and return federal operations to the private sector of the states. In essence, they promoted greater local jurisdictional freedom in providing funds, by consolidating twenty-one health programs into four block grants.

The Omnibus Budget Reconciliation Act of 1981 collapsed programs into five areas—one of which is health—and created a system of block grants to be awarded to individual states for allocation. This act also decreased overall budgetary allocations vis-à-vis the block grant programs by an average of 25 percent.

Funding for the block grants began in 1982, with a budget of 79.1 million dollars. In 1994 the funding was 152 million dollars. This means that among the fifty states, the District of Columbia, two Native American tribes, and all U.S. territories, $152 million was divided and proposed to fund state-selected areas from categories created by the Healthy People 2000 initiative.

Block Grant Programs

Originally, four block grants were associated with health care: (1) maternal and child health, (2) preventive health and health services, (3) alcohol and drug abuse and mental health services and, (4) primary care. While alcohol and drug services and primary care services are fairly specific it may be interesting to look at the great variety of services covered by maternal and child care and preventive health services:

1. Maternal and Child Health included: adolescent pregnancy programs, childhood diseases, genetic diseases, Sudden Infant Death Syndrome (SIDS), hemophilia, family planning, genetic testing, lead poisoning, well-child clinics, and handicapping conditions.

2. Preventive Health and Health Services included the following categories from among which states may determine which and how much of their block money will be spent (a few programs are required to be funded federally): home health, rodent control, water fluoridation, health education and risk reduction, health incentives, emergency medical services, rape crisis, hypertension programs, dental health, tuberculosis, environmental issues, chronic diseases, Hepatitis B, breast and uterine cancers, injury control, and disability.

In 1992 the federal government modified the Block Grant program to move the state funding from the four designated areas to thirty-four group areas based upon the objectives of Healthy People 2000.

Some believe that block grants give states flexibility, however, without adequate funding there is often less flexibility and fewer health programs. Two caveats for the state are: (1) Funds must be matching and (2) no money can be transferred from one block to another. Ultimately, the result has been a cut in state Medicaid funding and/or eligibility to cover block grant deficits; a reduction in screening programs; and cuts in licensing, family planning, surveillance, and mental health.

To continue receiving block grant money, states must provide data for the federal government that include the number of persons served through the grant, the types of services provided, the health care providers that delivered the services, and the cost of the services. States are required to include the public health objectives that they expect to achieve through the use of block grants. Finally, states are required to match $3.00 in funds for every $4.00 in federal funds.

Summary

Health care in the beginning of the twenty-first century is primarily provided by what is called Managed Care. Health care is paid for either privately or by on-the-job health insurance, by state resources for the poor and uninsurable called Medicaid, or through federal resources for older Americans called Medicare. As this suggests, providing health and safety is fractured, multi-tiered, expensive, and influenced by an economic system that tends to reward those who have the most voice and visibility within these overlapping systems.

CYBERSITES RELATED TO CHAPTER 3

Medicare
> www.medicare.gov
> www.medicarewatch.org

Medicaid
> www.hcfa.gov/medicaid/medicaid.htm

QUESTIONS

1. What are the pros and cons of federal block grants to states? Who is served best? Who is served least?

2. How will health care reform change the face of Medicare and Medicaid?

3. Why does poverty create a "death zone"?

EXERCISE

From the four block grants, take three issues from each and then create a list of priorities from most important to least important for your community. How does your list compare to other students'? Upon what criteria did you create your list?

INTERNET INTERACTIVE ACTIVITY

Determining If You Are Eligible for State Medicaid Assistance

The Center for Budget and Policy Priorities is a national organization that provides information on eligibility for Medicaid by state. Its homepage provides a document, "A State-by-State Analysis of the Number of Low-Income Working Parents Who Lack Health Insurance" by Jocelyn Guyer and Cindy Mann, that can help a community health educator determine their state's Medicaid eligibility.

Exercise
1. Go to the homepage for the Center for Budget and Policy Priorities: www.cbpp.org/2-9-99mcaid.htm

2. Go through the document's links and answer the following questions based on information you retrieve for your state.

   - Number of working parents below 200 percent of poverty?
   - Number without health insurance?
   - Percent without health insurance?
   - Number of working poor parents?
   - How much can a working parent who is applying for Medicaid earn and still be eligible for coverage?
   - Does your state cover two-parent families to the same extent as single-parent families?
   - How much can a working parent already enrolled in Medicaid earn and still retain eligibility for coverage?

3. Now go to State by State information provided at:

   www.mcare.net/1115/usaregns.htm and www.kff.org/docs/state/

4. Click on your state and determine the total spending by category on social services.

5. Compare your state's expenditures and benefits with two other states in different parts of the country. What does your research suggest about your state?

REFERENCES

1. Summary of Health Care Financing Administration FY 1999 Annual Performance Plan. www.hcfa.gov/stats/apps1999.htm 1998.

2. *USA Today* (1998). 1 in 6 Americans now lack protection; who's next? October 1, page 14A.

3. *Managed Care* (2000). An industry matures. www.managedcaremag.com/archives/0011/011.outlook

4. Lasker, Roz. D. (1997). *The current predicament. medicine and public health: The power of collaboration.* New York: N.Y. Academy of Medicine.

5. Schneider, Mary-Jane (2000). *Introduction to public health.* Gaithersburg, MD: Aspen Publishers

6. Ibid.

7. Ibid.

8. USN&WR (1995). Database, July 31, p. 13.

9. Chollet, D. (1988). Uninsured in the United States: The non-elderly population without health insurance, 1986. Employee Benefit Research Institute, Washington, D.C.

10. Black, Douglas (1991). Inequalities in health. *Public Health,* Vol. 105:23–27.

11. U.S. Department of Housing and Urban Affairs.

12. *New York Times* (1992). Health care: Four Plans. January 12.

13. Gorlick, Carolyne A. (1991). Unemployment and poverty: Correlates of

morbidity and mortality. In *Horrendous death, health and well-being,* edited by Leviton, Daniel (1991). New York: Hemisphere Publishing Corporation.

14. Ibid.

15. Ibid.

16. *USA Today,* op. cit.

17. Schneider, op. cit.

18. Butler, Sandra (1994). *Middle-aged, female and homeless.* New York: Garland Publishing.

19. (National Law Center on Homelessness and Poverty, 1999). nch.ari.net//numbers.html

20. Butler, op. cit.

21. U.S. Department of Housing and Urban Affairs, op. cit.

22. Caton, Carol (1990). *Homeless in America.* New York: Oxford University Press. pp. 96–109.

23. Ibid.

24. Chollet, D. (1988). Uninsured in the United States: The non-elderly population without health insurance, 1986. Employee Benefit Research Institute, Washington, D.C.

25. Grant, Murray (1987). *Handbook of community health.* Philadelphia: Lea & Febiger.

26. Ibid.

27. *US News,* op. cit.

28. Statistical Abtracts of the United States (2000). U.S. Census.

29. Rosenbaum, Sara, Hughes, Dana, & Johnson, Kay (1991). Legislative applications and interventions: The U.S. experience. In *Oxford textbook of public health,* pp. 29–44.

30. Ibid.

31. Doress, Paula Brown (1987). *Ourselves growing older.* New York: Simon and Schuster.

32. www.hcfa.gov.op. cit.

33. U.S. Department of Human Services (1999). MEDICARE. SSA Publication No.05.

34. Rosenbaum, op. cit.

35. USDHR (1993), op. cit.

36. U.S. Health Care Financing Adminstration (2000). Statistical Report on Medical Care Eligibles, Payments, and Services.

37. Ibid.

38. www.aspe.os.dhhs.gov/cfda/p93774.htm. Medicare.

39. Welch, William (1995). Medicaid: The bill-payer of last resort. *USA Today,* August 29, p. 4A.

40. Rosenbaum, op. cit.

41. Friedman, Bernard (1999). Tracking the states health insurance program with national baselines. Medical Care Research and Review, December, Vol. 56, No. 4.

42. Ibid.

CHAPTER 4

The Global Community and Its Health Care Issues

Community Health in the 21st Century
Malawi and many other developing countries are really still part of the
18th or 19th century. Basic issues of housing, sanitation, clean water,
immunization and feeding the people are still basic to public health. AIDS
and malaria will continue to be major health problems in the 21st century.

—Betsy Hipple, M.S. Health Education,
Peace Corps volunteer, Malawi, Africa

The day will come when nations will be judged not by their military or eco-
nomic strength, nor by the splendour of their capital cities and public build-
ings, but by the well-being of their peoples: by their levels of health, nutrition
and education; by their opportunities to earn a fair reward for their labours;
by their ability to participate in the decisions that affect their lives; by the
respect that is shown for their civil and political liberties; by the provision
that is made for those who are vulnerable and disadvantaged; and by the
protection that is afforded to the growing minds and bodies of their children.

—UNICEF Executive Director Carol Bellamy discussing
the themes of *The Progress of Nations,* 1999

Chapter Objectives

The student will:

1. acknowledge his or her role as a member of the global community.

2. give examples of health problems associated with meeting the carrying capacity.

3. discuss the similarities in health issues in both developed and less developed countries.

4. list the primary health issues of developing countries.

5. give five reasons why discrimination against women impacts world health.

6. identify the health implications of urbanization in developed and developing countries.

7. list methods for reducing health risks from environmental pests.

8. state the health implications of war.

Population Growth

The world's population more than doubled from 1954 to 2000 from 2.5 billion to 6 billion. It is expected to be 7.5 billion people by the year 2025 as shown in Figure 4.1. Every time your heart beats, three more persons are added to the world's population. By this time tomorrow, there will be about 266,000 more people on our planet; 248,000 in less developed countries (some of which are given in Table 4.1) and 18,000 in more developed countries (industrialized countries). Despite these numbers, with the exception of much of sub-Saharan Africa, perhaps the most dramatic change in most of the developing world over the past twenty-five years is not the birth rate, but the rapidly declining fertility rates.[1] This means that all national populations are aging. Life expectancy in

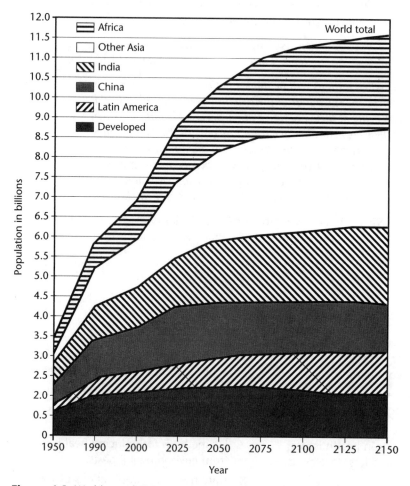

Figure 4.1 World population growth in developing (LCD) and developed (MDC) countries.

(*Source:* United Nations Population Division. In *World population: Turning the tide: Three decades of progress.* London: Grahm & Trotman, Martinus Nijhoff. Reprinted by permission of Kluwer Academic Publishers)

Table 4.1 The United Nations list of least developed countries (1995).

Afghanistan	Angola	Bangladesh	Benin
Bhutan	Burundi	Burkina Faso	Cambodia
Cape Verde	Chad	Central Africa	Comoros
Djibouti	Eritrea	Equatorial Guinea	Ethiopia
Gambia	Guinea	Guinea Bissau	Haiti
Kiribati	Lao	Lesotho	Liberia
Madagascar	Malawi	Maldives	Mali
Mauritania	Myanmar	Mozambique	Nepal
Niger	Rwanda	Sao Tome	Samoa
Solomon Islands	Somalia	Sudan	Togo
Tuvalu	Uganda	Tanzania	Vanuatu
Yemen	Zaire	Zambia	

(*Source:* UNCTAD, 1995. *Least Developed Report,* United Nations Publication. No E.95.II.D.2)

Table 4.2 World population dynamics.

	Population mid–1999 (millions)	Births per 1,000 pop.	Deaths per 1,000 pop.	Natural Increases (annual, %)	"Doubling Time" in Years at Current Rate	Projected Population 2010	2025 (millions)
World	5,981.7	23	9	1.4	49	6,883	8,054
More developed	1,181.2	11	10	0.1	583	1,216	1,241
Less developed	4,800.5	26	9	1.7	40	5,667	6,613
Less developed (Excl. China)	3,546.4	29	9	2.0	35	4,272	5,251

(*Source:* The World Bank. Health, Nutrition, and Population. http://devdata.worldbank.org/hnpstats/)

Table 4.3 World population over 60 years.

	Population aged 60 years or older					
	Number (thousands)		Percentage of total population		Percentage 80 years or older	
Country or area	1999	2050	1999	2050	1999	2050
World total	593,111	1,969,809	10	22	11	19
More developed regions	228,997	375,516	19	33	16	27
Less developed regions	364,133	1,594,293	8	21	9	17
Least developed countries	30,580	180,983	5	12	7	10

(*Source:* United Nations. www.un.org/esa/socdev/ageing/agewpop1.htm)

more developed countries is seventy-four years, and in less developed countries it is sixty-three years. World ppopulation dynamics are given in Table 4.2. Table 4.3 shows the differences in the population over age 60 for different regions of the world. In a study among population experts, the emerging issues for world population growth are given in Figure 4.2.

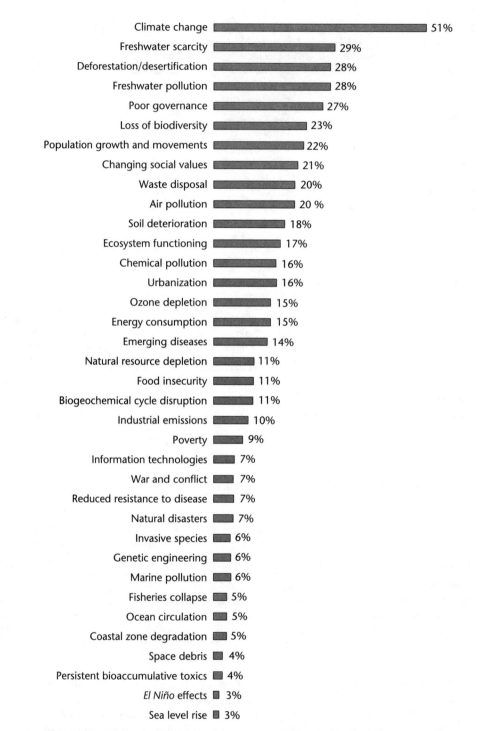

Figure 4.2 Percentage of respondents mentioning emerging international issues.

Discussion: Should fertility control be required of countries where most people live in poverty? Should fertility control be required of people who live in poverty in the United States? How would you feel if the state controlled your ability to reproduce?

The increase in world population is directly related to the decrease in the planet's forests, grasslands, wetlands, topsoils, wild animal species, fossil fuels, and clean air. It is not enough to just document the reduction in these natural resources. Humans on the planet live in a very delicate relationship with the diversity of other life forms. When the natural resources disappear or become so polluted as to be useless to the planet, the health of both the planet and all living things on the planet is in jeopardy. The maximum population of individuals or a species that a specific environment can support without harmfully affecting these resources is called the environment's **carrying capacity.** The carrying capacity has already been met in many countries. For example, over 2,000 years ago, northern Africa was a fertile land that supplied the expanding Roman empire with grain. Today, this region is mostly desert, and half of its own grain supplies are imported.[2] Carrying capacity becomes difficult to adequately define when working with the human species because of the modifiable factors of technology, levels of physical and human capital, political infrastructure, international and regional trade, and cultural needs of a population.[3]

Look at the world population grow by the second at this address: www.metalab.unc.edu/lunarbin/worldpop

In 1983, three international organizations estimated the population-supporting capacities of 117 countries, excluding China, in the year 2000. The estimates were based on both the level of farming technology employed and the physical potential of the land to produce food, taking into account such factors as the type of soil, available moisture, and the length of the growing season. For all countries in the study, the estimated carrying capacity was 5.7 billion people with a low level of technology, 14.4 billion with an intermediate level and 32.3 billion with a high level.[4] This study does not include economic analysis of gain or loss due to trade between regions or countries. In short, although there are many uncertainties and little to go on, the reality is that population seems to be increasing at a significant rate. Health and survival are two important questions to be addressed as a result of population growth.

Ninety percent of the world's growth occurs in poor or newly developing countries, with the increase in the number of persons sixty and over being three times that of the population in general (Table 4.2). Although developing countries seem to demonstrate more dramatically the health consequences of world population growth without ecological or economic balance, developed countries such as the United States are only marginally behind.

About half the U.S. population lives within fifty miles of the coastline. Coastal wetlands are gobbled up at an extraordinary rate by population growth that ruins bays and estuaries through increased sewage, industrial waste water, and runoff from cities and farms that are now dangerously close to the breeding grounds and nurseries for fully 75 percent of commercial seafood species. Louisiana, for example, loses about fifty square miles of piscatorial breeding ground annually. In California, only 9 percent of the state's original 3.5 million acres of coastal wetlands remain.[5] Wetlands are extremely important because of their interface between land and water, and they are among the most productive ecosystems on the planet. From 60 percent to 80 percent of the world's commercial marine fish depend upon wetlands. Wetlands help protect inlands against erosion and flood damage and they provide cash crops such as timber, rice, cranberries, and shellfish.[6]

Note in Figure 4.3 that the United States was the fourth most populous country in the world with an ever-increasing aging population in 2000. Figure 4.4 gives the projected demographic characteristics of the U.S. population in the year 2025, showing this increase in median age.[7]

Humans are not the only life form affected by overpopulation. Every hour, four of the Earth's wild species are driven into permanent extinction. In the United States there are 3,900 species on the candidate endangered species list

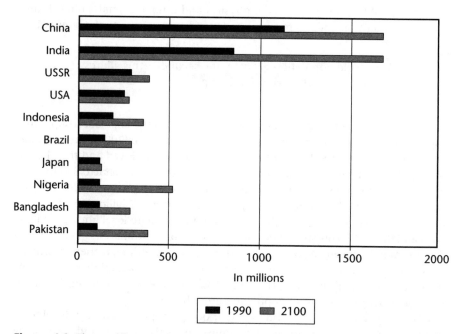

Figure 4.3 The world's ten most populous countries in 1990 with projections of population in 2100.

(*Source:* World Bank: (1990). Baltimore: John Hopkins University Press)

that will inevitably become extinct unless industrial and agricultural development is examined. In 1996, 25 percent of the world's approximately 4,630 mammal species and 11 percent of the 9,675 bird species were at significant risk of total extinction.[8]

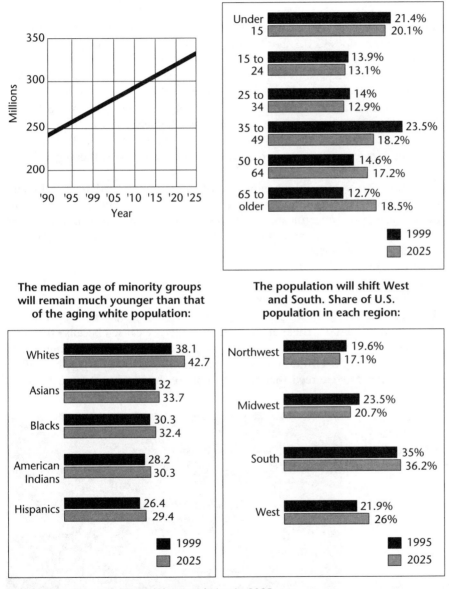

Figure 4.4 Characteristics of the population in 2025.

(*Source:* U.S. Census Bureau)

Community Health Issues Associated with Population Growth

An estimated one billion people on the Earth suffer from malnutrition caused by famine, resource depletion, and war. On the planet, one out of five persons lacks clean drinking water and bathes in water contaminated with deadly, disease-causing organisms. Even in the United States, only 74 percent of community drinking water systems meet clean drinking water standards. There are still whole communities in U.S. border towns without running water, electricity, or sewage systems.

One out of five persons worldwide also has inadequate housing and an estimated 150 million people—100 million of them children—are homeless. Government census figures in 1999 put the number of homeless in the United States at about 700,000+/night; 2 million/year homeless in the United States. In 1997, the National Coalition for Homelessness estimated that 12 million of the adult residents of the United States have been homeless, literally, at some point in their lives.[9]

Homelessness is a serious public health issue in its own right. In addition, homeless people suffer from associated conditions such as mental illness, alcoholism, drug use, tuberculosis, and substantial excess of deaths. Homelessness is a symptom of deeper and more serious changes in society regarding health care, housing, employment, and education.[10]

Furthermore, more than half of humanity lack sanitary toilets. Migrant workers hoeing, weeding, and gathering the produce that the non-hungry Americans are eating, still work under conditions that lack sanitary toilets, bathing, or drinking water. Every day, about 10,000 people in the world die unnecessarily from diarrheal disease. Their deaths are caused because they and their families, along with 70 percent of the people of the developing world, have no access to even the most basic sanitation services. Many gatherings of world leaders have agreed that a safe supply of drinking water and hygienic

Shanty towns lacking in-home water, electricity, or toilet facilities often surround some of the most urban areas of the world.

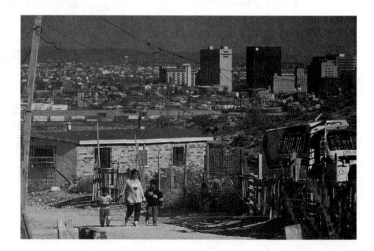

Table 4.4   Percentage of global population without water
or sanitation (2000).

Region	Percent Without Water	Percent Without Sanitation	
Global	18%	40%	(89%)*
Africa	38	40	(55%)*
Asia	18	52	(94%)*
Latin America	15	22	(59%)*
Oceania	14	7	(85%)*
Europe	4	8	(44%)*
North America	0	0	(99%)*
* regional population represented			

(*Source:* WHO. Global Water Supply and Sanitation Assessment 2000 Report.
www.who.int/water_sanitation_health/Globassessment/Global2.1.htm#Table 2.2)

means of sanitation are basic human needs. Yet the situation continues to get worse. The percentage of the population outside the United States without water or sanitation is given in Table 4.4.

> *Discussion:* What are the health implications of communities without proper sanitation? Does anyone in your community live without proper sanitation?

One out of three persons on the planet has poor health care and not enough fuel to keep warm or to cook food. Even in the United States, 47 million people have no health insurance, which results in no health care or marginal health care. The number in poverty (a family of four earning less than $17,603 a year in 2001) is 31 million.[11] By race, 33.3 percent of the poor are black, 29.3 percent are Hispanic, and 11.6 percent are white. By age, 21.9 percent are under 18 years, 12.9 percent are over 65 years, and 11.7 percent are between eighteen and sixty-four years. Of those living in poverty, 40.3 percent work full time.[12]

More developed countries such as the United States, Canada, Japan, Australia, and western European countries, which have 22 percent of the world's population and command 80 percent of the world's wealth, might at first appear to epitomize health and stability. However, the same personal and community health issues that are devastating less developed countries do in fact exist, and their negative consequences are increasing.

It is not enough to just control population; both developed and developing countries must invest in the populations they produce. Shortsighted economic policies pursued by governments of both industrial and developing countries encourage the wasteful use of energy, water, and forests. Economic policies of the past fifteen years in particular have favored industry over rural occupants of the planet. Flooded farmland created by dammed reservoirs has displaced whole communities of rural peoples. Besides the displacement of millions, misguided development projects have neglected environmental factors and local needs.

The Aswan Dam in Egypt is a good example of the effect of a dam on a land-based people. Among the many consequences, there were necessary and difficult changes in irrigation and farming for 60 percent of the population. Communicable disease increased because of the change of the ecosphere, especially schistosomiasis, a parasitic disease that is now found in the majority of the Egyptian population. The dam also caused an increase in sleeping sickness because the fly lost much of the game that it once lived on and instead fed on human blood, thus passing on the disease.

Birth and Death Rates

Demographers, or population specialists, normally use the annual crude birth rate and crude death rate rather than total number of live births and deaths to describe population change. The **crude birth rate** is the number of live births per 1,000 persons in a population in a given year. The **crude death rate** is the number of deaths per 1,000 persons in a population in a given year. Since the base is equal (1,000), comparison of different populations can be made that

---

BOX 4.1 Facts from the World Health Report, 1998[13]

- Life expectancy at birth was just 48 years; in 2025 it will be 73 years.
- Infant mortality was 148 per 1,000 in 1955; 59 in 1995, and will be 29 in 2025.
- Maternal mortality—over 500,000 women die each year from causes related to pregnancy and childbirth.
- Overall deaths—50 million people die worldwide each year; 17 million due to infectious and parasitic diseases; 15.3 million due to circulatory diseases; 6.2 million due to cancer; 2.9 million due to COPD; and 3.6 million due to perinatal conditions. Among the most common infections in the world are 1,000 million roundworm infections (*Ascaris*); 900 million have hookworm.
- *Dracunculiasis,* or guinea worm, will be eradicated by 2025 if national commitment is maintained; however, malaria cases are increasing and 1,700 million

people are at risk for developing tuberculosis.
- Diarrheal diseases remain a major cause of morbidity and mortality in infants and young children. Cholera is becoming endemic in Latin America and the Caribbean.
- About 50 percent of deaths among children under 5 are associated with malnutrition.
- Sexually transmitted diseases are increasing. There are 250 million cases of major STDs every year. There are 1 million newly infected HIV cases each year. In 1997, 590,000 children under age 15 became infected with HIV.
- About 7 million new cancer cases occur each year, half of them in developing countries. Two-thirds of all cancers are attributable to lifestyle and the environment.

would be impossible using only the total number of births. Table 4.5 shows the crude birth rates and death rates of various groups of countries in 2000.

Discussion: What factors encourage the disparity in birth and death rates seen in Africa?

When the birth rate of an area is greater than the death rate, its population grows. When the crude birth rate equals the crude death rate, population size remains stable or **Zero Population Growth (ZPG).** The United Nations Fund for Population Activities believes that ZPG cannot be reached worldwide until the year 2110. The 1999 crude birth rate for the world was twenty-six per 1,000 and the crude death rate was nine per 1,000. Needless to say, the world's population grew exponentially in 1999, creating a **Vital Index** of eighteen. The vital index is the birth rate minus the death rate. A vital index of eighteen is exceptionally high. When a nation's vital index begins to approach two, that nation's population is thought to be nearly stable.[14]

There are some important social factors that affect the birth and death rates and ultimately the population in developing countries. The most important factors affecting birth rates include: (1) average levels of education, especially of women; (2) importance of children as a part of the family labor force; (3) urbanization; (4) education and employment opportunities for women; (5) infant mortality rates; (6) availability of reliable birth control; and (7) religious and cultural norms. These issues were discussed at the United Nations International Conference held in Cairo in September 1994. The conference, which was convened to design a twenty-year plan to control world population growth, did have its share of critics. Some nations opposed plans that would include abortion services as part of reproductive rights and family planning. Ultimately, factual information supported the social factors mentioned above, which impact high birth rates worldwide. The greatest worldwide emphasis will be directed toward literacy programs for women and basic human rights for women and female children. For example, we know an average of 6.9 children are born in developing countries to women with no schooling, while 3.9 are born to women with seven or more years of schooling. Chances are, in fact, that ninety-three of every one hundred babies born in 2000 were born in a less developed country.[15]

Factors that influence death rates include: (1) nutrition; (2) sanitation, clean water and personal hygiene; (3) improvements in medical and public health technology including antibiotics and immunization. (Please see Chapter 5 for a detailed description of **rates.**) As shown in Figure 4.5, the greatest cause of death worldwide is infectious and parasitic diseases (32 percent), followed by diseases of the circulatory system (19 percent), and unknown causes (16 percent).

All of the factors mentioned above can be impacted by a worldwide commitment to public health. Even in the United States, the infant mortality rate is among the highest in the developed world, with twenty-two other developed countries having lower rates. Factors that could reduce the infant mortality rate

Table 4.5   Birth and death rates for selected countries.

Country or Area	Crude Birth Rate[1]		Crude Death Rate[2]		Expectation of Life at Birth (years)		Infant Mortality Rate[3]		Total Fertility Rate[4]	
	1996	2000, proj.	1996	2000, proj.	1996	2000, proj.	1996	2000, proj.	1996	2000, proj.
Slovakia	12.6	15.5	9.4	9.5	73.0	73.5	10.7	10.2	1.65	1.95
Somalia	44.2	41.7	13.2	12.0	55.5	57.0	121.1	111.6	7.01	6.53
South Africa	27.9	25.5	10.3	11.6	59.5	57.2	48.8	46.6	3.43	3.13
Spain	10.0	12.0	8.9	9.1	78.3	79.1	6.3	5.7	1.26	1.51
Sri Lanka	17.9	16.9	5.8	5.9	72.4	73.2	20.8	18.7	2.05	1.95
Sudan	41.1	38.8	11.5	10.3	55.1	56.8	76.0	69.2	5.89	5.47
Sweden	11.6	10.5	11.4	11.1	78.1	78.5	4.5	4.4	1.72	1.60
Switzerland	11.4	11.2	9.6	9.5	77.6	78.1	5.4	5.2	1.47	1.59
Syria	39.6	36.1	5.9	5.3	67.1	68.4	40.0	35.2	5.91	5.19
Taiwan[5]	15.0	14.4	5.5	5.7	76.0	77.3	7.0	6.3	1.76	1.75
Tajikistan	33.8	34.5	8.4	8.3	64.5	65.1	113.1	104.1	4.38	4.47
Tanzania	41.3	39.8	19.5	20.9	42.3	40.0	105.9	101.4	5.67	5.31
Thailand	17.3	16.2	7.0	7.2	68.6	69.4	33.4	28.3	1.89	1.80
Tunisia	24.0	22.5	5.2	5.1	72.6	73.6	35.1	30.1	2.92	2.68
Turkey	22.3	20.4	5.5	5.2	71.9	73.8	43.2	33.3	2.58	2.35
Uganda	45.9	43.1	20.7	21.8	40.3	38.1	99.4	95.6	6.61	6.24
Ukraine	11.2	13.2	15.1	14.9	66.8	67.8	22.5	21.2	1.60	1.87
United Kingdom	13.1	12.1	11.2	10.9	76.4	77.1	6.4	6.0	1.82	1.79
Uzbekistan	29.9	28.9	8.0	7.7	64.6	65.2	79.6	77.5	3.69	3.56
Venezuela	24.4	21.5	5.1	4.9	72.1	73.3	29.5	25.5	2.87	2.53
Vietnam	23.0	20.0	7.0	6.5	67.0	68.5	38.4	33.7	2.69	2.31
Yemen	45.2	43.3	9.6	7.9	59.6	62.6	71.5	57.9	7.29	6.86
Zaire	48.1	46.5	16.9	15.6	46.7	48.1	108.0	98.9	6.64	6.39
Zambia	44.7	43.8	23.7	25.8	36.3	33.7	96.1	97.6	6.55	6.28
Zimbabwe	32.3	29.3	18.2	21.6	41.9	38.2	72.8	72.2	4.09	3.50

[1] Number of births during 1 year per 1,000 persons (based on midyear population). [2] Number of deaths during 1 year per 1,000 persons (based on midyear population). [3] Number of deaths of children under 1 year of age per 1,000 live births in a calendar year. [4] Average number of children that would be born if all women lived to the end of their childbearing years and, at each year of age, they experienced the birth rates occurring in the specified year. [5] See footnote 2, table 1325. [6] Serbia and Montenegro have asserted the formation of a joint independent state, but this entity has not been recognized by the United States. Data in this table are for Serbia alone.

(*Source:* U.S. Census Bureau, unpublished data)

in the United States include: (1) prenatal care; (2) providing drug treatment programs for pregnant women; (3) access to family planning services; and (4) reducing teen pregnancies.

Miller (1992)[16] and other demographers and public health activists believe that the most important method of improving life on earth is by improving the

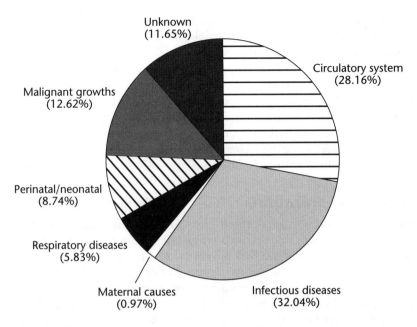

Figure 4.5 Primary causes of death worldwide (2000 estimates).

(*Source:* World Health Report, WHO. With UNAIDS estimates)

socioeconomic-political conditions of women in developing and developed countries. Today, women do most of the world's domestic work and child care, mostly without pay. They also do more than half the work associated with growing food, gathering fuelwood, and hauling water. Women also provide more health care with little or no pay than all the world's organized health services put together. The worldwide economic value of women's work at home is estimated at $4 trillion annually. This unpaid labor is not included in the GNP of countries, making the value of women in an economy unrecognized and unrewarded.

Despite their vital economic and social contributions, most women in developing countries do not have a legal right to own land or to borrow money. Many women are legally abused, raped, or beaten by their husbands. When birth control is available it is at the behest of male governments that are trying to control their economies, not care for the health and welfare of women.

Given the legal and social position of women worldwide, it is impossible to believe that population growth can be controlled by uneducated, disempowered women who lack inexpensive, available birth control. Attempts by countries such as India and Thailand to have men participate in birth control through vasectomies have not been very successful.

Numerous studies have shown that increased education is a strong factor leading women to have fewer children. Educated women are more likely to be employed outside the home, to marry later, lose fewer infants to death, and have access to birth control.[17] Educated women seem to have greater self-esteem and a more positive sense of personal power.

Each year, 1.3 million women die from reproductive health-related problems. A woman in Italy has a one in 17,000 chance of dying from the complications of reproduction verses a one in sixteen chance in Zaire (compared to a one in 5,600 chance in the United States). The United Nations World Conference on Women, held in Beijing in September 1995, focused much of its program on the goal of improving the second-class health status of women, and the goal of medical equality for women and men.[18]

Health and Urbanization

As economies shift from a rural subsistence to an urban industrial basis, changes such as improved sanitation and refrigeration help reduce the risks of communicable disease. Urban dwellers have increased proximity to and use of health services. However, half of the urban population of developing countries live in slums and shanty towns. In such urban environments there is an increase in industrial and vehicular accidents, and an increase in incidence of environmentally related morbidity. While access to food is increased and malnutrition may be curbed, different dietary regimes can increase the risks of death due to obesity, hypertension, atherosclerosis, and diabetes.[19]

Hunger

The World Commission on Environment and Development of the United Nations concluded that the problem of global hunger is now primarily social and political, not technological. The 1992 Commission believed that the agricultural resources and the technology needed to feed growing populations were available. What is lacking are policies to ensure that food is produced where it is needed and in a manner that sustains the rural poor.

Despite massive relief efforts from Europe and North America, more than 300,000 people died of hunger-related causes during the Ethiopian famine of 1983–1985. As horrifying as this was, and continues to be throughout the famine stricken parts of the planet, this tragedy pales beside the figures of 148 earlier famines. The Ukrainian famine of 1921–1922 may have taken 9 million lives and the famous Bengal famine of 1770 claimed 10 million lives.

Amazingly, most hunger related deaths do not occur in famines. They happen daily, quietly, largely unchronicled, all around the world. The Hunger Project (1985) estimated the annual death rate from hunger at 13 to 18 million. The United Nations estimated the number of hungry people in the world grew by 15 million from 1970 to 1980, to a total of 475 million in 1990 and those with inadequate diets rose from 650 million to 730 million. Several million of these hundreds of millions die each year.[20]

Time magazine, in 1974, described eloquently and succinctly how hunger kills:

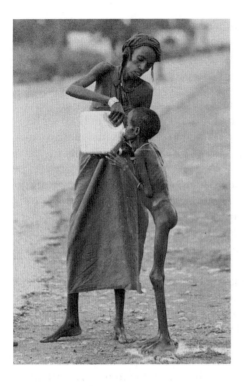

A Somali mother gives her starving daughter a drink outside an international aid agency feeding center.

The victim of starvation burns up his or her own body fats, muscles, and tissues for fuel. The body quite literally consumes itself and deteriorates rapidly. The kidneys, liver, and endocrine system often cease to function properly. A shortage of carbohydrates, which play a vital role in brain chemistry, affects the mind. Lassitude and confusion set in, so that starvation victims often seem unaware of their plight. The body's defenses drop; disease kills most famine victims before they have time to starve to death. An individual begins to starve when he or she has lost about a third of his normal body weight. Once this loss exceeds 40 percent, death is almost inevitable (p. 68).[21]

Although adult males often do die of hunger during a famine, the majority of deaths, whether from famine or from chronic undernutrition, occur among preschoolers, with pregnant and lactating women at substantial risk, though less so than children.

Africa is the only continent on which poverty is expected to rise during the twenty-first century. As a result of declining food security, the number of undernourished people in Africa nearly doubled from 100 million in the late 1960s to nearly 200 million in 1995.

Undernutrition

Undernutrition is the primary killer of children worldwide. Throughout the world, including the United States, children suffer undernutrition or malnutrition in a multitude of ways. They may be crippled by vitamin D deficiency (rickets), blinded from Vitamin A deficiency (xerophthalmia), or stunted from lack of protein (kwashiorkor). The most common form of child undernutrition results simply from lack of sufficient calories.

In the United States, researchers estimate that 13 million children, more than one-fourth of all children under the age of 12, have a difficult time getting all the food they need. In the United Kingdom, children and adults in poor families have been found to face increased risks due to poor diet, including premature births, low birthweights, anemia, dental diseases, diabetes, obesity, and hypertension.[22]

Undernutrition diminishes the body's immune response, contributing to more frequent and longer episodes of sickness. For school children this means decreased attentiveness and learning while attending school as well as fewer days spent in school due to illness. Undernutrition is a major public health concern, yet, despite this serious problem, school breakfast and lunch programs have lost federal and state funding during the past ten years as economic hard times have impacted social service programs.

In developing countries, the most cost-effective way of prolonging the lives of children at risk to undernutrition or severe diarrhea is to teach mothers about **oral rehydration therapy.** In 1948, nutrition specialists found that certain combinations of sodium and glucose can be absorbed through the intestine, even though severe diarrhea may be present. Oral rehydration is the process of replacing life-supporting nutrients that have been lost due to undernutrition or diarrhea. It was not until 1985 that the American Academy of Pediatricians began to emphasize immediate rehydration therapy as an easy and important treatment for dehydration of children and the elderly.

Oral rehydration combines a mixture of 1.5 g/l calcium chloride, 3.5 g/l sodium, and 20 g/l glucose with 2.5 g/l sodium bicarbonate. After twenty-four hours of oral rehydration, rice water and wheatgerm can be added. This is not a difficult process, and the United Nations Children's Fund (UNICEF) is vigorously promoting this for developing countries to combat dehydration due to diarrhea. Diarrheal diseases remain a major cause of morbidity and mortality in infants and young children in developing countries. They cause 1,500 million episodes of illness and more than 4 million death each year in children under five years.[23]

Housing

As the nightly news brings pictures of refugees from war-torn nations fleeing their communities and entering previously uninhabited safety zones, the issues of housing, infestation, and germ control take on meaningful images. Imagine rearing a large family of small children in the open, without roof or refuge, surrounded by disease, decay, death, and fecal material. While even the bleakest of housing degradation in the United States probably compares minimally to refugee housing in Rwanda, Sudan, or Afghanistan, United States examples may begin to illustrate the problems.

Even early colonists knew the importance of good housing. In 1626, the Plymouth colony passed a law stating that new houses must be roofed with board. In 1648, wooden or plastered chimneys were prohibited on new houses in New Amsterdam. In 1657, New Amsterdam prohibited rubbish and filth thrown into the streets or canals, and in 1657, living in caves was made illegal in Pennsylvania.[24]

An example of the impact of public policy on health may be drawn from the housing sector. We spend two-thirds of a twenty-four-hour day in our homes. Housing is our most basic physical environment. Housing conditions are closely associated with health status, and housing tenure correlates with mortality. In Britain, people in all social classes who live in houses they own experience lower mortality than people who rent in public housing.[25] Overcrowding contributes to increases in respiratory diseases, stress, violence, and lower overall levels of health and well-being.

Housing and the hygiene of housing have sometimes been artificially separated from other environmental concerns in the structure of government programs, even though housing has the most abiding environmental impact on human life. The poorest of our population still live in dilapidated and unsanitary housing surrounded by accumulations of garbage, filth, and squalor that encourage the propagation of rodents and other pests. Poor housing aggravates the risk of air and water pollution, pest-borne diseases, bites, and toxic substances.[26]

There are approximately 12 million crowded substandard dwellings in the United States. This comprises about 15 percent of all available housing. Four million are in such poor condition that they cannot be refurbished without major repairs. This contributes to 25 million home accidents each year due to faulty appliances, electrical connections, poor lighting, broken furniture, and stairs, floors, and walls in need of repair. There are an estimated 60,000 rat bites each year. Accidental poisoning causes 3,000 deaths and 1 million injuries. Poor housing increases the incidence of infectious diseases, chronic diseases, and environmental diseases. Over 400,000 children have high levels of soft lead in their blood. The Hurricane Andrew tragedy of 1992 showed the nation the poor quality of housing construction. Recently constructed new homes just blew away when the hurricane hit. Deserted homes become dilapidated, vandalized, and havens for transient homeless. They become dumping places for garbage, breeding places for roaches, mice, and rats, and meeting places for drug addicts and criminals.

Housing quality includes climate control, numbers of people per room, running water, toilet facilities, safe environment, fire prevention, accident reduction, working electricity, and pest control. Noise control, ventilation, waste and refuse disposal, and drainage are part of community health requirements for adequate housing. In community housing projects all of the above plus the addition of green spaces, playgrounds, and parking are part of a healthy environment. Sadly, one-third of all urban populations in big cities of developed countries live in slums that do not provide the conditions for good health mentioned above.

Vector Control

In countries that have poor pest abatement programs or no programs at all, insects and small mammals are a major source of disease and infection. In some countries, animal-borne illnesses are endemic and are a daily part of living.

Poor, dilapidated housing, cluttered yards, and garbage areas are breeding grounds for many disease carrying **vectors.** Among the diseases spread by insect and rodent vectors are typhus, plague, Rocky Mountain spotted fever, typhoid, malaria, yellow fever, amebic dysentery, and tetanus. Rat bites are still a major health problem in crowded, urban public housing. It has been said that in the major cities of the United States, the rat population may be measured by assuming that there is roughly one rat for each human resident in the city.[27] Urban rats are described as "superbreeders," and produce an average of ten young every six to seven weeks.[28]

Prevention of insects and rodents includes:

1. Reduction of rat harborage by rat proofing buildings.
2. Making food supplies unavailable by proper disposal of garbage.
3. Eradication by the use of rodenticides and insecticides and by trapping and gassing.
4. Elimination of breeding sites such as stagnant water.
5. Control of infected animals which may carry an insect vector.
6. Protection of human hosts through immunization.[29]

Rats

Each year more than 43,000 people in the United States are estimated to be bitten by rats and mice. Approximately two-thirds of rat bite victims are children under the age of ten. The brown, or Norway rat, is found most frequently near commercial and residential places where garbage and solid waste accumulate and where food is prepared or stored. It often inhabits poorly maintained houses as well as warehouses and dumps. Historically, the flea carried on rats was the cause of the Black Plague. An outbreak of plague occurred in India in 1994 due to flooding that sent rats into urban areas. A combination of crowding, mobility and travel, unsanitary conditions, and lack of immediate public health control combined to create an environment conducive to the outbreak of this epidemic and its inevitable spread throughout Asia and the Near East.

Globally, the World Health Organization reports 1,000 to 3.000 cases of plague every year. In North America, plague is found in certain animals and their fleas from the Pacific Coast to the Great Plains, and from southwestern Canada to Mexico. Most human cases in the United States occur in two regions: (1) northern New Mexico, northern Arizona, and southern Colorado; and (2) California, southern Oregon, and far western Nevada. Plague also exists in Africa, Asia, and South America.

The two most common rats are the black *rattus* and the larger, brown *Rattus norvegicus*. The black rat carried the infamous plague that killed scores of millions of people during the Middle Ages. In addition to spreading many diseases, including leishmaniasis, scrub typhus, hemorrhagic fever, and Lyme disease; rats damage sewers by chewing through lead pipes.[30]

Brown rats destroy and pollute food supplies in famine-stricken parts of the world. A single rat left free to roam a warehouse for one year will eat about twenty-seven pounds of food and deposit 25,000 droppings to spoil much more.

Mosquitoes

Mosquitoes are the primary vectors of encephalomyelitis, malaria, and yellow fever. Although these are not endemic in the United States, they may be introduced into a population through immigration or foreign travel and may proliferate in poor housing conditions.

Malaria is one of the major tropical diseases occurring in many parts of the poorly developed tropics and subtropics. Malaria is transmitted by the bite of an infected female anopheline mosquito. In order to prevent malaria, environmental improvements and personal precautions must include sanitary improvements and biological control with larvivorous fish that eat mosquito larva.[31]

Flies

The housefly feeds upon human and animal waste, garbage, and other filth and debris. It then travels to other food sources and feeds again, dropping pathogens carried on its body parts to consumable food. Diseases carried by flies include cholera, dysentery, typhoid, and pinworm. The best prevention is good screening of windows and doors and frequent disposal of waste and food products. Diarrhea, often caused by the spread of waste products through fly contamination, is one of the major public health problems worldwide. It is estimated that about one thousand million episodes of diarrhea occur annually in children under five years old, with 4.6 million deaths in developing countries.

Mice

The house mouse inhabits most modern buildings of all cities if food is available. The increase of mice is correlated with the increase in rickettsial pox in humans. The deer mouse has been the most recent vector for Hantavirus that was first found in Korea and last found in the southwest United States in 1994.

Pigeons, Sparrows, and Starlings

Pigeons, house sparrows, and starlings live in urban areas all over the world, scavenging for food in streets and yards. Disease is spread through bird droppings. An increase in diseases caused by yeast and fungi that are cultured in the excreta of birds has been noted since the beginning of the AIDS epidemic because of low immune resistance to fecal-carried pathogens. Increased cases of **histoplasmosis,** caused by inhalation of dried bird feces is also possible among those who keep birds as pets.

Cats and Dogs

Cats and dogs that run free may frequent abandoned buildings, which accounts for large accumulations of fleas in these areas. Where there are large populations of dogs in cities and town, the parks and streets may become littered with feces. Tapeworms that ordinarily infest dogs, cats, and rats are occasionally transmitted to humans through animal feces deposited on human food or accidentally ingested.

Although rabies is relatively rare in domestic animals, it can be passed from raccoons, skunks, or bats to dogs that are running loose. Cases of rabies are increasing as cities move closer to the homes of forest and mountain mammals.

Head Lice, Mites, and Fleas

Crowding is one of the most significant environmental factors associated with **ectoparasites**—lice, mites, and fleas. Typhus is transmitted to humans primarily by the feces of lice and fleas deposited on human skin and then rubbed into the skin when the person scratches the bite of an arthropod. It is then spread from person to person. Flea bites are most common in developing countries, but fleas bite worldwide.

Scabies is a disease caused by human infestation with the itch mite **(Sarcoptes scabiei).** Females burrow into tunnels in the upper epidermis of the human skin, lay eggs that hatch in three to five days, and cause an itching irritation.

Current International Objectives

During the past three decades, establishing targets in public health as a national effort has been undertaken by many countries. In 1971, the Federal Republic of Germany issued a planning document that linked health policy with economic policy, cultural attitudes, and political values. Special emphasis was given to prevention, health maintenance, and care of the sick and handicapped. The Soviet Five-Year Plan of 1971 called for a general improvement in mental and physical health and a lowering of many sources of morbidity and mortality, especially those associated with alcohol abuse. The ten-year plan for the Americas, issued by the Pan American Health Organization in 1971, had a special emphasis on emerging chronic diseases such as chronic lung diseases and arthritis. In 1974, the Canadian health care system renewed its five-pronged health strategy on health promotion, regulatory protection, research, efficiency of health care services, and goal setting.[32]

Perhaps the most visible international effort of the 1980s was the World Health Organization (WHO) **Health For All** project. WHO member nations agreed to pursue the health efforts of their social and economic sectors and to report their progress every three years using a common framework to describe intersector collaboration, managerial processes and mechanisms, citizen health status, and availability of primary health care. WHO states:[33]

Health For All by the Year 2000 does not mean that disease and disability will no longer exist, or that doctors and nurses will be taking care of everybody. What it does mean is that resources for health will be evenly distributed, and that essential health care will be accessible to everyone with full community involvement. It means that health begins at home, in school, and at the work-place and that people will use better approaches for preventing illness and alleviating unavoidable disease and disability.[34]

The ultimate hope and goal of Health For All in the twenty-first century is a means of allowing people throughout the world to lead socially and economically productive lives. The barriers to reaching this goal are suggested in Box 4.2. The emphasis was to be redirected from curative medicine to primary health care and preventive health. A consideration of social problems relating to hunger, poverty, and overpopulation became worldwide objectives. The two major goals that surpassed all others were providing safe drinking water for everyone on the planet and the immunization of all children in the world against major childhood infectious diseases. (Immunization rates for childhood infections are given in Figure 4.6.) Incidently, it was not until 1993 that President Bill Clinton first articulated comprehensive childhood immunization as a political goal in the United States.

The twenty-first century world health problems are those that must be tackled by all nations. Poverty is probably the greatest factor associated with attaining health. Sadly, poverty did not ease globally in the 1990s and is projected to become worse in the twenty-first century. Hunger has been discussed at length as a worldwide health concern, along with the problems of food storage and distribution, and overpopulation. Other focuses for world health

---

BOX 4.2 *Evaluation of Health for All, 1979–1996*

In many countries, progress toward HFA is hampered by:

- insufficient political commitment to the implementation of HFA;
- failure to achieve equity in access to all PHC elements;
- the continuing low status of women;
- slow socioeconomic development;
- difficulty in achieving intersectoral action for health;
- unbalanced distribution of, and weak support for, human resources;
- widespread inadequacy of health promotion activities;

- weak health information systems and no baseline data;
- pollution, poor food safety, and lack of safe water supply and sanitation;
- rapid demographic and epidemiological changes;
- inappropriate use of, and allocation of resources for, high-cost technology;
- natural and human-made disasters

(Based on three major evaluations of the Global Strategy for Health for All)

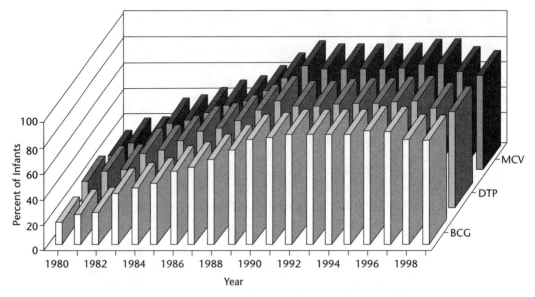

Figure 4.6 Global immunization coverage for Diphtheria/Pertussis/Tetanus (DPT), Measles (MCV) and Tuberculosis (BCG).

(*Source:* WHO. Vaccines, Immunization and Biologicals, 2001)

include housing, pest control, water supply, and desertification. Parasitic infections are still destroying populations of people in less developed countries. A sad but vivid example occurred in 1994 during the internal war in Rwanda, Africa. Thousands of desperate people were forced to scoop up muddied, fecal-contaminated water for use as a drinking supply. Unsanitary conditions bred cholera and the disease quickly took its toll on starving, malnourished people who did what they needed for a chance at survival. Other drinking water sources were shared with animals and livestock and became contaminated from organisms in urine and feces.

Desertification is another worldwide health concern. This is the destruction of land for any viable use due to overgrazing of livestock, shifting rainfall patterns, and overpopulation. Much of the continent of Africa, for example, once flourishing with vegetation, has been overused to the point of being a vast, useless desert. Inhabitants, who had little resources, raised animals for income and food, and in turn destroyed their land. People then moved on, leaving more sand in their place.

Many organizations are fighting to preserve what precious resources we have left, while trying to improve the health of world peoples and prevent diseases. Two leading international organizations, both previously mentioned, are the World Health Organization (WHO) and the United Nations Children's Fund (UNICEF).

World Health Organization

WHO was founded as an agency of the United Nations in 1948. Its motto is to "help nations help themselves" and it works toward the betterment of health for all nations, especially less developed countries. WHO developed our universally accepted definition of health as "optimal well-being and not just the absence of disease." Although safe drinking water and immunization of the world's children are two priority concerns, WHO also advocated for other community health causes. Every year on December 1, WHO sponsors World AIDS Day, in which each nation is encouraged to recognize the problems with HIV at home and abroad. Perhaps WHO's greatest past achievement was the eradication of small-pox, and its greatest future endeavor is to eradicate polio from the earth.

The World Health Organization operates through public health campaigns, worldwide data collection, and epidemic control; financing international research and training for all types of community health professionals who work in the field. WHO's headquarters is in Geneva, Switzerland, but there are regional offices throughout the world, including Washington, D.C.

United Nations Children's Fund

The United Nations Children's Fund (UNICEF) has undergone name changes over the years, but the organization's purpose has remained true: to help the world's children. UNICEF has various projects throughout the world, but concentrates on less developed countries. The agency is concerned with many health issues, including communicable diseases, malnutrition, breast feeding, immunization, and oral rehydration therapy.

BOX 4.3   A Summary of the Year 2000 Goals Agreed to by Almost All Nations at the 1990 World Summit for Children

- Reduction of infant and under-5 child mortality rates by one-third of the 1990 levels, or to 50 and 70 per 1,000 live births respectively, whichever is less.
- Reduction of the 1990 maternal mortality rates by half.
- Reduction of severe and moderate malnutrition among under-5 children by half of the 1990 levels.
- Universal access to safe drinking water and to sanitary means of excreta disposal.

- Universal access to basic education and completion of primary education by at least 80 percent of primary school age children.
- Reduction of the adult illiteracy rate (the appropriate age group to be determined in each country) to no more than half its 1990 level, with emphasis on female literacy.
- Improved protection of children in especially difficult circumstances.[35]

Voluntary Organizations for World Health

There are numerous private and church-related organizations that depend upon a paid administration and a minimally or unpaid volunteer staff to work with world health and education problems. Among these groups are the United States Peace Corps and the Maryknoll Brothers and Sisters of the Catholic Church. Many other churches also have missions and outreach programs to developing countries.

Summary

Some believe that the greatest ecological and health danger on the planet is overpopulation. When the carrying capacity of a location is reached, all well-being becomes affected vis-à-vis loss of resources, land, water, housing, oil, and balance. Others, because of religious, political, or economic beliefs, oppose efforts to curb population growth.

Although the community health issues of developing countries appear to be more serious and more significant than those in developed countries, a careful analysis will show that crowding, population growth, and limited resources create the same problems everywhere; housing needs, sanitation needs, pest control, adequate food, noise, waste disposal, water, and solid waste disposal.

CYBERSITES RELATED TO CHAPTER 4

Population Index
   popindex.princeton.edu

Unicef
   www.unicef.org

Peace Corps
   www.peacecorps.gov/indexf.cfm

QUESTIONS

1. Is there an ethical, moral, and nonracist way to control the population of the planet? How?

2. Without further damaging the planet, how might we accommodate greater population growth?

3. Why and how has food been used as a weapon of war?

EXERCISE

You are the director of the Peace Corps. You send volunteers for two-year commitments to various less developed countries around the world. Based on your reading, what would be your three priority objectives for increasing the quality of the world's health?

INTERNET INTERACTIVE ACTIVITY

THE WHO DATABANK

The WHO database contains the cancer mortality data provided by the WHO databank. This databank can provide a community health educator with prevalence of cancer by year, by country, or by type of cancer. The homepage is:

www-dep.iarc.fr/dataava/infodata.htm

Example

For this exercise the community health educator will determine all malignant neoplasms for men and women in Canada in 1997.

1. Go to www-dep.db.larc.fr/
2. Click on **Cancer Mortality database**
3. Make appropriate selections. (You can highlight more than one age and period.)
4. Click **Execute**

You can now determine the number of deaths, the mortality rate, the age standardized rate (ASR)* for men and women in Canada in 1997.

Exercise

Using **WHO DATABANK** compare the ovarian coancer rates and the breast cancer rates for women in three different parts of the world for the most recent year data are available. Select a very developed country, a moderately developed country, and a poor developing country.

Build a table that reflects the rates for your countries.

What reasons might you give for the difference in the rates of ovarian cancer for the three countries you have selected?

REFERENCES

1. Leslie, Joanne (January, 1993). *Women's lives and women's health: Using social science research to promote better health for women.* Berkeley, CA: Pacific Institute for Women's Health.
2. Kime, Robert E. (1992). *Environment and health.* Guilford, CT: Dushkin Publishing.
3. Cohen, Joel E. (1992). How many people can earth hold? *Discover,* November, p. 114.

---

* An age-standardized rate (ASR) is a summary measure of a rate that a population would have if it had a standard age structure. Standardization is necessary when comparing several populations that differ with respect to age, because age has such a powerful influence on the risk of cancer. The most frequently used standard populations are the World and European standard populations. The calculated incidence or mortality rate is then called the World age standardized or European age standardized incidence or mortality rate. They are expressed as a rate per 100,000.

4. Ibid.

5. Database. (USNWR, June 22, 1992).

6. Koren, Herman (1991). *Handbook of environmental health and safety.* Vol. I. 2nd ed. Chelsea,MI: Lewis Publishers.

7. *USA Today* (1999). In the future, diversity will be the norm. Sept. 7, p. 13A.

8. www.nch.ari.net/numbers.html (1999).

9. www.grida.no/geo2000/ov_e/0003.htm

10. *American Journal of Public Health* (1994). Editorial: Homelessness in America. December, Vol. 84, No. 12, p. 1885.

11. Appleby, Julie (2001). Report: More had health coverage in 2000. *USA Today,* Sept. 28, p. 6B.

12. U.S. Dept. of Commerce (1992). *Population and health transitions.* Bureau of the Census P/92-2, December.

13. World Health Organization (1998). www.who.int/whr/1998/factse.htm

14. Green, Lawrence W. (1990). *Community health.* St. Louis, MO: Times Mirror/Mosby.

15. *US News and World Report* (1994). September 1, p. 12.

16. Miller, G. Tyler Jr. (1992). *Living in the environment.* Belmont, CA: Wadsworth.

17. Miller, Dean (1992). *Dimensions of community health,* 3rd ed. New York: Wm C. Brown.

18. Laurence, Leslie (1995). Medical Care: Women get the short shrift. *Salt Lake Tribune,* Aug. 10, p. C2.

19. U. S. Dept of Commerce, op. cit.

20. Foster, Phillips (1991). Malnutrition, starvation and death. In *Horrendous death, health and well-being* by Daniel Leviton. pp. 205–218.

21. *Time Magazine* (1974). How hunger kills. Nov. 11, p. 68.

22. www.unicef.org/pon99/stat1.htm

23. Foster, op. cit.

24. Baum, Frances (1995). Can health promotion and primary health care achieve Health For All without a return to their more radical agenda? *Health Promotion International,* Vol. 10, No. 2, p. 149.

25. Koren, op. cit.

26. Turshen, Meredeth (1989). *The politics of public health.* New Brunswick, N.J.: Rutgers University Press.

27. Committee on Urban Pest Management (1980). *Urban pest management.* National Academy Press, Washington, D.C.

28. Koren, op. cit.

29. Grant, Murray (1987). *Handbook of community health,* 4th ed. Philadelphia: Lea & Febiger.

30. World Health Organization Special Programme for Research and Training in Tropical Diseases. ICD-9 084—Malaria.

31. Grant, op. cit.

32. WHO op. cit.

33. Ibid.

34 Ibid.

35. World Summit for Children (1990). www.unicef.org.wsc.goals.htm

CHAPTER 5

Epidemiological Methods and Language

Community Health in the 21st Century
"Much of the public has grown to mistrust results of epidemiological studies into disease causation. I believe this mistrust is born out of the media's efforts to turn research results directly into news packets for the general public, providing an appearance of contradictory and confusing recommendations. Great efforts must be undertaken to restore faith in the scientific process.

—Robert Greenlee, M.P.H.,
Public Health Epidemiologist

Chapter Objectives

The student will:

1. speak the language of epidemiology.

2. identify the demographic characteristics of a given population exposed to a communicable disease and describe how one would test an hypothesis of cause for such an outbreak.

3. be able to show the relationship among the host, agent, and environment in view of the nature of the epidemic.

4. calculate the morbidity and mortality rates for selected vital statistics.

5. list the vital statistics collected by the National Center for Health Statistics.

6. list the most common vital statistics collected by state agencies.

7. distinguish between incidence and prevalence rates.

8. compare the health status of any two states based on the eighteen health indicators established by the CDC.

History of Epidemiology

John Snow, a London physician in 1854, is thought to be the father of epidemiology after solving *"The Case of the Broad Street Pump."* After an epidemic outbreak of cholera in a London neighborhood in 1854, Dr. Snow plotted the individual cholera deaths on a simple map shown in Figure 5.1 to try to determine why the

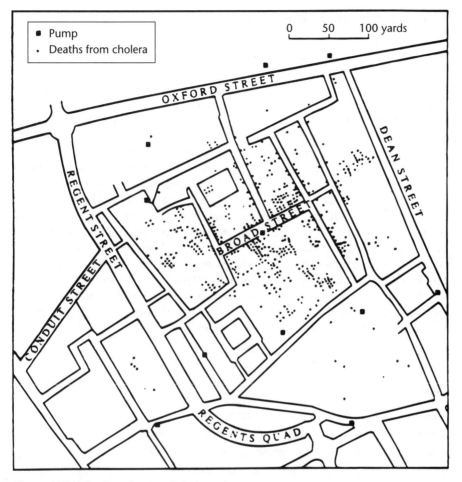

Figure 5.1 John Snow's map of cholera.

(*Source:* Vignette Figure 1-1, in Melinda S. Mead, John W. Florin, and Wilbert M. Gesler, *Medical geography.* New York: The Guilford Press, 1988, p. 20)

cholera outbreak was occurring in this neighborhood. As he looked at the picture that his plotted map revealed, he determined that cholera death rates were eight to nine times higher in areas served by the Broad Street water pump. The suspicious pump was found to be contaminated with sewage dumped by the city into the Thames River. Snow stopped the cholera epidemic by removing the handle from the Broad Street pump, preventing the use of contaminated water by the population and hence, stopping the spread of this dreaded disease. This simple act is thought to be the birth of modern epidemiology even though it was thirty years before the pathogen causing cholera was discovered.

The Science of Epidemiology

Epidemiology is the core science of public and community health and preventive medicine. The word epidemiology comes from the Greek *epi, demos,* and *logos,* which literally translated means the study (*logos*) of what is among (*epi*) the people (*demos*). Classical epidemiology was concerned almost entirely with the behavior of a communicable disease within a population or population of hosts. Chronic diseases have been the more frequent health issues of the past forty years, and have required epidemiology to develop new expertise. To study either communicable or chronic diseases requires similar, internationally recognized, methodological techniques. Epidemiology represents a philosophical and scientific method of studying a health problem, ranging from transmission of an infectious disease to the design of a new strategy of health care delivery within a population. The collection and interpretation of these data are reported in universal terms. Usually epidemiology compares a healthy group of people to a group that either has a disease or has been exposed to a harmful substance. The comparisons are made by plotting numbers of cases, locations, times, and variations in the cases to help to determine the cause (**etiology**) and distribution of a condition. The major factors involved in the analysis are distribution of the illness, population dynamics, occurrence, affected population, place characteristics, and disease determinants.

BOX 5.1 Pioneers of Epidemiology

Hippocrates (460–377 BCE)	Hot and cold diseases
John Graunt (1620–1674)	Mortality recording
Bernadino Ramiazzini (1633–1714)	Occupational injuries
James Lind (1700s)	Nutritional deficiencies
Marie Jonet-Duges (1730–1797)	Statistical use in obstetrics
Edward Jenner (1749–1823)	Smallpox vaccine
John Snow (1813–1858)	Etiology of cholera
Florence Nightingale (1820–1910)	Hygienic standards
Robert Koch (1843–1910)	Identified microorganisms
Anna Wessels Williams (1863–1954)	Diphtheria immunization; rabies vaccine
Alice Hamilton (1869–1970)	Etiology of typhoid; industrial poisons
Gladys Dick (1881–1975)	Etiology of scarlet fever; streptococcus
Lemual Shattuck (late 1800s)	Sanitation and public health
Margaret Pittman (b. 1901)	Pertussis vaccine
Edgar Syndensticker (early 1900s)	Morbidity classifications
Frances Kelsey (b. 1911)	Alerted public about thalidomide

A good example of this process was the 1993 outbreak of a mystery illness in the Four Corners area of the United States (Colorado, Utah, Arizona, and New Mexico). A deadly outbreak of respiratory distress in young Navahos living on or near the Four Corners Navaho Reservation attracted worldwide attention when no immediate cause or cure could be found. Within a day or so of flu-like symptoms, young, seemingly healthy people were dead. The first cases were only young Navahos under the age of thirty, living in a sparsely populated 25,000 square mile reservation. Within days the Centers for Disease Control and Prevention, state health agencies, and national expert epidemiologists, were given the task of identifying this mysterious illness, its etiology, prevention, and cure. The job was not as simple as it was hoped it would be. Here's how epidemiologists used their craft to solve this problem:

Population Characteristics: Fatalities included young Navahos of both genders. Two weeks into the epidemic there were some non-Navaho cases among those who lived in proximity to the infected area. Cases began to include some older people. All the victims had similar symptoms—fever that did not exceed 103 degrees, muscle aches, a cough, and some also had conjunctivitis. Within one to four days their lungs filled with fluid until breathing stopped and they literally drowned.

Assumption: It was assumed that there was a common source of infection, isolated in a relatively vast area, infecting people of great similarity.

Tests: Autopsies were done to test tissue and fluids, and cells were cultured to try to identify a common organism. Blood and tissue cultures showed no apparent growth of an unexplained organism. This did not necessarily mean bacteria was not present; some bacteria are very difficult to grow in culture, and other diseases kill by means of a toxin produced by a bacteria that is not recognized in culture. This was a problem faced by the CDC. Using many testing means, the CDC began a process of elimination and would eliminate more than two dozen bacteria, viruses, fungi, and parasites from their list of suspects.

When bacterial tests failed to identify an **agent,** new tests were begun to see if the agent was a virus, a **pathogen** more difficult to detect.

While still uncertain, a preliminary finding suggested that the agent may be an exotic virus called Hantaan, named after a river in Korea. Hantaan does not cause symptoms like those seen in this epidemic, but it was thought a new strain, a mutant strain, or a variation of the Hantavirus, may be involved. After introducing this possible agent as the cause, new tests on patients found antibodies to the Hantavirus in blood samples from three victims. The finding of antibodies means the person has been exposed and the body has tried to resist infection.

How did this occur? Hantaviruses are not common in the United States, but much like plague, it exists in some form in many locations without causing a problem. It is theorized that the 1993 winter had more rain than usual, causing excessive piñon nut production. More piñon nuts meant more rodents, such as field mice, who live on them. In a very rural community where there is no electricity, running water, or other public health safety measures or precautions, it is thought that infected mice, multiplying rapidly and living in dusty holes in wooden homes, excreted the virus in feces that were swept out of the home producing inhalable dust that infected those in contact.

Cultural Considerations: An interesting facet of this epidemiological process was the collaboration with Navaho Medicine Men and Women. The indigenous healers helped with the survey, the data collection process, and encouraging reluctant Navahos to come to the clinics, speak with the non-Indian experts, and assess their lifestyle in view of the epidemic.

Conclusion: In September 1993, with thirty confirmed deaths, the Hantaan virus was verified as the pathogen causing this "Hantapulmonary virus" disease.

Epidemiology is concerned with populations rather than individuals and is based on the relationship among causative **agents, hosts, and environments** (Figure 5.2). The epidemiologist considers health to represent a general balance among these three forces. Health problems occur when the balance is threatened by changes in the agent, host, or environment. Prevention is the major goal derived from exploring this model.

The **host** may be a person, an animal, or a plant. Host factors relate primarily to personal resistance to disease through biological immunity, instruction and knowledge, behavior modification, screening, and personal power. Susceptibility or resistance is influenced by age, sex, socioeconomic status (SES), ethnicity, genes, behavior, nutritional state, previous exposure, and other factors.

Agent factors are the biological or mechanical means of causing disease, illness, or disability. They include pathogens, drugs, automobiles, radiation, and

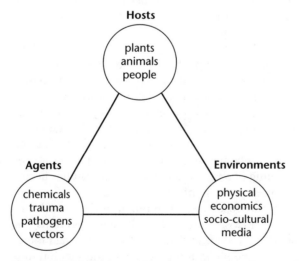

Figure 5.2 The balance of host, agent, and environment.

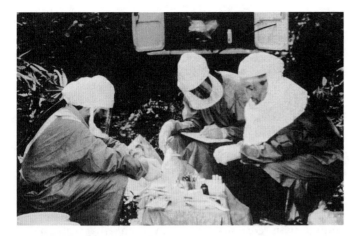

When the Ebola virus broke out in Zaire, epidemiologists from the Centers for Disease Control in Atlanta were immediately sent to find the host and stop the spread of this epidemic.

chemicals, and are influenced by biology, marketing, engineering, regulation, and legislation.

The **environment** is the world in which we live, including physical, socio-cultural, sociopolitical, and economic components. These environmental conditions are influenced by media, greed, beliefs, occupation, climate, housing, sex roles, technology, and more.

Changes in any one of these three factors may result in loss of health. For example, the host may be compromised as a result of treatment with steroids, making him or her more susceptible to agents that do not ordinarily cause disease. The environment may also be changed, for example, by a breakdown in the water supply system. This kind of environmental change occurred when the main water supply of New Delhi was drastically reduced by drought. This caused water with fecal matter infected with Hepatitis A to be not properly purified, resulting in an epidemic of this disease. Finally, some agents may become more or less virulent (severe) over time, thereby disturbing the dynamic balance among agent, host, and environment."[2]

BOX 5.2 *Life in the Real World*

Epidemiologists, CDC, Atlanta

Epidemiologists were the first scientists on the scene of the Ebola virus outbreak in Zaire in 1995. As epidemiologists, the "disease busters," or "disease cowboys," had to do everything they could to contain one of the scariest microbes on the planet, find the source of infection and prevent its spread.

Community Health in the 21st Century

"In the real world, staffs are shrinking, labs are deteriorating, and adminstrators worry about the day when two Ebola-like emergencies happen at the same time and they find themselves short of heroes."[1]

Epidemiology can be used to provide many pieces of data and information. Epidemiology may:

1. describe the spectrum of disease
2. describe the natural history of a disease
3. identify factors that increase the risk of acquiring a disease
4. predict disease trends
5. elucidate mechanisms of disease transmission
6. test the efficacy of intervention strategies
7. evaluate intervention programs
8. identify the health needs of a community.

An epidemiologist is actually a detective who proceeds from the known to the unknown, beginning with curiosity about an event that cannot be explained by chance, such as the flu-like, respiratory symptoms experienced by thousands of Gulf War veterans returning from the Mideast in 1991. The epidemiologist then attempts to identify the factors that are essential or contributory to the occurrence. Soldiers from the Gulf War believed they had been exposed to chemical agents. The Pentagon denied this, and others suggested crowded living conditions and extremes of weather, sandflies, food pathogens, airborne pollutants from the Kuwait oil fires, or other unknown agents. Ordinarily, after looking at all the possible host, agent, and environmental factors and analyzing their relationship amid the clues, there is a conclusion—the mystery is solved, the case is closed. In the case of the Gulf War veterans, however, the mystery is yet to be solved, although research is pointing more clearly toward either a reaction to prophylactic drugs given to soldiers before their departure, or to exposure to chemicals.

The Language of Epidemiology

There are many terms unique to the science of epidermiology:

Ecological Fallacy: The danger in confusing correlation (a relationship) with causation when interpreting a collection of statistics. A correlation is when two factors happen to rise and fall in tandem; causation is when one factor makes the other rise or fall. An example of ecological fallacy occurred in 1852 when William Farr observed that areas of London at higher altitudes had less cholera mortality than those at sea level. He inferred from the inverse correlation of elevation and death that **miasma** (bad smells) was rising from the swamps and marshes and causing the disease. Two years later John Snow found the real cause, not the correlation, at the Broad Street pump.

Endemic: A condition that persists within a particular population and within a particular geographical area. For instance, enteric (intestinal) diseases are endemic in most developing countries. There are also wooded areas of the United States where plague is endemic to small mammal populations.

Epidemic: Epidemic describes a condition from a common etiology that affects a large number of people. Although ten cases of measles might not seem to be an epidemic, when previous incidence has been zero, an outbreak of ten in a population may be epidemic. When three deaths from *E.coli*-infected hamburgers occurred in Seattle in 1993, the result was an epidemic. This was an extraordinary occurrence isolated to a particular area.

Pandemic: An epidemic that becomes nationwide, continentwide or worldwide is pandemic, AIDS being the most recent. The fear of pandemic influenza still motivates most countries to immunize against an anticipated influenza virus.

Eradication: To eradicate a disease is to extinguish it, to make it extinct so that it disappears absolutely, utterly, and entirely from the world. On October 26, 1979, the Director General of WHO participated in a ceremony in Nairobi, Kenya, to mark the anniversary of the eradication

---

BOX 5.3 *Milestones in Disease Eradication*

1892   Contagious pleuropneumonia of cattle declared eradicated in the United States.

1896   Rabies eradicated from England.

1901   Yellow fever eradicated from Havana.

1907   Rockefeller Foundation established sanitary commission for eradication of hookworm.

1915   Rockefeller Foundation establishes Yellow Fever Commission.

1937   Eradication of TB in the United States close.

1947   Pan American Organization adopts proposal for eradication of *A. aegypti* from the Americas.

1951   Malaria eradicated from Sardinia.

1954   Yaws eradication goal declared by WHO.

1955   World Health Assembly adopts goal of global malaria eradication.

1958   World Health Assembly adopts goal of global smallpox eradication.

1969   WHO changes malaria eradication policy to malaria control.

1970   Smallpox eradicated from the Americas.

1977   Smallpox eradicated worldwide.

1978   United States goal of measles elimination by 1982 announced.

1985   PAHO sets goal of poliomyelitis elimination from Americas by 1990; Europe sets goal of measles elimination by 2000.

1991   WHO declares goal of global dracunculiasis eradication by 1995; last case of indigenous poliomyelitis in the Americas occurs in Peru.

(*Source:* CDCP. (1993). Recommendations of the International Task Force for Disease Eradication. MMWR Vol. 42 (No. RR-16) pp. 6–7)

of the smallpox virus from the planet, the first and only successful eradication program in the world. The World Health Organization has set its sights on leprosy as the next public health problem that can be eradicated by the end of the century. An investment of $420 million would eliminate the disease through multi-drug therapies (MDT). At the beginning of 2000, 750,332 leprosy cases were registered for treatment in the world as reported by seventy-six countries. Worldwide, 2.3 million cases are currently receiving MDT treatment.[3]

Etiology: The cause of disease or condition.

Event: Events such as deaths, accidents, or outbreaks of disease occur at a **point** in time. They must be interpreted over a **period** of time, and be reported continuously. Frequencies of events are expressed as **event rate or attack rate or incidence,** which is usually expressed per unit time per 1,000 population.[4]

Population: A population is an assemblage of organisms of the same species that occupies a defined point or points in place or time. Characteristics of a population can never prove the cause of an individual's mortality or morbidity. The population being studied for Gulf War syndrome is all soldiers who served in the Mideast. The Four Corners mystery population was about 95 percent of the Navahos living on the reservation.

Surveillance: Surveillance is the epidemiological foundation for modern public health. In 1963, Alexander D. Langmuir defined disease surveillance as "the continued watchfulness over the distribution and trends of incidence through the systematic collection, consolidation, and evaluation of morbidity and mortality reports and other relevant data" together with timely and regular dissemination to those who need to know. Surveillance is important for the planning, implementation, and assessment of disease control. In contrast to archival (public records) health data, surveillance methods are dynamic. They include the ongoing, regular collection, and use of health data. Unfortunately, surveillance for environmental hazards and occupational exposures is quite inadequate and lags behind surveillance of chronic and infectious diseases.

Surveillance systems involve information loops, with data flowing from local to central agencies and back. They keep prevention and control activities moving rapidly and in the right direction. New attention to surveillance of recreational water, toxic dumps, and radiation exposure is beginning to be a major part of community health analysis.

Trends: Trends are determined by using a simple linear regression of incidents or rates and the sequence number of the time periods.

Demography

The goals of public health workers at every level are the same: improving the quality of life for individual human beings. Improvement requires knowledge of

---

BOX 5.4 *Flow of Surveillance Information*

Surveillance depends on the sequential flow of information through the full surveillance cycle.

Planning

- Reporters from all sectors of health care systems
- Proper forms for collecting detailed information
- Regular reporting ranging from daily to annually
- Aggregation of data as opposed to individual data
- Timely transmission of data using electronic formats

Data Management and Dissemination

- Updating records through follow-up and reclassification

- Proper tabulation
- Detailed published reports—simple and easy to understand using graphs, tables, and maps
- Confidentiality

Data Collection

- Notification systems
- Health care provider networks
- Laboratory surveillance
- Disease registries
- Vital records
- Medical examiner and coroner reports
- Medical records
- Insurance records and workers compensation
- Surveys of health behavior and physician utilization
- Hazard and exposure surveillance

(*Source:* Healthy People 2010)

---

what has been, what is happening at present, and what may happen in the future. **Demography** is the study of this dynamic nature of population changes and includes the vital statistics of **person, place, time, climate, or season.** Demographic characteristics that are most commonly reported as associated with chronic and acute disease are age, race, gender, economic status, and education.

Vital Statistics

All countries collect data about the resources they provide for health care, the patients treated, and their conditions. Despite the inaccuracies, incomplete nature, and often out-of-date data that are collected, routine data are very important to the understanding of the health status of a group, a locality, a state, or nation. The importance of vital statistics is to determine if there is a statistical significance that the number of cases of a disease or number of deaths observed in a population would be the number expected under normal conditions. Expected deaths are either the known death rate over time or the number that would have occurred if the location had the same mortality rate as the United States as a whole. The greater the gap between the observed and the expected (as measured by a Chi square statistic), the less probable it is that a difference is due to chance. Since mortality (death) and birth are easily determined and are fairly universal measures, comparison of mortality and birth rates among countries or communities can improve health professionals' means of assessing need and providing programs.

Under the law, the National Center for Health Statistics (of the CDC) has been authorized to collect data on:

1. The extent and nature of illness and disability of the population of the United States.
2. The impact of the illness and disability of the population on the economy of the United States.
3. Environmental, social, and other health hazards.
4. Determinants of health.
5. Health resources, including physicians, dentists, nurses, and other professionals, the supply of services by hospitals and other health institutions.
6. Utilization of health care.
7. Health care costs and financing.
8. Family formation, growth, and dissolution.

Vital statistics are concerned with people: their births, deaths, marriage, divorce, adoption, and related data. It is the bookkeeping of public health. Vital statistics are compiled and recorded in numerical form through official records on standard certificates provided by the National Center for Health Statistics and approved by state legislatures. The data that are collected are expressed in the form of rates, such as the number per 100,000 population, and not as individual cases. This is primarily to protect privacy, while providing sufficient comparable data to establish intervention priorities, determine allocation of funds, and plan and evaluate health programs. Commonly used vital and health statistics include the annual **crude live birth rate, crude death rate, infant mortality rate,** and specific **morbidity** and **mortality rates** as shown in Table 5.1.

Why Are Rates Important?

Rates represent the number of events (birth, death, morbidity, etc.) in a specific population over a given period of time, per a specific number, usually 1,000 or 100,000. This gives the community health educator the ability to make comparisons. For example, if you wish to compare the number of new HIV cases in one year in Community A with 250,000 people with Community B of 500,000 people, you would calculate the rate:

Size	New HIV Cases	Rate
(A) 250,000	150	$150/250,000 \times 100,000 = 60$ per 100,000
(B) 500,000	275	$275/500,000 \times 100,000 = 55$ per 100,000

Since each community reports its rate per 100,000 you know that even though there are fewer new HIV cases in Community A, the rate of infection is higher.

The most common statistical division of the population used in the United States is income, however, this measure does not really describe the barriers or privileges of social class. A proxy for social class most frequently used in the United States is race, which is the political category that has become more refined over time. It is disturbing to many public health analysts that some so-called races

Table 5.1   Commonly used vital and health statistics.

Name of Rate	Definition		Remarks
1. Crude Birth Rate	$=\dfrac{\text{no. of live}}{\text{estimated midyear population**}}$	$\times 1,000$	Useful as a crude measure of population growth
2. Premature Birth Rate	$=\dfrac{\text{no. of premature births}}{\text{no. of live births}}$	$\times 1,000$	
3. Crude Death Rate	$=\dfrac{\text{no. of deaths*}}{\text{estimated midyear population**}}$	$\times 1,000$	Useful as a crude measure of population decrease due to natural causes.
4. Age-Specific Death Rate	$=\dfrac{\text{no. of deaths of specified age}}{\text{estimated midyear population of that age group**}}$	$\times 1,000$ or $100,000$	May also be specific with sex, which increases utility as measure of risk
5. Cause-Specific Death rate	$=\dfrac{\text{no. of deaths from specified cause*}}{\text{estimated midyear population**}}$	$\times 1,000$	Can be presented as specific for age and sex which increases utility as measure of risk.
6. Infant Mortality	$=\dfrac{\text{no. of deaths under 1 year of age*}}{\text{no. of live births one calendar year}^\dagger}$	$\times 1,000$	Widely used as an indicator of health and general well-being. Also indicator of the effectiveness of medical care and public health programs
7. Neo-natal Mortality Rate	$=\dfrac{\text{no. of deaths under 28 days of age*}}{\text{no. of live births}^\dagger}$	$\times 1,000$	Usually accounts for 80% of total infant mortality most often result of prematurity. Reflection on quality of prenatal care etc.
8. Postneonatal Mortality	$=\dfrac{\text{no. of deaths from 28 days to end of*}}{\text{no. of live births}^\dagger}$	$\times 1,000$	These deaths are clearly preventable. Indicates real failure of health care delivery. Most deaths due to problems of prematurity have occurred in 1st month of life.
9. Fetal Mortality Rate	$=\dfrac{\text{no. of fetal deaths*}}{\substack{\text{no. of live births plus fetal deaths}\\ \text{(of 20 weeks or 28 weeks}\\ \text{or more gestation)}^\dagger}}$	$\times 1,000$	Can be broken down further by period + 20 weeks or more gestation or 28 weeks or more.
10. Fertility Ratio	$=\dfrac{\text{no. of children under 5 years of age}}{\substack{\text{no. of women in pop. (midyear)}\\ \text{of childbearing age (15–44)}}}$	$\times 1,000$	Indicates population trends
a. Fertility Rate	$=\dfrac{\text{no. of live births*}}{\substack{\text{estimated number of females}\\ \text{aged 15–44 at midyear**}}}$	$\times 1,000$	
11. Sex Ratio	$=$ no. of men per* 100 women		High ratio indicates large male population. Decreases with age— 105 at birth. Overall sex ratio in U.S. is 98.
12. Maternal Mortality Rate	$=\dfrac{\text{no. of deaths from maternal conditions*}}{\text{number of live births}^\dagger}$	$\times 1,000$	

*Occurring in a defined population during a given calendar year.
**Refers to population and given calendar year in which event occurred.
†In the population in which event in the numerator occurred.

such as Hispanic are often classified with whites, often to seemingly better equalize the enormous disparity between people of color and others in the United States. Often, significant "races" such as Pacific Islanders, Native Americans by nation, or Hispanic by origin such as Mexico, Puerto Rico, or South America, are lumped together as "other" or included as gross aggregates.

Internationally, there has been an attempt to standardize the primary indicators of health so cross-cultural comparisons can be made. As yet this standardization is not universal.

The vital statistics that are recorded by agencies and organizations can then be used as measurements of health, most often called **morbidity** and **mortality rates** and interpreted as **prevalence** and **incidence**.

Sources of Vital Statistical Morbidity and Mortality Data

Most health professionals seek morbidity and mortality data from standardized sources that utilize the same formulas for determining rates and the same means of data collection. This provides the ability to compare data across geographical, population, time, and agency differences. The most common sources of standardized data are found in local and state health departments of vital statistics, and in the published sources below:

1. **The United States Census**—taken every ten years with some mid-decade analysis. Congress is debating the controversial counting method for census taking.

2. **Monthly Vital Statistics Report**—published by the NCHS. This report is a collection of statistical summaries of vital records and major life events.

3. **Statistical Abstracts of the United States**—a standard summary of social, political, economic, health, educational, law, and environmental data published annually.

4. **Morbidity and Mortality Weekly Report (MMWR)**—CDC's weekly review of the reportable illnesses throughout the United States. This publication offers special editions devoted to new developments in health and weekly alerts about disease outbreaks. The MMWR was the first official word of the impending AIDS epidemic in June, 1981.

5. **National Surveys**—Some surveys are conducted by national agencies while others are conducted through government funding by academic institutions. Survey data often look at such things as nutrition, youth risk, breast cancer, lifestyle indicators, sexuality.

6. **Sentinel Surveillance**—this surveillance includes a wide range of activities that focus on key health indicators in a population. A sentinel event is a preventable disease, disability or untimely death. NIOSH has created the Sentinel Event Notification System for Occupational Risk.

7. **Chronic Disease Registries**—Chronic disease registries are a means of collecting data on chronic diseases that are not otherwise reported to public health agencies. Registries are generally maintained by hospitals and clinics. In 1992, Congress established the national program of cancer registries that by 1996 established data collection in forty-six states.

Morbidity

Morbidity data are the numerical frequencies of a recognized new occurrence of a particular illness or condition in a population in a given period of time (**incidence**), or the relative frequency of a disease or other attribute in a group at a specific time (**prevalence**). For instance, the morbidity rate for children out of school with the influenza may be reported as the number missing from school during the winter semester (prevalence) or the number of new cases of children out with the influenza during any given week during the winter semester (incidence). Incidence rates reflect the number of new occurrences of a condition in ratio to the population at risk over a specific period of time.

Like the example above, if 500 women develop breast cancer in a year in a population of 342,000, the incidence rate is 500 divided by 342,000 × 100,000 or 146 per 100,000 population.

When incidence rates are compared by year, for instance, it is a means of determining if new cases are greater than would be expected. Incidence rates are most commonly used to describe **acute diseases,** such as measles or chicken pox, since these usually have a beginning and end point that is within a determinable range.

The prevalence of a disease in a population at any point in time depends on the prior incidence of new cases and the average duration of the disease from onset to recovery or death. While one could simply count the number of cases of an illness on any given day, the prevalence rate can give the researcher a rate that can be compared. In other words, the rate of those giving birth in one community can be compared to the rate of births in a different community. If frequency and not a rate were used, the raw numbers may not reflect the difference in number of women of reproductive age and thus give an inaccurate picture of the maternal or obstetric needs of each community. Prevalence rates are most useful for looking at **chronic diseases**, such as cancer or diabetes, since these diseases last over a long time as opposed to seasonal diseases such as the flu.

A point prevalence rate is the prevalence of a disease at a specified point in time over the population at that time, multiplied by 1,000. In other words it resembles a morbidity rate, but it is specific in time.

An **attack rate** is a unique incidence rate that is calculated for a single disease outbreak and is expressed as a percent. For example, if people become ill after a community event that involved food, you might be able to determine the percent or attack rate of those who were ill by family groups or ethnic groups and see if there was a common food item that was related to that family or ethnic group which may be the source of the foodborne illness.

Usually ill health is described by type (diagnosis), by severity, duration, distribution in place and time, and by demographic characteristics. There are two general categories of sources for morbidity data: the records routinely compiled and accumulated by various agencies, clinics, or persons and special surveys made to obtain information on particular issues.

In July 1991, the Centers for Disease Control and Prevention released a list of eighteen health status indicators, in response to Objective 22.1 of Healthy People 2000.[5] The CDC attempted to develop a set of health status indicators that would be small in number, allow a comprehensive measure of community health, include general and specific measures of community health, be measurable at federal, state, and local levels, be readily and uniformly understandable, be measurable using available data, imply specific interventions compelling action, and be outcome oriented. These vital statistics give a picture of how one community, local or state, might compare with the same measure at the United States level. The eighteen indicators are:

1. Race/ethnicity specific infant mortality
2. Total deaths
3. Motor vehicle crash deaths
4. Work-related injuries
5. Suicide
6. Homicides
7. Lung cancer deaths
8. Female breast cancer deaths
9. Cardiovascular disease deaths
10. Reported incidence of Acquired Immunodeficiency Syndrome
11. Incidence of measles
12. Incidence of tuberculosis
13. Incidence of primary and secondary syphilis
14. Prevalence of low birth weight
15. Births to adolescents
16. Perinatal care
17. Children in poverty
18. Proportion of persons living in counties exceeding EPA standards for air quality

In general, while mortality indicators are monitored, only 75.5 percent of the states monitor work-related injury deaths. Further, only 47 percent of the states monitor poor air quality and only 59 percent monitor childhood poverty.[6] Monitoring the indicators are very important for assessing the health status of a population and for area-wide health planning and allocation of health resources. Morbidity data are very difficult to collect accurately, or to compare across countries. In the twentieth century, essentially all countries adopted some form of compulsory notification of certain illness, however, the laws vary from country to country about who should report, when the report should be made, and what conditions should be reported.

In 1971, the International Health Regulations went into effect, defining the diseases that are officially reportable by all health authorities to the World Health Organization. These include cholera, plague, and yellow fever, which must be reported within 24 hours of diagnosis. The International Sanitary Regulations, which have been in effect since 1950, require international reporting of the three WHO diseases plus relapsing fever, typhus, influenza, malaria, and poliomyelitis which have now been shifted to "under surveillance" and not necessarily reportable. All reports appear in the Weekly Epidemiological Record of the WHO.

Morbidity data are very difficult to collect accurately, or to compare across countries. In the twentieth century, essentially all countries have adopted some form of compulsory notification of certain illness, however, the laws vary from country to country about who should report, when the report should be made, and what conditions should be reported.

Mortality

"Health is measured by its opposite—mortality."[7] In the middle of the seventeenth century, a London cloth merchant, John Graunt, began a study of the **Bills of Mortality,** church parish registers of births and deaths. He is considered the father of vital statistics because of these early studies of the birth and death records of 1603 to 1662. From his work, inferences about the London population and the groundwork for epidemiology were set. The result of Graunt's work, published in 1662, was to show that human life conforms to certain predictable statistical patterns. This publication also signaled the beginning of the development of analytical methods, such as the life table method, for using vital statistics and mortality data to examine public health issues.

Mortality data, the amount of death by cause, are the primary means for making comparisons among countries or peoples. The primary advantage of mortality statistics over other statistics relating to health is mainly that they are more generally available, they are relatively unambiguous, and they provide a basis for hypotheses concerning differential causes of death.[8]

The primary source of mortality data comes from death certificates that were standardized by WHO in 1940 and are revised periodically. Improvements made in 1989 include better clarification of cause of death, occupation of the deceased, and whether the deceased is of other ethnicity, not just Caucasian or non-Caucasian. The parts of the standard death certificate are:

Part I—Demographic data and place of death
Part II—Medical cause and other significant conditions related to death
Part III—Certification of death by authorized individual
Part IV—Where buried

Table 5.2   Leading causes of death in the United States (1998).

Rank	Causes of Death	Number	Rate
All causes		2,338,075	865.0
1.	Diseases of heart	724,269	268.0
2.	Malignant neoplasms	538,947	199.4
3.	Cerebrovascular diseases	158,060	58.5
4.	Chronic obstructive pulmonary diseases	114,381	42.3
5.	Pneumonia and influenza	94,828	35.1
6.	Accidents and adverse effects	93,207	34.5
	Motor vehicle accidents	41,826	15.5
	All other accidents and adverse effects	51,382	19.0
7.	Diabetes mellitus	64,574	23.9
8.	Suicide	29,264	10.8
9.	Nephritis, nephrotic syndrome, and nephrosis	26,295	9.7
10.	Chronic liver disease and cirrhosis	24,936	9.2
11.	Septicemia	23,643	8.7
12.	Alzheimers disease	22,824	8.4
13.	Homicide and legal intervention	17,350	6.4
14.	Atherosclerosis	15,424	5.7
15.	Hypertension with or without renal disease	14,216	5.3
	All other causes	**375,857**	**139.1**

(*Source:* Healthy People 2010)

One copy of the certificate is sent to the local health department, one is sent to the state file where the deceased is a resident, and one copy is sent to the National Death Registry.

Mortality Rates

The basic measure of mortality is the **crude death rate,** determined by dividing the number of deaths during the year by the mid-year population. The crude death rate is expressed per 1,000 population. The leading causes of death and their crude death rates are given in Table 5.2.

Infant Mortality Rates The WHO has strongly promoted infant mortality rates as an international health status indicator. These may be the most sensitive measure of the health of a people because they reflect many adverse social, economic, and environmental factors and the synergy among factors such as nutrition, infection, literacy, and development.[9] Infant mortality is measured as the number of infant deaths under one year of age per 1,000 births. From 1980 to 2000, there was a decline in the United States infant mortality rate from 12.6 to 7.2/1,000.

The major correlates of infant mortality are low birth weight, maternal age, birth order, number of pregnancies, interval since previous birth, maternal education, and ethnicity.

Perinatal Mortality Rates The number of infant deaths under one month old per 1,000 births is considered the perinatal mortality rate. Race, social class, age, and parity are all known to influence this rate. Many researchers believe that a more sensitive measure would be birthweight specific mortality rates for particular demographic groups.

In developing countries, the identification of specific, preventable perinatal causes of death, such as neonatal tetanus, can be clear markers of one aspect of effective antenatal care. However, Opit (1991) reminded us that the interpretation of crude perinatal mortality rates as a measure of health service outcome is not without difficulty.[10]

Maternal Mortality Maternal deaths are defined as the death of a woman while pregnant or within forty-two days of termination of pregnancy. Maternal deaths are subdivided into two groups: direct obstetrics deaths resulting from birthing complications, and indirect deaths aggravated by the physiological effects of pregnancy. Unlike other rates of mortality, maternal mortality is expressed as a ratio per 100,000 live births.

The world total of maternal deaths is often estimated at 500,000 per year, but the actual number is unknown because "most of those who die are poor, live in remote areas, and their deaths are accorded little importance. In those parts of the world where maternal mortality is highest, deaths are rarely recorded and even if they are, the cause of death is usually not given."[11]

Abortion In the United States, states are now required to report induced and spontaneous abortion rates. Induced termination of pregnancy has been defined as "the purposeful interruption of pregnancy with the intention other than to produce a liveborn infant or to remove a dead fetus."

Epidemiological Research Studies

Research is the key component of epidemiology. As in any research study, certain factors must be considered:

1. A population exists that needs to be analyzed in some way vis-à-vis all persons in the population or a sample of those persons.

2. A relationship between an independent variable such as age or gender is compared with the dependent variable, which may be incidence or traffic accidents at a certain intersection or outbreaks of an infectious disease. This relationship is posed as an **hypothesis,** a prediction of outcome based upon known facts.

3. The hypothesis is tested by either a nonexperimental means such as a survey or observation, or by an experimental means such as an experimentally designed manipulation of a variable in one group as compared to another group.

Nonexperimental Studies

When the independent variable or the population being studied is not manipulated in any way, such as injection with a vaccine, given a prevention intervention, or being put under some experimental condition, the analysis of the problem is nonexperimental. Nonexperimental studies often use **observation** that follows a **cohort** (a group related by some similar demographic variable such as age, gender, or occupation) in its natural setting (the workplace, school) for a given time through past records, at the immediate time through observational notes or surveys, or into the future recording relevant changes in incidence of morbidity or mortality. Thus, there are three kinds of observational, or nonexperimental studies: **prospective, retrospective,** and **cross-sectional.**

Prospective Studies A prospective study, also known as a **longitudinal study,** follows a **cohort,** a particular group of individuals studied as a group because of their similarity in a common experience, usually generational. The prospective (cohort) study attempts to study the relationship between a purposed cause and the subsequent risk of developing a disease before the development of a condition occurs. In this type of study there is no attempt to manipulate the exposure to any given factor, but merely to determine at the end of the study how the cohort has responded to a variety of variables such as stress, cholesterol, harassment, radiation, and other factors.

The Tremin Trust study now being conducted at the University of Utah has followed approximately 1,000 women since the 1940s who have recorded changes in their life associated with their menstrual histories. This analysis begins to assess the effect of the menstrual cycle on other life and body events.

The most well-known and important prospective, cohort study in public health is **The Framingham Study.** In 1948, the United States Public Health Service decided to study the factors associated with the development of atherosclerotic and hypertensive cardiovascular diseases. They decided that a long-term surveillance of the adult population of Framingham, Massachusetts, would give them the information they sought. Framingham was, at that time, a small town of about 28,000 people, eighteen miles west of Boston. After careful analysis, it was estimated that between 5,000 and 6,000 men and women between the ages of thirty to fifty-nine, would be needed to participate in what was projected to be a twenty-year longitudinal study. Town residents were first categorized according to family size and then arranged alphabetically. Then, every third family was eliminated, resulting in a list of 6,507 initial subjects. These people were examined for preexisting cardiovascular conditions.[12]

After eliminating people with coronary heart disease, 5,127 men and women were left in the study, who then participated in biannual physical examinations. These exams included medical histories, blood tests, physical exams, and laboratory work that would eventually include cholesterol levels. Hypotheses were tested regarding the relationship of physical activity, dietary intake, and stress to the development of coronary heart diseases. After seven years there was enough data to conclude that, in fact, the variables that were being tested were related to the development of heart disease.[13]

Framingham has taken two new directions since its success with cardio-vascular disease. In 1978, the subjects began to be given neurological exams in an investigation of the development of Alzheimer's disease.[14] The second direction is the Framingham Offshoot Study.

For the last two decades, 5,100 of the children of the original participants have also been studied. The Framingham offspring, now middle aged, are in many respects significantly healthier than their parents were when they entered the study forty-four years ago, with lower blood pressure and cholesterol levels. The men however, are heavier and less active and both men and women have much higher rates of diabetes than their parents did at comparable ages.[15]

The results of this longitudinal study have been very important in identifying the etiology of and risks for cardiovascular illness. As with most prospective studies, the cost has been great, and research is time consuming. A large sample size was necessary to prevent statistical error due to a loss of subjects over time because of death or disinterest.

Another well-known longitudinal cohort study is the Nurses Health Study, which has followed 120,000 married female nurses, looking for factors that may be related to breast cancer and other diseases. The study has found that nurses had a 50 percent higher risk of breast cancer while they were taking oral contraceptives, but the risk was normal after they stopped taking the medications.[16]

The disadvantages of prospective cohort studies are their cost and the time it takes to complete them. Persuading participants to remain in a cohort study for long periods of times is both difficult and expensive. For this reason, cohort studies are usually done primarily to confirm an association that has been well established on the basis of descriptive, cross-sectional and/or case-control studies.

Retrospective Studies   The retrospective study is an observational analysis of data collected about a cohort with or without a particular disease. The past history of this cohort or certain individuals is used to determine if any exposure to certain pathogens or environmental agents have subsequently been the cause of a present condition. The investigation of the Gulf War veterans, mentioned earlier in this chapter, is a good example of a retrospective study. Each soldier who has been diagnosed with an unexplainable disability, skin rashes, bronchitis, joint pain, short-term memory loss, or chronic fatigue contracted soon after service in the Gulf War is now being studied retrospectively for exposure to chemical, pathological, or food-borne agents. The first tests showed infection with *Leishmania tropica,* a parasite transmitted through the bites of infected sandflies. More soldiers, however, tested negative. A study of respiratory disease among 2,598 male soldiers found that these symptoms were probably due to housing conditions and crowding.[17] However, this study does not address the chronic, debilitating symptoms of many other veterans of this war. These soldiers' symptoms are now being compared to soldiers from the same areas who have not experienced severe debilitating reactions and symptoms. The hope is that evaluating, retrospectively, the similarities and differences between these two cohorts will give the epidemiologist the key to the etiology of this mystery.

Cross-Sectional Studies Cross-sectional surveys or studies are concerned with the prevalence of a situation existing at a given time in a group or population, or set of groups or populations. Cross-sectional surveys require information relating to the state of the individual at two or more points in time. They can be expensive since they require the collection of data from a very large sample. Cross-sectional studies document the co-occurrence of disease and suspected factors not only in the population, but also in specific individuals within the population. It is a useful tool for the study of chronic disease since prevalence is more measurable by this method than incidence. They are not useful for studying diseases that have a low prevalence rate.

Today's malls offer the consumer marketing researcher an interesting environment to study the opinions of shoppers through cross-sectional survey data collection. The cross-sectional study asks a cohort (those shopping in a given mall on a given day) questions that are designed to obtain an opinion or determine the state or condition of a person's life. It is a survey of present status or opinion and can be used as polling exit interviews or measures of a community's opinion about school health education, gays in the military, or their current health status. These studies do not show cause, but may identify differences in particular cohorts or give a picture of demographic variables that may be impacting a given health condition.

Case-Control Studies A case study is the study of an individual and his or her relationship to exposure and disease. Unlike an ecological study that shows how a single factor is distributed in the population and establishes trends between two or more populations, the case-control study is used primarily to assess risks and to study the etiology of disease in general. Data cannot be generalized within a population.

In a **case-control study** deaths from disease currently under study can always be considered as cases, but advanced disease is sometimes used as a substitute. However, early disease should be excluded from the cases to remove lead-time bias. Like a cohort study, it is difficult to find controls who are not somehow exposed to similar interventions or historical perspective as the experimental group.

Compared to cohort studies, case-control studies are relatively inexpensive and easy to do. Participants are seen only once, and no follow-up is necessary. The case-control study is particularly useful for exploring relationships noted in observational studies.

Experimental Studies

Experimental studies require that the researcher set controls around the manipulation of variables in a study. Animal studies used to determine the efficacy of AZT on a Simian virus would give specifically measured amounts of AZT to genetically similar primates for exactly the same period of time, under identical laboratory conditions. These primates would then be compared with primates from the same gene pool, kept under identical conditions but without the experimental drug, AZT. If humans are the subjects, similar control must be maintained over all experimental conditions to insure validity and reliability of research results. The purpose of experimental research is to determine cause and effect with statistical confidence.

Experimental community health epidemiology are usually **clinical studies** requiring control of variables. Clinical studies compare two types of groups, those with the disease (**cases**) and those without (**controls**). The source population from which cases and control are drawn are known as the **target population.** If the prevalence of a factor is significantly different in cases than it is in controls, this suggests that the factor is associated with the disease.

Clinical studies may include clinical trials of experimental drugs for certain health conditions such as AIDS or Alzheimer's, intervention techniques that might reduce conditions such as high blood pressure, and prevention techniques such as vaccines. Clinical studies are expensive and require maximum control of all variables. They require experimental groups that are available, randomly similar and willing to participate in the study for extended periods of time. A recent university study to reduce stress in HIV positive patients using group counseling or biofeedback was not statistically meaningful because the morbidity and mortality rate was so high in the control and experimental groups, that by the end of the eight-week study there were not enough participants to make a statistical comparison of the two experimental interventions.

A **randomized preventive trial** is the experimental method most preferred for research. Unfortunately these studies are very expensive and difficult to control for social science research variables. Most experimental methods require controlled laboratory conditions.

Environmental Epidemiology

The incidence of cancer among those exposed to toxins or other chemicals has become a major concern of community health education. Environmental epidemiology is a branch of traditional epidemiology that attempts to determine the agents causing diseases such as cancer or toxic poisoning. It is an attempt to find out why some people get sick and some do not when exposed to similar agents over similar time periods or locations.[18]

Risk Assessment

Probably the most talked about addition to epidemiology and particularly environmental epidemiology is risk assessment. A risk is the possibility of loss or injury. It is a function of the hazard involved (exposure and toxicity), the dose response from the person, and the situation in which the person is exposed. Once it is determined that a chemical is likely to cause a specific health problem, it is then necessary to establish the relationship between the amount of the exposure (dose) and the effect produced.

Exposure assessment is a determination of how much of a chemical in question is available to individuals. The degree of exposure may vary from chemical to chemical. Risk characterization is the exposure time, multiplied by the potency, multiplied by the unit or the individual risk. For noncarcinogens the evaluation of the margin of safety (MOS) is estimated by dividing the NOAEL (No Observed Adverse Effect Level) by the estimated daily human dose. For carcinogens, the MOS is estimated by multiplying the actual human dose by the risk per unit of dose projected in dose-response models. Risk assessment for carcinogens is particularly difficult because cancer may take from fifteen to forty years after onset of exposure to manifestation. The site of a malignant tumor may vary from portal of entry or site of biotransformation. Most risk assessments are for individual chemicals, however, in reality people are exposed to many multiple chemicals.

To summarize risk analysis one must: (1) determine the source of the chemical and how long it has been released into the environment; (2) determine the pathways through which the chemical travels through the environment; (3) the behavior of the substance in the body and the pathways that the chemical takes during metabolism, as well as the toxicity of the metabolite products; (4) estimate the concentration or dose at the specific site in the organs and how long the organ is exposed; (5) determine the persistence of the substance in the environment; (6) determine the relationship between the dose the individual gets and the effect on the individual; and (7) estimate the risk to the exposed population.

Dose Response Curve

A scientific study to determine risk of contamination is sometimes called a **dose response rate,** the amount of a pollutant to which an individual is exposed in relation to the amount of damage to the organism. The **dose response curve** is a relationship between the potential toxicity inherent in a given chemical and the kind of symptoms exhibited when the chemical interacts with the living biological system. A chemical may be extremely toxic, but safe in a given situation in which no contact with a living organism occurs. However, a chemical may be mildly toxic, yet problematic, if is comes in constant contact with a living organism.

Dose is usually expressed as: (1) the amount of the substance actually in the body; (2) the amount of the material entering the body as in food or water; or (3) the concentration in the environment.[19]

Most dose amounts are difficult to measure because the body generally does not retain all of the ingested or inhaled pollution; some is excreted, exhaled, or converted to less toxic forms. Another confounding variable in measuring dose response is the length of time of exposure, and chronic versus acute exposure. Response, or health damage, can be measured in many different ways:

1. The likelihood that a person exposed to a pollutant will, as a result of the exposure, contract a particular disease during her or his lifetime.

2. The likelihood the exposed person will contract a specific disease and eventually die of it.

3. The average number of days of work that a person will miss because of exposure.

4. The decrease in some measure of performance as a result of exposure.

Finally, a difficult concept in environmental epidemiology is understanding the probability of risk. When one has a 1 percent chance of developing a cancer from exposure this does not mean that out of a group of 100 people only one person will develop the cancer. The percentage is actually the average of all cancer incidence within many groups. Like cohort studies, accuracy becomes more specific when exposed groups are compared to similar groups with no exposure. Subtracting the percentage of exposure of the nonexposed from the exposed groups gives the estimate of the **attributable risk** to the toxin.

Actual hazard assessment requires the combined scientific efforts of environmental epidemiology and investigative toxicology in a controlled laboratory environment. Toxicology gives epidemiology the LD_{50} of a toxin, the dose that causes immediate death in 50 percent of animals exposed. LD_{50} is often used as the marker for permissible levels of exposure to humans. Unfortunately, there are limitations to this method.

Obviously, humans cannot be used for testing toxic substances. Therefore, mice and rats are tested instead. While the use of non-human species to investigate human physiology has a long history, and though there are many similarities between other animals and humans, there are some caveats. One potential problem is the issue that laboratory testing frequently uses dosages far greater than the concentrations to which people are ordinarily exposed, which may mask the issue of latency or duration of exposure in humans and begs the question of whether the high dose itself causes the disease. Second, the metabolism of mice and rats is much different than humans and may confound real-life exposure. Third, laboratory mice and rats are genetically engineered to eliminate confounding variations. Variations in metabolism, sensitivity, immune response, previous exposure, and lifestyle cannot be entered into equations of toxic risk to humans in the laboratory study.

Summary

To treat the planet and its people there must be a common, universally understood language to describe the problems and suggest solutions. The use of epidemiological data and demographic vital statistics gives world health professionals a basis upon which to build theory and test hypotheses. It is unfortunate that some countries do not have the economic resources to continually and consistently collect data that are as accurate as more affluent nations, but their efforts are appreciated and comparisons can still be made with the sensitivity to bias, selectivity, and underreporting.

CYBERSITES RELATED TO CHAPTER 5

Epidemiology
 chanane.ucsf.edu

Vital Statistics
 www.cdc.gov/nchswww/currpubs.html (type in vital statistics)
 www.census.gov

QUESTIONS

1. What might trigger an endemic disease to become epidemic?

2. Why is infant mortality the primary indicator of the health of a community?

3. Give an example of how season and climate affect disease patterns.

4. What are three new environmental conditions of the past decade that need to be put into the epidemiological equation?

EXERCISE

Using the first letter of your last name, select a state in the United States that begins with that letter. Using the resources of vital statistics data in the library, describe the demography and health status of your state and compare your state to the same data for the nation.

INTERNET INTERACTIVE ACTIVITY

THE NATIONAL VITAL STATISTICS REPORT (NVSR)

The National Vital Statistics System is responsible for the nation's official vital statistics. These vital statistics are provided through state-operated registration systems. The registration of vital events—births, deaths , marriages, divorces, and fetal deaths—is a state function.

The community health educator may link to her or his own state health department by starting at this web page at the CDC:

 www.cdc.gov/nchs/about/major/natality/sites.htm

Example.   The community health educator wants to know the status of the eighteen health indicators for the state of Oklahoma during the past year and compare them to ten years ago.

1. Go to www.cdc.gov/nchs/about/major/natality/sites.htm

2. Click on Oklahoma

3. The homepage gives the health educator a number of ways to get the health indicators. You may do a search using **"health indicators"** as the search term and receive profiles by county. Or, you may click on the **State of the State's Health 2000** which will lead you to another document with additional links.

Exercise

1. Using the CDC link page,

   www.cdc.gov/nchs/about/major/natality/sites.htm

   click on your home state and follow the directions on your state health department's homepage to determine the status of the health indicators for your state. Search by clicking on links or doing a search with "health indicators" as a key phrase.

2. Compare your state health indicators with national data that are usually provided by your own state health department.

3. If after you have searched your state health department's site, if you have been unable to access the data that describe the health indicators for your state, call your state health department and obtain the information you need to access these data on a computer or have the data sent to your home.

REFERENCES

1. Preston, Richard (1994). *Hot zone*. New York: Random House.

2. Detels, R. (1997). Epidemiology, the foundation of public health. In *Oxford textbook of public health*, Vol. 2, pp. 501–505. New York: Oxford University Press.

3. WHO. Leprosy Fact Sheet #101. www.who.int/inf-fs/en/fact101.htm

4. Knox, E. G. (1991). Spatial and temporal studies in epidemiology. In *Oxford textbook of public health*, Vol. 2, pp. 95–105. New York: Oxford University Press.

5. Office of Surveillance and Analysis (1993). *Healthy People 2000 health status indicators*. Utah Department of Health, May.

6. Zucconi, Sharon L., & Carson, Catherine (1994). CDC's consensus set of health status indicators: Monitoring and prioritization by state health departments. *AJPH* Oct. Vol. 84 (10), 1644–1646.

7. Goldman, Benjamin A. (1991). *The truth about where you live*. New York: Times Books, Random House.

8. Ibid.

9. Opit, L. J. (1991). The measurement of health service outcomes. In *Oxford textbook of public health* (pp. 159–172). New York: Oxford University Press.

10. Ibid.

11. Basch, Paul (1990). *Textbook of international health*. New York: Oxford University Press.

12. Shurtleff, Dewey (1992). An overview of the Framingham study. *Journal of Epidemiology and Community Health*. Vol. 46.

13. Sorlie, Paul (1987). An epidemiological investigation of cardiovascular disease. DHEW Publication No. (NIH) 77-1247.

14. Shurtleff, op. cit.

15. Brody, Jane E. (1994). Heart diseases persist in study's 2d generation. *The New York Times*, January 5, p. B7.

16. Garland, M., Hunter, D. J., et al (1998). Menstrual cycle characteristics and history of ovulatory infertility in relation to breast cancer risk in a large cohort of US women. *Am J of Epidemiology* 147: 636–643.

17. Office of Surveillance, op. cit.

18. Miller, G. Tyler (1992). *Living in the environment.* Belmont, CA: Wadsworth.

19. Harte, John, Holdren, Cheryl, & Schneider, Richard (1991). *Toxics A to Z.* Berkeley: University of California Press.

Section II

The Leading Causes of Death: Looking Toward the Future

The Centers for Disease Control and Prevention have listed the ten leading causes of death for all people in the United States. Chapters 6 through 8 discuss these causes of death and their implications for community health education. Readers will notice that almost all of the leading causes of death can be reduced or eliminated through individual behavior changes or compliance with community health prevention and promotion programs.

CHAPTER 6

Cardiovascular Diseases, Cancer, and Cerebrovascular Diseases

Community Health in the 21st Century
"There will be a renewed focus on caring for the caregivers of those with long-term chronic illnesses. Helping people to cope with professional and personal health demands an ongoing change. There will probably be more violence in our society."

—Jerry Braza, Ph.D. Health Education;
Private consultant—healing resources

Chapter Objectives

The student will:

1. distinguish between chronic and communicable diseases.

2. list those risk factors associated with cardiovascular diseases and cerebrovascular diseases.

3. name the three most prevalent cancers associated with women.

4. name the three most prevalent cancers associated with men.

5. list from one to ten the leading causes of death in the United States.

6. discuss why smoking is such an important, preventable risk factor associated with health.

Unlike communicable diseases that were the major killers of the population prior to the discovery of penicillin, chronic or long-term debilitating diseases are the major killers of the population today. As the name implies, chronic diseases get progressively worse over time, often require constant care and rehabilitation, are costly, and generally irreparable. Although public health often focuses on infectious diseases that can cause immediate health emergencies, the prevention and control of chronic illnesses are ongoing efforts of community health educators.

Nearly 90 percent of all deaths in the United States are currently attributable to the ten leading causes of death. Although the leading causes of death change slightly every year, there has been minimal change in the top six or seven killers for the past few decades. Table 6.1 indicates that in 1998, the lead-

Table 6.1   Ten leading causes of death (1998).

Rank	Causes of Death	Number	Rate
All causes		2,338,075	865.0
1.	Diseases of heart	724,269	268.0
2.	Malignant neoplasms	538,947	199.4
3.	Cerebrovascular diseases	158,060	58.5
4.	Chronic obstructive pulmonary diseases	114,381	42.3
5.	Pneumonia and influenza	94,828	35.1
6.	Accidents and adverse effects	93,207	34.5
	Motor vehicle accidents	41,826	15.5
	All other accidents and adverse effects	51,382	19.0
7.	Diabetes mellitus	64,574	23.9
8.	Suicide	29,264	10.8
9.	Nephritis, nephrotic syndrome, and nephrosis	26,295	9.7
10.	Chronic liver disease	24,936	9.2

(*Source:* Healthy People 2010)

ing causes of death in the United States were heart disease, cancer, cerebrovascular disease, chronic obstructive pulmonary disease, unintentional injuries, pneumonia/flu, diabetes, suicide, kidney disease, and liver disease. Table 6.2 on pages 136–137 breaks down deaths within age groups for 1998. As one might note, four of the top five killers are chronic illnesses, and certainly unintentional injuries—when not fatal—may create chronic, long-term disability.

Although the ten leading causes of death changed in the 1990s with the reduction in HIV/AIDS deaths and community interventions to reduce homicide deaths, the first seven leading causes of death have not changed dramatically in three decades despite public and private health initiatives. Community health prevention programs are intended to help people decrease their risks for these causes of death. The messages for prevention of chronic diseases are quite simple—change habits, lifestyle, behaviors—the reality of Americans making these changes is much more complex and frustrating.

Readers will notice that discussion about the leading causes of disease and mortality will often vary in describing the ten leading causes of death. Leading causes of death can change every year, with the most variation around diseases such as AIDS or influenza/pneumonia, where education and pharmaceutical intervention have dramatically changed mortality rates every year. Additionally, some major killers, such as accidents or chronic obstructive pulmonary diseases, have mortality rates so similar that unforseen events can change one killer from being fourth to fifth in one year and back to fourth in the next. The reader should not be concerned about the actual ranking of a leading cause of death from year to year, but note that in general the leading eight or ten causes of death have remained consistent for almost fifty years. It is the combination of public health commitment, resources allocated to combating specific diseases, changes in medical technology, and sometimes legislation that reduce deaths within categories in different years or decades. It appears that those ten killers of the population in the United States will remain as such, in various forms, for the beginning decades of the twenty-first century.

Further, a report by McGinnis[1] suggests that there are clear factors that impact all of the leading causes of disease:

- Tobacco: 19 percent of all deaths
- Diet/activity patterns: 4 percent of all deaths
- Alcohol: l5 percent of all deaths
- Microbial agents: 4 percent of all deaths
- Toxic agents: 3 percent of all deaths
- Firearms: 2 percent of all deaths
- Sexual behavior: 1 percent of all deaths
- Motor vehicles: 1 percent of all deaths
- Illicit use of drugs: <1 percent of all deaths

Until these factors are dramatically challenged by health and science, the leading causes of death will remain relatively stable.

The next few chapters are dedicated to the major killers of the population. In this chapter, the three leading causes of death—cardiovascular diseases, cancer, and cerebrovascular diseases—are discussed, along with their causes, risk factors, and prevention.

Cardiovascular Diseases (CVD)

In the twentieth century, cardiovascular diseases (diseases of the heart and blood vessels) have come to overshadow all others as a cause of death in industrialized populations. Over 57 million Americans have one or more types of CVD. This disturbing fact reflects changes in lifestyle and environment whose origins are social, cultural, and economic. In western countries, cardiovascular diseases are responsible for over 30 percent of deaths in men and 25 percent of deaths in women. Cardiovascular disease is the primary killer of both genders, black or white (Figure 6.1, page 138).

The major cardiovascular diseases include heart disease, hypertension, atherosclerosis, stroke, and rheumatic heart disease. Other kinds of cardiovascular disease are usually the secondary result of a major health problem such as alcoholism or diabetes. Since a great deal is known about the variables that increase risk for cardiovascular diseases, a great deal of medical science, community health and personal health efforts have been directed toward reducing cardiovascular disease morbidity and mortality. For example, it is known that quitting smoking, reducing fat intake, controlling weight and blood cholesterol levels, reducing stress, and exercising regularly all promote a healthy cardiovascular system. The Framingham Study, a longitudinal study of heart disease discussed in Chapter 5, has been one of the greatest sources of proof of those prevention suggestions. It

Table 6.2   Ten leading causes of death by age groups (1998—all races, both sexes).

Rank	<1	1–4	5–9	10–14	15–24	25–⌐
1	Congenital Anomalies 6,212	Unintentional Injury & Adv. Effects 1,935	Unintentional Injury & Adv. Effects 1,544	Unintentional Injury & Adv. Effects 1,710	Unintentional Injury & Adv. Effects 13,349	Uninten Injury & Effec 12,0⌐
2	Short Gestation 4,101	Congenital Anomalies 564	Malignant Neoplasms 487	Malignant Neoplasms 526	Homicide & Legal Int. 5,506	Suici⌐ 5,36
3	SIDS 2,822	Homicide & Legal Int. 399	Congenital Anomalies 198	Suicide 317	Suicide 4,135	Homici⌐ Legal 4,56
4	Maternal Complications 1,343	Malignant Neoplasms 365	Homicide & Legal Int. 170	Homicide & Legal Int. 290	Malignant Neoplasms 1,699	Malign⌐ Neopla 4,38⌐
5	Respiratory Distress Syndrome 1,295	Heart Disease 214	Heart Disease 156	Congenital Anomalies 173	Heart Disease 1,057	Heart D⌐ 3,20⌐
6	Placenta Cord Membranes 961	Pneumonia & Influenza 146	Pneumonia & Influenza 70	Heart Disease 170	Congenital Anomalies 450	HIV⌐ 2,91⌐
7	Perinatal Infections 815	Septicemia 89	Bronchitis Emphysema Asthma 54	Bronchitis Emphysema Asthma 98	Bronchitis Emphysema Asthma 239	Cerebrov⌐ 670
8	Unintentional Injury & Adv. Effects 754	Perinatal Period 75	Benign Neoplasms 52	Pneumonia & Influenza 51	Pneumonia & Influenza 215	Diabe⌐ 636⌐
9	Intrauterine Hypoxia 461	Cerebrovascular 57	Cerebrovascular 35	Cerebrovascular 47	HIV 194	Pneumo⌐ Influen⌐ 531
10	Pneumonia & Influenza 441	Benign Neoplasms 53	HIV 29	Benign Neoplasms 32	Cerebrovascular 178	Liver Dis⌐ 506

con⌐

(*Source:* Centers for Disease Control. National Center for Injury Prevention and Control Homepage)

Continued.

Rank	35–44	45–54	55–64	65+	Total
1	Malignant Neoplasms 17,022	Malignant Neoplasms 45,747	Malignant Neoplasms 87,024	Heart Disease 605,673	Heart Disease 724,859
2	Unintentional Injury & Adv. Effects 15,127	Heart Disease 35,056	Heart Disease 65,068	Malignant Neoplasms 384,186	Malignant Neoplasms 541,532
3	Heart Disease 13,593	Unintentional Injury & Adv. Effects 10,946	Bronchitis Emphysema Asthma 10,162	Cerebrovascular 139,144	Cerebrovascular 158,448
4	Suicide 6,837	Liver Disease 5,744	Cerebrovascular 9,653	Bronchitis Emphysema Asthma 97,896	Bronchitis Emphysema Asthma 112,584
5	HIV 5,746	Cerebrovascular 5,709	Diabetes 8,705	Pneumonia & Influenza 82,989	Unintentional Injury & Adv. Effects 97,835
6	Homicide & Legal Int. 3,567	Suicide 5,131	Unintentional Injury & Adv. Effects 7,340	Diabetes 48,974	Pneumonia & Influenza 91,871
7	Liver Disease 3,370	Diabetes 4,386	Liver Disease 5,279	Unintentional Injury & Adv. Effects 32,975	Diabetes 64,751
8	Cerebrovascular 2,650	HIV 3,120	Pneumonia & Influenza 3,856	Nephritis 22,640	Suicide 30,575
9	Diabetes 1,885	Bronchitis Emphysema Asthma 2,828	Suicide 2,963	Alzheimer's Disease 22,416	Nephritis 26,182
10	Pneumonia & Influenza 1,400	Pneumonia & Influenza 2,167	Septicemia 2,093	Septicemia 19,012	Liver Disease 25,192

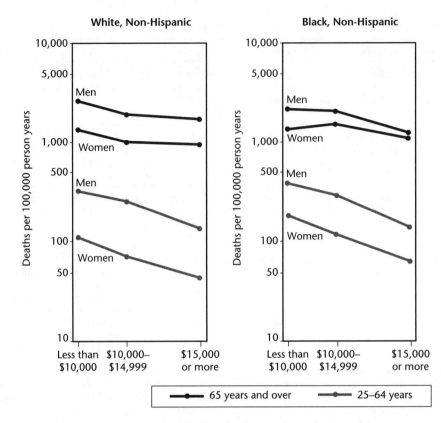

Figure 6.1 Cardiovascular disease mortality by gender and race and income.

(*Source:* Centers for Disease Control. Health, United States, 1998 with Socioeconomic Status and Health Chart Book.)

is known that the offspring of the subjects in the Framingham study, today in their forties, are heavier, less active, eat fattier foods and have higher rates of diabetes and cardiovascular illnesses than their parents did at comparable ages. Although there are many diseases within the scope of cardiovascular problems, heart disease and stroke are highlighted as they are the most prevalent. Other contributing cardiovascular diseases are mentioned within the context of heart disease and stroke to show their contribution to the potential problem.

Heart Disease

The importance of the coronary arteries in supplying oxygenated blood to the myocardium, the heart muscle, cannot be understated. When blockage occurs in the small vessels, less oxygen is supplied to portions of the heart which may result in heart damage. The result and damage that occurs from lack of oxygen may produce sudden results such as a heart attack (a coronary thrombosis or myocardial infarction) or it may be more chronic, producing reduced energy and inability for the body to function properly.

Figure 6.2 shows the mortality rates for coronary heart disease among men and women in many industrialized countries. What is most important for the community health educator to understand is that heart disease is preventable and reversible through the modification of risk factors including elevated blood lipids, elevated blood pressure, cigarette smoking, and sedentary lifestyle. Entire populations are at risk because of risk factors enhanced by culture, economic factors, and the environment.[2]

Healthy People 2010 Objective: Reduce Coronary Heart Disease Deaths

Target: 166 deaths per 100,000 population.

Baseline: 208 coronary heart disease deaths per 100,000 population in 1998 (preliminary data; age adjusted to the year 2000 standard population).

Public Health experts call the Southeast United States the "enigma area" because nine of the ten states with the highest rates of heart disease mortality are in the South.[3] Blood pressure is higher in the South among men, women, blacks, whites, and children. The southeastern counties with the highest rates of heart disease are rural and among the poorest areas in the nation. Within metropolitan areas, heart disease is much higher in industrial inner cities than in suburbia. Household incomes in counties with the highest rates of heart disease mortality are 13 percent below the national average and poverty is 50 percent higher.

Preventing Heart Disease   Heart disease has both modifiable and nonmodifiable risk factors. You cannot control your age, race, sex, or genetic inheritance, which may be risks for heart disease. You can, however, modify or control sev-

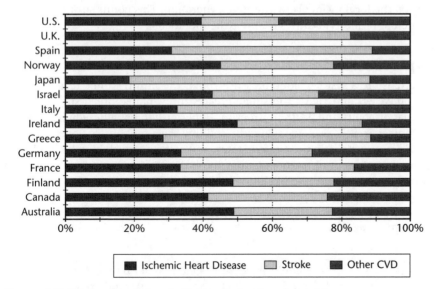

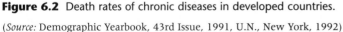

Figure 6.2 Death rates of chronic diseases in developed countries.

(*Source:* Demographic Yearbook, 43rd Issue, 1991, U.N., New York, 1992)

eral other risk factors for heart disease: atherosclerosis, hypertension, cholesterol (and other fats) level, cigarette smoking, lack of exercise, diabetes mellitus, weight, personality traits, and stress.[4]

Atherosclerosis

Atherosclerosis is the progressive obstruction of coronary artery blood flow, a condition where cholesterol rich, fibro fat is deposited under the intima of the larger arteries. It is a progressive disorder that begins in childhood and is aggravated by hypertension, lack of exercise, heavy smoking, poor nutrition, and stress. Coronary heart disease, the number one killer of the population, is caused in 85 percent of the cases by atherosclerotic conditions. Atherosclerosis is the fifteenth leading cause of death with a 6.6 per 100,000 death rate.

By the fourth or fifth decades of life, the deposition of this fatty plaque causes a diminution of blood flow to primary organs, especially the heart. When oxygen loss to this muscle is decreased, many coronary conditions can disable or kill a person. In 20 percent of all cases, ventricular fibrillation with oxygen depletion **(ischemia),** also known as **angina pectoris,** is one of the first recognized symptoms. When plaque blocks vessels and valves, myocardial infarction (death of the heart tissue, or heart attack) occurs.

All of the causes of atherosclerosis are not known, but various risk factors have been identified. Foremost among the suspected factors is the high proportion of saturated fat in the U.S. diet, smoking, high blood pressure, and the level of cholesterol circulating in the blood.

Various nationalities of the world, such as the Japanese, have a low incidence of atherosclerosis, but when they migrate to the United States, they develop the local incidence within one generation. This points strongly to environmental or lifestyle causes that may be modifiable.

Hypertension

Hypertension, a systolic blood pressure above 140 mm Hg and a diastolic pressure above 90 mm Hg, is the single greatest preventable precursor of cardiovascular disability and death in America. Hypertension has a hereditary propensity, however, it is also aggravated by sodium consumption that averages four to ten grams per day in the United States, and being overweight, which is found in about 20 percent of the population. Too little calcium or too little potassium also appear to increase the likelihood of hypertension.

Healthy People 2010 Objective: Reduce the Proportion of Adults with High Blood Pressure

Target: 16 percent.

Baseline: 28 percent of adults aged 20 years and older had high blood pressure in 1988–1994 (age adjusted to the year 2000 standard population).

Over 50 million people in the United States have hypertension in some form. This number reflects 20 percent of the adult population. Since there are no visible signs or symptoms, many people are not aware that they have high blood pressure; in fact, it is known as "the silent killer." Those at highest risk for hypertension are males, people over fifty years old, and people of color. Lack of access to primary care is an important predisposing factor for severe uncontrolled hypertension in disadvantaged populations that have been studied. Educational level and social class are powerful predictors of health outcome treating hypertension.[5]

Hypertension can be reduced with medication, although often just a change in lifestyle may reduce blood pressure. A change in diet that reduces cholesterol and fat and a regular exercise program will often reduce blood pressure.

Cholesterol

Cholesterol is a fatty substance that contributes to plaque buildup in the arteries. This substance is manufactured within the body, in addition to that of which we consume through animal products. At a general level, cholesterol is divided into two types: LDL (low-density lipoproteins) and HDL (high-density lipoproteins). LDL is referred to as "bad cholesterol." HDL is "good cholesterol" in that this transports LDL in the blood. The goal is to have optimal levels of HDL (which can be raised by regular exercise) and to minimize the level of LDL in the blood (which can be lowered with dietary changes).

The National Cholesterol Education Program, of the National Heart, Lung, and Blood Institute, recommends that an adult's cholesterol level be below 200 mg/dl of blood. For optimal prevention, everyone should be familiar with his or her cholesterol level. The National Institutes of Health advise that in addition to cholesterol testing, people should also have their individual HDL level checked. The higher the HDL the lower the cardiovascular risk. It is thought that 35 milligrams per deciliter (mg/dl) is the cut-off point. Lower than 35 mg/dl HDL will put a person at risk even with a safe cholesterol level range of less than 200 mg/dl of blood.

Healthy People 2010 Objective: Reduce the Mean Total Blood Cholesterol Levels Among Adults

Target: 199 mg/dL.

Baseline: 206 mg/dL was the mean total blood cholesterol level for adults aged 20 years and older in 1988–1994 (age adjusted to the year 2000 standard population).

Smoking   No country has yet taken action against tobacco commensurate with the cost it poses. The global use of tobacco has grown nearly 75 percent over the past two decades. In China tobacco use has doubled, and in only four countries are fewer cigarettes smoked now than in 1964. In the United States, the

Table 6.3   Percentage of smokers by state in 1999.

Alabama	24.6	Louisiana	25.5	Oklahoma	23.8
Alaska	26.0	Maine	22.4	Oregon	21.2
Arizona	21.9	Maryland	22.4	Pennsylvania	23.8
Arkansas	26.0	Massachusetts	20.9	Rhode Island	22.7
California	19.2	Michigan	27.4	South Carolina	24.7
Colorado	22.8	Minnesota	18.0	South Dakota	27.3
Connecticut	21.1	Mississippi	24.1	Tennessee	26.1
Delaware	24.5	Missouri	26.3	Texas	22.0
Washington D.C.	21.6	Montana	21.5	Utah	14.2
Florida	22.0	Nebraska	22.1	Vermont	22.4
Georgia	23.7	Nevada	20.4	Virginia	21.2
Hawaii	19.5	New Hampshire	23.3	Washington	21.4
Idaho	20.3	New Jersey	19.2	West Virginia	27.9
Illinois	23.1	New Mexico	22.6	Wisconsin	23.4
Indiana	26.0	New York	24.3	Wyoming	22.8
Iowa	23.4	North Carolina	24.7	USA	22.9
Kansas	21.2	North Dakota	20.0		
Kentucky	30.8	Ohio	26.2		

(*Source:* Centers for Disease Control)

Many cities are banning smoking inside public buildings. The result is many smokers getting a little "fresh air" a few times during their work day.

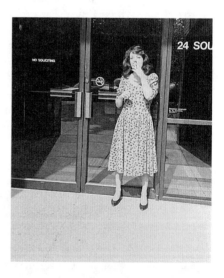

percentage of adults who smoke has fallen from forty-three to twenty-seven percent, but more tobacco is used, and the United States now ranks eleventh in the world in per capita cigarette use.[6] As cigarette smoking has declined, cigar smoking has increased. In 1999, 39 percent of Americans had tried a cigar; 5.2 percent had smoked a cigar in a previous month.[7] National smoking percentages by state are given in Table 6.3. How does your state's smoking rate compare to the highest and lowest rates in the country?

Table 6.4   International rates of smoking by selected countries (1999).

Country	Percent of Male Smokers	Percent of Women Smokers
Korea	68	7
Russian Federation	67	30
China	61	7
Poland	51	29
Fiji	59	31
Cuba	49	25
Israel	45	30
Argentina	40	27
Iraq	40	5
France	40	27
Egypt	40	1
Italy	38	26
Switzerland	36	26
Canada	31	29
Australia	29	21
United States	28	23
United Kingdom	28	26
Sweden	22	24

(*Source:* Physicians for a Smoke-Free Canada. www.smoke-free.ca/factsheets/pdf/worldprev1.PDF)

Smoking is an epidemic growing at 2.1 percent per year, faster than the world population. Growth in tobacco use slowed briefly in the early 1980s, but is resuming its rapid increase. Worldwide, over a billion people now smoke, consuming almost 5 trillion cigarettes per year. Korea leads the world in per capita cigarette consumption, followed by the Russian Federation, China, and Poland. The United States dropped from second in 1982 to eleventh in 1998. Eastern-bloc countries, in general, smoke more heavily than Westerners and twice as much as people in developing countries.[8] Table 6.4 compares some smoking rates around the world by gender.

There have been declines in the number of smokers since the 1990s in the United States. However, there are increasing numbers of smokers among teens, especially girls, and among women. Sadly, the decline in smoking among adults is now very minimal. A survey of 35,816 adults nationwide in 1997 reported that one of four adults smoke on a regular basis, 28 percent of men and 22 percent of women. Only 12 percent of college-educated adults smoke. Changes in smoking patterns among young adults are shown in Figure 6.3.

There were sixteen national health objectives set by the Public Health Service for the year 2000 associated with tobacco use. Substantial progress has been made in achieving these goals, however, the pressure of the tobacco lobby is a major barrier to full attainment of the objectives. One objective was to reduce the proportion of adults who smoke to less than 20 percent. The proportion remains about 30 percent today.

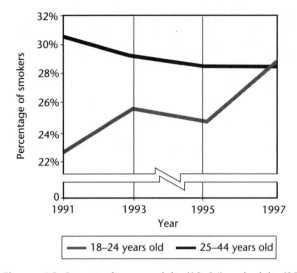

Figure 6.3 Percent of young adults (18–24) and adults (25–44) who smoke every day or some days (1991–1997).

(*Sources:* Centers for Disease Control. Youth Tobacco Surveillance)

Healthy People 2010 Objective: Reduce Tobacco Use by Adults Aged 18 and Older

Target: 12 percent.

Baseline: 24 percent of adults aged 18 and older smoked cigarettes or cigars, chewed tobacco, or used other tobacco products in 1997 (age adjusted to the year 2000 standard population).

Healthy People 2010 Objective: Reduce Tobacco Use by Adolescents Grades 9 through 12

Target: 21 percent.

Baseline: 43 percent of adolescents in grades 9 through 12 used tobacco products in 1997 (age adjusted to the year 2000 standard population).

The evidence linking tobacco use with disease, disability, and premature death is extensive. This body of information continues to grow as research reveals more about the health effects of tobacco use. Smoking is a prime risk factor for heart and blood vessel disease, chronic bronchitis, and emphysema. Cigarette smoking is also responsible for more cancers and more cancer deaths than any other known agent.

In addition, pregnant women who smoke are more likely than nonsmokers to experience complications during pregnancy and deliver babies who are born prematurely, are small or underweight, have respiratory and cardiovascular problems, or die within the first year of life.[9]

Healthy People 2010 Objective: Increase Smoking Cessation during Pregnancy

Target: 30 percent.

Baseline: 12 percent smoking cessation during the first trimester of pregnancy in 1991 (age adjusted to the year 2000 standard population).

Data from the National Center for Health Statistics show that at the beginning of their pregnancy more than one-third of mothers under twenty-five years of age and about one-fourth of older mothers smoke. Fortunately, the public education about pregnancy and smoking has been extensive and reductions are being realized.[9]

Tobacco affects children beginning with exposure before they are born. Nicotine, toxic chemicals, and radioactive polonium may all interfere with fetal development as they are received by the fetus through the mother's blood when she smokes or chews tobacco. Studies in MDC and LDCs show that smoking by pregnant women reduces infants' weight at birth by roughly one-tenth. Low birth weight has been associated with tobacco chewing in India, where 39 percent of women chew tobacco.[10] Nicotine has been implicated in spontaneous abortions, prematurity, and birth complications.[11]

Studies of 132 children in a day care center found that exposure to passive smoke appears to increase the frequency and duration of middle ear infection among young children. One theory for this increase is that smoke causes an abnormal increase in cells and mucus secretion in the respiratory tract, Eustachian tube, and middle ear. Middle ear infection, the most common illness diagnosed by pediatricians, costs between $1 to 2 billion a year to treat.[12]

Children with parents who smoke experience much higher rates of respiratory illness, bronchitis, asthma, and pneumonia. Parents who smoke may also reduce the intellectual development of their children. Learning ability of eleven-year-olds whose mothers smoke has been shown to lag by six months.

Other Forms of Tobacco After the Marlboro Man quit selling cigarettes, baseball players started chewing Red Man and dipping Skoal, encouraging young people to do as they do, not as community health educators say. The World Health Organization describes smokeless tobacco use as a "new threat to society" estimating that there are now 12 million users of snuff and loose leaf chewing

BOX 6.1 Suing the Tobacco Industry

On June 25, 1992, the U.S. Supreme Court determined that an individual has the right to sue the tobacco industry for health complications incurred from tobacco use. It upheld that a New Jersey Federal District Court found internal tobacco industry documents showing how some cigarette companies have developed strategies to mislead the public about the health risks of smoking.

tobacco in the United States. By 1981, several major studies had linked smoke-less tobacco to various cancers and diseases of the gums and tooth decay.[13]

The NIH estimates that at least 3 million of all United States users are under age twenty-one. Surveys in Massachusetts, Texas, Oregon, and Oklahoma indicate that approximately 30 percent of teenage males are chewing or dipping. The CDC found that 17 percent of 5-year-old girls and 10 percent of 5-year-old boys in Alaska use smokeless tobacco, while 21 percent of Arkansas children used smokeless tobacco. These frightening numbers contribute to the 27,000 deaths each year from oral cancer.

A well publicized case in point was the death of Sean Marsee, a high school athlete and regular user of Copenhagen snuff. Marsee began using snuff at age 12. At age 18 he was diagnosed with tongue cancer in the spot where the "quid" touched his tongue. In 1984, after a series of disfiguring operations including partial removal of his tongue, Marsee died at age 19.[14]

Exercise

As a result of the Framingham results, the American Heart Association has included sedentary lifestyles as a major risk factor for heart disease, along with hypertension, high cholesterol, and smoking. In fact, the CDC has stated that sedentary living is *the* leading culprit in deaths from heart attacks.[15] Exercise is extremely important in maintaining cardiovascular health. To obtain and maintain heart health, aerobic exercise (with oxygen) should be performed three to four times per week, twenty to thirty minutes per session.

Diabetes Mellitus

Diabetes is a disease of the endocrine system that increases the risk for heart disease and stroke. Diabetes can be controlled in most cases through diet and exercise, but some will have to regulate it with medication. It does run in families, therefore, knowledge of family history would be a step in prevention. Diabetes, itself a leading killer in the United States, is discussed in more detail in Chapter 7.

Weight

Obesity has been implicated as a risk factor for many chronic diseases, including heart disease. It is always best to maintain the ideal weight for your height and body type. Through exercise and proper nutrition, one can reach his or her ideal body weight and reduce risks for several chronic conditions. Forty-three states had populations with over 15 percent obese in 1999. Overweight and underweight percentages for selected countries are given in Figure 6.4.

Stress and Personality Traits

Some stress in your life is actually good. We wouldn't be alive without it. However, once we become overloaded with stress, it affects us in psychological and

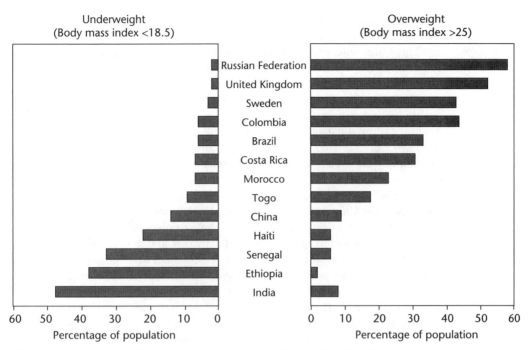

Figure 6.4 Percentage of population underweight and overweight in selected countries, around 1993.

(*Source:* World Health Organization)

physical ways. It is understood that two personality types exist, Type A and Type B. Type A personalities, those very driven and task oriented, were once determined to be at higher risk for chronic conditions, including heart disease. Recent studies have suggested, however, it is not necessarily having Type A characteristics that put an individual at risk, but how these persons deal with emotions like frustration and anger. Those Type A individuals who manage these emotions may not have any higher risk for heart disease than Type B individuals,[16] who are more calm, easy going, and less prone to stress.

Prevention Programs

Today, many communities and businesses have set health goals of reducing CVD by promoting behavior change programs within institutions such as government, schools, and private businesses. Community health educators are being hired to plan, conduct, and evaluate these programs with the goal of reducing health costs for organizations through health promotion. Several research and demonstration projects are underway or completed in the United States and Europe. Three major U.S. studies addressing cardiovascular risk reduction currently in progress are: the Stanford Five-City Project, the Pawtucket Heart

Health Program and the Minnesota Heart Health Program. The largest of these studies in the United States is the Minnesota Heart Health Program (MHHP).[17]

The Minnesota project was started in 1980 and involves approximately 400,000 persons in six communities in the Upper Midwest. Selected communities were given risk reduction education intervention programs over an extended period of time. The interventions included advocating hypertension prevention, healthy eating patterns for lower blood cholesterol and blood pressure, non-smoking, and regular physical activity. Individual, group, and community level programs were initiated with a wide range of strategies and theories. Mass media techniques were used to increase community exposure to the programs and community leaders spread the word about activities and programs.[18] This large-scale intervention program has been replicated in less extensive ways in many communities in the United States and Europe. Unfortunately, results from the MHHP study show only modest and time limited improvements in exposure to coronary heart disease risk reducing messages and activities, and in coronary heart disease risk factors. What is now important is for professionals to determine why such an extensive education program did not work in these communities and to take those components of risk reduction programs that are effective and modify and expand upon them. The future of community-based cardiovascular disease studies may lie in targeting specific groups within a large population and address interventions to the specific characteristics of subpopulations.

Cancer

Recognized in some of their forms since antiquity, cancers today represent a public health problem of major dimensions in economically developed countries and an emerging problem in developing countries. It is the second leading cause of death in the United States. Cancer is a collective name for more than a hundred clinical diseases that affect various sites of the body in different ways. As a group, cancers rank among the first three causes of death in all countries for which data are available. The rise in cancer has been concurrent with a steady decrease in death from cardiovascular diseases over the past four decades.[19] In fact, it was predicted that by the year 2010 cancer would be the leading cause of death in this country.[20] Sites of new cancer cases and deaths by gender are given in Table 6.5.

Despite this prediction, cancer incidence and death rates for all cancers combined and for most of the top ten cancer sites declined between 1990 and 1995, reversing an almost twenty-year trend.[21] The incidence rates declined for most age groups, for both men and women, and for most racial and ethnic groups with the exception of black males for whom the incidence rate increased, and Asian and Pacific Islander females whose rates remained level. Despite this overall decline, both incidence and mortality from non-Hodgkin's lymphoma and melanoma skin cancer are on the rise. The previous decline in uterine cancer has leveled off.[22]

Worldwide, one of every ten deaths is due to cancer. Figure 6.5 contrasts the incidence of cancer in developed and developing countries. The numbers of

Table 6.5   Leading sites of new cancer cases and deaths (2000 estimates).

Cancer Cases by Site and Sex		Cancer Deaths by Site and Sex	
Male	Female	Male	Female
Prostrate 180,400	Breast 182,800	Lung & bronchus 89,300	Lung & bronchus 67,800
Lung & bronchus 89,500	Lung & bronchus 74,600	Prostrate 31,900	Breast 40,800
Colon & rectum 63,600	Colon & rectum 66,600	Colon & rectum 27,800	Colon & rectum 28,500
Urinary bladder 38,300	Uterine corpus 36,100	Pancreas 13,700	Pancreas 14,500
Non-Hodgkin's lymphoma 31,700	Non-Hodgkin's lymphoma 23,200	Non-Hodgkin's lymphoma 13,700	Non-Hodgkin's lymphoma 12,400
Melanoma of the skin 27,300	Ovary 23,100	Leukemia 12,100	Ovary 1,400
Oral cavity 20,200	Melanoma of the skin 20,400	Esophagus 9,200	Leukemia 9,600
Kidney 18,800	Urinary bladder 14,900	Liver 8,500	Uterine corpus 6,500
Leukemia 16,900	Pancreas 14,600	Urinary Bladder 8,100	Brain 5,900
Pancreas 13,700	Thyroid 13,700	Stomach 7,600	Stomach 5,400
All Sites 619,700	All Sites 600,400	All Sites 284,100	All sites 268,100

*Excludes basal and squamous cell skin cancer and in situ carcinomas except urinary bladder.

(*Source:* © 2000, American Cancer Society, Inc., Surveillance Research)

new cases for sixteen cancers are about evenly divided, 49.3 percent in developed countries and 50.7 percent in developing countries. However, the distribution of the cases by cancer site is quite different. Lung, prostrate, breast, and colorectal cancers rank first in developed countries. Cancer of the cervix, stomach, mouth-pharynx, and esophagus rank first in developing countries.[23]

If you look at the lifestyle behaviors indicative of developed and developing countries, the cancer patterns become quite understandable. In westernized countries, foods with toxins and chemicals, cigarette smoking, low fiber foods, and high fat foods that are typical of developed countries are all major risks. In developing countries, the extraordinary number of smokers, high incidence of sexually transmitted diseases, and polluted waters that ultimately get into food chain probably account for high cancer rates. Measures of industrial toxins are more frequently associated with geographic variation in cancer mortality than any other cause of death.

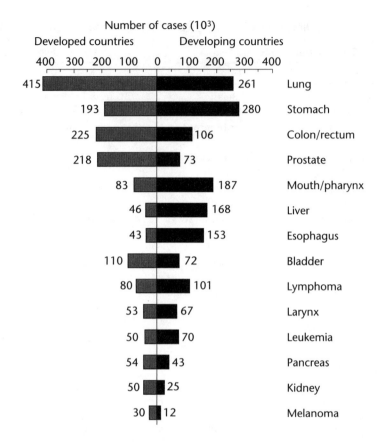

Number of cases (10^3)

Developed countries   Developing countries

| 400 | 300 | 200 | 100 | 0 | 100 | 200 | 300 | 400 |

415 ▮▮▮▮▮ ▮▮▮▮▮ 261   Lung

193 ▮▮▮▮ ▮▮▮▮▮ 280   Stomach

225 ▮▮▮▮ ▮▮▮ 106   Colon/rectum

218 ▮▮▮▮ ▮▮ 73   Prostate

83 ▮▮ ▮▮▮▮ 187   Mouth/pharynx

46 ▮ ▮▮▮▮ 168   Liver

43 ▮ ▮▮▮ 153   Esophagus

110 ▮▮ ▮▮ 72   Bladder

80 ▮▮ ▮▮▮ 101   Lymphoma

53 ▮ ▮▮ 67   Larynx

50 ▮ ▮▮ 70   Leukemia

54 ▮ ▮ 43   Pancreas

50 ▮ ▮ 25   Kidney

30 ▮ 12   Melanoma

Figure 6.5 New cases of cancer by site: Developing and developed countries (1994).

(*Source:* GloboCan. International Agency for Research on Cancer)

About 552,200 Americans were expected to die of cancer in 2000, more than 1,500 people a day. In the United States, one of four deaths is from cancer. Nearly 5 million lives have been lost to cancer since 1990. In 2000, about 1,220,100 new cancer cases are expected to be diagnosed.[24]

Cancer will strike about 1 million Americans this year, and one of every three men and one of every two women now living will eventually have some type of cancer. On the average, one person dies from cancer every 66 seconds in the United States.

Geographical trends for cancer mortality in the United States are markedly different from other causes of death. Cancer rates in rural areas are catching up to those in urban areas and there is a concentration of mortality in the Northeast, especially New Jersey, Connecticut, and parts of New York. Researchers have found significant associations between chemical waste sites and cancer rates in New Jersey. White male cancer mortality tracks the Ohio and Mississippi rivers with clusters in the Louisiana delta. White female cancer mortality is particularly high in upper New York and northern California. The north-

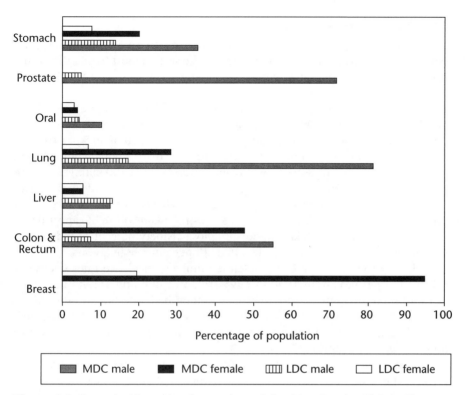

Figure 6.6 Cancer Incidence rates by gender and site: More Developed Countries (MDC) and Less Developed Countires (LDC) (2000).

(*Source:* GloboCan 2000. www.dep.iarc.fr/globocan/)

south difference between the sexes parallels differences in smoking prevalence among men and women.[25]

Minorities have the highest rates of cancer in the Midwest, with clusters in the Northwest and Northeast. In the 1950s, cancer mortality among black men was about 20 percent lower than for white men in the United States. Now black men have the highest cancer mortality rates in the country, which parallels the beginning of the smoking habit among blacks. Asians suffer highest from liver cancer, whites from breast cancer, and blacks from prostate cancer.

The bad news is that a white man of the "baby boom" generation has about twice the risk of developing cancer as his grandfather, and a white woman of the same age has about a 50 percent greater risk than her grandmother of developing cancer. The good news is that almost 50 percent of Americans under age 75 who get cancer can now be cured, compared with only 38 percent in 1960. This has happened mostly because of a combination of early detection and improved use of surgery, radiation, and drug treatments. Thus, the preeminent status of cancer will not endure. The continuing battle against cancer should bring major victories within the next thirty or so years.[26]

The Most Prevalent Cancers

Lung Cancer Lung cancer is the leading cause of death from cancer in men and women. After prostate cancer, lung cancer is the second most frequently occurring cancer in men, and after breast, colon, and rectal cancers, the third most frequently occurring cancer in women.

Lung cancer is rising to epidemic proportions. There were an estimated 164,100 new cases in 2000, accounting for 14 percent of cancer diagnoses. The incidence rate is declining significantly in men, from a high of 86.5 per 100,000 in 1984 to 70.0 in 1996. In the 1990s the rate of increase among women began to slow. In 1996 the incidence rate in women was 42.3 per 100,000. There were an estimated 156,900 deaths in 2000, accounting for 28 percent of all cancer deaths. Since 1987, more women have died each year of lung cancer than breast cancer, which, for over forty years, was the major cause of cancer death in women.[27] Lung cancer has a poor prognosis. Ninety percent of individuals with lung cancer will die from it; less than 15 percent live five years.

Although lung cancer is in epidemic numbers, incidence rates decreased 1.1 percent per year from 1990 to 1995. This was due primarily to decreased rates for men. In contrast, only Hispanic women had a decline in lung cancer mortality from 1990 to 1995.[28] In 1997, there were an estimated 178,100 new cases of lung cancer and 150,400 lung cancer-related deaths. There were 1 million new cases worldwide.[29]

Only 1–6 percent of patients with lung cancer are younger than forty years. Race has been found to be an important factor in lung cancer deaths; mortality rates are higher in black men than white men, although rates are comparable among women. Access to health care and early diagnosis may be more of a variable than race. The state-by-state pattern for lung cancer mortality is very similar to smoking rates, however, the South claims seven of the eight states with the highest lung cancer mortality rates, but only three of the eight states with the largest percentages of smokers.[30] Why do you think this is?

Several factors are involved in the etiology of lung cancer, however, tobacco smoking is the primary risk factor for lung cancer in the United States. Current and former smokers comprise the most clearly defined group at risk for lung cancer.[31] Lung cancer is a rare cause of death in nonsmokers; however, involuntary smoking can cause lung cancer from the presence of carcinogens in sidestream, secondhand smoke.

In fact, a recent concern of health care professionals is the risk of lung cancer from exposure to passive smoke. **Mainstream smoke** (smoke actively inhaled) and **sidestream smoke** or **secondhand smoke** (smoke released in ambient air from burning cigarettes) have similar compositions, including the presence of established carcinogenic chemicals. Sidestream smoke releases fifty times the amount of carcinogens inhaled by the user into the surrounding air. It contains several thousand other compounds, many of which cause irritation and allergic reactions in the eyes and nose.

Over twenty epidemiological studies have suggested a causal link between sidestream smoke and lung cancer, with an apparent excess risk of 30–40 percent for nonsmoking women exposed under average conditions in the home. Ambient tobacco smoke causes more cancer deaths than all regulated industrial air pollutants combined. The cost in lives may be as high as 5,000 nonsmokers per year. Although smoke-free environments are being created in schools, workplaces, and public buildings, about 60 percent of U.S. workers are exposed to tobacco smoke.

Environmental deterioration may also be contributing to lung cancer. Urban areas frequently show an excess of lung cancer compared to nonurban areas. It is thought that air pollution contributes to this increase as well, although the data are inconclusive. Another possible relationship is population density, which manifests in the socioeconomic factors associated with early diagnosis and primary care. There are, however, proven environmental causes of lung cancer—radon, steroids, asbestos, and tobacco smoke. Lung cancer may also be caused by hazardous dusts such as asbestos or coal. When these dusts are combined with inhaled tobacco, the result is deadly.

Breast Cancer Among women, breast cancer is the most frequently occurring cancer and the second leading cause of cancer deaths (after lung cancer). The rate of breast cancer in the United States rose by about 1 percent every year since the mid-1930s until 1990 when it began to level off. Among women ages thirty-five to fifty-five years, breast cancer is the leading cause of death. Cancer of the breast accounts for 28 percent of all cancers in women. New cases are diagnosed in about 180,000 women annually, and 45,000 women die each year from breast cancer. It is thought that breast cancer rates are changing because of widespread breast cancer screening as part of routine medical care, and the increased use of adjuvant treatments.

White and African American women have the highest rates of breast cancer, but it is increasing dramatically among Native Americans. Since 1995, however, mortality has dropped for white and Hispanic women. Breast cancer death rates remain level for black women and may be on the rise for Asian and Pacific Islander women.[32]

A number of personal characteristics have been associated with higher risks of breast cancer: family history, late childbearing, having no or few children, early menarche, late menopause, obesity, and/or a high-fat diet. These factors account for only 25 to 30 percent of all breast cancer cases; the rest remain a medical mystery. Newest research is suggesting that environmental risk factors such as pollutants and pesticides may be part of the mystery.[33] Women with higher socioeconomic status (SES) are more likely to get breast cancer, but women with lower SES are more likely to die from it. Early diagnosis is a major determinant of survival.[34]

At all ages, breast cancer mortality is higher among urban residents in the Northeast than among rural residents in the South. There are also clusters of high rates in a number of Midwestern and Western states, especially among white women. Among women over forty, whites have higher rates than blacks, whereas among women under forty, whites have lower rates than blacks.

BOX 6.2 National Breast and Cervical Cancer Early Detection Program

In 1990 Congress passed the Breast and Cervical Cancer Mortality Prevention Act. This legislation authorized the CDC to establish the National Breast and Cervical Cancer Early Detection Program. This program includes:

- Community-based screening services
- Paid screening for low-income women
- Education programs
- Quality assurance standards for testing
- Cancer control partnerships among organizations

Researchers suggest this may be due to reproductive behavior such as delayed childbearing and contraceptive use.

Not preventable is the risk associated with the so-called "breast cancer genes," BRCA-1 and BRCA-2. When functioning properly, these genes are thought to help suppress the growth of cancerous cells. Over 200 variations of BRCA genes have been identified. Some appear to be linked to an increased risk of breast and ovarian cancer. A woman born with one damaged version of BRCA gene has only one working set of "brakes" for uncontrolled cell growth. Inherited mutations appear to play a role in only about 5 percent of breast and ovarian cancer cases. It is now possible to test women to see if they have inherited an altered BRCA gene. There is still some controversy as to whether or not testing women for a defective BRCA gene is advantageous.[35]

Colon and Rectal Cancers Colon and rectal cancers (colorectal cancers) are a major cause of cancer deaths (12.5 percent). There were an estimated 130,200 cases in 2000, including 93,800 of colon cancer and 36,400 of rectal cancer. Rates are reported on Table 6.5. Colorectal cancers are the third most common cancers in men and women. There were approximately 56,300 deaths (47,700 from colon cancer, 8,600 from rectal cancer) in 2000, accounting for about 11 percent of cancer deaths. Colorectal cancers account for 14 percent of all cancers in men and 15 percent of all cancers in women. Although the incidence rate has been rising gradually over the past thirty-five years, the mortality rates for colorectal cancer have also declined for men and women over the past twenty years. The declines in colorectal rates are not well understood, although increased removal of polyps and better treatments may be contributing.[36]

Certain risk factors are known to increase a person's chances of developing colon or rectal cancer: family history, being over age forty, an urban lifestyle, and high-fat diets. Black men have the highest mortality rates of colon and rectum (27.8 per 100,000), lung and bronchus (100.8 per 100,000), and prostate cancer (54.8 per 100,000).

Prostate Cancer Prostate cancer is now the second leading cause of death in men. It represents 21 percent of all cancers in men. There were 180,400 new cases diagnosed in 2000 with 31,900 deaths.[37] You will notice from Table 6.5 that the mortality numbers are about the same as breast cancer deaths for women.

Prostate cancer is most common in men over 60, but has also been found in young adults. Thus, aging appears to be the most common risk factor associated with prostate cancer. Incidence of prostate cancer declined from 1990 to 1995 for white men and is beginning to decline among black men, although inidence rates are 66 percent higher in black men when compared to white men. Mortality is two times greater for black men. Death rates from prostate cancer have decreased for all except Hispanic men. The decline in prostate cancer rates is not well understood. The change is likely due to several interacting factors that include the increased use of prostate-specific antigen (PSA) testing in the late 1980s and early 1990s. This more accurate test caused an increase in diagnoses during those years. At the beginning of the twenty-first century, the incidence rate may be dropping to a rate that better reflects the true incidence in the population. Another part of the decrease in incidence may be that since PSA testing is easily done in outpatient settings, there may be incomplete or delayed reporting of the diagnoses.[38] Community health efforts to encourage more PSA testing and reporting is underway.

Prior to the early 1990s, the only sure means of detection was through a rectal examination of the prostate gland by a clinician. By the mid-1990s the use of prostate-specific antigen testing (PSA) increased diagnosis and early treatment of previously undetected cancers.[39] If detected early it is relatively easy to cure.

The incidence of prostate cancer increases with age; more than 75 percent of all prostate cancers are dignosed in men over age 65.[40] Black American men have the highest prostate cancer incidence rates in the world; the disease is common in North America and Northwestern Europe and is rare in Asia, Africa, and South America. Recent genetic studies suggest that strong familial predispositon may be responsible for 5–10 percent of prostate cancers. International studies suggest that dietary fat may also be a factor.

Skin Cancer There are approximately 1.3 million cases a year of highly curable basal cell or squamous cell skin cancers. They are more common among individuals with lightly pigmented skin. The most serious form of skin cancer is melanoma, which is expected to be diagnosed in about 47,700 persons in 2000. Since the early 1970s the incidence rate of melanoma has increased significantly, on average 4 percent per year from 5.7 per 100,000 in 1973 to 13.8 in 1996. Incidence rates are more than ten times higher in whites than in blacks. Other important skin cancers include Kaposi's sarcoma and cutaneous T-cell lymphoma.[41] There were an estimated 9,600 deaths in 2000; 7,700 from melanoma and 1,900 from other skin cancers.

Community health prevention programs are targeting parents of young children, in hopes that preventing overexposure and severe sunburns in early childhood will prevent skin cancers in adults.

Preventing Cancer

Cancer prevention uses three major approaches: education, regulation, and host modification. Education is intended to reduce the cancer-causing behaviors of individuals and practices of society through the translation of scientific findings into sound, practical advice.

Early detection of cancer is one of the best means of preventing cancer death. However, the single most preventable measure to stopping the occurrence of cancer is eliminating smoking from your behaviors. Today, education includes the provision of anti-smoking messages.[42] Tobacco smoking has been shown in over 50,000 epidemiological studies to be causally associated with cancers at several sites in humans and animals and other hazardous health effects. Smoking is related to 40 percent of all cancers and is the primary risk factor for lung cancer in the United States. Smoking causes more death and suffering among adults than any other toxic material in the environment. In 1992, the Marlboro Man died of lung cancer after years of getting paid to encourage others to smoke as he did. In his last painful years, he spent many hours speaking to school-aged young people about the risks they faced every time they lighted up. (See information on smoking provided earlier in this chapter.)

Heredity   For many types of cancer, having a family history can increase one's risk of developing that cancer (i.e., breast cancer). Knowing your family history can help you to establish for which cancers you may be at risk.

Race   Race has been a risk factor for some types of cancer. As was stated earlier, it isn't necessarily one's skin color or genetics that determine risk. Overall, blacks are more likely to develop cancer than persons of any other racial and ethnic group. During 1990–1996, incidence rates were 442.9 per 100,000 among blacks, 402.9 per 100,000 among whites, 275.4 per 100,000 among Hispanics, 279.1 per 100,000 among Asian/Pacific Islanders, and 153.4 per 100,000 among Native Americans. During these same years, cancer incidence rates decreased among whites (–1.2 percent per year), Hispanics (–1.7 percent per year), and Native Americans (–0.7 percent per year), and remained relatively stable among blacks and Asian/Pacific Islanders.[43]

The incidence rate of female breast cancer is highest among white women (113.2 per 100,000) and lowest among Native American women (33.9 per 100,000). Black women have the highest incidence rates of colon and rectum (44.9 per 100,000) and lung and bronchus cancer (46.2 per 100,000) followed by whites, Asian/Pacific Islanders, Hispanics, and Native Americans.[44]

Socioeconomic status, access to health care, public information brochures written only in the English language, lack of awareness, and fear are only a few of the factors that make one's ethnicity a possible risk.

Environmental Agents   While tobacco is the most pervasive carcinogen to which most of us are exposed, there is substantial evidence to indict many other environmental agents as carcinogens. Earliest evidence of this information dates from about 1880. Figure 6.7 illustrates the historical development of evidence of cancer in humans and its association with environmental agents since 1880.[45] Occasionally the agents are single substances. More often they are complex, uncharacterized mixtures of substances.

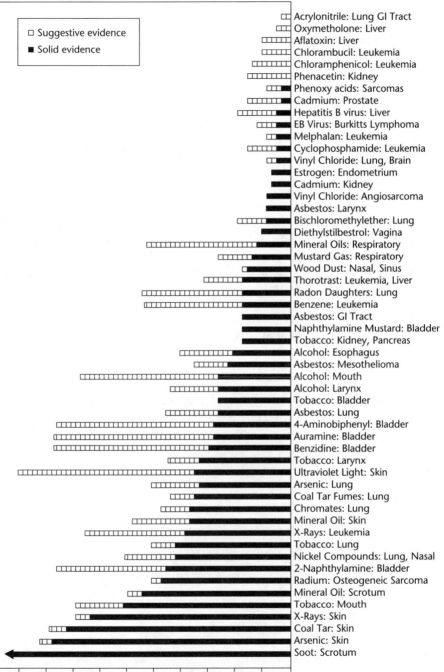

Figure 6.7 Environmental cancers: historical development in humans.

Environmental agents generally refer to any influence other than that of the genetic material inherited from one's parents. Using this rough definition, it is estimated that as much as 90 percent of all cancer is environmentally induced. A good example of an environmentally induced cancer may be melanoma. Melanoma is a cancer of the melanocyte, or pigmented cells of the skin. This cancer has increased steadily for decades. According to the Society, the incidence of melanoma has grown about 4 percent each year since 1973. Although research has not found the specific etiology of melanoma, it appears that severe sunburns as children may contribute more to adult melanoma than the total amount of time a person spends in the sun. Studies on mice now suggest that sunscreens may not protect against skin cancer, although they may reduce other types of skin damage.[44]

Nutrition and Diet   Scientific evidence suggests that about one-third of the cancer deaths that occur in the United States each year is due to the adult diet, including its effect on obesity, while another third is due to cigarette smoking. Therefore, for the majority of Americans who do not use tobacco, dietary choices and physical activity become the most important modifiable determinants of cancer risk. The evidence also indicates that although inherited genes do influence cancer risk, heredity alone explains only a fraction of all cancers. Behavioral factors such as tobacco use, dietary choices, and physical activity modify the risk of cancer at all stages of its development. The introduction of healthful diet and exercise practices at any time from childhood to old age can promote health and probably reduce cancer risk.

Many dietary factors can affect cancer risk: types of foods, food preparation methods, portion sizes, food variety, and overall caloric balance. Cancer risk can be reduced by an overall dietary pattern that includes a high proportion of plant foods (fruits, vegetables, grains, and beans), limited amounts of meat, dairy, and other high-fat foods, and a balance of caloric intake and physical activity.

Personal Prevention through Detection   The American Cancer Society has listed seven warning signs for cancer. Please consult your health care provider should you experience any of the following:

BOX 6.3 *Attributable Risk Factors for Cancer Deaths*

Tobacco use	30%	Reproductive factors	3%
Adult diet, obesity	30%	Alcohol use	3%
Sedentary lifestyle	5%	SES	3%
Occupation	5%	Pollution	2%
Family history	5%	Ultraviolet radiation	2%
Virus	5%	Prescriptions	1%
Perinatal factors	3%	Food additives	1%

(*Source:* Harvard University School of Public Health)

1. Change in bowel or bladder habits

2. A sore that doesn't heal

3. Unusual bleeding or discharge

4. Thickening or lump in the breast, testis, or elsewhere

5. Indigestion or difficulty swallowing

6. Obvious change in a wart or mole

7. Nagging cough or hoarseness

Cerebrovascular Disease (Stroke)

Cerebrovascular disease is the third most common overall cause of death in virtually all developed countries and is becoming increasingly important as a cause of death in developing countries.

Cerebrovascular disease can result in stroke, a rapidly developing, severe impairment of the body brought on by a disruption in the flow of blood to the brain. It may be a focal or at times global disturbance of cerebral function, lasting for 24 hours or more or leading to death with no apparent cause other than vascular origin. Almost as many people die or are disabled when a blood vessel in the brain bursts (aneurysm), or a clot blocks the flow of blood to the brain as die from heart attacks. Both of these life-threatening conditions are called "stroke" or "apoplexy." Despite the fact that stroke is highly preventable and treatable, most adults do not know the warning signs nor do they seek medical help for symptoms until a stroke has occurred.

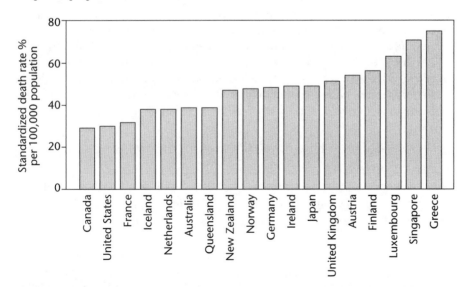

Figure 6.8 Cerebrovascular disease mortality by selected countries.

(*Source:* Health of Queenslanders: Status Report
www.health.qld.au/publications/sr2/images/attachment4d.gif)

Table 6.6   Comparison of heart disease and stroke deaths.

	Heart Disease	Stroke Deaths
Total Population, 1997	**Rate per 100,000**	**Rate per 100,000**
Total	216	62
Race and Ethnicity		
Native American or Alaska Native	134	39
Asian or Pacific Islander	125	55
Native Hawaiian and other Pacific Islander	DNC	DNC
Black or African American	257	82
White	214	60
Hispanic or Latino	151	40
Non-Hispanic or Latino	219	63
Gender		
Female	170	60
Male	276	64
Education Level (aged 25 to 64 years)		
Less than high school	95	22
High school graduate	81	17
At least some college	40	8

(*Source:* Healthy People 2010)

Strokes usually occur in middle-aged or elderly adults. Two-thirds of the over 500,000 people who have strokes are over age sixty-five. Worldwide, stroke is the most important cause of healthy years lost in late adulthood. The next most common age group for stroke is young to middle-aged adults. Figure 6.8 shows the great variability in mortality rates among industrialized countries.[45]

There is evidence of a marked improvement in long-term stroke survival over the past thirty years, and there has been a steady decline in the incidence of stroke over the past several decades in developed countries. This may be due to better detection and better control of diastolic blood pressure.

> *The Healthy People 2010 Objective:* Reduce Stroke Deaths
>
> *Target:* 48 deaths per 100,000 population.
>
> *Baseline:* 60 deaths from stroke per 100,000 population in 1998 (preliminary data; age adjusted to the year 2000 standard population).
>
> *Target setting method:* 20 percent improvement.

A decline in mortality rates has been reported over different times in the United States but stroke remained the third leading cause of death in 2001. The "stroke belt" along the southeastern coastal plain has recently declined in incidence while clusters along the Mississippi and Ohio Rivers have become more pronounced. Excess stroke deaths are particularly high in western Pennsylvania, as well as in population centers throughout the country.

In all instances, within the United States, morbidity and mortality rates in men have been higher than those in women, and Caucasian rates have been shown to be lower than those for African Americans who have the highest rates of heart disease and cardiovascular diseases of any other racial group in the United States (Table 6.6). In England, socioeconomic status is a variable in cardiovascular mortality, with manual workers reported as having the higher standardized mortality rates.[48]

While four in five stroke patients survive, stroke is still the number one cause of disability among older Americans and lags only behind Alzheimer's disease as a cause of dementia.

Risk Factors

As in coronary heart disease, increased arterial blood pressure is a very important risk factor for men and women. The higher level of either systolic or diastolic pressure measured in middle age, the higher is the risk of stroke in later years. Knowledge of the risk factors of stroke is not as complete as it is for coronary heart disease. Stroke generally occurs later in life, so cohort studies have been difficult to achieve. Among what is known is that stroke is strongly linked to age. It is 20 to 30 percent higher in men than women and there is some evidence to suggest a familial predisposition. It is highest among U.S. blacks compared to U.S. whites although the covariate of environmental conditions is unknown. The Framingham study has shown that persons with diabetes mellitus are at increased risk, especially those who have poorly controlled diabetes. Climate may be another factor, since stroke mortality is higher in cold climates (Figure 6.9).

BOX 6.4 *Treatable Medical Risk Disorders for Stroke*

High blood pressure	Heavy drinking
Heart disease	Being overweight
High cholesterol level	Lack of exercise
Smoking	Birth control pills (especially over age 30)[49]

BOX 6.3 *Carotid Endarterectomy*

In 1994 a study sponsored by the National Institutes of Health found that male patients benefited from a surgical procedure that removed fatty deposits that clog neck arteries, called carotid endarterectomy. This surgery produced a 69 percent reduction in relative stroke risk in men and a 16 percent reduction in women. The surgery costs about $15,000, but insurance is willing to cover this cost given the outcome and the difference in cost of long-term stroke care.[50]

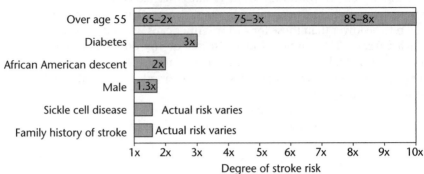

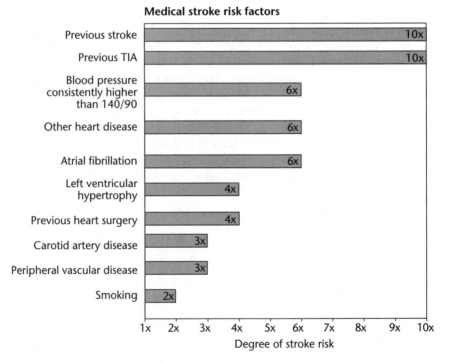

Figure 6.9 Risk factors for stroke.

(*Source:* National Stroke Association)

Prevention

Many of the prevention efforts previously mentioned for reducing risk of heart disease will also reduce risk for stroke. Stopping smoking, getting one's blood pressure under control, eating foods low in fat and cholesterol, and avoiding obesity can all reduce risk for stroke.

Summary

The major causes of death, cardiovascular diseases, cancers, and cerebrovascular diseases (stroke) are all preventable through behavior changes. Changes in personal health habits associated with nutrition, exercise, smoking, stress, and preventive diagnostic tests can reduce these deaths substantially. Despite this, millions of Americans die each year primarily from neglect of their own health. The cost of such neglect is overwhelming the health care system of the United States and the work and family communities in which people participate. More community health efforts are spent in trying to promote healthful behaviors associated with these causes of death than all other causes combined. Despite such efforts, little headway has been made.

CYBERSITES RELATED TO CHAPTER 6

Cardiovascular Diseases
> amhrt.org

Cancer
> www.acor.org
> cancer.med.upenn.edu

QUESTIONS

1. What are your personal behaviors that contribute to the three leading causes of death? What do you perceive is your risk of suffering from one of these diseases in the next ten to twenty years?

2. What preventive programs would you suggest to the community in which you live that would reduce the incidence of the three leading killers?

3. What would be the most motivational reasons for you to begin a healthy lifestyle program? How could that be achieved?

EXERCISE

Do a personal health history that includes the health history of your family members at least two generations back. Interview your grandparents, aunts, and uncles about their health history. Based upon the data you find, what is your hereditary risk for death by the three leading causes of death in America?

INTERNET INTERACTIVE ACTIVITY

DevCan—Surveillance, Epidemiology, and End Result

DevCan takes cross-sectional counts of incident cases from the standard areas of the Surveillance, Epidemiology, and End Results (SEER) Program conducted by the National Cancer Institute and mortality counts for the same areas from data collected by the National Center for Health Statistics by five-year age groups and uses them to calculate incidence and mortality rates using population estimates from census data for these areas.

About SEER Cancer Data   The incidence data delivered with DevCan originates from the National Cancer Institute's Surveillance, Epidemiology, and End Results (SEER) program. The SEER program is a collection of population-based cancer registries in the United States that collects and submits cancer incidence and follow-up data to the National Cancer Institute.

The homepage for the DevCan program is:

srab.cancer.gov/DevCan/

To use this data anaylsis system you must first download the DevCan program.

1. Go to the Homepage for **DevCan**

   www-dccps.ims.nci.nih.gov/SRAB/DevCan/index.html

2. Click on **Download DevCan Software** to download DevCan

3. After you have a password, return to the homepage and download **DevCan Installation Program [Setup.exe(2.1 MB)] - password required**

4. Once you have installed the DevCan program you are able to look for cancer-related death and incidence data.

Example.   The community health educator wants to know the incidence on breast cancer among black women between 1993–1995.

1. Execute the **DevCan** program

2. Click on **File**
   New Program

3. Click **Data**
   Select Data Base

4. Select
   SEER database

5. Click **Session**
   Select Output Options
   Number in 100,000

6. Under **Parameters**
   Year -1993–1995
   Race - Black
   Sex - Female
   Site - Breast invasive

7. Click **Session**
   Execute

8. Click on the following to read cancer tables related to your parameters:

   Life Table Developing
   Age Conditional Developing
   Life Table Dying
   Age Conditional Dying
   Raw Data

From the tables you now know that the probablity of dying from cancer if you are now forty years old and black is 0.01021105.

Among twenty-year-old black women, the number who will develop breast cancer by age thirty-five is 218.

The number of black women between the ages of twenty-five and twenty-nine who died from cancer during 1993–1995 is 1,026.

Exercises

1. Determine the incidence and probabilities of testicular cancer among men of both races for the years 1995–1997.

    a. Describe the age and race of men at most risk of developing testicular cancer.

    b. Describe the age and race of men at most risk of dying from testicular cancer.

2. Using the DevCan program investigate five other sites of cancer incidence and mortality for men, women, black and white. What do the data tell the community health educator about program development of risk reduction programs?

REFERENCES

1. McGinnis, J. Michael (1993). Actual causes of death in the United States. *JAMA*, November 10, Vol. 270, No. 18, p. 2207.

2. Luepker, Russell V. et al. (1994). Community education for cardiovascular disease prevention: Risk factor changes in the Minnesota Heart Health Program. *AJPH*, Vol. 84 (9), p. 1383.

3. Goldman, Benjamin A. (1991). *The truth about where you live.* New York: Times Books, Random House.

4. Hales, D. (1994). *An invitation to health,* 6th ed. Redwood City, CA: The Benjamin/Cummings Publishing Company, Inc.

5. Stockwell, David H., Madhavan, Shantha, et al. (1994). The determinants of hypertension awareness, treatment and control in an insured population. *APHA*, November 84 (11), p. 1768.

6. Pilcher, James (1999). Report shows that little has changed in rates of smokers. *USA Today*, November 19, p. 3A.

7. Ibid.

8. Chandler, William U. (1986). Banishing tobacco. *Society*, May/June.

9. Janson, D. (1988). *The health of America's children.* Washington, D.C.: Children's Defense Fund.

10. Chandler, op. cit.

11. Ibid.

12. Janson, op. cit.

13. Wolfe, Rachel (1987). Smokeless tobacco: The fatal pinch. *Multinational Monitor,* July/August.

14. Ibid.

15. Hales, op. cit.

16. Healthy lives: A new view of stress (1990). *Wellness Newsletter,* University of California, Berkeley, June.

17. Luepker, op. cit.

18. Ibid.

19. Baby boomers more likely to get cancer? (1994) *The Washington Post,* February 9.

20. Cancer prevention: Accomplishments and prospects. (1994). *APHA Journal, 84*(1), pp. 8–9.

21. Schellenback, Joann (1998). New report on declining cancer incidence and death rates. *Cancer Research,* Washington, DC: CDC.

22. Ibid.

23. Goldman, op. cit.

24. www.cancer.org/statistics/index.html

25. Goldman, op. cit.

26. Cancer prevention, op. cit.

27. National Vital Statistics reports (1999). Deaths: Final data for 1997. Vol. 47, No. 19.

28. Schellenback, op. cit.

29. American Cancer Society (1997). *Cancer facts.*

30. Brody, Jane E. (1994). Heart diseases persist in study's 2nd generation. *The New York Times,* January 5, p. B6.

31. Mulshine, James L. (1993). Initiators and promoters of Lung Cancer. *Chest, 103,* pp. 45-95.

32. Schellenback, op. cit.

33. Breast cancer's deadly masquerade? (1994). *U.S. News and World Report,* February 7, p. 59.

34. Ibid.

35. Boston Women's Health Book Collective (1998). *Breast cancer genes: Myths and facts.*

36. Schellenback, op. cit.

37. American Cancer Society (1997). *Cancer facts & figures—2001.* Atlanta, GA.

38. www.cancer.org/statistics/index.html

39. Cancer prevention, op. cit.

40. National Vital Statistics, op. cit.

41. Maclure, K. Malcolm (1980). An epidemiologic perspective of environmental carcinogenesis. *Epidemiological Reviews,* Vol. 2, 1980.

42. Cancer prevention, op. cit.

43. National Vital Statistics, op. cit.

44. Ibid.

45. Maclure, op. cit.

46. Mouse study raises doubts on sunscreens. (1994). *The New York Times,* January 25. p. B6.

47. Garraway, Michael (1991). Cerebrovascular disease. In *Oxford textbook of public health,* Vol. II (pp. 207–228). New York: Oxford University Press.

48. Ibid.

49. National Stroke Association (1988). Stroke: Questions and answers. Denver.

50. Podelsky, Doug (1994). Surgery that staves off strokes. *U.S. News and World Report,* October 17, p. 90.

CHAPTER 7

Chronic Obstructive Pulmonary Disease, Pneumonia and Influenza, Unintentional Injuries, and Diabetes

Community Health in the 21st Century
If trends continue, intentional and unintentional injuries will still be major contributors to mortality and morbidity, especially in the area of violence.

—Cherilynn Soderquist, M.S. Health Promotion; Family Health Services, Child Injury Prevention Program

Chapter Objectives

The student will:

1. identify the greatest accident risks associated with different age groups.

2. list engineering agents associated with motor vehicle accidents.

3. name the host factors associated with motor vehicle accidents.

4. explain why falls occur so often in the home among older Americans.

5. describe ten ways to improve community awareness to prevent accidents among children.

6. give an example of each of the ten leading work-related injuries.

7. know the risk factors for adult onset diabetes.

8. compare the differences in risk factors for diabetes among people of color.

9. be able to give educational information to interested persons about how to prevent COPD, pneumonia, diabetes and influenza.

Chronic Obstructive Pulmonary Disease

It sometimes appears that community health gives little discussion to the fourth leading cause of death in the United States, **chronic obstructive pulmonary disease** (COPD), although its mortality rate is increasing. Perhaps this is because death from lung damage may come from a variety of sources, most preventable,

168

and many are addressed in discussions of cancer. Further, these lung diseases are usually chronic, meaning it takes many years of progressive degeneration to ultimately end in death, such as among people with emphysema. Death is usually later in life and does not occur early in one's life, under mysterious circumstances, and without specific prevention.

Asthma, a chronic obstructive pulmonary disease, and obstructive sleep apnea (OSA), however, are a significant public health burden to the United States. Several behaviors and diseases that affect the respiratory system, such as tuberculosis, acquired immunodeficiency syndrome (AIDS), pneumonia, and occupational lung disease, are other important respiratory diseases that are often not seen by communities as public and community health issues. Their omission, however, is not a reflection on the magnitude of the health problems associated with them.[1]

The most common contributing behavior associated with COPD is smoking. Between 80 and 90 percent of COPD is attributable to cigarette smoking. However, not all smokers develop COPD, and not all patients with COPD are smokers or have smoked in the past. Population studies have shown that chronic exposure to air pollution has an independent adverse effect on lung function. A multi-year study of the respiratory effects of long-term exposure to environmental tobacco smoke and air pollution reported that both long-term ozone and childhood exposure to maternal tobacco smoke were associated with diminished lung function in college students. Viral infections also may contribute to susceptibility to COPD, and they are considered to play a role in the onset of airflow obstruction.

Chronic obstructive pulmonary diseases are any chronic conditions that lead to permanent airflow obstruction in the lungs. COPD occurs most often in older people. As much as 10 percent of the population sixty-five years of age and over is estimated to have COPD.[2] COPD has a major impact on health care, illness, disability, and death in the older population, and the magnitude of the problem is growing. Since 1980, the prevalence and age-adjusted death rate for COPD increased more than 30 percent. Any decline in the proportion of persons with COPD is unlikely without substantial changes in risk factors, mainly reductions in cigarette smoking. This is important for both men and women, given the modest decline in cigarette smoking rates.[3] Death rates for persons with COPD are reported in Table 7.1.

The three primary chronic lung diseases discussed in this text are **chronic bronchitis**, a prolonged irritation of the moist linings of the lungs; **asthma**, a hypersensitivity to various allergens; and **emphysema**, the destruction of the alveoli of the lungs. Bronchitis and emphysema are more prevalent among males and higher among whites than blacks.

Bronchitis

Chronic bronchitis is a confusing condition that is seldom a primary entity, but rather a complication of some pre-existing condition such as chronic heart dis-

Table 7.1   Death rate for chronic obstructive pulmonary disease (1998).

Race		Death Rate per 100,000
All		41.7
Native American	Male	17.7
Native American	Female	15.6
Asian/PI	Male	11.9
Asian/PI	Female	6.4
Hispanic	Male	9.3
Hispanic	Female	7.4
Black	Male	24.7
Black	Female	17.5
White	Male	42.7
White	Female	45.7
All Males		43.2
All Females		40.0

(*Source:* National Vital Statistics System)

ease or prolonged smoking. Its mortality is higher in unskilled laborers, which suggests the aggravation of environmental irritants such as particulate matter in the air.

Chronic bronchitis affects an estimated 5 percent of the population or 14 million people in the United States. The prevalence rate of chronic bronchitis has been consistently higher in females than in males. Chronic bronchitis affects people of all ages, but is higher in those over forty-five years old.[4]

Emphysema

Emphysema is one of the most important and most common pulmonary diseases. The word actually means "over inflation." The lungs become filled with stale air high in carbon dioxide. This air cannot be adequately exhaled to allow oxygen to enter. The patient experiences a suffocating feeling and great distress from the inability to breathe.[5]

Emphysema is neither a contagious nor an infectious disease, but one of chronic lung obstruction and destruction. Emphysema may be one of the most disabling physical conditions over time because a person with emphysema does not die quickly, but after many years of painful, disabling distress. A person with emphysema may have to breathe 20,000 times in twenty-four hours. Each breath is painful and does not fill the lungs with adequate air.

Currently there are about 2 million Americans in the United States who have emphysema. Emphysema ranks fifteenth among chronic conditions that contribute to activity limitations: Almost 44 percent of individuals with emphysema report that their daily activities have been limited by the disease.

Many of the people with emphysema are older men, but the condition is increasing among women. Males with emphysema outnumber females by more than 54 percent.[6]

The pathogenesis of emphysema is still not completely known, but it is a fact that one of the greatest precursors to this condition is smoking. Air pollution and long-term exposure to irritants of the respiratory tract also seem to be factors of its etiology. Despite what tobacco companies would have us believe, smoking is a major contributor to premature death in this country.

Asthma

About 20 percent (15 million people) of the U.S. population suffer from **asthma**, an inflammation of the airways that results in wheezing and shortness of breath. It is the most common chronic disease among children. Bronchial asthma is not inherited, but there is a hereditary factor involved. A predisposition for hypersensitivity to various allergens is inborn.

Asthma cases and deaths have increased at least 50 percent since 1982. The reasons for this increase probably include increases in air pollution, airtight homes, and windowless offices as well as more exposure to pollens, cat dander, cigarette smoke, marijuana, and dust mites. A National Institutes of Health study found that 36 percent of inner-city asthmatic children are sensitive to cockroaches and 77 percent are exposed to cockroaches in their home.[7]

The National Cooperative Inner-City Asthma Study found that a higher proportion of children test positive to cockroach allergen than to dust mite and cat dander, and thus have a higher sensitivity to asthma-related health problems when compared to other children.[8] A study conducted at Mount Sinai Medical Center found that asthmatic children are more likely to be overweight than others. This study also linked asthma with risks for diabetes and heart disease in later life.[9] Asthma deaths by groups are given in Table 7.2.

Healthy People 2010 Objective: Reduce Asthma Deaths

Age Group	1998 Baseline	2010 Target
	Rate per Million	
Children under age 5 years	1.7	1.0
Children aged 5 to 14 years	3.2	1.0
Adolescents and adults aged 15 to 34 years	5.9	3.0
Adults aged 35 to 64 years	17.0	9.0
Adults aged 65 years and older	87.5	60.0

Table 7.2   Asthma death by groups (1997).

Select Age Groups	Asthma Death				
	Children Under Age 5 years	Children Aged 5 to 14 years	Persons Aged 15 to 34 Years	Persons Aged 35 to 64 Years	Persons Aged 65 Years and Older
	Rate per Million				
TOTAL	1.8	2.1	6.2	18.9	85.9
Race and ethnicity					
Native American or Alaska Native	DSU	DSU	DSU	DSU	DSU
Asian or Pacific Islander	DSU	DSU	DSU	22.3	141.2
Black or African American	7.6	9.7	17.4	52.7	120.2
White	DSU	1.8	4.3	14.3	81.5
Hispanic or Latino	DSU	DSU	4.8	17.1	81.8
Non-Hispanic or Latino	2.2	3.4	6.4	19.1	86.1
Gender					
Female	DSU	2.8	5.2	23.5	99.5
Male	2.3	3.3	7.2	14.2	66.3
Education (aged 25 to 64 years)					
Less than high school	NA	NA	12.5	30.6	NA
High school graduate	NA	NA	10.5	23.4	NA
At least some college	NA	NA	4.3	11.1	NA

DSU = Data are statistically unreliable.

(*Source:* Healthy People 2010)

In 1998, the asthma rate was 50.2 per 1,000 persons. The death rate for asthma rose 40 percent since 1988 to 18.8 per 1 million people or about 5,000 deaths a year.

New studies are showing an inordinately high rate of asthma among inner-city Hispanics, especially Puerto Ricans. Although exposed to similar levels of environmental insults as blacks and whites, it appears that an underlying genetic predisposition puts Hispanics at greater risk for asthma.[10] Although blacks and whites have similar incidence rates of asthma, 38.1 percent of asthmatic deaths were among blacks versus 15.1 percent among whites.[11]

Influenza and Pneumonia

Few Americans realize that influenza- and pneumonia-related diseases are the sixth leading cause of death in the United States. Most of these deaths occur among people over the age of sixty-five and children under four years.

Influenza

Influenza, or "the flu," is a common, viral, respiratory illness. There are three primary types of influenza that concern community health educators: Types A, B, and C. Many different strains of these three types may exist. Symptoms of each type have a sudden onset and may include fever, muscle aches, congestion, runny nose, cough, sore throat, and general fatigue. Nausea, vomiting, and diarrhea may occur, especially in small children. Influenza symptoms range from mild to fatal, depending on the person infected. Transmission is predominantly airborne among people in enclosed spaces, however, transmission can also occur by droplet spread. Since the virus can live for hours in dried mucus, contact from inanimate objects may also occur. Persons with the flu usually take two to seven days to recover. Treatment for influenza includes bed rest and perhaps nonprescription pain relievers and decongestants for flu symptoms.[12]

Most Americans do not realize there is an immunization available to prevent the flu. Influenza shots are recommended for people considered "high risk": adults and children with chronic and debilitating disease, those receiving immunosuppressive therapy, adults over 65 years old, residents of nursing homes and other chronic care facilities, and those health care providers who work with at-risk groups. Side effects may occur from the influenza vaccine, but are rare. Unfortunately, immunity to one strain of influenza does not protect a person from another strain and there is no cure.

Community health initiatives have highlighted the need to focus vaccination resources on adults. Vaccination is an effective strategy to reduce illness and deaths due to pneumococcal disease and influenza. Current levels of coverage among adults vary widely among age, risk, and racial and ethnic groups. Any new universally recommended vaccine should be at a 60 percent coverage level within five years of recommendation. Influenza and pneumococcal vaccines are covered by Medicare; thus vaccinating greater numbers of adults aged sixty-five years and older is feasible. High-risk adults aged eighteen to sixty-four years may not have insurance coverage for influenza and pneumococcal vaccines.[13]

Pneumonia

Pneumonia causes an inflammation of the lung, and fills the air chambers with fluid. It has both viral and bacterial causes. Sometimes pneumonia is a secondary disease to other infections like influenza or bronchitis, and can occur in one lung or both (double pneumonia). Symptoms may vary, but those of classic bacterial pneumonia include fever, shortness of breath, cough, and general weakness. Pneumonia's duration and treatment, much like its symptoms, depend somewhat on the type of pneumonia a person contracts, since there may be gradual or acute onset. Pneumonia immunizations are recommended for those at highest risk, including older adults, the chronically ill, people who have had previous pneumonia infections, and those with compromised immune systems. A rare type of pneumonia that has gained attention is *Pneumocystis carinii.* It is a classic opportunistic infection associated with AIDS, and was seen in few circumstances until the onset of the HIV/AIDS epidemic.

Unintentional Injuries

Unintentional injuries are the single, most common type of traumatic death for persons of any age. They were the sixth leading cause of death for adults in the United States and the fourth leading cause of death for children in 1998. Each year approximately 2.6 million people are hospitalized for nonfatal injuries and 37.2 million are treated in emergency rooms. Injury is the leading cause of death during the first half of life in most countries of the world. Approximately 400,000 of these deaths are caused by road accidents, and it is estimated that there are ten serious injuries and thirty minor injuries for every death.[14] Incidence of deaths due to unintentional injuries are, in descending order, motor vehicle accidents, firearms, poisoning, falls, suffocation, drowning, fire/burn, and cut/piercing.

The term *injury* has replaced *accident* as the public health reporting term. Because unintentional injuries occur by chance and public health initiatives can, in fact, prevent the chance occurrence of an accident, injury prevention and data collection more accurately reflect the nature of intentional and unintentional injury.[15] **Injury** is any physical damage to a person or host due to mechanical, chemical, thermal, or energy agents within the environment. Injury may be the result of the effect of the agent on the host, or the behavior of the host manipulating the environment in an unsafe manner. While unintentional injuries and fatalities are unplanned, intentional injuries may include suicide, homicide, and planned violence such as hate crimes, domestic violence, and assault. Accidents are one type of unintentional injury and will be discussed as appropriate below. The epidemiology of injury is displayed in Figure 7.1.

Death by injury is premature, tortuous, and without redeeming value. The Surgeon General's Report on Health Promotion and Disease Prevention (1980) identified unintentional injuries as one of the most important health problems facing our nation. Even after that warning, there are still about 100,000 unintended injury fatalities and about 9 million disabling injuries that occur each

---

BOX 7.1 *The Cost of Unintentional Injuries*

The total cost of unintentional injuries in 1998, $480.5 billion, includes estimates of economic costs of fatal and nonfatal unintentional injuries together with employer costs, vehicle damage costs, and fire losses. Wage and productivity losses, medical expenses, administrative expenses, and employer costs are included in all four classes of injuries:

Motor-Vehicle Crashes	$191.6 billion
Work Injuries	$125.1 billion
Home Injuries	$113.5 billion
Public Injuries	$66.3 billion

(*Source:* National Safety Council)

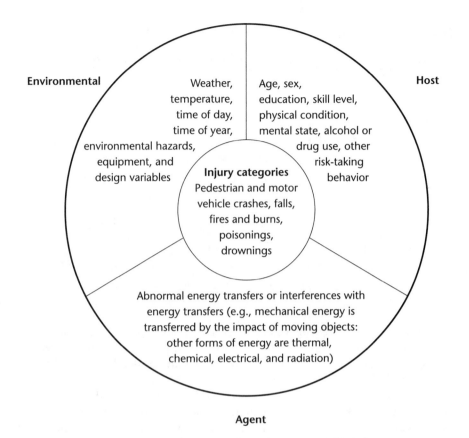

Environmental

Weather,
temperature,
time of day,
time of year,
environmental hazards,
equipment, and
design variables

Age, sex,
education, skill level,
physical condition,
mental state, alcohol or
drug use, other
risk-taking
behavior

Host

Injury categories
Pedestrian and motor
vehicle crashes, falls,
fires and burns,
poisonings,
drownings

Abnormal energy transfers or interferences with
energy transfers (e.g., mechanical energy is
transferred by the impact of moving objects:
other forms of energy are thermal,
chemical, electrical, and radiation)

Agent

Figure 7.1 Common epidemiological variables of unintentional injuries.

year in the United States. Death by unintended injury ranks first in terms of years of life lost prematurely, killing 92,300 people in 1998 in the United States, and injuries are the number one cause of death for ages 1 to 38. The death rate for 1998 was 34 per 100,000.[16]

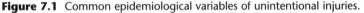

Healthy People 2010 Objective: Reduce Deaths Caused by Unintentional Injuries

Target: 20.8 deaths per 100,000 population.

Baseline: 33.3 deaths per 100,000 population were caused by unintentional injuries in 1998.

Motor Vehicle Accidents

In 1998, there were approximately 215 million registered motor vehicles in the United States. These cars traveled an estimated 2.5 trillion miles and consumed almost 150 billion gallons of fuel.

Table 7.3   Deaths in passenger vehicles per 100,000 people (1998).

Age	Male Drivers	Male Passengers	Female Drivers	Female Passengers
<13	0.0	2.7	0.0	2.5
13	0.3	2.9	0.2	3.3
14	1.0	4.3	0.2	5.7
15	2.3	6.8	1.5	6.9
16	14.0	10.4	9.4	9.8
17	19.3	11.2	10.7	9.3
18	27.3	14.6	11.5	8.6
19	23.3	12.1	9.0	7.4
20–24	23.4	9.3	7.1	4.8
25–29	16.4	4.8	6.3	2.6
30–64	11.5	2.1	5.2	2.3
65–74	14.2	2.3	6.1	5.4
≥75	24.9	5.0	7.7	7.8

(*Source:* Insurance Institute for Highway Safety)

Given the number of vehicles on the road, accidents are probably inevitable. However, recent years have shown that reductions in motor vehicle accidents are possible as shown by the 1992 mileage death rate of 2.0 per 100,000 miles driven, the lowest rate on record.[18]

In 1998 there were 41,200 traffic accident fatalities, one death every twelve minutes (Table 7.3). Another 3 million people were injured.[19] Among these fatalities and injuries were 1,772 children aged less than fifteen years who were killed, and 274,000 who were injured while riding in motor vehicles in the United States. The National Highway Traffic Safety Administration considers this to be an epidemic. Although the United States has the greatest number of motor vehicle accidents, our accident rate is not the highest (Table 7.4). Worse drivers are found in countries such as Korea, Brazil, Spain, and Greece. In 1995, New Zealand led the international rate of motor vehicle deaths among males aged 15–24 with a rate of 62 per 100,000, followed by the United States with 41 per 100,000 and France with 39 per 100,000.

When a moving vehicle decelerates very rapidly in a crash or sudden stop, unrestrained occupants continue to move at the pre-deceleration speed until they contact interior or exterior surfaces. The extent of injury is a function of the speed, the amount of energy absorbed outside the passenger compartment, the energy-absorbing or energy-concentrating characteristics of the contacted surfaces, and the energy-absorbing ability of the organism.[20]

Healthy People 2010 Objective: Increase Use of Child Restraints

Target: 100 percent.

Baseline: 92 percent of motor vehicle occupants aged 4 years and under used child restraints in 1998.

Table 7.4   Motor-vehicle deaths and rates by nation.

Nation	Year	Number	Rate[a]	Nation	Year	Number	Rate[a]
		Motor-Vehicle Traffic Deaths				Motor-Vehicle Traffic Deaths	
Hong Kong	1991	335	5.8	Czechoslavakia (former)	1991	2,174	13.9
Egypt	1987	3,248	6.6	Austria	1992	1,177	14.9
Chile	1989	941	7.3	Mauritius	1992	159	15.1
Norway	1991	321	7.5	Italy	1990	9,123[c]	15.8
Iceland	1992	20	7.7	Puerto Rico	1991	581	16.3
Israel	1990	366	7.9	Mexico	1991	14,126	16.4
United Kingdom	1992	4,681	8.1	France	1991	9,397[e]	16.5
Netherlands	1991	1,240	8.2	Yugoslavia (former)	1990	3,970	16.7
Thailand	1987	4,441	8.3	Kuwait	1987	343	18.3
Sweden	1990	747	8.7	United States	1990	45,827[b]	18.4
Argentina	1990	2,942	9.1	Belgium	1989	1,830[c]	18.4
Singapore	1991	258	9.3	Poland	1992	7,357	19.2
Australia	1992	1,881	10.8	Luxembourg	1992	76	19.4
Switzerland	1992	752	10.9	New Zealand	1991	657	19.5
Denmark	1992	575	11.1	Ecuador	1988	2,037	20.0
Finland	1992	570	11.3	Spain	1990	7,989[d]	20.5
Japan	1992	14,547	11.8	Venezuela	1989	3,905	20.7
Ireland	1991	425	12.1	Greece	1991	2,246	22.0
Uruguay	1990	375	12.1	Hungary	1992	2,346	22.7
Bulgaria	1992	1,066	12.5	Brazil (reporting areas)	1989	22,100	22.7
Canada	1991	3,463[b]	12.7	Portugal	1992	2,774	28.1
Costa Rica	1991	415	13.3	Korea, Republic of	1991	13,143	30.4
Germany	1991	10,899	13.6				

[a]Deaths per 100,000 population.

DEATH DEFINITION: In general, deaths are included if they occur within thirty days after the accident, but other time periods are as follows: [b]one year. [c]at accident scene only. [d]24 hours. [e]three days.

(*Source:* Motor-vehicle traffic deaths—World Health Organization. Vehicle registrations—American Automobile Manufacturers Association. *Motor Vehicle Facts and Figures, 1994 Edition.* Used with permission.)

Prior to 1993, there had been a decline in fatal injuries on the road. The Insurance Institute for Highway Safety credited drunken driving laws, better built cars, and more widely available safety devices such as air bags.

Many of the victims in traffic accidents are not in vehicles. Pedestrians account for 14 percent of all motor vehicle-related deaths. In 1998, 5,220 pedestrians were killed in traffic accidents and 82,000 were injured. In the 1990s, pedestrian deaths dropped 24 percent as a result of stricter law enforcement, public service campaigns, and better signaling at crosswalks. Figure 7.2 reports the pedestrian fatality rates.[21] More than one-third of all children between the ages of five and nine years who were killed in traffic accidents were pedestrians and one-fourth of the fatalities under age sixteen were pedestrians. Even so, the highest number of pedestrians killed in traffic fatalities are among those seventy years and older. In 1998, persons aged seventy years and older made up 9 percent of the population but accounted for 14 percent of all traffic fatalities and 18 percent of all pedestrian fatalities. Compared with the fatality rate for drivers

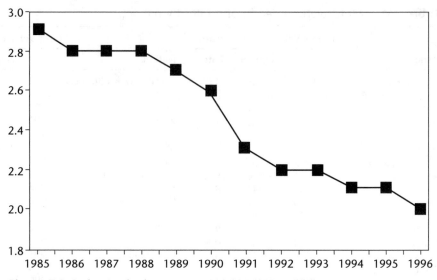

Figure 7.2 Pedestrian fatality rates per 100,000 (1985–1996).

(*Source:* Insurance Institute for Highway Safety)

Table 7.5   Distribution of pedestrian deaths by time period (1996).

Time Period	Percentage
12:01 AM to 3:00 AM	11
3:01 AM to 6:00 AM	7
6:01 AM to 9:00 AM	8
9:01 AM to noon	6
12:01 PM to 3:00 PM	8
3:01 PM to 6:00 PM	13
6:01 PM to 9:00 PM	25
9:01 PM to Midnight	22

(*Source:* Insurance Institute for Highway Safety)

aged twenty-five through sixty-nine years, the rate for drivers in the oldest group is nine times higher.[22]

Men are twice as likely to be killed walking as women, and alcohol is involved in more than half of adult pedestrian deaths. In 1997 the National Institute of Aging reported that only one in a hundred older pedestrians manages to cross the street in the time allocated by traffic lights. Table 7.5 shows the distribution of pedestrian deaths by time period.

Interestingly, the lowest child pedestrian rates are in the Scandinavian countries, with rates less than 1 per 1,000. The rate is 4.9 in Portugal and between those rates is the United States, with 1.6 per 1,000 in 1996.[23]

Healthy People 2010 Objective: Reduce Pedestrian Deaths on Public Roads

Target: 1 pedestrian death per 100,000 population.

Baseline: 2 pedestrian deaths per 100,000 population occurred on public roads in 1997.

Prevention Intervention Suggestions

Community prevention programs for pedestrian safety have included pedestrian islands in the center of busy highways or streets, longer "Walk" signals, improved ways for drivers to see pedestrians, slower speed limits on streets with heavy pedestrian traffic, and more supervision for young children crossing the street. Other communities are installing runway lights, radar sensors, and electronic eyes along pedestrian crossways, and they are using countdown signs instead of flashing "Walk/Don't Walk" signals. Technology may become an important preventive medium for a variety of community health issues in the twenty-first century.

Each highway fatality in 1998 cost the nation more than $700,000 in expenses and economic losses from accident death. Total motor vehicle crashes cost the nation $200.3 billion in 1997, more than 3% of the gross domestic product.[24]

Healthy People 2010 Objective: Reduce Deaths Caused by Motor Vehicle Crashes

Target: 9.0 deaths per 100,000 population and 1 death per 100 million vehicle miles traveled (VMT).

Baseline: 15.0 deaths per 100,000 population were caused by motor vehicle crashes in 1998 (preliminary data; age adjusted to the year 2000 standard population) and 2 deaths per 100 million VMT were caused by motor vehicle crashes in 1997.

Contributing Factors   Major contributing factors in traffic accidents are alcohol, speed, vehicle and roadway conditions, and driver error. A common fallacy about accidents is that they stem from only one cause. Traffic accidents are often the unexpected effect of many variables, a wet road, psychological stress, bad tires, or several beers. Any one of these factors will probably not cause an accident by itself, but each added variable increases the likelihood of an accident (Figure 7.3).

Human or host factors are by far the greatest contributors to motor vehicle accident death, and in fact, 85 percent of all motor vehicle accidents have human error as a contributing factor. Alcohol consumption is involved in approximately 50 percent of all traffic fatalities. Driving at an unsafe speed is involved in 25 percent of all accidents. Three public health initiatives have dramatically influenced the host factors in motor vehicle accidents:

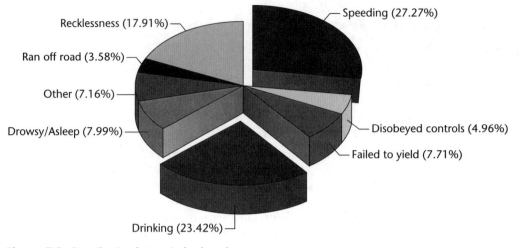

Recklessness (17.91%)

Ran off road (3.58%)

Other (7.16%)

Drowsy/Asleep (7.99%)

Speeding (27.27%)

Disobeyed controls (4.96%)

Failed to yield (7.71%)

Drinking (23.42%)

Figure 7.3 Contributing factors in fatal crashes.

(*Source:* National Highway Traffic Safety Administration)

1. A twenty-one-year-old drinking age

2. Seat belt legislation

3. Legislation that prohibits a blood alcohol level higher than .10 as the threshold of intoxication in most states

Enforcement of these three initiatives directly affects the number one factor in motor vehicle injuries and fatalities—a drunk driver.

Preventive Factors More than 215 million cars are on U.S. roads today. About 4 percent or 6 million cars have air bags; most only on the driver's side. Air bags protect occupants in ways that seat belts alone cannot. They spread out the violent impact of a crash and keep even a belted occupant from smashing against the steering wheel, dashboard, or windshield.[25] The first federal study of automobile air bags in actual traffic accidents found that air bags are far more effective than seat belts alone in preventing death. In a head-on collision, air bags reduced the risk of death by 26 percent and in all serious accidents reduced death by 13 percent. It is estimated that air bags saved at least 2,400 lives between 1990–1995.[26]

It was projected in 1987 that even without air bags, if all vehicle occupants wore safety belts, 12,000 to 15,000 fewer people would die each year in the United States alone.[27] In 2001 forty-nine states had mandatory seat belt laws and all fifty states had mandatory child safety seat laws. (New Hampshire has no seat belt law.)

Bicycle Accidents

The first bicycle accident in the United States occurred in New York City on May 30, 1896. Motorist Henry Wells, driving a Duryea motor wagon, hit bicyclist Evylyn Thomas. Thomas suffered a broken leg while Wells spent the night in jail.[28] In 1990, 42 percent of adults bicycled, 75 percent of adults owned a bicycle, and one in every sixty rode a bike to work.[29] Approximately 1,000 fatalities a year occur to bicycle riders, and in 1998, there were 53,000 reported bicycle-injury-related accidents.[30] The average age of a bicycle fatality victim in 1999 was twenty-seven years. Each year approximately 530 children under nineteen years and 430 adults die, while 443,000 children and 115,000 adults are treated in emergency departments for injuries occurring in bicycle crashes.[31]

Bicyclists are most seriously injured in collisions with motor vehicles. About one in four injuries involving bicycle-motor vehicle collisions results in hospital admission of the bicyclist compared with one in twenty bicycle injuries not involving motor vehicles. Almost 40 percent of fatalities occur when the driver runs up on a bicyclist from the rear and 27 percent occur from bicycles darting out. Brain injury has been found to be the primary cause of death in about three-quarters of bicyclists' deaths.[32]

> *Healthy People 2010 Objective:* Increase the Number of States and the District of Columbia with Laws Requiring Bicycle Helmets
>
> *Target:* All states and the District of Columbia.
>
> *Baseline:* Eleven states had laws requiring bicycle helmets for bicycle riders under age fifteen years in 1999.

Use of helmets by bicyclists is suggested as one strategy to reduce severe injury. Bike paths away from the road, enforcement of traffic laws for bicyclists, and changes in the front ends of motor vehicles from energy-concentrating points and edges to energy absorption would probably also reduce severe injuries. Certainly better driver education should include more awareness of bicycles and motorcycles on the road. Further, two-wheeled vehicles must obey

---

BOX 7.2 The More Health Bicycle Safety Project

More Health is an innovative community health education program originally developed by the Hillsborough County, Florida Junior League, and currently managed by a local public hospital and sponsored by various local businesses, community, and health organizations. The program allows school children in grades K–12 to experience hands-on activities related to health and science in the classroom. The Bicycle Safety program was designed to increase helmet use through education and reduced-price bicycle helmets. The targeted population for this program were grades K–2. The curriculum includes use of a model of the human brain, helmet demonstrations, traffic lights demonstrations, examination of protective gear for roller blades, puppet shows, and song presentation. Continuing education included community support of posters, public service announcements, and billboards. Early results of this community health program show that helmet use increased in the intervention schools, but that most children do not wear bicycle helmets.

the same traffic laws as four-wheeled vehicles. Mandatory helmet laws appear to be the major way to achieve this objection.

Other Recreational Activities

Bicycles are not the only recreational source of accidents. There were 3.9 million visits to hospital emergency departments (ED) in 1997 by those engaging in a sporting or recreational activity. Sport-related injuries accounted for 11.2 percent of ED injury visits. The top ten recreational activities with reported injuries are basketball, baseball, bicycle riding, football, soccer, roller skating, swimming, volleyball, fishing, and horseback riding.[33]

Motorcycles

There were 4 million motorcycle registrations in 1998, a reduction of 27 percent since 1982. The National Highway Traffic Safety Administration said 2,216 motorcycle riders died in 1998; 55,000 were injured. Of those deaths, 43 percent were intoxicated and 85 percent were men. The National Highway Traffic Safety Administration also indicated that 57 percent of injuries were due to collisions with other motor vehicles, while 21 percent resulted from noncollision accidents and 15 percent were the result of collisions with a fixed object.[34]

> See your state's motor vehicle mortality rate at
> www.insure.com/auto/injury/statefate1099.html

It is believed that helmet laws in many states are an important factor in this decline. Also, more riders are taking hands-on classes, riders tend to be older, and the recession buying in the 1980s slowed motorcycle purchases. States that do not adopt helmet laws now must also reallocate their federal transportation money away from highway repair to safety education. The result was 490 lives saved in 1996; a 29 percent effectiveness in preventing fatalities and 67 percent effectiveness in preventing brain injuries.[35]

> *Healthy People 2010 Objective:* Increase the Proportion of Motorcyclists Using Helmets
>
> *Target:* 79 percent.
>
> *Baseline:* 67 percent of motorcycle operators and passengers used helmets in 1997.

Recreational Vehicles

Americans spend more time, effort, energy, and money on recreational pursuits today than at any other time in history. As healthy as these pursuits are, when skill development, safe behavior, and equipment maintenance are substandard, the risk of accidental injury and death have increased. Among those recreational "toys" that pose the greatest risks are snowmobiles, all-terrain vehicles (ATVs), boats, and skis. The Consumer Product Safety Commission has estimated that more than 20,000 people a year are injured as a result of snowmobile accidents. Each winter about 6 million people ski resulting in over 100,000 injuries or a rate of 4.5 per 1,000 skiers. There are approximately 1,500 boating fatalities each year, mostly drownings.[36]

Like motor vehicle accidents, most recreational accidents could be prevented by community education programs, proper use and maintenance of equipment, and adherence to safety rules and regulations. In 1997, four-wheeled ATVs injured 31,290 people. Trail bikes injured an additional 25,275 people. In the early 1990s three-wheeled ATVs (motorized, gasoline-powered vehicles with oversized, low-pressure tires used for off-road, non-paved terrain) were outlawed by the federal government due to their lack of safety and the high cost in human life that was being reported. Sales of adult size four-wheeled ATVs were banned to anyone under 16. Manufacturers and dealers agreed to provide warnings, safety instructions, and rider training. In 1992, casualties declined to 198 deaths and 65,300 injuries. Children less than 16 years, however, still accounted for 40 percent of ATV deaths in 1997. The American Academy of Pediatrics has recommended age requirements for ATV riders, licensing of ATV riders, and mandatory helmet use. As of September 1998, twenty-one of thirty-one states had laws associated with these public health recommendations.[37]

Other motorized vehicles that have increasing rates of fatalities and injuries are jet skis and other "wet bikes." In 1996, among 760,000 jet ski owners, there were 55 fatalities and 12,110 injuries reported. Adoption of laws that enforce minimum operating age, required use of life jackets, and safety education classes have reduced the number of fatalities in those states with such laws.

Falls

Falls are the second leading cause of accidental death in America but the leading cause of nonfatal injury. Falls cause more deaths per year than drowning and fires combined. The 1990 national objective was to reduce deaths from falls to no more than 2 per 100,000. Unfortunately, the 1990 rate was 5.0 per 100,000 and increased to only 5.6 in 1997 as shown on Table 7.5. The shift in age distribution of the U.S. population is a factor influencing our inability to achieve this objective.

Table 7.5   Death from falls (1997).

Total: 5,200; Death Rate: 1.9

Age Group	0–4	5–14	15–24	25–44	45–64	65–74	75+
Deaths	30	30	140	400	500	400	3,700
Rates	0.2	0.1	0.4	0.5	0.9	2.2	23.1

(*Source:* Healthy People 2010)

Healthy People 2010 Objective: Reduce Deaths from Falls

Target: 2.3 deaths per 100,000 population.

Baseline: 4.5 deaths per 100,000 population were caused by falls in 1998 (preliminary data; age adjusted to the year 2000 standard population).

The population group at highest risk for fatal falls, those persons over seventy-five years of age (65 per 100,000), is becoming an ever-increasing proportion of the population. Impairments such as poor vision, unsteady gait, and chronic medical conditions may predispose an individual to fall or contribute to the death once a fall occurs. Numerous host, environmental, and agent risk factors contribute to the high rate of fatal and nonfatal falls in this age group.

Most deaths from falls occur in the home (28,200 in 1997).[38] Since most older adults are home a great deal of the time and many suffer from age-related debilities that put them at risk for falls, a major community health initiative should be planned to improve home safety through education and modification of high risk areas in the home, such as the kitchen, bathroom, and stairs. Environmental factors such as stairway design and disrepair, inadequate lighting, and slipping and tripping on water, ice, clutter, loose rugs, or electrical cords may also play a key role in the occurrence of a fall.

During their middle-aged years, males are at greater risk than females of dying from a fall. The larger number of men working in hazardous occupations, such as construction, may increase their risk of falling from heights and sustaining more severe injuries than females. But as females continue to enter nontraditional careers, their injuries will increase.

Poisoning

Accidental deaths from solid and liquid poisoning is the third most common cause of accidental deaths in the nation. Total human poisoning exposures, both fatal and nonfatal, were more than 2.1 million cases in 1999, according to the American Association of Poison Control Centers.[39] Most poisoning occurs among children under the age of five as a result of curiosity combined with an inability to read. Since the 1960s childproof caps and "Mr. Yuk" warning stickers resulted in a 60 percent reduction in childhood poisonings. Child poisoning deaths from aspirin declined 80 percent from 1965 to 1975 when manufacturers voluntarily adopted container caps difficult for children to remove. There were complaints initially from adults who had difficulty opening childproof caps, and new caps have been designed for easier adult use, while still protecting children. There were thirty poisoning fatalities among children under four in 2000.

Several drugs, household solvents, corrosives, and caustics continue to result in child poisoning. Hospitalization rates of five to twelve per 100,000 children per year are average for each category of product. There exists a need to "safety proof" homes so that children are not exposed to household chemicals and for adults to be aware of the potentially toxic substances found in everyday use.

Table 7.6   Deaths from drowning (1997).

Total: 2,400; Death Rate: 0.9

Age Group	0–4	5–14	15–24	25–44	45–64	65–74	75+
Deaths	120	260	500	800	400	120	200
Rates	0.6	0.7	1.3	1.0	0.7	0.7	1.2

(*Source:* Healthy People 2010)

Community poisoning prevention efforts including community outreach seminars, school curriculum seminars, retail outreach efforts, distribution of educational materials, and publicity in media have been associated with declines in emergency room visits for poisonings. Use of Maternal and Child Health block grant funds as well as state and local funds for education has been undertaken in the United States, but no systematic evaluation of the effects of specific efforts has been conducted. Unfortunately, poisoning deaths by solids and liquids increasead in 1997 to 8,600.

Healthy People 2010 Objective: Reduce Deaths Caused by Poisonings

Target: 1.8 death per 100,000 population.

Baseline: 5.8 deaths per 100,000 population were caused by poisonings in 1998 (preliminary data; age adjusted to the year 2000 standard population).

The abuse of drugs is a significant source of unintentional poisoning. Poisoning mortality is predominately a problem among young adults, particularly men twenty to thirty-nine years of age. The highest mortality rates of unintentional poisoning for both blacks and whites were for young adult men. Cocaine has been the most frequently reported drug involved in emergency visits, and heroin/morphine and cocaine each were involved in more than one-third of deaths. Most of the fatal poisonings by other liquids were due to alcohol ingestion. An emerging trend is binge drinking on college campuses that occasionally induce fatal alcohol poisoning.

Drowning

More than 4,000 persons a year die from drowning as was seen in 1997 when 4,631 deaths occurred. After motor vehicle accidents, drowning is the leading cause of accidental death from ages one through forty-four years. More than 60 percent of all drowning fatalities are under twenty-five years and the majority are male with a ratio of male-to-female drowning rates of 12:1 (Table 7.6). Alcohol is a major contributing factor. Alcohol use can reduce body temperature and through its effect on the central nervous system, can impair swimming ability. Because alcohol affects balance, movement, and vision, its use represents risk for injury and death for swimmers as well as boat operators and passengers.

Drowning rates for black children were almost twice those for white children in 1996. In the first six decades, other races had drowning rates between those of blacks and whites, however, after age sixty-four, drowning death rates for other races were higher than those for blacks and whites. In all states, up to 90 percent of drowning among children occurred in residential swimming pools. Drowning death rates for men (2.8) is higher than for women (0.72).

Healthy People 2010 Objective: Reduce Drowning

Target: 0.9 drowning per 100,000 population.

Baseline: 1.6 drowning per 100,000 population in 1998 (preliminary data; age adjusted to the year 2000 standard population).

People drown in a variety of collections of water including bathtubs, buckets, swimming pools, lakes, rivers, flood waters, and rarely, oceans. Drowning associated with children is all too common. Prevention may include teaching children as young as toddlers to swim. Requiring fences and childproof gates around pools will dramatically reduce children wandering into unsupervised swimming pools, and a change in pool design will allow children easier exit from a pool.

Fire

Half the nation's fires occur in the home. Fires are the fifth leading cause of accidental death in America, and over 75 percent of all deaths from fires occur in residential fires. Residential fires are most often associated with smoking, cooking, home heating, or electricity. Other factors include defects in the building, lightning, hazardous storage of flammable products, and inadequate or absent sprinkler systems, smoke detectors and/or fire extinguishers.

Healthy People 2010 Objective: Reduce Residential Fire Deaths

Target: 0.6 deaths per 100,000 population.

Baseline: 1.2 deaths per 100,000 population were caused by residential fires in 1998 (preliminary data; age adjusted to the year 2000 standard population).

Most deaths from heat energy and accompanying smoke and toxic fumes occur in house fires, while major nonfatal injuries occur from scalding burns and contact with hot surfaces. The leading source of ignition in house fires (30 to 45 percent) is the cigarette, usually dropped in a bed, couch, or chair and left to smolder as the smoker sleeps.[40]

Most brands of cigarettes have design characteristics and additives that promote continued burning for up to forty minutes when dropped. The feasibility of modifications to make cigarettes self-extinguish when dropped has been studied, but no federal agency has the authority to require manufacturers to make this modification. Thanks in part to the pro-tobacco lobby, the Consumer

Table 7.7   Deaths from fires (1999).

Total: 200; Death Rate: 0.1

Age Group	0–4	5–14	15–24	25–44	45–64	65–74	75+
Deaths	10	10	20	60	40	30	30
Rates	0.1	NA	0.1	0.1	0.1	0.2	0.2

(*Source:* Healthy People 2010)

Product Safety Commission and the FDA are specifically prohibited from regulating cigarettes.

Ironically, economic factors can act as either an incentive or a disincentive to fire prevention. In the United States, the purchase of fire insurance is encouraged, blame for fires is discouraged, and the United States has one of the highest fire incidence rates in any industrialized nation. Japanese society views fire accidents as a disgrace to the fire victim and has one of the lowest fire incidence rates of all industrialized countries.[41] The United States 1990 objective was to reduce residential fire deaths to no more than 4,500 people. This objective was met in 1990 and decreased further to 4,050 deaths in 1998, the lowest rate of fire-related deaths in 20 years (Table 7.7).

The reductions in fire-related death rates are associated with great increases in the installation of smoke detectors in residences. Unfortunately, most people do not check smoke detectors regularly to see if they are working. It has been suggested that batteries in smoke detectors be changed every year when changing to Daylight Savings Time. Even with good community health education, the fact that smoke detectors require little attention by the consumer is probably a stronger factor in use than preventive education programs.

Burns

Overheated tap water is a major source of children's burns. The 1990 national objective was to reduce the number of tap water scald injuries to no more than 2,000 a year, from the approximately 3,133 cases in 1984. Standards for maximum temperatures for new water heaters could be set. Utility companies could offer periodic checks of water temperatures during routine meter reading. Insulation of other heat sources such as heating registers, stoves, and fireplaces could be increased. The ban on fireworks with particular heat, diffusion of heated particles, or explosive characteristics has reduced childhood injury in many states.

Occupational Accidents

The 1990 national objective for less than 3,750 workplace accidents per year was met in 1984; however, the achievement may not be permanent. The reduction in OSHA inspectors and an increase in standards during the 1980s has put workers at increased risk for accidents. An analysis of fatal accidents that occurred in 1994 and 1995 found that 75 percent of the work sites where accidents occurred had not been inspected in the five previous years. "Two key reasons OSHA did not make advance visits to these lethal work sites are a shortage of inspectors and its mandate to follow up all worker complaints, no matter how routine."[42]

The toll of workplace injuries and illnesses is significant. Every five seconds a worker is injured in the United States. This is one in every fifteen workers who are injured more commonly with back and hand injuries. Almost one in every five workers had suffered a week or more of back pain and 22 percent had trouble with his or her hands, including carpal-tunnel syndrome.[43]

Every ten seconds a worker is temporarily or permanently disabled. Each day, an average of 137 persons die from work-related diseases, and an additional seventeen die from injuries on the job. Although youth (persons aged 18 years and under) represent only 2 percent of the total workforce, each year 74,000 require treatment in hospital emergency departments for work-related injuries, and seventy die of those injuries. In 1996, an estimated 11,000 workers were disabled each day due to work-related injuries. In 1996, the National Safety Council estimated that on-the-job injuries alone cost society $121 billion, representing the sum of lost wages, lost productivity, administrative expenses, health care, and other costs.[44]

In 1997, there were 117,400,000 workers, 6,218 on-the-job deaths and 3 million disabling injuries.[45] The injury rate was 12.5. Work days lost should be

---

BOX 7.3 Ten Leading Work-Related Injuries

1. **Occupational lung diseases**
   Asbestosis, byssinosis, silicosis, coal workers' pneumoconiosis, lung cancer, occupational asthma

2. **Musculoskeletal injuries**
   Disorders of the back, trunk, upper extremity, neck, and lower extremity, traumatically induced Raynaud's phenomenon

3. **Occupational cancers (other than lung)**
   Leukemia, mesothelioma, cancers of the bladder, nose, and liver

4. **Severe occupational traumatic injuries**
   Amputations, fractures, eye loss, lacerations, traumatic deaths

5. **Occupational cardiovascular diseases**
   Hypertension, coronary artery disease, acute myocardial infarction

6. **Disorders of reproduction**
   Infertility, spontaneous abortion, teratogenesis

7. **Neurotoxic disorders**
   Peripheral neuropathy, toxic encephalitis, psychoses, extreme personality changes (exposure-related)

8. **Noise-induced loss of hearing**

9. **Dermatological conditions**
   Dermatoses, burns (scaldings), chemical burns, contusions (abrasions)

10. **Psychological disorders**
    Neuroses, personality disorders, alcoholism, drug dependence

(*Source:* National Institute for Occupational Safety and Health)

reduced to 55 per year per 100 workers; however, in 1989 the rate was 66.8 per 100 workers. The cost to Americans was $63.8 billion. The ten leading work-related injuries according to the National Institutes of Occupational Safety and Health (NIOSH) are given in Box 7.3. The five leading occupational deaths in 1997 were from (1) highway accidents (1,387); (2) assaults and violent acts (1,165); (3) being struck by an object (1,034); (4) falls to lower levels (715); and (5) nonhighway transportation accidents (377).[46]

The greatest number of occupational injuries are reported during the first year of employment for any worker and are traced to first-year workers who have not been trained to do their job safely. Other occupational hazards include slippery or uneven surfaces, unguarded machinery, impeded means of egress, and exposures to hazards such as toxic chemicals, asbestos, cyanide or carbon tetrachloride, radiation, noise, and extremes of heat and cold.

Healthy People 2010 Objective: Reduce Deaths from Work-Related Injuries

	1998 Baseline	2010 Target
	Deaths per 100,000 Workers Aged 16 Years and Older	
All industry	4.5	3.2
Mining	23.6	16.5
Construction	14.6	10.2
Transportation	11.8	8.3
Agriculture, forestry, and fishing	24.1	16.9

Consumer Product Safety Act

In 1972 Congress passed the Consumer Product Safety Act. This act was designed to provide the consumer with a reasonable amount of assurance that a product is safe and reliable, and passage created the Consumer Product Safety Commission. Injuries associated with consumer products in 1993 are given in Table 7.8.

The purposes of the Consumer Product Safety Act are to:

1. Protect the public against unreasonable risks of injury associated with consumer products.

2. Assist consumers in evaluating the comparative safety of consumer products.

3. Provide for the development of uniform safety standards.

4. Minimize conflicting state and local regulations.

5. Promote research and investigation into the causes and prevention of product-related deaths, illness, and injuries.[47]

Table 7.8   Injuries with consumer products (1992 and 1993).

Product	1992	1993	Product	1992	1993
Home maintenance:			General household appliances:		
Noncaustic cleaning equip.[1]	26,654	27,184	Cooking ranges, ovens, etc.	53,401	51,243
Cleaning agents (except soap)	43,758	42,426	Irons, clothes steamers	17,266	17,888
Paints, solvents, lubricants	23,383	21,071	Refrigerators, freezers	35,895	33,895
Misc. household chemicals	24,679	23,709	Washers, dryers	22,590	22,786
Home workshop equipment:			Misc. household appliances	34,941	31,314
Power home tools, except saws	31,742	30,200	Heating, cooling equipment:[4]		
Power home workshop saws	97,606	89,177	Chimneys, fireplaces	26,664	23,256
Welding, soldering, cutting tools	20,686	23,678	Fans (except above)	17,050	20,661
Workshop manual tools	125,780	122,221	Heating stoves, space heaters	37,805	31,005
Misc. workshop equipment	46,407	44,797	Pipes, heating and plumbing	23,216	23,335
Household packaging and containers:			Home entertainment equipment:		
Cans, other containers	239,521	238,081	Pet supplies, equipment	26,703	(NA)
Glass bottles, jars	63,170	32,342	Sound recording equip.[5]	46,022	43,898
Paper, cardboard, plastic products	47,495	46,358	Television sets, stands	42,000	42,988
Housewares:			Personal use items:		
Cookware, pots, pans	36,700	31,110	Cigarettes, lighters, fuels	23,547	20,737
Cutlery, knives, unpowered	468,587	460,248	Clothing	142,457	148,136
Drinking glasses	130,200	127,111	Grooming devices	31,991	32,918
Scissors	34,602	29,381	Jewelry	55,142	55,677
Small kitchen applicances	43,453	38,789	Paper money, coins	30,274	28,592
Tableware and accessories	120,940	110,526	Pencils, pens, other desk supplies	49,226	46,376
Misc. housewares	61,201	60,789	Razors, shavers, razor blades	43,365	44,147
Home furnishing:[2]			Sewing equipment	29,814	(NA)
Bathtub, shower structures	166,327	161,673	Yard and garden equipment:		
Beds, mattresses, pillows	400,732	395,268	Chains and saws	38,692	40,149
Carpets, rugs	112,763	127,341	Hand garden tools	36,374	44,835
Chairs, sofas, sofa beds	413,759	407,472	Hatchets, axes	16,760	16,929
Desks, cabinets, shelves, racks	228,676	223,309	Lawn garden care equipment	51,324	62,708
Electric fixtures, lamps, equipment	54,097	58,213	Lawn mowers	85,202	78,553
Ladders, stools	189,210	189,596	Other power lawn equipment	21,598	24,929
Mirrors, mirror glass	24,928	20,261	Sports and recreation equipment:		
Sinks, toilets	61,281	60,557	Bicycles, accessories	649,536	603,946
Tables	345,271	329,573	Exercise equipment	95,127	91,238
Other misc. accessories	57,555	59,030	Mopeds, minibikes, ATV's[6]	132,271	122,615
Home structures, construction:[3]			Nonpowder guns, BB's, pellets	34,552	29,502
Cabinets or door hardware	24,876	25,908	Playground equipment	290,382	268,915
Ceilings, walls, inside panels	262,572	262,316	Skateboards	44,068	27,718
Counters, counter tops	36,888	36,896	Toboggans, sleds, snow disks, etc.	43,273	59,698
Fences	123,014	126,714	Trampolines	43,665	46,215
Glass doors, windows, panels	216,193	215,284	Miscellaneous products:		
Handrails, railing, banisters	42,965	42,876	Dollies, carts	45,257	46,549
Nails, carpet tacks, etc.	239,711	233,507	Gasoline and diesel fuels	19,205	20,386
Nonglass doors, panels	357,149	349,080	Nursery equipment	112,732	110,498
Porches, open side floors, etc.	129,152	131,475	Toys	177,061	164,379
Stairs, ramps, landings, floors	1,879,029	1,912,743			
Window, door sills, frames	60,147	59,146			
Misc. construction materials	95,147	88,684			

NA Not available. [1]Includes detergent. [2]Includes accessories. [3]Includes materials. [4]Includes ventilating equipment. [5]Includes reproducing equipment. [6]All-terrain vehicles.

(*Source:* National Safety Council, Itasca, IL. Accident Facts, 1994)

The influence of big business lobbies is evident in what is **not** covered by the Act:

1. Tobacco and tobacco products
2. Motor vehicles or motor vehicle equipment
3. Aircraft
4. Boats
5. Foods, drugs, and cosmetics

The Consumer Product Safety Act requires public input into the development of mandatory standards. Both consumer and professional groups have the opportunity for input when a product is being assessed for its risk. After the community gives its technical and experiential input and the economic and environmental impact of a safety standard is evaluated, regulations are established for those products. This community process has established safety regulations for as many as 367 consumer product classifications including cribs, bicycles, toys, space heaters, televisions, swimming pool slides, firecrackers, and children's bed clothing.

The Commission has the ability to enforce regulation. If a product is found to be "imminently hazardous" its future production may be banned and current merchandise may be seized. Over 1,800 toys have been banned as being dangerous. If a consumer product poses an "unreasonable risk" in injury or death, mandatory standards can be issued. Products may be recalled, replaced, or repurchased if found defective after their sale.

In-line skating is also a popular recreational pastime that has many risks for the estimated 12.6 million people who own in-line skates. The Consumer Product Safety Commission projected that there would be 83,000 in-line skating injuries requiring hospital emergency room visits in 1994, up from 37,000 in 1993. Almost 60 percent of those injuries would be among children under fifteen years.[48] Probably the best prevention is protective gear—helmet, padding, and reflective clothing.

Prevention of Unintentional Injuries

Training of the host, engineering improvements of the agent, and modifying the environment are three means of preventing accidents. Some say engineering is the primary means of prevention, but even perfect engineering cannot compensate for a poorly trained worker or a safety conscious consumer.

Safety education of the host, school age children, workers, older citizens, drivers, and others should introduce sound behavioral practices and adherence to laws and safety regulations. Skill development is an important educational tool for accident prevention, especially among children and new workers. When preventive behavior is not possible, environmental factors can still be altered to help dissipate the harmful consequences of accidents. For example, the United States Highway Safety Act, enacted in 1966, improved highway design by adding impact attenuators: barrels filled with water or sand to dissipate the force of a crash, guard rails that bring cars to safe stops, and breakaway light poles that break off their stanchions with the force of impact.[49]

Engineering agent factors can also be improved to prevent, reduce, or mitigate the consequences of accidents. Sadly, even with technological knowledge and scientific data to substantiate their need, installing compulsory seat belts in all U.S. cars was fought by the auto industry to the Nixon administration; air bags were fought by the auto industry to the Reagan administration; in the 1990s shatterproof windshields were fought by the auto industry to the Bush and Clinton administrations. In all cases, the economic cost seemed too great to the manufacturer in relationship to the perceived human cost in terms of lost wages, medical expenses, and damaged property to the potential victim.

Encouraging personal responsibility must also be supplemented with institutional policies, workplace safety standards, and local enforcement to reduce risks. Unsafe and preventable acts such as smoking in bed or unsafe conditions such as poorly lit parking lots put people at risk unnecessarily, and are therefore, community health problems, not just individual problems. Speeding and drinking are the two leading contributing factors associated with traffic fatalities (Figure 7.3). Both can be significantly reduced by the combined efforts of education, enforcement, and personal responsibility. Community, economic, legal, and governmental actions all can make a significant impact on the accident problem. The perceived initial cost of safety prevention must be weighed against the overwhelming social, personal, and economic losses in the overall system.

A major barrier to preventive action is the mistaken belief that accidents are uncontrollable events. On the contrary, studies have shown that people who act to protect themselves against accidents by wearing seat belts and obeying the law live eleven years longer on the average than those who fail to adopt automobile safety behavior. Not all accidents are the result of human failure. Often accidents occur as a result of mechanical failure such as the parachute that fails to open, or natural physiological processes that begin to fail with age. This is true as one grows older, as there is loss of visual and auditory acuity. To anticipate any of these predisposing factors, accident prevention must stress three initiatives—education, engineering and enforcement, and should involve the relationship among host, agent, and environment.

Diabetes

Diabetes, the seventh leading cause of death in the United States in 2000, may be defined as a group of vascular as well as metabolic diseases, because much of the morbidity of diabetes, such as coronary heart disease and stroke, is caused by vascular complications of diabetes. Diabetes is the body's failure to process blood sugar properly. Diabetes poses a significant public health challenge for the United States. Some 800,000 new cases (2,200 per day) are diagnosed each year. The changing demographic patterns in the United States are expected to increase the number of people who are at risk for diabetes and who

Table 7.9   Prevalence of diabetes (1998).

Men	7.5 million	8.2% of all men
Women	8.1 million	8.2% of all women
Age 65 or older	6.3 million	18.4% of this age group
Age 20 or older	15.6 million	8.2% of this age group
Under 20	123,000	.16% of this age group
White	11.3 million	7.8% of nonHispanic whites
Black	2.3 million	10.8% of blacks
Mexican American	1.2 million	10.6% of Mexican Americans
Hispanic/Latino	Twice as likely to have diabetes as nonHispanic whites	
Native American and Alaska Native	5–50% of Native Americans and Alaska Natives	
Asian/Pacific Islander	NA	

(*Source:* Adapted from National Diabetes Information Clearinghouse)

eventually develop the disease. Diabetes is a chronic disease that usually manifests itself as one of two major types: type 1, mainly occurring in children and adolescents eighteen years and younger, in which the body does not produce insulin and thus insulin administration is required to sustain life; or type 2, occurring usually in adults over thirty years of age in which the body's tissues become unable to use its own limited amount of insulin effectively. Treatment for type 2 diabetes usually consists of a combination of physical activity, proper nutrition, oral tablets, and insulin. Type 1 diabetes has been sometimes referred to as juvenile or insulin-dependent diabetes; and type 2 diabetes has been referred to as adult-onset or noninsulin dependent diabetes.[50]

In 1998 there were 11.3 million diagnosed and approximately 6 million undiagnosed Americans.[51] It is the leading cause of kidney failure and new blindness in people under sixty-five in the United States. Since the mid-1980s, the number of global diabetes cases has more than tripled, affecting at least 100 million people worldwide with a projection of 300 million by 2025. In developing countries, diabetes is about to explode. The CDC and WHO are now working on low-cost treatment options and international diabetes control programs.

The toll of diabetes on the health status of people in the United States is expected to worsen before it improves, especially in vulnerable, high-risk populations—African Americans, Hispanics, Native Americans or Alaska Natives, Asians or other Pacific Islanders, elderly persons, and economically disadvantaged persons.[52] Prevelence of diabetes is given in Table 7.9. Evidence suggests that Asians, in particular, may have a genetic predisposition toward diabetes. Once Asians and others in developing countries adopt Western eating habits and diets, diabetes becomes rampant.[53]

Several factors account for this chronic disease epidemic, including behavioral elements (improper nutrition, for example, increased fat consumption; decreased physical activity; obesity); demographic changes (aging, increased growth of "at-risk populations"); improved ascertainment and surveillance systems that more completely capture the actual burden of diabetes; and the relative weakness of interventions to change individual, community, or organizational behaviors. Several other interrelated factors influence the present and future burden of diabetes, including genetics, cultural and community traditions, and socioeconomic status. [54]

Type I insulin dependent diabetes (juvenile diabetes) affects about 1.4 million people in the United States. Diabetes is a metabolic disorder caused when the pancreas stops secreting insulin, a hormone that enables the cells of the body to extract glucose from the bloodstream for energy and growth. Untreated diabetes extracts a terrible toll in premature death, blindness, urinary and kidney problems, and stroke.

Type II diabetes (adult) is a form of diabetes caused by insufficient insulin rather than a lack of insulin. It can often be prevented and managed through diet, weight control, and regular exercise. As diabetics age, however, they increase their risk for blindness, kidney disorders, and nerve damage that ultimately may result in amputation.

The number of people in the United States diagnosed with diabetes has increased sixfold since 1960 to 11.3 million people in 1998. Approximately 6 to 8 million more people are thought to have the disease but are as yet undiagnosed.[55]

However serious diabetes is in the general population, the astronomical rate of diabetes among Native Americans takes an even greater toll. Mortality from diabetes mellitus is 166 percent higher among Native Americans than all other races within the population. As a result of non-native food being imposed on these people, one of every 1,000 members of the Tohono O'odham tribe near Tucson, Arizona, dies of diabetes. Among the Colorado Ute Indians, one-fourth of those older than forty-five have diabetes. The Pima Indians who live near Phoenix, Arizona, have the highest rate of diabetes in the world. More than half of all Pimas over thirty-five are severely diabetic.[56] Although the U.S. government spent less than 15 percent of its diabetes research budget on minorities, taxpayers spent nearly $70 million in 1991 to provide dialysis, surgery, and medicine to treat Native Americans, and the bill is rising. Figure 7.4 indicates the prevalence of Type II diabetes worldwide, and the age and ethnic distribution in the United States in 1991.

Healthy People Objective: Prevent Diabetes

Target: 2.5 new cases per 1,000 persons per year.

Baseline: 3.1 new cases of diabetes per 1,000 persons (3-year average) in 1994–1996.

The Division of Diabetes Translation (DDT) at the Centers for Disease Control and Prevention (CDC) supports a rapidly expanding national and state-based program to reduce the burden of diabetes in the United States. CDC's framework includes four major components: (1) defining the diabetes burden (public

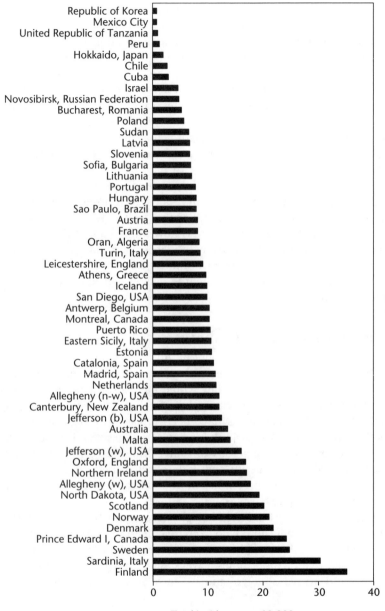

Total incidence per 10,000 person-years

Figure 7.4 Worldwide prevalence of Type II diabetes (1991).

(*Source: Prevention of diabetes mellitus.* Report of a WHO study group. Geneva, World Health Organization, 1994 (Technical Report Series, No. 844)

health, surveillance), (2) developing state-based diabetes control programs, (3) conducting applied translational research, and (4) implementing the National Diabetes Education Program (NDEP). The DDT appropriation from Congress has grown from $7 million in 1992 to $46 million for 1998. Over $20 million of this will be disseminated to state health department diabetes control programs now in all fifty states and eight U.S. territories.

Public health activities of the CDC in diabetes are guided by the following assumptions: Diabetes prevention and control is linked closely to lifestyle-related health behaviors concerning diet-weight management, physical activity, and vaccinations for influenza; federal, state, and local public health agencies to be maximally effective must work closely with partners in the communities they serve, including health care providers, persons and families with diabetes, payers and purchasers, and community organizations; the burden of diabetes is greater for some racial and ethnic groups; many people with diabetes are unaware they have the disease; much more is now known about the prevention of diabetes complications, but many with diabetes are not receiving adequate care; and the most important point of impact for reducing the diabetes burden is in reshaping the health care system to deliver high-quality care and services to those with diabetes.

Prevention/Treatment of Diabetes

First, public health money needs to be spent on nutrition education for Native Americans. Research suggests that tribes such as the O'odham seem to have evolved the ability to store fat so that they would have a source of calories in lean times. This survival mechanism has proven fatal as native foods such as prickly pear, carob, and cholla cactus have been replaced by high-fat, high-sugar foods that are common to our junk food culture. These foods pose a risk to all, but they are especially dangerous to Native Americans, whose genetic makeup predisposes them to obesity and early-onset diabetes. Obesity itself increases one's risk of diabetes three times more than those who were within 20 percent of their ideal weight.

A five-year study of 21,271 diabetes-free physicians, mostly men, ages forty to eighty-four, has found that those who exercise at least once a week were 36 percent less likely to get diabetes than those who exercised less often. If the physicians exercised five or more times a week their risk was reduced by 42 percent. A similar Harvard study of nurses, mostly women, found similar results.

In 1993, diabetes researchers believed they discovered the most important treatment advance since the discovery of insulin. Instead of maintaining blood-sugar levels by injecting insulin once or twice a day, the new findings show that up to four injections a day can reduce complications from diabetes and save millions in health care costs. Diabetics who followed the strict regimen suffered 60 percent less nerve damage, 50 percent less kidney problems, and 76 percent less blindness.

Summary

Most injuries can be prevented through risk reduction by human behavior, structural changes, alteration in the environment, or compliance with legislation. Although the United States has come a long way to reduce death, disability, and injury from accidents, more preventive steps are needed. Although many accidents involve motor vehicles, bicycles, motorcycles, and other recreational vehicles are also involved in needless deaths. Other common accidents include falls, drownings, fires, and occupational accidents.

This chapter described various prevention devices and programs in place to protect the public, including the Consumer Products Safety Commission. Although the Commission has extensive responsibilities for protecting human health, there are still many harmful products out there that do not fall under their jurisdiction.

COPD continues to increase in the U.S. population; the death rate from these chronic conditions parallel lung cancer deaths. Further attention to these lung diseases cannot be overlooked.

Lastly, diabetes was mentioned as the seventh leading cause of death in the general population. This condition also contributes to other chronic killers—making it a risk factor as well as a killer. Specific measures to control diet and increase exercise should be suggested, along with proper medical care, to those millions of people who live with diabetes.

CYBERSITES RELATED TO CHAPTER 7

COPD
   www.copdprofessional.org

Pneumonia
   www.lungusa.org/diseases/lungpneumoni.html

Diabetes
   www.diabetes.org

Influenza
   www.fluwatch.com

QUESTIONS

1. What variables would you use to determine the level of safety of your community?

2. What behaviors make teens at greatest risk for accidental death?

3. What changes could be made to improve safety in three local community locations of which you are familiar?

4. What is your family risk for diabetes? Do you know your family health history? What should a person do to prevent diabetes?

5. How would you promote influenza vaccination in your community?

EXERCISE

Take a walk around your college or university. Assess the safety of your campus. Look at traffic, lighting, accessibility, indoor air, obstructions, classroom conditions, sanitation, and related factors. Make one suggestion for improving campus safety and submit this suggestion to your campus safety department.

INTERNET INTERACTIVE ACTIVITY

THE WONDERS OF WISQARS™

WISQARS™ (Web-based Injury Statistics Query and Reporting System), pronounced "whiskers," is an interactive system that provides injury-related mortality data useful for research and for making informed public health decisions. You can use Injury Mortality Reports to determine injury deaths and death rates for specific external causes of injuries. You can use Leading Causes of Death Reports to determine the number of injury-related deaths relative to the number of other leading causes of death in the United States or in individiual states. The homepage address for WISQARS is:

www.cdc.gov/ncipc/osp/data.htm

1. Go to the following address by clicking on **Injury Mortality Rates**

   webapp.cdc.gov/sasweb/ncipc/mortrate.html

2. Choose from the data options

   pedal cycle

   C0lorado

   all races

   both sexes

   1997

3. CLick **submit**

   Your response should be

1997, Colorado
Pedal Cyclist Deaths and Rates per 100,000
All
races,
Both Sexes, All Ages
E800-E807(.3), E810-E825(6), E826.1,.9, E827-E829(.1)

Number of Deaths	Population	Crude Rate	Age-Adjusted Rate**
14*	3,892,644	0.35*	0.39*

You now know that there were fourteen deaths among all races and all genders in Colorado in 1997. The death rate for bicycles was .35 per 100,000.

Use WISQARS to determine an injury rate for a population of your choice and compare your results by

1. another state in a different part of the United States

2. by gender

3. between 1987 and 1997

What do your results tell you?

REFERENCES

1. www.health.gov/healthypeople/Document/HTML/Volume2/ 24Respiratory.htm#_Toc471904419

2. Ibid.

3. Ibid.

4. www.lungusa.org/diseases/lungemphysem.html#how

5. Mulvihill, Mary Lou (1991). *Human diseases.* Norwalk, CT: Appleton & Lange.

6. www.lungusa.org/diseases/lungemphysem.html#how

7. Levy, Doug (1995). Hispanics may be inclined to asthma. *USA Today,* May 23, p. 6D.

8. *Digest of Health Care for Poor and Disabled* (1998). National study reveals the prominent role of cockroach allergens. Oct, p. 18.

9. Levy, op. cit.

10. Ibid.

11. Ibid.

12. Mulvihill, op. cit.

13. www.health.gov/healthypeople/Document/HTML/Volume2/ 24Respiratory.htm#_Toc471904419

14. The Associated Press (1995). Asthma cases, deaths are skyrocketing. *Salt Lake Tribune,* April 2.

15. www.nsc.org/lrs/statinfo/99078.htm

16. National Safety Council (1997). *Accident facts.* nsc.org/lrs/statinfo/af78.

17. Ibid.

18. Kime, Robert E. (1992). *Environment and health.* Guilford, CT: Dushkin Publishing.

19. www.nsc.org/lrs/statinfo/99078.htm

20. Robertson, Leon (1991). Traumatic injury. In *Oxford textbook of public health,* Vol. II (pp. 501–513). New York: Oxford University Press.

21. Castaneda, Carol (1997). South a danger spot for walking. *USA Today,* April 9, p. 3.A.

22. National Safety Council, op. cit.

23. Preston, Barbara (1995). Cost effective ways to make walking safer for children and adolescents. *Injury Prevention,* Vol. 1, p. 188.

24. National Safety Council, op. cit.

25. *New York Times.* June 26, 1992.

26. The Safety Advocate (1993). *Safe driving 2000: A public/private partnership.* Advocates for Highway and Auto Safety, Washington, DC, Fall.

27. Ibid.

28. U.S. Department of Transportation. (19932). *Traffic Safety Facts: Pedalcyclists.*

29. Database (1992). *U.S. News and World Report,* May 6.

30. NHTSA (2000). State legislature fact sheet: Bicycle helmet use laws.

31. Insurance Institute For Highway Safety (2000). Fatality facts: Bicycles. www.hwysafety.org

32. Robertson, op. cit.

33. Burt, Catherine W. (1998). Emergency visits for sport-related injuries. APHA Annual Meeting presentation. Washington, DC.

34. National Center for Health Statistics (1996). Traffic safety facts: Motorcycles. Washington, DC.

35. NHTSA (1997). Motorcycle traffic safety facts. Washington, DC.

36. Robertson, op. cit.

37. CDC (1999). ALl-terrain vehicle-related deaths. www.cdc.gov/epo/mmwr/preview/mmwrhtml.

38. National Safety Council, op. cit.

39. Ibid.

40. Robertson, op. cit.

41. Dixon, Marian (1991). Accidents. In *Horrendous death, health and well-being,* Daniel Leviton, pp. 219–225. New York: Hemisphere Publishing.

42. Eldridge, Earle (1995). Study links job deaths to OSHA failure. *USA Today,* September 5, p. D1.

43. Associated Press (1995). One in fifteen suffered job injuries in year's time. *Salt Lake Tribune,* July 29, p. A11.

44. www.health.gov/healthypeople/Document/HTML/Volume2/20OccSH.htm

45. National Census of Occupational Injuries (1998). www.bls.gov/special.requests/

46. Ibid.

47. Miller, Dean (1992). *Dimensions of community Health,* 3rd ed. New York: Wm. C. Brown.

48. Dreyfuss, Ira (1994). In-line skating offers enjoyment and danger. *Salt Lake Tribune,* October 11, p. B8.

49. Dixon, op. cit.

50. USHHS (1998). National diabetes fact sheet, Nov. 1.

51. Ibid.

52. Kotulak, Ronald (1995). Deadly diabetes. *Salt Lake Tribune,* March 2.

53. Ibid.

54. Brownson, Ross C. (1998). Chronic disease epidemiology and control. American Public Health Association.

55. Public Health Reports (1997). New diagnosis guide. Sept/Oct. p. 359.

56. Caplan, Arthur (1992). Old world diet habits unhealthy for natives. *The Oregonian,* July 3, p. C9.

CHAPTER 8

Suicide, Nephritis, Chronic Liver Disease, HIV/AIDS

Community Health in the 21st Century
Hopefully, public health institutions and activists will be responding to the
increasing health needs of the poor by addressing the structural (economic
and political) causes of the differential distribution of illness and disease.
There will still be a need for AIDS advocacy and program development for
women, especially sex workers, women of color, lesbians, incarcerated women,
and drug users.

—Nancy Stoller, Ph.D., Sociology; Director of Educational
Materials Development and Distribution, San Francisco
AIDS Foundation; Coordinator of the Women's AIDS
Network of Northern California

Chapter Objectives

The student will:

1. identify those behaviors that put one at risk for being infected with HIV.

2. distinguish between the incubation period and the latency period for HIV.

3. give the CDC definition of AIDS.

4. explain why a person is a carrier of HIV during the window period.

5. give examples of HIV prevention programs implemented worldwide.

6. list those factors that contribute to suicide.

7. explain what social factors directly and indirectly contribute to homicide and suicide among African American men.

8. identify those populations most at risk for suicide.

9. differentiate between chronic kidney disease and end stage kidney failure.

10. recognize the relationship between hepatitis C and chronic liver disease.

Suicide

Mental disorders generate an immense public health burden of disability. The World Health Organization, in collaboration with the World Bank and Harvard University, has determined the "burden of disability" associated with the whole range of diseases and health conditions suffered by people throughout the world. A striking finding of the landmark *Global Burden of Disease* study is that the impact of mental illness on overall health and productivity in the United States and throughout the world often is profoundly under-recognized. Today, in established market economies such as the United States, mental illness is on a par with heart disease and cancer as a cause of disability.[1] Suicide is a major public health problem in the United States and the eighth leading cause of death in 1999. It occurs most frequently as a consequence of a mental disorder. Mental health will be discussed more fully in Chapter 16, but this chapter will discuss suicide as a leading cause of death.

A frequent result of chronic depression and the lack of mental health services by a community is suicide. The incidence of suicide is aggravated by the social pathology of our society. In a society marked by alcohol and drug abuse, family violence, unemployment, crime, gangs, and instability, the risk of depression, loss of self-esteem, and sense of worthlessness can be expected. Individual illness becomes a community's malaise as these social pathologies escalate and become more overwhelming to the resources of a community. Suicide is both a symptom and a personal attempt at "treatment" for the social pathologies of the twenty-first century.

A suicide occurs in America every seventeen minutes. During these same seventeen minutes there are eight to twenty attempts. Suicide is not a new act of personal violence. The oldest recorded suicide note was written 4,000 years ago on Egyptian papyrus. In 1999, Jack Kevorkian was convicted of murder in Michigan for lethally injecting a terminally ill man. Essentially, this was a type of suicide, **euthanasia.** The bioethical question of euthanasia has become even more important as many terminally ill or irreversibly debilitated people suffering from AIDS to cancer, from Alzheimer's to multiple sclerosis, make the very difficult choice to commit suicide rather than experience the worst possible quality of life.

Among those fifteen to twenty-four years and sixty-five to seventy-four years suicide is the third leading cause of death with a rate of 13.5 per 100,000 and 10.1 per 100,000 respectively. Suicide and homicide cause about 22 percent of deaths in childhood and adolescence and 35 percent of all injury deaths. The risk for engaging in suicidal behaviors also differs by gender. A history of physical or sexual abuse appears to be a serious risk factor for suicide attempts in both women and men. Women attempt suicide more often than men, but men's risk of completed suicide is on average 4.5 times higher than women's. White males account for 73 percent of all suicides with a rate of 25.2/100,000 for men twenty to thirty-four years and a rate of 46.1 for white men over sixty-five years. Table 8.1 reports the suicide rate by race and age in 1998. Together, white males and white females account for more than 90 percent of all suicides in the United States. The suicide gender gap begins in adolescence and grows through middle and later life.[2] The 1998 gender ratio for this age group was 7:1 (males: females).

Disturbingly, numbers are increasing for young women, blacks, Native Americans, and older Americans (please refer to other chapters in this text for more information on suicide among certain groups of people). During the

Table 8.1   Suicide in the United States (1998).

Characteristic	Number	Rate per 100,000
Total	30,575	11.31
White	27,648	12.40
Black	1,977	5.74
Native American	310	13.14
Asian	640	6.09
Hispanic	950	7.38
Males	24,538	18.58
Females	6,037	4.37
Age 10–14	303	1.6
Age 15–19	1,802	9.5
Age 20–24	2,384	13.6
Age >85	801	65.0

(*Source:* www.cdc.gov/ncipc/osp/mortdata.htm)

period 1979–1992, suicide rates for Native Americans (a category that includes American Indians and Alaska Natives) were about 1.5 times the rate for the general population. There were a disproportionate number of suicides among young male Native Americans during this period, as males fifteen to twenty-four accounted for 64 percent of all suicides by Native Americans.[3]

Suicide incidence is two times greater in whites than blacks; however, Native American suicide exceeds the general population rate though the rate varies among tribes. Among all Indian Health Service populations the rate is 16.2 per 100,000. The suicide rate is three to four times greater in men than women, but women are more likely to attempt suicide. It is thought that suicide is a leading cause of death among gay teens. Suicide rates peak in the spring and on Mondays, go down during wars, and rise during economic crises. A comparison of international suicide rates is given in Table 8.2.

The variables most associated with suicide are feelings of hopelessness and depression linked to perceived loss, previous attempts, access to a lethal weapon, and exposure to suicide. For example, cluster suicides are often reported in high schools after one student commits suicide. Psychological autopsies have begun to show some important preventive information about potential suicide. Suicide more often resembles the eruption of a long, simmering volcanic process than the sudden strike of a lightning bolt. In several large-scale studies, 92 percent or more of victims were found to be suffering from diagnosable, often long-standing, mental disorder at the time of their deaths. Among these were depression, alcoholism, and psychosis. For most suicide victims, the decision to die emerges out of a broad context of psychic upheaval. There is always something more than mental illness. There may be a period of intense stress, a state of exhaustion or sleep deprivation, a shift to a new environment, a divorce, death, or other loss. In rare cases, the immediate trigger is dramatic, such as public exposure of wrongdoing.[4] Alcohol is associated with 25–50 percent of all suicides.

Table 8.2   International suicide rates (1994).

Country	Suicide Rate per 100,000
Estonia	40.9
Hungary	39.1
Denmark	31.6
Brazil	25.3
France	20.8
Japan	16.6
Germany	15.6
Canada	13.2
Australia	12.7
Italy	8.0
Israel	7.1
UK	8.0
Mexico	2.9
Kuwait	1.7

(*Source:* International Violent Death Rates www.guncite.com/gun_control_gcvintl)

Two-thirds of suicide victims give clues to their intentions, expressing despondency, making jokes about suicide, asserting that the world would be a better place without them, or explicitly stating a wish to die. Sadly, the signs and symptoms of impending suicide are often ignored or misunderstood. For many suicidal people, no one knows that they are so despondent, so they do not get immediate emotional support. Community education may help people hear and react to warning signs, and community programs may help those at risk find support.[5]

Suicide is a complex behavior usually caused by a combination of factors. Research shows that almost all people who kill themselves have a diagnosable mental or substance abuse disorder or both, and that the majority have depressive illness. Studies indicate that the most promising way to prevent suicide and suicidal behavior is through the early recognition and treatment of depression and other psychiatric illnesses. Sometimes the ability to distinguish between an accident and a suicide is painfully difficult. Certainly many high-risk behaviors are "suicidal," such as cycling without a helmet, drinking and driving, diving into unknown water, using drugs, or even smoking. However, planned death is a violent act of desperation. It is thought that there is one successful suicide for every ten attempts and about 5 percent of those who fail are repeaters.

Healthy People 2010 Objective: Reduce the Suicide Rate

Target: 6.0 suicide deaths per 100,000 population.

Baseline: 10.8 suicide deaths per 100,000 population in 1998 (preliminary data; age adjusted to the year 2000 standard population).

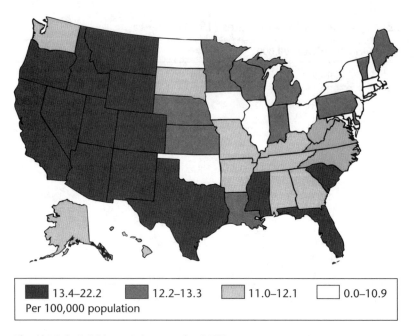

| ■ 13.4–22.2 | ■ 12.2–13.3 | ▨ 11.0–12.1 | □ 0.0–10.9 |

Per 100,000 population

Figure 8.1 Suicide rates by state for 1997.

(*Source:* Regional Variations in Suicide Rates. MMWR, August 29, 1997. 46(34); 789–793)

Research suggests that one in five high school students says he or she seriously considered suicide within the past year. Suicide incidence rates by state for 1997 are given in Figure 8.1.

Nephritis

Nephritis, or chronic kidney failure, became one of the ten leading causes of death in the United States in 1998. It is now the ninth leading cause of death. It was not included in the Healthy People 2000 goals and objectives; however, because of the tremendous increase in the rate of death, it now is included in the 2010 goals. Regrettably, there is not much that community health can do to prevent nephritis specifically. Most prevention programs will target aggravating conditions such as diabetes and cardiovascular disease.

When kidney function has deteriorated and is no longer adequate to sustain life and the process is considered irreversible, renal replacement therapy (RRT), dialysis, or transplantation, becomes necessary to maintain life. Treated chronic kidney failure, also called end-stage renal disease, is the most feared consequence of kidney disease. Chronic renal insufficiency, however, is more common than treated chronic kidney failure and can also severely affect health and well-being. Therefore, ideally, programs should be directed at preventing the development of chronic renal insufficiency and its subsequent progression to end-stage renal disease (ESRD).[6]

Unfortunately, chronic renal insufficiency is usually asymptomatic, and the exact number of people affected is unknown. The best available estimates are based on national surveys. Current estimates indicate approximately 10 million persons aged twelve years and older have some form of chronic kidney disease. People with end-stage kidney failure represent a small fraction of all individuals with chronic kidney disease. A significant proportion of people with chronic kidney failure progress to end-stage as shown in Figure 8.2. The challenge is to initiate effective programs to prevent progression of established kidney disease and to institute methods to assess the progress of such initiatives.

In 1998, 87,334 new cases of end-stage kidney failure were reported. Virtually all of these patients became permanently dependent on renal replacement therapy to stay alive.

Dialysis and kidney transplantation are the two methods of treatment available to people with kidney disease when they reach end-stage. In 1998, 259,182 people in the United States depended on either dialysis or transplants to replace the function of their own failed kidneys. Although these treatments are life-saving, dialysis and transplants have substantial limitations. Neither treatment restores normal health, and both are expensive. The rates of illness, disability, and death experienced by individuals with treated chronic kidney failure are substantially higher than those of the general population.[7]

In most instances, terminal kidney failure develops as the result of progressive damage to the kidneys over a decade or more. A number of underly-

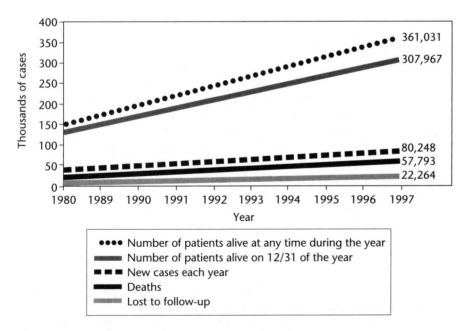

Figure 8.2 End-stage renal disease—trends (1988–1997).

(*Source:* NIH. U.S. Renal Data System. *1999 Annual Data Report*)

ing diseases can cause progressive kidney failure. The two most important of these are diabetes, which in 1998 accounted for 40 percent of the new cases of chronic kidney failure, and high blood pressure, which was responsible for 20 percent of the new cases.

Chronic kidney failure affects people of all ages. The number of new cases peaks in the sixth decade of life, but 25 percent of persons arriving at end-stage in 1998 were under age forty-five, and 1.5 percent, nearly 1,100, were under age twenty. Kidney failure is particularly devastating in childhood, often resulting in impaired growth and development.

A worrisome increase in the number of new cases of kidney failure occurred between 1987 and 1998. The rate increased from 142 per million population in 1987 to 296 per million population in 1997, representing an increase in the annual number of new cases from 34,797 to 87,534 respectively.[8]

This relentless growth in new cases of kidney failure has occurred in spite of the fact that death rates from other diseases, especially cardiovascular diseases, have declined. The increase has not been confined to a single age group. Although the rates of new cases have grown slightly more rapidly for individuals aged seventy-five and older, sizable increases have been noted in every age group.[9] There is a slight preponderance of kidney failure in men. In 1998, the incidence of treated chronic kidney failure was 322 per million population in men, compared with 271 per million in women.[10]

The causes of these increases are not completely understood, but one major factor appears to be an increase in the number of new cases of diabetes, particularly Type II diabetes. In 1987, the rate of new cases of treated chronic kidney failure due to diabetes was 45 per million population. By 1998, the rate had increased to 124 per million population.[11]

Kidney disease has a disproportionate impact on certain racial and ethnic groups, especially African Americans and Native Americans or Alaska Natives. African Americans have the highest overall risk of chronic kidney disease. The reasons are not entirely explained by the higher number of persons in this population who have diabetes and high blood pressure. On average, African Americans develop end-stage kidney failure at an earlier age than whites (55.8 years compared to 62.2 years). Native Americans or Alaska Natives have a much higher risk of chronic kidney disease due to diabetes than whites. Overall, the rates of new cases are 4 times higher in African Americans and Native Americans or Alaska Natives and 1.5 times higher in Asians or Pacific Islanders than in whites.[12] A description of renal disease by race, gender, and age is given in Table 8.3.

End-stage renal disease rates are also greater in certain racial and ethnic populations than in white populations. Rates of new cases are increasing by 7 percent per year for African Americans, 10 percent per year for Native Americans or Alaska Natives, and 11 percent for Asians or Pacific Islanders, compared to 6 percent per year for whites. Two communities of an American Indian tribe, the Zuni Pueblo in New Mexico and in Sacaton, Arizona, may have the highest rates of chronic kidney failure in the world, at 12.6 and 14.0 times the overall

Table 8.3   Incidence of end-stage renal disease (1999).

Total Population, 1999	New Cases of End-Stage Renal Disease Rate per Million
TOTAL	317
Race and ethnicity	
Native American or Alaska Native	652
Asian or Pacific Islander	386
Black or African American	953
White	237
Hispanic or Latino	260
NonHispanic or Latino	325
Gender	
Female	290
Male	346
Age	
Under 20 years	15
20 to 44 years	119
45 to 64 years	603
65 to 74 years	1,317
75 years and older	1,434

(*Source:* Healthy People 2010)

average U.S. rate, respectively. Projections indicate that increases in the rates of new cases will continue in Native Americans or Alaska Natives.[13]

Healthy People 2010 Objective: Reduce the Rate of New Cases of End-Stage Renal Disease (ESRD)

Target: 217 new cases per million population.

Baseline: 289 new cases of end-stage renal disease per million population in 1997.

Chronic Liver Disease and Cirrhosis

The tenth leading cause of death in the United States in 1999 is chronic liver disease and cirrhosis. It appears that diseases associated with death from liver pathology have increased dramatically as a result of the new epidemic of hepatitis C, a viral infection that is spread primarily from sharing infected needles. Hepatitis C is often spread while sharing drugs, or through the misuse of dirty needles used for tattooing, piercing, and branding, popular behaviors among teens and young adults. There are some who believe that hepatitis C may also

---

BOX 8.1 Facts on the Symptoms of Kidney Disease

- People can lose more than half their normal kidney function before they start to notice the symptoms of kidney disease. These symptoms include nausea, vomiting, tiredness, and loss of appetite.
- In many cases, kidney function gets worse, even with the best possible treat-

ment. As kidney failure worsens, the symptoms of chronic renal failure (CRF) also get worse.
- When kidney function is very limited (this is called end-stage renal disease, or ESRD), dialysis is usually prescribed. Some people choose to have a kidney transplant instead of long-term dialysis.

BOX 8.2 Kidney Transplant Statistics

Number of Kidney Transplants (by year)
  1997: 12,399 1996: 12,248 1987: 8,620

Number of Kidney Transplants (by type, 1997)
  From cadaver: 8,523
  From living related donor: 3,217
  From living unrelated donor: 705

People Awaiting Transplants (September 15, 1999)
  Kidney (only): 43,114
  Kidney and pancreas: 1,966

(*Source:* Healthy People 2010)

---

be spread through sexual intercourse, although sexual transmission of hepatitis C between monogamous partners appears to be uncommon. Whether hepatitis C is spread by sexual contact has not been conclusively proven, and studies have been contradictory.

The hepatitis C virus (HCV) is a major cause of both acute and chronic hepatitis in the United States. Hepatitis C, previously known as "non-A, non-B hepatitis," affects between 1 and 2 percent of Americans, and chronic infection with HCV is probably the single most important cause of chronic liver disease, cirrhosis, and liver cancer in the Western world. Not all cases of hepatitis C are severe or progressive. Many patients are asymptomatic and are only diagnosed when they are found to have abnormal liver tests following a blood donation or routine evaluation for another problem. Yet, chronic hepatitis C can be insidious and slowly progressive and lead to cirrhosis and liver failure after years or decades of infection.

HCV accounts for about 20 percent of acute viral hepatitis, 60 to 70 percent of chronic hepatitis, and 30 percent of cirrhosis, end-stage liver disease, and liver cancer. Almost 4 million Americans, or 1.8 percent of the U.S. population, have antibody to HCV (anti-HCV), indicating ongoing or previous infection with the virus. Hepatitis C causes an estimated 8,000 to 10,000 deaths annually in the United States.[14]

BOX 8.3 *Clinical Features of Cirrhosis*

Once a patient develops cirrhosis or if the patient has severe disease, symptoms and signs are more prominent. In addition to fatigue, the patient may complain of muscle weakness, poor appetite, nausea, weight loss, itching, dark urine, fluid retention, and abdominal swelling. Physical findings of cirrhosis may include

1. Enlarged liver
2. Enlarged spleen
3. Jaundice
4. Muscle wasting
5. Excoriations
6. Ankle swelling

Chronic hepatitis C can cause cirrhosis, liver failure, and liver cancer. About 20 percent of patients develop cirrhosis within ten to twenty years of the onset of infection. Liver failure from chronic hepatitis C is one of the most common reasons for liver transplants in the United States. Hepatitis C might be the most common cause of primary liver cancer in the developed world. In Italy, Spain, and Japan, at least half of liver cancers could be related to HCV. Men, alcoholics, patients with cirrhosis, people over age forty, and those infected for twenty to forty years are more likely to develop HCV-related liver cancer.

Prevention

At present, the only means of preventing new cases of hepatitis C are to screen the blood supply, encourage health professionals to take precautions when handling blood and body fluids, and inform people about high-risk behaviors. Programs to promote needle exchange offer some hope of decreasing the spread of hepatitis C among injection drug users. Vaccines and immunoglobulin products do not exist for hepatitis C, and development seems unlikely in the near future because these products would require antibodies to all the genotypes and variants of hepatitis C. Nevertheless, advances in immunology and innovative approaches to immunization make it likely that some form of vaccine for hepatitis C will eventually be developed.[15]

Acquired Immune Deficiency Syndrome

Although deaths from Acquired Immune Deficiency Syndrome (AIDS) have dropped dramatically in the past five years, and it is no longer among the ten leading causes of death in the United States, AIDS remains an incurable epidemic and will be considered in this chapter.

Age-adjusted death rates from HIV infection in the United States declined an unprecedented 47 percent from 1996 to 1997, and HIV infection fell from eighth to fourteenth among leading causes of death in the United States over the same time. For those aged twenty-five to forty-four, HIV dropped from the leading cause of death in 1995 to third-leading in 1996 and fifth-leading in 1997. The age-adjusted HIV death rate of 5.9 deaths per 100,000 is the lowest rate since 1987, the first year mortality data were available for the disease.

Table 8.4   Persons living with HIV infections and AIDS by state and age group (1998).

U.S. state of residence (Date HIV reporting initiated)	Cumulative Totals			U.S. state of residence (Date HIV reporting initiated)	Cumulative Totals		
	Adults/ adolescents	Children <13 years old	Total		Adults/ adolescents	Children <13 years old	Total
Alabama (Jan. 1988)	6,710	59	6,769	New Hampshire	416	3	419
Alaska	212	2	214	New Jersey (Jan. 1992)	23,766	594	24,360
Arizona (Jan. 1987)	5,494	42	5,536	New Mexico (Jan. 1998)	937	8	945
Arkansas (July 1989)	2,864	42	5,536	New York	43,884	781	44,865
California	38,054	210	38,264	North Carolina (Feb. 1990)	10,897	149	11,046
Colorado (Nov. 1985)	7,593	34	7,627	North Dakota (Jan. 1988)	96	1	97
Connecticut (July 1992)[5]	4,960	167	5,127	Ohio (June 1990)	7,066	96	7,162
Delaware	936	10	946	Oklahoma (June 1988)	3,175	24	3,199
District of Columbia	4,730	86	4,816	Oregon (Sept. 1988)	1,717	23	1,740
Florida (July 1997)	34,026	630	34,656	Pennsylvania	8,287	149	8,436
Georgia	8,357	79	8,436	Rhode Island	786	5	771
Hawaii	786	4	770	South Carolina (Fen. 1986)	9,500	131	9,631
Idaho (June 1986)	426	3	429	South Dakota (Jan. 1998)	209	6	215
Illinois	7,391	111	7,502	Tennessee (Jan. 1992)	7,721	61	7,782
Indiana (July 1988)	5,295	39	5,334	Texas (Fen. 1994)[5]	19,640	381	20,021
Iowa	493	4	497	Utah (April 1989)	1,483	12	1,495
Kansas	790	4	794	Vermont	150	2	152
Kentucky	1,171	11	1,182	Virginia (July 1989)	10,925	161	11,086
Louisiana (Feb. 1993)	10,008	149	10,157	Washington	3,405	14	3,419
Maine	363	8	371	West Virginia (Jan. 1989)	841	4	845
Maryland	7,452	156	7,808	Wisconsin (Nov. 1985)	3,327	41	3,388
Massachusetts	4,469	77	4,546	Wyoming (June 1989)	118	2	120
Michigan (April 1992)	7,463	116	7,579	Subtotal	339,162	4,898	344,060
Minnesota (Oct. 1985)	3,517	34	3,551	U.S. dependencies, possessions, and associate nations			
Mississippi (Aug. 1988)	5,042	69	5,111	Guam	7	—	7
Missouri (Oct. 1987)	7,260	62	7,322	Pacific Islands, U.S.	2	—	2
Montana	138	—	136	Puerto Rico	7,712	168	7,878
Nebraska (Sept. 1995)	734	10	744	Virgin Islands, U.S.	182	7	189
Nevada (Feb. 1992)	4,122	35	4,157	Total	347,305	5,074	352,379

1. Includes only persons reported with HIV infection who have not developed AIDS.

2. Persons reported with vital status "alive" as of the last update. Excludes persons whoe vital status is unknown.

3. Includes only persons reported from states with confidential HIV reporting. Excludes 1,777.

(*Source:* CDC: Divisions of HIV/AIDS Prevention Serv. Report Vol. 10, No. 1)

Reductions in AIDS deaths have been due to increased prevention efforts and the use of protease inhibitors in treating HIV infection, but the outlook for those infected with the virus is still not positive; most will die from complications of this disease. Tables 8.4 and 8.5 report the number of HIV/AIDS cases in the United States in 1998.

Human Immunodeficiency Virus (HIV), the virus thought to be the cause of AIDS, was first recognized by American and French virologists in 1981. AIDS is a viral pandemic that is causing immune system failure and ultimately, death,

Table 8.5   AIDS cases by age, gender, and exposure category (1998).

Adult/adolescent exposure category	Males July 1997– June 1998 No. (%)	Males Cumulative total No. (%)	Females July 1997– June 1998 No. (%)	Females Cumulative total No. (%)	Totals July 1997– June 1998 No. (%)	Totals Cumulative total No. (%)
Men who have sex with men	18,893 (45)	317,862 (57)	— —	— —	18,893 (35)	317,862 (48)
Injecting drug use	9,050 (22)	122,933 (22)	3,634 (30)	45,075 (43)	12,684 (23)	168,008 (26)
Men who have sex with men and inject drugs	2,116 (5)	42,093 (8)	— —	— —	2,116 (5)	42,093 (6)
Hemophilia/coagulation disorder	153 (0)	4,559 (1)	13 (0)	222 (0)	166 (0)	4,781 (1)
Heterosexual contact:	2,796 (7)	21,855 (4)	4,419 (37)	40,744 (39)	7,215 (13)	62,599 (10)
Sex with injecting drug user	751	7,728	1,332	17,548	2,083	25,276
Sex with bisexual male	—	—	200	3,009	200	3,009
Sex with person with hemophilia	2	42	22	371	24	413
Sex with transfusion recipient with HIV infection	26	361	28	553	54	914
Sex with HIV-infected person, risk not specified	2,017	13,724	2,837	19,263	4,854	32,987
Recipient of blood transfusion, blood components, or tissue	182 (0)	4,752 (1)	158 (1)	3,559 (3)	340 (1)	8,311 (1)
Other/risk not reported or identified	8,894 (21)	38,994 (7)	3,713 (31)	14,428 (14)	12,608 (23)	53,423 (8)
Adult/adolescent subtotal	42,084 (100)	553,048 (100)	11,937 (100)	104,028 (100)	54,022 (100)	657,077 (100)

(*Source:* CDC: Divisions of HIV/AIDS Prevention Serv. Report Vol. 10, No. 1)

among citizens of all countries of the world. By 2000, more than 208 countries and all 50 states, the District of Columbia, and U.S. dependencies and possessions had reported cases of AIDS. By the end of 2000, more than 775,000 cases of AIDS had been reported, and nearly 448,800 people had died from HIV disease or AIDS. Disparities in the rate of infection among certain racial and ethnic groups, particularly African American and Hispanic populations, remain a challenge. Recently introduced therapies for HIV/AIDS have reduced illness, disability, and death due to HIV/AIDS; however, access to culturally and linguistically appropriate testing and care may limit progress in this area.

The WHO estimates that as many as 20+ million people worldwide may be infected with HIV, which is thought by most experts to cause AIDS. This number may grow to 40 million plus by the year 2010.[16] In most nations the number of reported AIDS cases is doubling every six to twelve months. The distribution of worldwide AIDS cases is described by selected countries in Table 8.6.

Table 8.6   Adult HIV infections (1995–2000).

Geographic Area	1995 high estimate	2000 high estimatae
North America	1,495,000	8,940,000
Western Europe	1,186,000	2,331,000
Oceania	40,000	45,000
Latin America	1,407,000	8,554,000
Sub-Sahara Africa	11,449,000	33,609,000
Caribbean	474,000	6,962,000
Eastern Europe	44,000	20,000
S.E. Mediterranean	59,000	3,532,000
Northeast Asia	80,000	486,000
Southeast Asia	1,220,000	45,059,000
World	17,454,000	109,538,000

(*Source:* CDC: Divisions of HIV/AIDS Prevention)

HIV is a retrovirus that requires replication within a host cell, in this case a T_4 lymphocyte. As HIV replicates, it destroys the T_4 helper cells, which in turn reduces the immune system's ability to produce B cells and fight off antigens or pathogens. When the immune system shuts down, or slows down, a myriad of opportunistic diseases are able to get by the immune system and infect the body. In 1993, the Centers for Disease Control and Prevention announced that a diagnosis of AIDS required: (1) infection by HIV, (2) a T-cell count of less than 200 cells or a CD4+ percentage of less than 14, and/or (3) any of a number of clinical opportunistic diseases that may infect a person as shown in Table 8.7. This definition has helped broaden the diagnosis to women whose opportunistic infections include chronic vaginal yeast infections and invasive cervical cancer, two conditions not included in earlier definitions of the disease.[17]

Being HIV positive(+), or showing antibody exposure to HIV alone, is not a diagnosis of AIDS. There are many people who live years without any other contributing or disabling clinical condition other than seropositivity (testing positive for HIV antibodies). These people do not have AIDS. They are HIV positive, or **carriers**, able to infect others with the virus without showing any signs or symptoms of the disease itself. This is certainly one reason why HIV testing may be important. Those who are HIV positive but show no symptoms will need to be aware of their ability to infect others as well as the need to take care of their own health.

Unfortunately, the initial test for the HIV antibodies, the ELISA test, cannot measure antibodies to the virus until approximately six weeks to three months after exposure. Therefore, this **window period** is a time when a carrier may be infecting others without being able to know for sure if he or she is infected. The most common confirmatory test for HIV is called the Western Blot test.

AIDS can no longer be stigmatized as a male, homosexual disease. The male to female ratios of people infected with HIV in developed countries vary from 15:1 to 20:1, although the ratio is approximately 1:1 in African nations.[18] In

Table 8.7   CDC clinical definition of AIDS.

Summary of Diseases and Conditions

Effective January 1, 1993, the adult/adolescent AIDS case definition of the Centers for Disease Control and Prevention (CDC) was amended to include HIV infection and any of the following clinical conditions.

Candidiasis of bronchi, trachea, or lungs
Candidiasis, esophageal
*Cervical cancer, invasive, diagnosed by microscopy
Coccidioidomycosis, disseminated or extrapulmonary
Cryptococcosis, extrapulmonary
Cryptosporidiosis, chronic intestinal (>1 month duration)
Cytomegalovirus disease (other than liver, spleen, or nodes)
Cytomegalovirus retinitis (with loss of vision)
Encephalopathy, HIV-related
Herpes simplex: chronic ulcer(s) (>1 month duration); or bronchitis, pneumonitis, or esophagitis
Histoplasmosis, disseminated or extrapulmonary
Isosporiasis, chronic intestinal (>1 month duration)
Kaposi's sarcoma (KS)
Lymphoma, Burkitt's (or equivalent term)
Lymphoma, immunoblastic (or equivalent term)
Lymphoma, primary, of brain
Mycobacterium avium complex or *M kansasii,* disseminated or extrapulmonary
Mycobacterium tuberculosis, any site (*pulmonary or extrapulmonary), diagnosed by culture
Mycobacterium, other species or unidentified species, disseminated or extrapulmonary
Pneumocystis carinii pneumonia (PCP)
*Pneumonia, recurrent, diagnosed by both a) culture, and b) radiologic evidence of pneumonia
Progressive multifocal leukoencephalopathy
Salmonella septicemia, recurrent
Toxoplasmosis of brain
Wasting syndrome due to HIV

*CD4+ T-lymphocyte absolute count under 200/mm^3 or percent under 14 (see article on page 3)

(*Source:* Added in the 1993 expansion of the AIDS surveillance case definition, announced in the *Morbity and Mortality Weekly Report* (MMWR) December 18, 1992)

Rumania, health officials have reported over 1,000 cases of children infected with HIV. It is believed that HIV-contaminated blood was injected into Rumanian childrens' umbilical cords to stimulate growth. In China, AIDS, at one time, was thought to be "a foreign problem," but China now reports cases among injection drug users.[19]

In North America and Europe, the highest incidence of AIDS at the present time is among men who have sex with men, and injection drug users. In 2000, an estimated 13,562 AIDS cases were diagnosed among men having sex with men. This was a decrease from 1999 and is thought to be part of a continuing trend. Projected HIV cases are shown in Figure 8.3.

BOX 8.4 *Global Impact of AIDS*

- Global dollar loss from AIDS by year 2000—$514 billion
- In Thailand—1,000 new cases a day.
- In India—Within 5 years 30 percent of truckers will have HIV
- In Brazil—Ranks 4th in global AIDS cases

- In Dominican Republic—9 percent of sugar cane workers have HIV
- In Uganda—8.3 percent of the population has HIV
- In Zambia—The Copper Belt has 45 percent of AIDS cases

Studies of survival rates in New York City show that African American and Hispanic injection drug users die far more quickly on average than gay men. This finding suggests that poverty and access to health services may play an important role during the course of the disease.[20] The male-to-female ratio is between 20:1 to 15:1, and heterosexual transmission represents a small, though increasing, percentage of cases.[21]

In Africa (36 percent of the worldwide cases) and South America (12 percent of the worldwide cases), the highest incidence is among heterosexuals with almost equal numbers of women and men. African women with AIDS are often wrongly characterized as prostitutes. Prostitution is not more common in Africa than elsewhere, but rapidly declining economic conditions and lack of security

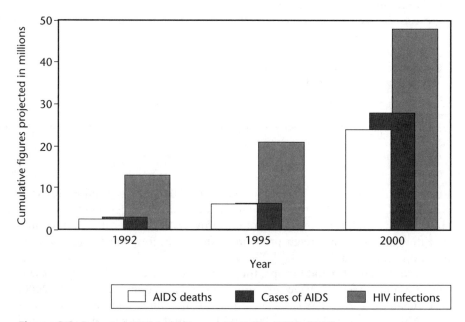

Figure 8.3 Projected HIV Morbidity and Mortality (1992–2000).

(*Sources:* Centers for Disease Control. National Center for Health Statistics)

Healthy People 2010 Objective: Reduce AIDS Among Adolescents and Adults

Target: 1.0 new case per 100,000 persons.

Baseline: 19.5 cases of AIDS per 100,000 persons aged 13 years and older in 1998. Data are estimated; adjusted for delays of AIDS in reporting.

in the war zones have led more women to barter or sell sexual services to meet their basic needs. A good deal of female sexual behavior in Africa can be viewed as economic survival and adaptation to patterns of male dominance.[22]

The origin of HIV is still unknown and its unique RNA nucleus and mutating properties are not well understood. All world health organizations agree that the most important control factors available to us at this time are AIDS-related information and education, ensuring a safe blood supply, and providing adequate care to those already infected.[23]

HIV infection rates appear to have stabilized since the early 1990s at about 40,000 new infections per year, which represents a slowing from growth rates experienced in the mid-1980s. About 750,000 to 900,000 persons in the United States are estimated to be infected with HIV, with over 200,000 to 250,000 persons who are not aware of their infection. About 250,000 persons are estimated to be in treatment with new antiretroviral treatment therapies, and another 250,000 are not currently in treatment.[24]

Significant changes in the epidemic have occurred over time. In 1992, AIDS became a leading cause of death among persons aged twenty-five to forty-four years, but by 1999 had dropped to the eighth leading cause of death in this age group. In 1997, HIV/AIDS remained the leading cause of death only for African Americans among persons in this age group. Between 1992 and 1997, the number of persons reported living with AIDS increased in all groups as a result of the 1993 expanded AIDS case definition and, more recently, improved survival rates due to new treatment. [25]

Some of these changes are reflected in the following:

1. Women accounted for just under 14 percent of persons over age thirteen years living with AIDS in 1992, compared with 20 percent in 1998.

2. By the end of 1998, the number of African Americans living with AIDS, which increased from 33 percent of the AIDS population in 1992 to 40 percent in 1998, was almost identical to the number of whites living with AIDS.

3. Persons living in the South accounted for 34 percent of AIDS cases in 1992 and 38.5 percent in 1998. Persons living in the Northeast accounted for 28.3 percent in 1992 and 31.0 percent in 1998. The proportion living in the West declined from 23.8 percent to 20.8 percent.

4. By December 1998, approximately 297,136 persons were reported to be living with AIDS, compared with 269,775 in 1997.[26]

Healthy People 2010 Objective: Reduce the Number of New AIDS Cases Among Adolescent and Adult Men Who Have Sex with Men

Target: 13,385 new cases.

Baseline: 17,847 new cases of AIDS in 1998 among males aged 13 years and older. Data are estimated; risk is redistributed; adjusted for delays in reporting.

AIDS is an obviously serious, sexually transmitted disease that is also passed through blood inoculation of needle sticks or transfusions, sharing injection drug "works," and organ, tissue, or sperm donation. Labor migration, transporting of goods, mobilization of armed forces, migration of peoples due to famine and drought, and overwhelming poverty, are dynamic means of spreading HIV across borders.

Among the many lessons that AIDS has taught public health, perhaps the most sobering is that the world can still be victim to pandemics that may destroy a significant part of our planet's population. It is understood that infection with HIV is lifelong, and that an individual may be an asymptomatic carrier of HIV for as many as ten years or longer (the incubation period) before experiencing the distinctive immune system failure that ultimately leads to numerous opportunistic infections that kill almost all persons with AIDS at this point in time.

HIV/AIDS in the United States

In the United States, African Americans and Hispanics have been affected disproportionately by HIV and AIDS, compared to other racial and ethnic groups. Through December 2000, 774,467 cases of AIDS had been reported among persons of all ages and racial and ethnic groups, including 331,160 cases among whites, 292,522 cases among African Americans, and 141,694 cases among Hispanics. Although 55 percent of the reported AIDS cases occurred among African Americans and Hispanics, these two population groups represent an estimated 13 percent and 12 percent, respectively, of the total U.S. population.[27]

In 2000, AIDS remained the leading cause of death for all African Americans aged 25 to 44 years; the second leading cause among African American females and the leading cause among African American males. In 1996, for the first time, African Americans accounted for a larger proportion of AIDS cases than whites, and this trend has continued. The AIDS case rate among African Americans in calendar year 1998 was 66.4 per 100,000 persons, or eight times the rate for whites (8.2 per 100,000) and over twice the rate for Hispanics (28.1 per 100,000).[28]

Among women with AIDS, African Americans and Hispanics have been especially affected, accounting for nearly 77 percent of cumulative cases reported among women by 2000. Of the 130,104 AIDS cases in women reported through December 2000, 77,624 cases occurred in African American women and 26,625 occurred in Hispanic women.

For young adults aged twenty to tweny-four years, 27,232 cumulative AIDS cases were reported through December 2000. Of this total, 11,603 (42 percent) occurred among African Americans, 9,432 (35 percent) among whites, and 5,833 (21 percent) among Hispanics. Overall, 73 percent of the AIDS cases in this age group occurred among males and 27 percent among females. Among African Americans in this age group, 63 percent were male, and 37 percent were female. Among Hispanics, 74 percent were male, and 26 percent were female. Because the time from initial infection with HIV to the development of AIDS is long and variable (often eight to ten years or more), many of these young adults likely acquired their infections while in their teens.[29]

Among teenagers aged thirteen to nineteen years, 4,061 cumulative AIDS cases had been reported through December 2000. In this age group, 1,147 cases (28 percent) occurred among whites, 2,041 (50 percent) among African Americans, and 809 (20 percent) among Hispanics. Overall, males accounted for 61 percent of the AIDS cases in this age group, and females accounted for 39 percent. Among African American teenagers with AIDS, 46 percent were male, and 54 percent were female. Among Hispanic teens, 67 percent of those with AIDS were male, and 33 percent were female. Among white teenagers with AIDS, 79 percent were male, and 21 percent were female.[30]

The disproportionate impact of HIV/AIDS on African Americans and Hispanics underscores the importance of implementing and sustaining effective prevention efforts for these racial and ethnic populations. HIV prevention efforts must take into account not only the multiracial and multicultural nature of society, but also other social and economic factors such as poverty, underemployment, and poor access to the health care system. These factors affect health status and disproportionately affect African American, Hispanic, Alaska Native, and American Indian populations.

Prevention

Global Perspective   The 1985 Global AIDS Strategy of the WHO had three objectives: (1) Prevent HIV transmission, (2) reduce the personal and social impact of HIV and AIDS, and (3) unify national and international efforts against the disease. In 1987, the General Assembly of the United Nations held a general session to encourage a network of organizations to work together under the guidance of the WHO to implement the Global AIDS Strategy objectives.[31]

Willingness and ability of governments to face the AIDS epidemic around the world vary greatly. Many African nations had been reluctant to acknowledge their AIDS rates because of the potential threat to tourism, a major economic base for some countries. Until the Soviet nations became independent, the USSR was reporting no cases of AIDS and doing little but warehousing their existing cases.

Brazil, with one of the highest prevalence rates in the world, has tried vigorous health education programs in an attempt to control this epidemic. Most European countries have followed suit with information programs in schools, media, and clinics.[32]

Most European governments have undertaken education programs. Switzerland (as did the United States) sent an educational brochure to every household. In the Netherlands and France, injection drug users are supplied with new, clean syringes and needles in exchange for used ones, and in some countries syringes are now sold over the counter. These public health efforts to prevent further injection drug use infection have been met, perhaps understandably, with criticism. Many people, generally outside public health, believe that having easy access to needles promotes injection drug use, not HIV prevention.[33] In 2000, an estimated 10,079 United States cases were diagnosed among adult men and women who injected drugs. This was a decrease from the previous year and part of a continuing trend.

U.S. Perspective   The same thinking—that information and supplies promote, rather than inhibit risky behavior—has been a major obstacle in early and preventive behavior in the United States. The United States was late off the starting block according to most experts. President Reagan did not mention the word, AIDS, until 1987, six years into the epidemic. The Surgeon General's information about AIDS was finally sent to every home in 1989, but it was thought to be too explicit by some because it discussed, in little detail, oral and anal sexual penetration, and homosexuality.[34]

The distribution of condoms, or even the discussion of condom use, a cornerstone of HIV prevention, is still controversial in many parts of the United States. Again, the basis of controversy is that if you give people (particularly teens) information or access to condoms they will then be inclined to become sexually active. Research does not support this premise. Those who are presently sexually active may be more inclined to use condoms if they are available (although there is still great resistance among adolescents), and those who are not sexually active at present will make their personal decision to do so based on many other considerations.

Although refraining from intercourse with infected partners remains the most effective strategy for preventing HIV infection and other STDs, the Public Health Service also has recommended condom use as part of its strategy. Latex condoms are highly effective for preventing HIV infection and other STDs when used consistently and correctly. Laboratory studies indicate that nonoxynol–9, a spermicide, inactivates HIV and other STD pathogens.[35] Laboratory studies indicate that the female condom (Reality™)—a lubricated polyurethane sheath with a ring on each end that is inserted into the vagina—is an effective mechanical barrier to viruses, including HIV.[36]

Internationally, condom distribution has met with some local resistance as well because of cultural, religious, "machismo," and economic reasons. The United States Agency for International Development has supplied about 500 million condoms annually worldwide, primarily for family planning. The strong role of the Catholic Church in many countries, which prohibits contraceptive use, has made condom acceptance by the public difficult to achieve.[37]

AIDS is probably the most perilous epidemic in modern time as may be seen by the increasing cases shown on Figure 8.3. It will require the complete cooperation of the international community, changes in beliefs, and a new look at sexual behavior by the people of the world to control and then eradicate this virus from the planet.

Summary

The emergence of liver diseases and kidney diseases among our leading causes of death in the United States demonstrates the complexity of the tasks before community health educators. These two health problems are somewhat unpreventable in the traditional sense that changes in behavior can prevent illness. They are often the result of a secondary infection or implication of a greater problem such as diabetes and hepatitis C. Therefore, it is important for health educators to work more closely with primary care givers to help patients interpret the conditions from which they suffer and help them make good life decisions that will improve quality of life and reduce the chance of a fatality associated with infection.

HIV/AIDS is a world community health concern. Trends show that HIV will not be eradicated anytime soon; therefore prevention and treatment of those infected needs to be a major focus despite the good news that AIDS is no longer among our ten leading causes of death. An important concept is that HIV is a disease of behaviors—not particular groups of people. Aims at reducing high-risk behaviors among all individuals should continue to be a community health prevention effort. If prevention behaviors become lax, as we are seeing among youth and young gay men, there is only one way for incidence of HIV to go.

Suicide is another leading cause of death, especially among those fifteen to twenty-four years, Native Americans, and older adults. Although the stresses of everyday life and the escalation of social ills seem oppressive and overwhelming to some, suicide is not a coping mechanism. It is permanent; social conditions and personal problems will change.

Cybersites Related to Chapter 8

AIDS
   hivinsite.ucsf.edu/InSite
   www.14aidsinfo.com
   www.aids101.com

Suicide
   www.suicidology.org
   www.afsp.org
   www.pbs.org/weblab/living/

Questions

1. Why are current public health efforts to prevent HIV still controversial in the United States? Why are they controversial in less developed countries?

2. Why was the United States so slow to respond to the AIDS epidemic? Why was it handled so differently than Legionnaires' disease?

3. What are the signs of depression that may lead to suicide?

4. What are the socioeconomic factors that contribute to homicide?

EXERCISES

1. Go to your local AIDS testing center and be tested for HIV. How does it feel to wait for the test results? Who will you tell that you are going for testing? To whom will you tell the results if you are positive? If you are negative?

2. Read your community newspaper for two weeks. Look for articles that report homicides or suicides. Now, pretend you are an epidemiologist. What are the demographic characteristics of those involved with these violent acts? What variables and interactions contribute to the host, agent, and environment of the incident? What community health interventions might have prevented these tragic acts of violence?

INTERNET INTERACTIVE ACTIVITY

THE EPIDEMIOLOGY OF HIV/AIDS

Epidemiological Fact Sheets contain the most recent country-specific data on HIV/AIDS prevalence and incidence, together with information on behaviors (e.g., casual sex and condom use) that can spur or stem the transmission of HIV. The data include prevention indicators originally developed by WHO's Global Program on AIDS, which aims to measure trends in knowledge of AIDS, relevant behaviors, and a host of other factors influencing the epidemic. The homepage for Epidemiological Fact Sheets is:

www.who.int/emc-hiv/fact_sheets/index.html

Exercise

In this exercise the community health educator will compare the epidemiology of HIV/AIDS in the United States with two other countries in the world.

1. Using the Epidemiological Fact Sheets, select two regions of the world and then a country in each region, and explore the epidemiology of HIV/AIDS in those two countries.

2. Describe the HIV/AIDS epidemic by building a table using these demographic characteristics:

age
gender
location
sexual orientation
mode of transmission
access to health care
condom availability and use
other significant variables

3. Now go to the CDC Division of HIV/AIDS Prevention homepage: www.cdc.gov/nchstp/hiv_aids/dhap.htm

4. Click on **Fact Sheets, Whats New, and Slide Sets**

5. Using the **view slides** icons, search through the CDC slide presentations and fill in your table with the HIV/AIDS demographic characteristics you used to describe your foreign countries.

   characteristics
   age
   gender
   location
   sexual orientation
   mode of transmission
   access to health care
   condom availability and use
   other significant variables

6. What are the primary differences and similarities in the HIV/AIDS epidemic among your three countries?

References

1. www.health.gov/healthypeople/Document/HTML/Volume2/18Mental.htm#_Toc471966636

2. www.health.gov/healthypeople/Document/HTML/Volume2/18Mental.htm#_Toc471966636

3. www.surgeongeneral.gov/library/calltoaction/fact1.htm)

4. *U.S. News and World Report* (1993). The mind in its despair. August 9, p. 58.

5. Ibid.

6. www.health.gov/healthypeople/Document/HTML/Volume1/04CKD.htm

7. www.niddk.nih.gov/health/kidney(2000). Kidney and Urology Statistics for the United States.

8. Ibid.

9. Ibid.

10. Ibid.

11. Ibid.

12. USRDS. (1999). ADR. Bethesda, MD: NIH, NIDDE, April. Tables A-1 and A-14.

13. www.niddk.nih.gov/health/kidney/pubs/kustats/kustats.htm

14. gi.ucsf.edu/ALF/info/chcniddk.html#A

15. Ibid.

16. Green, L. W., & Ottoson, J. M. (1994). *Community health.* St. Louis: Mosby.

17. CDC (1993). HIV/AIDS Surveillance report. Third quarter. *5*(3), October.

18. Shannon, G.W., Pyle, G.F., & Bashshur, R.L. (1990). *The geography of AIDS: Origins and course of epidemic.* New York: Guilford Press.

19. Ibid.

20. Cohen, F. L.(1993). HIV infection and AIDS: An overview. In F. L. Cohen & J. D. Durham (eds.), *Women, children and HIV/AIDS.* New York: Springer, pp. 3–30.

21. Mann, J. (1992). Health promotion against AIDS: A topology. In J. Sepulveda, H. Fineberg (Eds). *AIDS prevention through education: A world view.* New York: Oxford University Press, pp. 21–31.

22. Turshen, Meredeth (1989). *The politics of public health.* New Jersey: Rutgers University Press.

23. Cohen, op. cit.

24. www.health.gov/healthypeople/Document/HTML/Volume1/13HIV.htm

25. Ibid.

26. Ibid.

27. www.cdc.gov/hiv/stats/cumulati.html(2001). Basic Statistics.

28. Ibid.

29. Ibid.

30. Ibid.

31. Mann, op. cit.

32. Mann, J., Tarantola, D., & Netter, T. (1992). *AIDS in the world.* Cambridge: Harvard University Press.

33. Brown, P. (1992). World AIDS programme "lacks vision." *New Scientist 1086*(14).

34. Shilts, Randy (1988). *And the band played on.* New York: Penguin Books.

35. CDC (1993). Update: Barrier protection against HIV infection and other sexually transmitted diseases. MMWR, Vol. 43 (30). August 6. pp. 589–591.

36. Ibid.

37. Mann, op. cit.

Section III

Underserved Populations in Community Health

Chapters 9 through 13 explore the unique characteristics and behaviors, and the physical, cultural, and political implications of one's community that may put similar people at risk for health problems. These chapters attempt to introduce some of the primary target groups to community health educators. Knowing the people and their lifestyles assists community health educators when they initiate risk assessments, plan programs to prevent unhealthy behaviors or improve environments, and implement programs that are sensitive to diversity within any community. A health professional must adapt health programs and interventions to the specific qualities of the target population. The Internet sites referred to at the end of each chapter may help the reader explore in more depth the immediate perspectives and needs of the targeted groups.

CHAPTER 9

Infants, Children, and Adolescents

Community Health in the 21st Century
Access to health care, injury prevention, and domestic violence will still be major health issues in the 21st Century. Promoting early and regular prenatal and well-child care through public awareness activities, incentives, and health education will continue.

—Stephen P. McDonald, MSS; Baby Your Baby
Outreach Program Manager

Chapter Objectives

The student will:

1. compare the primary causes of infant death worldwide with infant death in the United States.

2. list the World Summit for Children's goals for the year 2000.

3. know the primary prevention measure for reducing infant death.

4. list the major health risks for adolescents.

5. discuss the implications of poverty on the health of children.

6. discuss the role and implication of gangs and violence on teen health.

The Children of the Planet

Looking at morbidity and mortality data, children and adolescents are healthier today than at any time in history. This good news does not negate the reality, however, that many preventable illnesses, traumas, abuses, and risks threaten the health and life of young people and a decline in overall health status may have begun. From birth until adulthood, families and society are directly responsible for the health of children and adolescents. Increased rates of chronic diseases, accidental death, and high risk behaviors suggest that we may not be doing our job in preventing unnecessary illness and death within this population.

The transition from childhood to adulthood is expected to be marked for many by potentially deadly "rites of passage" that are rather new to the end of

Table 9.1   Infant mortality rates in selected developed and developing countries (1998) (per 1,000).

Developing Countries	Rate	Developing Countries	Rate
Japan	4.4	Algeria	44.5
Finland	5.0	Egypt	54.2
Sweden	5.2	Tunisia	37.1
Hong Kong	5.8	Nigeria	73.0
China	38.0	Ghana	83.1
Canada	6.5	Tanzania	104.3
Germany	6.3	Rwanda	125.2
France	7.2	South Africa	48.3
Scotland	7.3	Iraq	95.4
Australia	6.0	Afghanistan	155.8
Israel	7.6	Bangladesh	78.9
Italy	7.6	India	76.4
United States	7.1	Yemen	103.5
Greece	8.2	Zaire	102.6
Puerto Rico	9.7	Cambodia	102.6
Costa Rica	86.0	Somalia	115.8
Chile	13.6	Nepal	82.5

(*Source:* www.unicef.org/sowc98/tab3.htm)

the twentieth and beginning of the twenty-first century. These include violence, handguns, delinquency, drugs, binge drinking, and HIV. Those youth growing up in urban areas are likely to be most at risk.[1]

Infant Mortality

Most epidemiologists believe the most important measure of the health of a community or nation is the infant mortality rate, the number of deaths of children under one year of age per 1,000 live births. In the nineteenth century, only three of ten newborn infants on the planet lived beyond the age of twenty-five. Of the seven who did not survive, two had died before they reached their first birthday. In 2000, only one in seven died before age one. In developing countries, almost one-fourth of children die before their fifth birthday due to preventable communicable illness and preventable socioeconomic and geopolitical distress.

Infant mortality rates for selected developed countries, contrasted with infant mortality rates of less developed countries, are given in Table 9.1. The dramatic differences in rates between these two populations should trigger a picture of the overall health of less developed nations.

Each hour almost 2,000 children worldwide die of illness and malnutrition. It is estimated that 210 million people worldwide (children and adults) do not have an adequate food supply and suffer from "wasting" malnutrition or thinness, while 1,300 million are "stunted" or abnormally short.[2] Disease and malnutrition contribute to lifelong physical and mental disability and lower life expectancy. In developing countries almost one-fourth of children die before their fifth birthday due to preventable communicable illness and preventable socioeconomic and geopolitical distress. Annually, at least 150 million episodes of diarrhea occur in children under the age of five. An estimated 4 million children die each year as a result. Difficulty in obtaining an adequate quantity of clean water and safe food, and the lack of basic sanitation, are major causes of diarrhea in young children. Despite an international effort to clean the planet's water, 1,131 million people in developing countries (excluding China) have no access to clean water. Further, 1,750 million people are without sanitation facilities.[3]

In 1990, seventy heads of state and representatives from 159 nations came together on behalf of the world's children. The World Summit for Children unanimously adopted a declaration to meet nine major goals by the year 2000. They agreed to:

1. reduce infant mortality by one-third

2. reduce child malnutrition by 50 percent

3. eliminate micronutrient deficiencies and empower women to breastfeed

4. reduce maternal mortality by 50 percent

5. obtain 90 percent immunization coverage

6. a 95 percent decrease in measles deaths and an end to polio and tetanus

7. create universal access to high-quality family planning services

8. provide safe water and sanitation for all families

9. insure at least a basic education for 80 percent of all children.[4]

The more developed countries were expected to contribute about one-third of the estimated $20 billion annual cost. The 1993 United States share was $510 million. This contribution to the children of the planet was taken from military and security assistance funding abroad, a reasonable reallocation of funds given the reduction of tension and the increase of child deprivation in the world.

Infant Mortality in the United States   In 1998, 28,045 infants died before their first birthday, which resulted in a record low infant mortality rate of 7.2 per 1,000 births. This improvement is probably a result of a major health initiative in the United States to improve birth weight through increased prenatal care. Other public health programs also decreased SIDS deaths. Despite these successes, as of 1998, the U.S. infant mortality rate ranked twenty-fifth among industrialized nations and the infant mortality rate for males (8.0 per 1,000) was still 21 percent higher than for females (6.6 per 1,000). Infant death rates by race are given in Table 9.2. African American infant deaths certainly are the target population for prevention.

The leading causes of death in 1998 for infants are listed in Table 9.3. The major causes of death continue to be congenital anomalies, low birth weight,

Table 9.2   Infant death rates by race (1998).

Characteristics	All races	White	Black	Native American	Asian/Pacific Islander
	— Race of Mother				
	Infant mortality rates per 1,000 live births in specific group				
Total	7.2	6.0	13.7	8.7	5.0
Age at death					
Total neonatal	4.8	4.0	9.2	4.5	3.2
Early neonatal (<7 days)	3.8	3.1	7.7	3.4	2.5
Late neonatal (7–21 days)	0.9	0.8	1.6	1.1	0.7
Postneonatal	2.4	2.1	4.5	4.2	1.8

(*Sources:* Centers for Disease Control. National Center for Health Statistics)

Table 9.3   Leading causes of infant death, all races (1998).

Cause	Number	Rate per 100,000
All causes	28,488	722.3
Congential anomalies	6,266	158.9
Disorders relating to short gestation and unspecified low birth weight	4,011	101.7
Sudden infant death syndrome	2,529	64.1
Respiratory distress syndrome	1,328	33.7
Newborn affected by maternal complications of pregnancy	1,328	33.7
Newborn affected by complications of placenta, cord, and membranes	932	23.6
Infections specific to the perinatal period	815	20.7
Accidents and adverse effects	726	18.4
Intrauterine hypoxia and birth asphyxia	459	11.6
Pneumonia and influenza	400	10.1
All other causes (Residual)	9,694	245.8

(*Sources:* Centers for Disease Control. National Center for Health Statistics)

SIDS, respiratory distress, and maternal complications of pregnancy. Because of birth defects—the leading cause of infant deaths—the infant mortality rate will be hard to reduce to meet national goals, according to a Centers for Disease Control (CDC) study. Whereas death from other causes was reduced, no one knows how to prevent most birth defects, which now total 23.2 percent of deaths of babies one year or younger. The other two major causes of infant mortality were low birth weight/prematurity/respiratory distress syndrome (18 percent), and sudden infant death syndrome (14 percent). Sadly, the Healthy People 2010 goal of reducing infant death from the current level of 7.2 per 1,000 to 45 per 1,000 is probably not attainable because deaths due to birth defects are poorly understood. Also, the death rate for infants who weigh below five pounds may be improved with proper nutrition and prenatal care, but unfortunately birth defects are often the underlying cause of death in these cases. To make major gains against infant mortality there needs to be a focus on understanding birth defects.[5]

Overall, in 1998 black babies in the United States had a far greater infant mortality rate (13.7 per 1,000 births) than white babies (6.0 per 1,000), Hispanic babies (6.3 per 1,000), Asian/Pacific Islanders (5.0 per 1,000) or Native American (8.7 per 1,000),[6] a fact previously thought to be due to lack of access to quality care by blacks. However, a study in the *New England Journal of Medicine,* in 1992, reported that even when poverty is no longer a factor, black babies still have a higher death rate. Researchers compared the death rates of more than 900,000 black and white children born to couples who were college educated. When controlling for socioeconomic standards, mortality rates among black infants were still 82 percent higher than among whites. Even with apparently similar prenatal care and similar birth weights for black infants, mortality is still higher. Public health must stop assuming the conventional wisdom that it is only poverty and poor medical care that are to blame for high black infant mortality. Something else, yet to be identified, needs to be addressed and prevented. Mortality surveillance, although crude, nevertheless shows a falling trend at early ages over this past century, particularly among more developed countries, and particularly in infants after the first week of life. Beyond these trends, the risk of early death varies markedly and consistently with other sociobiological characteristics of the mother, such as her age, number of births, and whether or not she is supported, as well as with disadvantageous personal habits like smoking or alcohol consumption.[7]

Healthy People 2010 Objective: Reduce Infant Deaths

Reduction in Infant Deaths	1998 Baseline	2010 Target
	Rate per 1,000 Live Births	
All infant deaths (within 1 year)	7.2	4.5
Neonatal deaths (within the first 28 days of life)	4.8	2.9
Postneonatal deaths (between 28 days and 1 year)	2.4	1.5

Discussion: Why are different populations given different target goals and objectives for infant mortality? Why isn't the goal no infant deaths?

Low Birth Weight

Other than congenital anomalies and Sudden Infant Death Syndrome (SIDS), the most important variable in infant mortality is low birth weight (less than about 5.5 pounds), which may reflect the effect of maternal deprivation and whether it was a single or multiple birth. Worldwide, 24 million low birth weight babies are born every year.

Healthy People 2010 Objective: Reduce Number of Low Birth Weight (LBW) and Very Low Birth Weight (VLBW) Infants

Reduction in Low and Very Low Birth Weight	1998 Baseline	2010 Target
	Percent	
Low birth weight (LBW)	7.6	5.0
Very low birth weight (VLBW)	1.4	0.9

It is known that four common pregnancy problems contribute to nearly all excess low birth weight infant mortality:

1. Rupture or infection of the amniotic membrane (38 percent)

2. Premature labor (21 percent)

3. High blood pressure (12 percent)

4. Uterine bleeding (10 percent)

All of these conditions are treatable, which suggests that reducing infant mortality lies in improving the overall health of women.

Smoking accounts for 20 to 30 percent of all LBW births in the United States. The effect of smoking on LBW rates appears to be attributable to intrauterine growth retardation rather than to preterm delivery. Very low birth weight is primarily associated with preterm birth, which may be associated with the use of illicit drugs during pregnancy.

Race also is a factor in birth weight, however, until more is known, it is more likely due to socioeconomic status than race. The marked gap in infant mortality rates between whites and blacks mirrors the over two-fold difference in the rate of low birth weight babies of whites (.93 percent) and blacks (2.55 percent).

When the nutrition of pregnant women is adequate, and prenatal care is complete, low infant birth weight can be averted. For Medicaid mothers making less than six prenatal visits, 18.5 percent indicate low birth weight; for those making over ten visits, only 9 percent of their babies indicate low birth weight. As the number of prenatal visits increase, the infant mortality rate for Medicaid mothers has decreased 40 percent, from 20.4 to 12.4 per 1,000 births.

The National Women's Health Network and the Black Women's Health Project have proposed a U.S. government increase in funding of prenatal education, care, and nutrition. These are the best preventive measures for infant mortality that could be provided. Improving birth weight will also reduce the approximately 21,000 babies who suffer major handicaps that begin in utero including cerebral palsy, some forms of blindness, deafness, and severe mental retardation. Research also shows that 15 percent to 25 percent of low birth weight children also suffer behavior problems, lowered IQ, attention disorders, and development problems. The community health implications of such a poor beginning of life are the long-term developmental, school-related, job-related and social relationship problems these children will face as they age.

The Healthy People objective for the year 1990 (which was not met) was a reduction in **perinatal death rates** (late fetal deaths over 28 weeks gestation plus infant deaths up to seven days old, expressed as a rate per 1,000 live births) to no more than 5.5 per 1,000. The perinatal death rate for high-risk, indigent women is 8.4 per 1,000. This may be due, in part, to reductions in funding for clinical sites for poor women.

Life Expectancy

In 2000, life expectancy at birth reached a record high in the United States of 76.9 years. The expectation of life at birth for 2000 represents the average number of years that a group of infants would live if the infants were to experience throughout life the age-specific death rates prevailing in 2000. Women currently outlive men by an average of 6.8 years, and white persons are expected to outlive black persons by an average of 6.9 years.[9]

It has been the majority opinion in public health that life expectancy has increased in the last century due to a reduction in infant disease, particularly communicable diseases. Communicable diseases such as smallpox, polio, TB, meningitis, and pneumonia have become less threatening as personal hygiene practices, immunization of children, and new treatment modalities evolved during the last sixty years. It is believed, however, that these developments actually contribute relatively little to increased life span. By 1900, before antibiotics and immunization, the death rate had dropped dramatically in the United States seemingly as a result in public health sanitation efforts. The decrease in the incidence of communicable diseases actually seems to be the result of reduced contact with the microorganisms that cause diseases such as cholera, typhoid, and TB due to purification of water, better sewage disposal, food hygiene, and pasteurization of milk. These public health measures, as well as community efforts to improve conditions in the home, at work, in the environment, and in the world that newborns face have caused a dramatic reduction in infant mortality since 1900.

Nutrition

Perhaps the greatest contributor to life expectancy and reduction in infant mortality is improved nutrition. An adequate diet that provides the necessary nutrients for good health also provides resistance to disease. As people started to eat a more nutritionally balanced meal around the turn of the century, there was also a reduction in childhood scarlet fever and measles due to the immune resistance to pathogens.

In developing countries nutrition is the most important factor in response to infection. The World Health Organization has reported that the best vaccine is an adequate diet. With massive malnutrition worldwide, it is no wonder that infant mortality in most developing countries is astronomical. The World Bank in 1984 estimated that infant mortality is ten to twenty times higher in the developing countries than in the West. Half of this increase is nutritionally related. In 1998, about 50 percent of deaths among children under five were associated with malnutrition.[10]

Family Planning

Finally, infant mortality is decreased by community or national programs that include accessibility to contraception and family planning. Unfortunately, high infant mortality rates often make parents in developing countries, where children are a measure of economic upward mobility, less responsive to family planning programs. In developing countries where seven of ten children die before adulthood there is a sense of urgency about continual pregnancy to create a large family. In spite of these health factors, it is difficult to convince some people to pay the economic, religious, and social costs of using birth control. Social and religious values must often be weighed against health and quality of life, and these are not easy decisions to make.

SIDS

Sudden Infant Death Syndrome (SIDS) hit a record low in 1998 with 2,866 crib deaths, down from 3,050 in 1996. Much research has shown that a non-prone sleeping position (that is, sleeping on the side or back rather than the stomach) greatly decreases the risk of SIDS among healthy full-term infants. However, healthy preterm infants have been shown to be more vulnerable to respiratory problems when put to sleep on their backs. The American Academy of Pediatrics has recommended that healthy full-term infants be put down to sleep on their backs. The National Institute of Child Health and Human Development and the Maternal and Child Health Bureau instituted the "Back to Sleep" campaign in 1994 to educate parents and physicians about this recommendation. While the percentage of infants put to sleep on their stomachs dropped dramatically between 1992 and 1997, much of the improvement was in the percentage of infants put to sleep on their sides. Although not as dangerous as the stomach, from this position infants may roll onto their stomachs. Therefore, the objective focuses on increasing the percentage of infants who are put down to sleep on their backs.[11] A NCHS study found that blacks and Southerners are more likely to put their babies to sleep on their stomach, which suggests that more education is required.

Healthy People 2010 Objective: Increase the Percentage of Healthy Full-Term Infants Who Are Put Down to Sleep on Their Backs

Target: 70 percent.

Baseline: 35 percent of healthy full-term infants were put down to sleep on their backs in 1996.

Children, Adolescents, and Young Adults

Since the health of a nation is most commonly measured by the infant mortality rate, it is not surprising that the health and welfare of children is probably one of the most important public health endeavors. It provides the opportunity of laying the foundations of good adult health and it is the best means of preventing future public health problems. Overall, the generation of school children born in the 1980s is the first to be less healthy and less cared for than their parents were at their age. The dramatic shift from communicable disease mortality (aside from AIDS) for young people is now in the direction of violence, abuse, and neglect.

Of the 37,000 young people who die each year, 30 percent are killed in car crashes, almost half of them linked to alcohol. Roughly 10,000 are murdered, commit suicide, or die from the complications of AIDS.[12]

Overall, substantial declines in U.S. childhood mortality have occurred in the past four decades, primarily due to decreases in mortality from unintentional injuries, cancer, pneumonia, influenza, and congenital anomalies. Internationally the primary causes of death among children are infectious diseases (63 percent), perinatal complications (20 percent), noncommunicable conditions (8 percent), and injuries (6 percent) (Figure 9.1). However, there has been a two-fold increase in suicide and homicide rates among children since 1968. Male, black, Native American, Hawaiian, and Puerto Rican children, and those in lower socioeconomic strata were at an increased risk of death.

Healthy People 2010 Objective: Reduce the Rate of Child Deaths

Reduction in Deaths of Children	1998 Baseline	2010 Target
	Rate per 100,000	
Children aged 1 to 4 years	34.2	25.0
Children aged 5 to 9 years	17.6	14.3

Decreases in mortality are a result of improvements in socioeconomic and living conditions, better nutrition, advances in medical knowledge and technology, improved medical care, and the introduction of Medicaid. There have been fewer accidents due to motor vehicle safety, mandatory use of seat belts, and efforts to curb drinking while driving. In 1998 there were 5,606 teen driver, crash-related deaths, which accounted for 14 percent of all highway deaths.

Childhood mortality continues to be higher in the United States than in most of its international peers due to higher cardiovascular disease, injury and violence, and suicide. In fact, the CDC has determined that 72 percent of all deaths among school-age youth and young adults ages five to twenty-four are from only four causes: accidents (30 percent), other unintentional injuries (12 percent), homicide (19 percent), and suicide (11 percent).[13] Other problems that commonly afflict this age group are one million adolescent pregnancies and

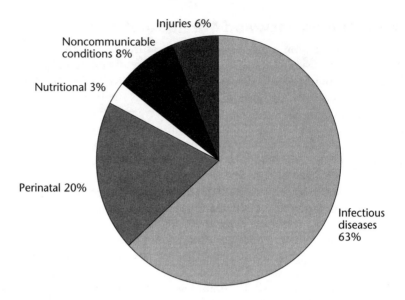

Figure 9.1 Leading causes of death among children worldwide one to four years (1998).

(*Source:* World Health Organization, 1998)

three million STDs a year. Unfortunately, bad habits are established in youth and extended into adulthood.[14]

Among morbidity problems cited by the Centers for Disease Control and Prevention are:

1. Sexually transmitted diseases
2. Lack of immunizations
3. Lead exposure
4. Asthma
5. Nutrition
6. Teen pregnancies

The leading causes of death for children five to fourteen years are given in Table 9.4 and for youth fifteen to twenty-four in Table 9.5.

Because among those over twenty-five years, 67 percent of all deaths and morbidity are from three causes—heart disease (35 percent), cancer (25 percent), and stroke (7 percent)—it is agreed that there are six high-risk behaviors that can be modified to reduce morbidity and mortality from adolescents through adulthood:

- Tobacco use
- Alcohol and drug use
- Sexual behaviors

Table 9.4   Leading causes of childhood death 5–14 years.

Cause	Number	Rate per 100,000
All causes	7,700	19.7
Accidents and adverse effects	3,115	8.0
Motor vehicle accidents	1,773	4.5
All other accidents and adverse effects	1,342	3.4
Malignant neoplasms, including neoplasms of lymphatic and hematopoietic tissues	1,025	2.6
Homicide and legal intervention	423	1.1
Congenital anomalies	355	0.9
Suicide	318	0.8
Diseases of heart	304	0.8
Chronic obstructive pulmonary diseases and allied conditions	145	0.4
Pneumonia and influenza	125	0.3
Benign neoplasms, carcinoma in situ, and neoplasms of uncertain behavior and unspecified nature	80	0.2
Cerebrovasular diseases	76	0.2
All other causes (Residual)	1,734	4.4

(*Source:* National Vital Statistics Reports. Vol. 47 #25, Oct. 1999)

Table 9.5   Leading causes of death 15–24 years.

Cause	Number	Rate per 100,000
All causes	30,211	81.2
Accidents and adverse effects	12,752	34.3
Motor vehicle accidents	9,635	25.9
All other accidents and adverse effects	3,117	8.4
Homicide and legal intervention	5,233	14.1
Suicide	4,003	10.8
Malignant neoplasms, including neoplasms of lymphatic and hematopoietic tissues	1,670	4.5
Diseases of heart	961	2.6
Congenital anomalies	429	1.2
Chronic obstructive pulmonary diseases and allied conditions	224	0.6
Pneumonia and influenza	211	0.6
Human immunodeficiency virus infection	208	0.6
Cerebrovasular diseases	182	0.5
All other causes (Residual)	4,338	11.7

(*Source:* National Vital Statistics Reports. Vol. 47 #25, Oct. 1999)

BOX 9.1   *National SAFE KIDS Campaign*

C. Everett Koop, Chair of the SAFE KIDS campaign noted that 8,000 kids fourteen and under are killed and 5,000 are permanently disabled from childhood injuries. SAFE KIDS is a nationwide coalition of children's advocates, health professionals, policy makers and others, working to raise awareness about childhood injury prevention. A child-safe house in Monroe, Wisconsin is an example of a community's effort to prevent injury death. The house has double hand rails—one for adults and one for children, fire escape hatch windows, windows with limited openings, electrical outlet plates that are considered safer than plastic outlet plugs, magnetic key locks, anti-scald faucets in tubs, showers and sinks, fire extinguishers, round edges on countertops and other selected safety features.[16]

- Unhealthy dietary behaviors
- Physical inactivity[15]

Healthy People 2010 Objective: Reduce Deaths of Adolescents and
  Young Adults

Reduction in Deaths of Adolescents and Young Adults	1998 Baseline	2010 Target
	Rate per 100,000	
Adolescents aged 10 to 14 years	21.8	16.8
Adolescents aged 15 to 19 years	69.7	43.2
Young adults aged 20 to 24 years	93.8	57.3

The CDC Youth Risk Behavior Surveillance System

The CDC Youth Risk Behavior Surveillance System was an effort to determine the health risks of youth in this country through national, state, and local surveys conducted in 1990, 1991, 1993, and 1998. In brief, the results are given in the charts on p. 239.[17]

While the percentages reported on page 239 above give an overall picture of the risk behaviors of today's youth, it should be noted that there are significant differences between males and females, among people of different ethnic groups, and in different age groups. In general, male students were most likely to report injury-related behaviors, smokeless tobacco use, and various types of drug use including binge drinking, marijuana use, steroid use, and injection drug use. Females were most likely to report suicide-related behaviors and weight loss attempts. White students were most likely to report tobacco use and some types of physical activity, while black students were most likely to report weapon carrying, physical fighting, and sexual behaviors. Hispanic students were most likely to report alcohol use, binge drinking, and cocaine and crack use.[18]

Carrying a weapon, physical fights, lack of condom use, and participation in physical activities occurred most frequently among students in grades 9 and 10. Cigarette smoking, alcohol and marijuana use, and sexual behaviors, except lack of condom use, occurred most frequently among students in grades 11 to 12.[19] Community health education must consider these unique differences in planning and implementing risk reduction and prevention programs.

Behaviors That Contribute to *Unintentional* Injuries[20]

Behavior	Rarely use seatbelt	Ever ride motorcycle	Rarely use motorcycle helmet	Ever ride bicycle	Rarely use bicycle helmet	Ever drink and drive
% of students	19.1	26.7	40.0	75.3	92.8	35.3

Behaviors That Contribute to *Intentional* Injuries

Behavior	Carrying a a weapon	Carrying a gun	Physical fight	Suicide attempt	Suicide ideation
% of students	22.1	7.9	41.8	8.6	24.1

Tobacco, Drug, Alcohol Use

Behavior	Cigarette use	Smokeless tobacco use	Alcohol use	Marijuana use	Cocaine use	Steroid use
% of students	69.5	11.5	80.9	32.8	4.9	2.2

Sexual Behaviors That Contribute to Unintended Pregnancy and STDs

Sexual Behavior	Lack of intercourse	condom use
% of students	53	52.8

Comparing Children's Health Risk Factors   All developed countries now have extensive sets of routinely collected demographic data about a population. In the field of child health, there are problems when comparing the definitions used within and between countries. The format of birth certificates or health notifications used by different countries varies, making it somewhat difficult to get accurate data regarding the international status of children. Further, some of the greatest risks to children's health—poverty, abuse, lack of education—are not easily measurable. However, enough is known to give a general picture of the health of the planet's children.

Table 9.6   Health issues facing elementary school children as reported by teachers.

Elementary School Teachers Reporting Health Problems Associated with Students (Grades K–6) (n = 500)			Single Most Serious Health Issue Facing Elementary School Children	
	% of Teachers Reporting			% of Teachers Reporting
Problem	Grades K–3	Grades 4–6	Issue	
Psychological/emotion	92	92	Psychological	30
Unhealthy lifestyle habits	74	82	Family problems	26
Family violence or abuse	75	80	Poor nutrition	22
Poor nutrition	71	71	Specific conditions	16
Violent behavior	60	66	Unhealthy habits	10
Lack of health care	54	62	Drugs/alcohol	9
Untreated illnesses	50	47	Lack of health care	6
Drugs/alcohol abuse	32	40	Don't know	4
Lack of immunizations	12	10	Violence/abuse	3

(*Source:* Porter/Novelli PR Agency, 1992. Health Care and a Child's Ability to Learn: A Survey of Elementary School Teachers, Chicago, Sept. ERIC File. Reprinted by permission of American Academy of Pediatrics)

A recent discovery is that **the feminization of poverty** reflects a pattern found not only in the United States but around the world that very negatively affects the well-being of children. The feminization of poverty refers to the low economic condition of increasing numbers of families headed by females as a result of divorce or out-of-wedlock births. Reducing poverty among single, female heads of households would probably occur if there were equal access to equal job opportunities, child care, and social support to these families. The definition of poverty, as set by the Bureau of the Census, is a family of four living on less than $17,029 a year. The fastest growth in child poverty in the United States is coming not from inner cities, but from the suburbs. The suburban poverty rates have increased by 76 percent in the past two decades.[21]

Additionally, a 1990 survey of elementary school teachers showed that more children come to grade school sick, disturbed, or abused than in years past. Half of surveyed teachers reported students suffering from untreated illnesses or problems with vision or hearing. Most teachers reported children with psychological and emotional problems, family violence and abuse, unhealthy lifestyles, poor nutrition, violent behavior, and lack of regular health care among their students as shown on Table 9.6.

Discussion: How can the health care system make children's health a priority? Why should we?

Table 9.7   Cardiovascular disease risk for school age children (1990).

Health Indicator	
Percentage of school age children with:	
1. Blood cholesterol	
greater than 170	41%
greater than 200	11%
2. Physical activity daily	
grades 1–12	36%
grades 9–12	42%

Cardiovascular Diseases

It often comes as a surprise that cardiovascular diseases are a common risk factor for school aged children. As indicated on Table 9.7, increases in blood cholesterol, being overweight, and decreases in physical activity have occurred during the past couple of decades. The result is the increased risk for cardiovascular problems for children and the subsequent adult problems that make cardiovascular diseases the number one killer among adults. Nutrition and thus weight may be the number one means of addressing cardiovascular disease in youth.

Secretary of Health and Human Services, Donna Shalala said, "It is clear that too many of our teenagers are overweight because they are inactive. . ."[22] While not necessarily obese, 22 percent of adolescent females are overweight and 20 percent of adolescent males are overweight.

Being overweight and obesity affect 55 percent of adults. Over two decades, the number of cases of obesity alone has increased more than 50 percent, from 14.5 percent of the adult population to 22.5 percent. Approximately 25 percent of U.S. adult females and 20 percent of U.S. adult males are obese.[23] The CDC reported in 1998 that nearly half of American adolescents are not active on a regular basis. It is no wonder, therefore, that the proportion of overweight adolescents in the United States had reached 21 percent.

Healthy People 2010 Objective: Reduce the Proportion of Children and Adolescents Who Are Overweight or Obese

Target and baseline:

Reduction in Overweight or Obese Children and Adolescents	1988–1994 Baseline	2010 Target
	Percent	
Aged 6 to 11 years	11	5
Aged 12 to 19 years	10	5
Aged 6 to 19 years	11	5

Maintenance of a healthy weight is a major goal in the effort to reduce the burden of illness and its consequent reduction in quality of life and life expectancy. Issues of weight begin in childhood, and if not corrected, become profound health risks in adults. The CDC uses the Body Mass Index (BMI) cut-point to establish the upper limit of the healthy weight range in relationship to risk factors for chronic disease or premature death. A BMI of less than 25 has been accepted by numerous groups as the upper limit of the healthy weight range, since chronic disease risk increases in most populations at or above this cut-point. The lower cut-point for the healthy weight range (BMI of 18.5) was selected to be consistent with national and international recommendations. Problems associated with excessive thinness (BMI less than 18.5) include menstrual irregularity, infertility, and osteoporosis. There is some concern that the increased focus on overweight may result in more eating disorders, such as bulimia and anorexia nervosa. However, no evidence currently exists that suggests the increased focus on overweight has resulted in additional cases of eating disorders.[24]

Overweight and obesity are caused by many factors. These factors reflect the contributions of inherited, metabolic, behavioral, environmental, cultural, and socioeconomic components. As weight increases, so does the prevalence of health risks. Simple, health-oriented definitions of overweight and obesity should be based on the amount of excess body fat at which health risks to individuals begin to increase. No such definitions currently exist. Whereas the relation of BMI to body fat differs by age and gender, it provides valid comparisons across racial and ethnic groups. However, BMI does not provide information concerning body fat distribution, which has been identified as an independent predictor of health risk. Thus, until a better surrogate for body fat is developed, BMI will be used to screen for overweight and obese individuals.[25]

Interpretations of data about overweight and obesity have differed because criteria for these terms have varied over time, from study to study, and from one part of the world to another. National and international organizations now support the use of a BMI of 30 or greater to identify obesity. However, the health risks associated with overweight and obesity are part of a continuum and do not conform to rigid cut-points.[26]

Unintentional Injury

In the past decade, unintentional injury has been recognized as the major cause of morbidity and mortality for children in communities throughout the United States. Children under the age of fifteen make up approximately 10 million emergency visits to hospitals due to injuries each year. In less developed communities, the injury rate is 846 per 100,000 compared to the United States rate of 656 per 100,000.[27]

One unique prevention program is The Safe Kids/Healthy Neighborhood Coalition Project in Central Harlem. This program targets an economically disadvantaged, predominantly black community where 29 percent of the population are younger than seventeen years. The injury reduction program promotes playground safety, reduction in assault, and motor vehicle safety. Parents help identify environmental and behavioral hazards, which include broken equipment and glass, poor lighting, drugs sold on the playground, alcohol use, or the absence of supervision. After identification, community interventions through activism of community coalitions help reduce risks. After one year of intervention there was a 15 percent decrease in major injury hospital admissions and a 12 percent decrease in emergency room visits for playground injuries.[28] The key to this success is community cooperation and coalition building.

Child Abuse

The 1997 Child Maltreatment Report from the States to the National Child Abuse and Neglect Data System found there were approximately 984,000 victims of maltreatment. The rate of child victims was 13.9 per 1,000 children in the general population in 1997.

There were 1,215 deaths as a result of abuse and neglect in 1995.[29] Among those demographic characteristics of families where abuse takes place, economic status is the greatest predictor of abuse. The findings regarding the types of maltreatment were as follows: 55.9 percent neglect, 24.6 percent physical abuse, 12.5 percent sexual abuse, and 6.1 percent emotional abuse. Physical abuse is the most common abuse *reported;* however, sexual abuse, verbal abuse, emotional abuse, and neglect are all parts of a horrific childhood problem. National survey data suggest a rate of fourteen abuse cases per one hundred children, which could put the incidence at 6.5 million cases a year. The disparity in data comes from trying to define child abuse and certainly from a reluctance to report child abuse. When does punishing a child become abusive? How can one accurately measure the nature of emotional abuse due to neglect and criticism?

The National PTA believes that increased abuse and neglect of children is in part a reflection of inadequate health insurance that does not cover routine preventive care. If children were seen more often by trained professionals, abuses and neglect would be documented more quickly, and parents under extreme stresses might be identified and referred for help before their children become their victims.

Adolescents

The fact that adolescents are relatively healthy does not mean that they do not come to the notice of health care agencies. The casualty rate of adolescents on

---

BOX 9.2 *Rates of Child Neglect*

Physical neglect	8.0 per 1,000
Educational neglect	4.5 per 1,000
Emotional neglect	3.0 per 1,000
Medical neglect	.05 per 1,000

(*Source:* U.S. Department of Health and Human Services, Children's Bureau. Child Maltreatment 1998: Reports from the States to the National Child Abuse and Neglect Data System. Washington, D.C.: U.S. Government Printing Office, 2000.)

many indices is high. Among adolescents, the social and personal problems that lead to health risks are:

1. Use of alcohol and other drugs
2. Aggressive behavior
3. Unprotected sexual activity
4. Depression and stress
5. Loneliness
6. Careless use of motor vehicles
7. Poor body image
8. Low self-esteem

The leading causes of death of young people ages fifteen to twenty-four are given earlier in Table 9.5. They are (1) injuries, (2) homicide, (3) suicide, (4) cancer, (5) heart disease, (6) congenital anomalies, (7) COPD, (8) pneumonia/influenza, (9) HIV and (10) stroke. It may be interesting to note that AIDs dropped from the leading causes of death in 1998.

Chronic diseases such as heart disease are increasing in frequency among young people. The percentage of schoolchildren with cardiovascular disease are given in Table 9.7.[24] The highest urban rates for cardiovascular diseases are found in New York City, Chicago, Detroit, Phoenix, and Riverside, California, and in rural areas of the central Midwest, the Appalachians, and the Hawaiian Islands.

Asthma deaths are on the increase after years of decline with the greatest increases among females, blacks, and economically disadvantaged children. Annual health care expenditures for asthma alone exceeded $4 billion in 1988.

Surprisingly, the most disturbing trend in U.S. mortality is the rise in deaths among older teens and young adults. While mortality for every other age group improved during the 1980s, death rates among young adults increased for the first time in the twentieth century when the United States was not engaged in a major war. AIDS and violence are the primary reasons for this ominous trend, but they may not be the only ones.

Mortality rate maps for young adult infectious diseases show highest rates in southern and central parts of the country; the high rate counties are rural and significantly poor, with large percentages of Hispanic and Native Americans, and significantly more violations of public water supply health standards than the rest of the country.[30] There seems to be a resurrection of an historical pattern of early mortality among urban and rural minority poor. Illness from tuberculosis, septicemia, measles, and syphilis were the leading causes of death in the United States at the start of the twentieth century and appear to be making a comeback with the introduction of AIDS as the twentieth century ends.

The increased morbidity and mortality among older teens and young adults can be traced to a host of diseases associated with immune deficiencies other than AIDS—chronic fatigue syndrome, multiple chemical sensitivity, Lyme disease, pelvic inflammatory disease, herpes, and lupus. Potential aggravators of immune deficiencies include pesticide residues on all of our food, 300,000 miles of high-voltage power lines, hundreds of military and civilian reactors routinely emitting low levels of electromagnetic and ionizing radiation, and the billions of pounds of toxins that industry spews into the air, water, and land each year. Epidemiologists remind us that the United States and the Soviets exploded the equivalent of 40,000 Hiroshima bombs from 1945 to 1962, releasing long-lived radioactive isotopes such as strontium 90 into the atmosphere. Some of it ended up in the milk of mothers and the bones of the very babies who, if they survived, are now young adults.[31]

These rather universal adolescent social problems lead directly to the primary health problems of the young; sexual identity confusion related to sexual orientation, sexually transmitted diseases, alcohol and other drug use and dependencies, suicide, accidents, unwanted pregnancy, eating disorders, and family stress. The National Adolescent Student Health Survey (NASHS), conducted in 1988 among 224 public and private schools, was the first major national study of adolescents' knowledge, attitudes, and behaviors related to health.

Healthy People 2010 Objective: Reduce Percent Tobacco Use by Adolescents

	1997 Baseline	2010 Target
Tobacco products (past month)	43	21
Cigarettes (past month)	36	16
Spit tobacco (past month)	9	1
Cigars (past month)	22	8

Sexuality

The World Health Organization has estimated that 100 million people worldwide have sexual intercourse daily. This sexual activity results in nearly 1 million conceptions and about 350,000 cases of sexually transmitted diseases. Worldwide, one out of twenty teenagers and young adults contract a sexually transmitted disease each year, while in the United States it is one in six. The increased education about HIV infection has prompted more condom use worldwide, which in fact has decreased STD risk, but condom use is still more common in industrialized countries, such as Japan, where it accounts for 70 percent of all contraception use, than in developing countries that have strong cultural, economic, and religious barriers to condom use.

In the 1990s most school systems came to consciousness about the need for sexuality education in the schools. Young people do not question the need for education. They almost unanimously are in agreement that they need to know more, especially given the reality of their sexual activity and sexual curiosity.

By age eighteen, 57 percent of teens have had sexual intercourse; and sadly, half of American teens at this age have had no sexuality or HIV education. Of those twelfth-grade teens who are sexually active, only 26 percent use condoms regularly. The initiatives of a previous Surgeon General to provide more sexuality education and the free distribution of condoms to sexually active teens was highly controversial and was met with great resistance by those who believe that priority should be placed on teen sexual abstinence. In an ideal world this might be realistic. In America in the second millennium, it is not enough and not realistic.

Teen Pregnancy

In spite of more available sexuality education and the availability of contraceptives, 20 percent (1 million) teenage girls in the United States become pregnant and have 25 percent of all abortions each year. Approximately 2 million adolescent women in developing countries undergo unsafe abortions each year, and a third of all women seeking hospital care for abortion complications are underage. Teen pregnancy, birth, abortion, and infant mortality rates are shown in Figure 9.2.

More than four out of ten young women become pregnant at least once before they reach the age of twenty; nearly 1 million a year. Eight in ten of these pregnancies are unintended and 80 percent are to unmarried teens. The good news is that there has been a ten-year decline in the teen birth rate, which was 51.1 per 1,000 in 1999. However, this is the highest rate in the industrial world.

Few young girls now marry because of pregnancy and few give up their child for adoption. Forty percent will choose abortion while approximately 470,000 will complete their pregnancy. The year 2000 national health objective was that there be no unintended births to girls fourteen years of age and under. Unfortunately, about 10,000 such births were reported in 1999.

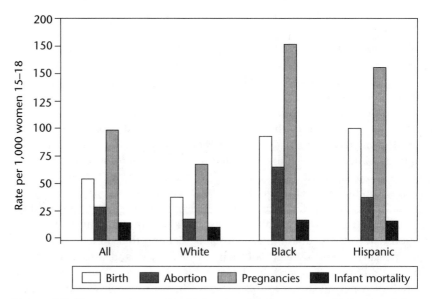

Figure 9.2 Teen pregnancy rates, birth rates, abortion rates, and infant mortality rates (1998).

(*Sources:* Centers for Disease Control. National Center for Health Statistics)

The teen birth rate has declined slowly but steadily from 1991 to 1996 with an overall decline of 12 percent for those aged fifteen to nineteen. The largest decline since 1991 by race was for black women. The birth rate for black teens aged fifteen to nineteen fell 21 percent between 1991 and 1996.

Hispanic teen birth rates declined 5 percent between 1995 and 1996. The rates of both Hispanics and blacks, however, remain higher than for other groups. Hispanic teens now have the highest teenage birth rates. Yet only 9 percent of all adolescent females are Hispanic. The combination of a conservative culture that makes it hard for Hispanic teens to talk about sexuality and a predominant Catholic religious background that makes contraceptive use a sin, may be the primary reasons for this disturbing increase in teens pregnancy among Hispanics.

Three public health initiatives that may decrease teen pregnancy include: (1) school-based sexuality education that would encourage postponing sexual activity, (2) contraceptive information for those teens who choose to be sexually active, and (3) confidential family planning services in Title X clinics for contraception, adoption, and abortion information. All three interventions have been opposed strongly by conservative groups and have not had the support of the federal government. Research points toward positive outcomes with these initiatives. There is less pregnancy when family planning services are available to teens, especially where contraceptive information, counseling, and prescriptions are available in the school.

Contraception

Of never married, sexually active teens fifteen to nineteen, 30 percent use no contraception. While no biomedical reasons exist to deny any contraceptive method based on young age alone, other factors may be important to consider. Good counseling helps sexually active young adults choose the most appropriate method.

Substantially fewer black teens use contraception and somewhat fewer Hispanic teens use contraception than their white peers. Of those teens who do use contraception, 60 percent use oral contraceptives, 25 percent use condoms, and 5 percent use an IUD or diaphragm. There has been an increased use of injectable Depo Provera (progesterone). Typical effectiveness of birth control methods in the United States is given in Table 9.8. Males are much less likely to know about contraceptive alternatives than females and less likely than females to want to use condoms.

Educating boys that reproductive health is not for women only is one of the goals of the Young Men's Clinic in the United States. Located in an urban neighborhood of New York, the clinic is part of a health facility that provides other services, including pediatric and obstetrical care. Dr. Bruce Armstrong of the clinic says family planning services were rarely being used by men. When health workers asked adolescents why they did not use these services, boys said they were embarrassed, and that it made them "feel not like a man" to visit a clinic that was primarily for women. The solution was to develop a clinic for

Table 9.8   Effectiveness of birth control methods in the United States.

Method	% of Women Experiencing an Accidental Pregnancy within the First Year of Use	
	Typical Use	Perfect Use
Chance	85	85
Spermicides	21	6
Periodic Abstinence	20	
Calendar		9
Ovulation Method		3
Sympto-Thermal		2
Post-Ovulation		1
Withdrawal	19	4
Cervical Cap		
Parous Women	36	26
Nulliparous Women	18	9
Sponge		
Parous Women	36	20
Nulliparous Women	18	9
Diaphragm	18	6
Condom Alone		
Female	21	5
Male	12	3
Pill	3	
Progestin Only		0.5
Combined		0.1
IUD		
Progesterone T	2.0	1.5
Copper T 380A	0.8	0.6
Depo-Provera	0.3	0.3
Norplant (6 capsules)	0.09	0.09
Female Sterilization	0.4	0.4
Male Sterilization	0.15	0.10

(*Source:* Hatcher, R. A. et al., 1994. *Contraceptive Technology,* 16th ed. New York: Irvington Publishers)

men and to provide a variety of health services, including physical exams necessary for work or school and screenings for disease, such as sickle-cell anemia. That way, men could come to the clinic without the fear that friends or neighbors might think they were seeking contraceptives. The clinic also sponsored sports events for men to encourage them to use services.[32]

A retrospective study of 8,450 women in the United States, ages fifteen to forty-four, examined the relationship between sex education and use of contraception at first intercourse. Women who received formal instruction on contraceptive use before their first sexual intercourse were more likely to use a

---

BOX 9.3 SIECUS Sex Education Concepts

SIECUS lists six key concepts that should be included in a comprehensive sex education program:

- Human development, which includes reproductive anatomy and physiology
- Relationships, which include relationships with families and friends, as well as relationships in dating and marriage
- Personal skills, which include values, decision making, communication, negotiation

- Sexual behavior, which includes abstinence as well as sexuality throughout the life cycle
- Sexual health, including contraception, STD and HIV prevention, abortion and sexual abuse
- Society and culture, which includes gender roles, sexuality and religion.

According to SIECUS guidelines, sex education should begin in early elementary school.[35]

---

method. Women were less likely to use a method if they received information on contraception the same year they began sexual activity. A survey, conducted among 1,800 fifteen- to nineteen-year-old males in the United States, found that among those who had received formal education about AIDS and family planning, there was a decrease in number of sexual partners and an increase in consistent use of condoms.[33]

The World Health Organization (WHO) recently published a review of 1,050 scientific articles on sex education programs. Researchers found "no support for the contention that sex education encourages sexual experimentation or increased activity. If any effect is observed, almost without exception, it is in the direction of postponed initiation of sexual intercourse and/or effective use of contraception."[34]

Sexual Orientation

Many estimates suggest that about 10 percent of the human population is homosexual. This same percentage exists among teens as well. Most recent research is pointing toward a biological-endocrine-genetic relationship to the natural differentiation in sexual orientation, although cause is not known at this time. Due to the many stresses related to sexual development, sexual behavior decision making, and the strong pressure to conform, gay male, lesbian, and bisexual teens often experience greater anxiety, increased isolation, fewer resources for discussing these stresses, and less support for personal decisions. Although research is limited, most studies of gay, lesbian, and bisexual youth indicate an increased risk for physical abuse, school problems, running away from home, pregnancy, depression, alcohol and drug abuse, and suicide.

A major contributor to gay male teen suicide is the lack of love and support for these teens by peers and those whom these young men respect. Lesbian teens are less inclined than gay male teens to attempt or commit suicide; however, self-destructive behaviors such as alcohol or drug abuse may be aggravated in this teen subgroup. In fact, suicide is the leading cause of death among gay, lesbian, and bisexual teens.

Sexual Abuse

It is hypothesized that one in four girls and one in eight boys will be sexually abused before the age of eighteen. Since most cases of abuse go unreported, the figure may be as high as one-quarter to one-third of all children who have had at least one sexual experience with an adult ranging from exhibitionism to sexual intercourse. **Incest** is a profound form of sexual abuse where members of one's own family are involved sexually with children. Seventy-five percent of prostitutes report having been victims of childhood sexual abuse; and as many as 75 percent of children on the street report having been victims of sexual abuse.

Survey data from 1994 indicate that 407,190 females aged twelve years and older were victims of rape, attempted rape, or sexual assault. Other surveys indicate that the problem is underestimated. For example, the National Women's Study, in conjunction with estimates based on the U.S. Census, suggests that 12.1 million females in the United States have been victims of forcible rape sometime in their lives.

Teen dating violence is a concern that may stem from childhood abuse or other experiences with violence. Battering in teen relationships is very different from intimate partner violence that occurs between adults. The issue of teen dating violence requires national attention and prevention efforts that need to continue focusing on adolescent violence within the larger context of family violence.[36]

The 1997 Child Maltreatment Report from the States to the National Child Abuse and Neglect Data System found a decrease from more than 1 million victims in 1996 in the fifty states, the District of Columbia, Puerto Rico, the Virgin Islands, and Guam. The rate of child victims was 13.9 per 1,000 children in the general population in 1997, which is slightly higher than the rate of 13.4 victims per 1,000 children in 1990. There were an estimated 1,196 fatalities due to child maltreatment in the fifty states and the District of Columbia. The findings regarding the types of maltreatment were as follows: 55.9 percent neglect, 24.6 percent physical abuse, 12.5 percent sexual abuse, and 6.1 percent emotional abuse. Based on data from thirty-nine states, 75.4 percent of the perpetrators were the victims' parents, 10.2 percent were relatives, and 1.9 percent were individuals in other caretaking relationships.[37]

> **Healthy People 2010 Objective:** Reduce Maltreatment and Maltreatment Fatalities of Children
>
> *Target:* 11.1 per 1,000 children under age 18 years.
>
> *Baseline:* 13.9 child victims of maltreatment per 1,000 children under age 18 years in 1997.

Table 9.9   Reported cases of STD by gender (1998).

Disease	Male	Female	Total
Total *Chlamydia Trachomatis*	104,435	501,128	607,602
Chlamydia PID	NA	3,099	31,03
Ophthalmia Neonatorum	116	202	318
Total Gonorrhea	175,233	179,651	355,642
Gonococcal PID	NA	4,013	4,019
Ophthalmia Neonatorum	20	19	39
Total Syphilis	19,739	18,179	37,977
Primary	1,878	541	2,420
Secondary	2,024	2,548	4,573
Early Latent	6,311	6,298	12,613
Late and Late Latent	9,157	8,406	17,570
Neurosyphilis	215	65	281
Congenital <1 year	369	386	801
Chancroid	112	76	189
Granudoma inguinale	1	2	3
Lymphogranuloma Venereum	62	24	86
Genital Herpes	3,019	4,894	7,918
Other and Nonspecified PID	NA	2,549	2,552
Nonspecific Urethritis in Men	26,818	NA	26,865

(*Source:* CDC. National Center for HIV, STD, and TB Prevention, 2001)

Healthy People 2010 Objective: Reduce Sexual Assault Other than Rape

Target: 0.2 sexual assaults other than rape per 1,000 persons aged 12 years and older.

Baseline: 0.6 sexual assaults other than rape per 1,000 persons aged 12 years and older in 1998.

Sexually Transmitted Diseases (STDs)

It is estimated that each year 3 million teenagers are infected with an STD. STDs have been shown to relate to a range of serious health problems. The National Adolescent School Health Study reports that 30 percent of teens do not know that most people get STDs by having sexual intercourse, and 25 percent did not know that using condoms is effective in avoiding STDs.

Table 9.9 reports STD cases by gender (1998). Selected international rates of STDs are given in Table 9.10.

Prevention   Sexually transmitted diseases (STDs), once called venereal diseases, are among the most common infectious diseases in the United States today. More than twenty STDs have now been identified (Box 9.4 lists some of them),

Table 9.10 Estimated prevalence and annual incidence rates of curable
STDs by region (1999).

Region	Population 15–49 per/1,000
North America	153
Western Europe	211
Australia	11
Latin America and the Caribbean	251
Sub-Saharan Africa	254
Northern Africa and Middle East	163
Eastern Europe and Central Asia	158
East Asia and Pacific	803
Total	2,946

(*Source:* World Health Organization)

and they affect more than 15 million men and women in this country each year.
The annual comprehensive cost of STDs in the United States is estimated to be
well in excess of $10 billion. The estimated annual incidence of curable STDs
(not including AIDS and other viral STDs) is 333 million cases worldwide.

Given the nature of STD spread and infection, education is probably one of
the most important prevention modalities available to community health professionals. There is no question that school and public education is the single best
means of preventing the spread of HIV/AIDS in the United States today, however,
it was not until almost eight years into the epidemic that federal and state legislatures began to understand and finance this endeavor. Much of the delay was
caused by the unwillingness of the public to discuss and educate about sexuality.

Prevention messages should be tailored to the teenagers, with consideration
given to their specific risks. Messages should include a description of measures, as
well as skill building that youth can take to avoid acquiring or transmitting STDs.[39]

There has always been interest in the possible protective role of various
contraceptive agents and methods in relation to STDs. Until the AIDS epidemic,
the public was loath to discuss, investigate, or encourage one of the best preventive STD methods, condom use. Even in the twenty-first century, many
school systems prohibit the discussion of condom use because of the fear of discussing sexual issues with teens (those most at risk for STD infection), and the
conservative vocal minority who prohibit the discussion of birth control.[40]

Barrier techniques have historically had a place as a prophylactic against
STDs and are still encouraged by health educators. The Swedes maintain that
their very remarkable decline in gonorrhea is a result of a condom use campaign in the 1970s.

Alcohol—the Drug of Choice

Because adolescence is a time for experimentation and the testing of adult attitudes and behaviors, many behaviors will be, if not intrinsically dangerous,

high risk. Alcohol and other drug use are good examples of both. Alcohol abuse remains the most serious problem facing U.S. high schools, according to high school leaders and their teachers. Of all teenagers who die each year, half die as a result of alcohol or other drug use.[41]

The Centers for Disease Control and Prevention conducted a national survey of 10,904 high school students in grades 9–12. This survey found that 80.4 percent of students had at least one drink of alcohol during their lifetime and that 51.6 percent of students had at least one drink of alcohol during the thirty days preceding a CDC survey. Students in grades 11 (53.7 percent) and 12 (56.5 percent) were significantly more likely than students in grade 9 (45.6 percent) to report current alcohol use. The survey found that 32.6 percent of students had five or more drinks of alcohol on at least one occasion during the 30 days preceding the survey (i.e., episodic heavy drinking). Males (36.2 percent) were significantly more likely than females (28.6 percent) to report episodic heavy drinking. Finally, white (81.7 percent) and Hispanic (82.9 percent) students were significantly more likely than black students (73.7 percent) to have had at least one drink of alcohol during their lifetime, to report current alcohol use, and to report episodic heavy drinking.[42]

BOX 9.4 *Sexually Transmitted Diseases and the Organisms Responsible*

Disease	Organism(s)
Acquired Immunodeficiency Syndrome (AIDS)	Human immunodeficiency virus
Bacterial vaginosis	*Bacteroides* *Gardnerella vaginalis* *Mobiluncus spp.* *Mycoplasma hominis* *Ureaplasma urealyticum*
Chancroid	*Haemophilus ducreyi*
Chlamydial infections	*Chlamydia trachomatis*
Cytomegalovirus infections	Cytomegalovirus
Genital herpes	Herpes simplex virus
Genital (venereal) warts	Human papillomavirus
Gonorrhea	*Neisseria gonorrhoeae*
Granuloma inguinale (donovanosis)	*Calymmatobacterium granulomatis*
Molluscum contagiosum	Molluscum contagiosum virus
Pubic lice	*Phthirus pubis*
Scabies	*Sarcoptes scabiei*
Syphilis	*Treponema pallidum*
Trichomoniasis	*Trichomonas vaginalis*
Vaginal yeast infections	*Candida albicans*

Almost half of all male deaths between the ages of fifteen and twenty-four years are caused by road accidents, with the largest contributing factor being alcohol. Data suggest that acute drinking among some adolescents is actually increasing in the United States. Factors contributing to acute drinking include peer pressure and the promotion of alcohol consumption through music and print media. A 1991 poll said that 73 percent of respondents agreed that alcohol advertising is a major contributor to underage drinking and most believe that the alcohol industry targets the youth.[43]

Healthy People 2010 Objective: Reduce Past-Month Use of Illicit Substances

Target: Increase the proportion of adolescents not using alcohol or any illicit drugs during the past thirty days to 89 percent.

Baseline: 77 percent of adolescents aged 12 to 17 years reported no alcohol or illicit drug use in past thirty days in 1997.

Monitoring the Future is an ongoing study of the behaviors, attitudes, and values of American secondary school students, college students, and young adults. Each year, a total of some 50,000 eighth, tenth, and twelfth grade students are surveyed (twelfth graders since 1975, and eighth and tenth graders since 1991). In addition, annual follow-up questionnaires are mailed to a sample of each graduating class for a number of years after their initial participation. Table 9.11 gives some of the results of this ongoing study.[44]

Other Drugs

Young adults aged eighteen to twenty-five continue to be the age group with the highest rates of illicit drug use. The most current CDC study of drug use indicates that past-month use of drugs increased among adolescents aged twelve to seventeen, and the 1997 rates of past month use of any illicit drug (11 percent) and marijuana (9 percent) were significantly higher than the 1996 rates of use by this age group (9 percent and 7 percent, respectively). Furthermore, past-month use of illicit drugs by youths was significantly higher in 1997 than at any time during the four years between 1991 and 1994. Past-month use of alcohol was about the same in 1997 as in 1996.[45]

The first goal of the 1998 National Drug Control Strategy is to "educate and enable America's youth to reject illegal drugs as well as the underage use of alcohol and tobacco." In response to this goal, specific targets for the reduction of drug use among adolescents aged twelve to seventeen have been established under the Youth Substance Abuse Prevention Initiative (YSAPI). These targets, which have a baseline of 1996 and goals for the year 2002 (seven years), are as follows:

1. Reverse the upward trend and reduce past-month use of marijuana among adolescents aged twelve to seventeen by 20 percent (1996 baseline: 7.1 percent; target: 5.7 percent in 2002).

Table 9.11 Various drugs for eighth, tenth, and twelfth graders (1999).

Any illicit drug		MDMA (Ecstacy)	
8th Grade	28.3%	8th Grade	2.7
10th Grade	46.2	10th Grade	6.0
12th Grade	54.7	12th Grade	8.0
Marijuana/Hashish		Cocaine	
8th Grade	22.0	8th Grade	4.7
10th Grade	40.9	10th Grade	7.7
12th Grade	49.7	12th Grade	9.8
Inhalants		Crack	
8th Grade	19.7	8th Grade	3.1
10th Grade	17.0	10th Grade	4.0
12th Grade	15.4	12th Grade	4.6
Halluccinogens		Amphetamines	
8th Grade	4.8	8th Grade	10.7
10th Grade	9.7	10th Grade	15.7
12th Grade	13.7	12th Grade	16.3
LSD		Steroids	
8th Grade	4.1	8th Grade	2.7
10th Grade	8.5	10th Grade	2.7
12th Grade	12.2	12th Grade	2.9

(*Source:* National Clearinghouse for Alcohol and Drug Information, 2001)

2. Reduce past-month use of any illicit drugs among adolescents aged twelve to seventeen by 20 percent (1996 baseline: 9.0 percent; target: 7.2 percent in 2002).

3. Reduce past-month use of alcohol among adolescents aged twelve to seventeen by 10 percent (1996 baseline: 18.8 percent; target: 16.9 percent in 2002).

Survey results report that 57 percent of all students have tried cigarettes (Table 9.12), 83 percent have tried an alcoholic beverage, 25 percent have used marijuana, and 6 percent report using cocaine. In general, there seems to be a downward trend in illegal drug use among high school seniors, although the use of LSD may be increasing. However, the absolute levels of drug use, especially in the lower grades, is a serious concern for community health educators. Drug use is estimated to be greater among youth in the United States than in any other industrialized country in the world.[46] Alcohol use in the past month by all ages is reported in Table 9.13.

Approximately 12.3 million, or 6 percent, of the 216 million persons surveyed in 1997 reported lifetime inhalant use. About 2.3 million persons (1 percent) used inhalants in the past year, and 883,000 persons (0.4 percent) used them in the past month. Among adolescents aged twelve to seventeen between 1996 and 1997, there was a significant increase in the lifetime rate of inhaling gasoline or lighter fluid fumes (from 1.9 percent in 1996 to 2.7 percent in

Table 9.12 Percentage of students in middle school (grades 6–8) and high school (grades 9–12) currently using tobacco products (1999).

	Sex		Race/Ethnicity			
	Male	Female	White	Black	Hispanic	Total
Type of Tobacco Product	%	%	%	%	%	%
Any Use						
Middle School	14.2	11.3	11.6	14.4	15.2	12.8
High School	38.1	31.4	39.4	24.0	30.7	34.8
Cigarette						
Middle School	9.6	8.8	8.8	9.0	11.0	9.2
High School	28.7	28.2	32.8	15.8	25.8	28.4
Smokeless tobacco						
Middle School	4.2	1.3	3.0	1.9	2.2	2.7
High School	11.6	1.5	8.7	2.4	3.6	6.6
Cigar						
Middle School	7.8	4.4	4.9	8.8	7.6	6.1
High School	20.3	10.2	16.0	14.8	13.4	15.3
Pipe						
Middle School	3.5	1.4	2.0	2.0	3.8	2.4
High School	4.2	1.4	2.6	1.8	3.8	2.8
Bidi						
Middle School	3.1	1.8	1.8	2.8	3.5	2.4
High School	6.1	3.8	4.4	5.8	5.6	5.0

(*Source:* National Youth Tobacco Survey)

1997), spray paint (from 1.4 percent in 1996 to 2.2 percent in 1997), and anesthetics, such as ether (0.2 percent in 1996 to 0.4 percent in 1997). Among adolescents, there were no significant differences between males and females in the use of inhalants.[47]

Overall, important age, racial and ethnic, and regional differences were found in the number of cases of inhalant use in 1997. Current use was highest among adolescents aged twelve to seventeen, whereas lifetime use was highest among the eighteen- to twenty-five-year age group. For both lifetime and past-year use, whites were more likely to report lifetime inhalant use than either blacks or Hispanics. Hispanics reported higher rates than blacks. Respondents living in metropolitan areas were significantly more likely to have used inhalants in the past year than those living in nonmetropolitan areas. Respondents in the West reported significantly higher levels of past-year inhalant use than did those in all other regions.

Discussion: What community education programs might prevent the experimentation of smoking among youth?

Table 9.13 Percentage reporting past-month use of alcohol.

Demographic Characteristic	12–17 1997	12–17 1998	18–25 1997	18–25 1998	26–34 1997	26–34 1998	35 and older 1997	35 and older 1998	Total 1997	Total 1998
TOTAL	20.5	19.1	58.4	60.0	60.2	60.9	52.8	53.1	51.4	51.7
Race/Ethnicity										
White, non-Hispanic	22.0	20.9	63.5	65.0	64.8	65.2	56.1	56.2	55.1	55.3
Black, non-Hispanic	16.3	13.1	46.6	50.3	51.0	54.8	40.9	38.3	40.4	39.8
Hispanic	18.8	18.9	48.5	50.8	51.6	53.1	42.8	47.7	42.4	45.4
Other, non-Hispanic	17.0	12.5	*	45.5	42.2	39.1	36.0	37.5	37.0	35.8
Gender										
Male	21.0	19.4	65.9	68.2	67.9	67.7	60.6	61.4	58.2	58.7
Female	19.9	18.7	50.8	51.7	52.6	54.2	46.0	45.8	45.1	45.1
Population Density										
Large Metro	21.4*	17.7	58.5	58.2	62.4	61.2	56.6	57.0	54.3	53.9
Small Metro	20.4	20.0	58.7	63.1	62.3	61.5	53.5	54.6	52.0	53.3
Nonmetro	19.0	20.1	58.0	57.4	51.0*	59.0	45.4	43.4	44.9	44.7
Region										
Northeast	19.3	22.1	59.9	64.3	60.3	62.4	56.7	57.7	54.0	55.8
North Central	23.4	20.6	68.0	72.1	66.6	67.9	55.3	58.7	55.6	57.8
South	19.3	17.5	55.1	54.4	57.9	58.3	47.7	45.6	47.4	45.8
West	20.3	17.4	53.3	53.0	56.8	56.5	55.7	55.0	51.7	50.9
Adult Education										
<High School	N/A	N/A	52.4	50.8	48.7	51.5	32.7	36.0	38.0	40.4
High School Grad	N/A	N/A	56.7	57.6	56.9	59.0	52.7	49.4	54.0	52.3
Some College	N/A	N/A	61.3	64.6	61.6	64.0	56.0	57.3	58.2	60.1
College Graduate	N/A	N/A	67.4	70.5	68.9	64.3	65.9	65.5	66.6	65.5
Current Employment										
Full-time	N/A	N/A	65.3	66.6	64.0	64.4	60.4	60.9	61.9	62.5
Part-time	N/A	N/A	51.5	56.0	59.9	59.9	58.4	59.1	56.6	58.4
Unemployed	N/A	N/A	55.8	63.3	55.7	54.5	61.7	59.8	58.8	59.7
Other	N/A	N/A	51.3	49.4	44.6	45.3	40.8	40.6	42.1	41.9

*Low precision; no estimate reported.
N/A: Not applicable.

(*Source:* CDC. Health, United States: 2000)

Drug use still shows class-related patterns of being more accessible and more utilized in lower socioeconomic groups where unemployment and school dropout rates are high among teens.

Health professionals in 2001 are suggesting that drug treatment may be preferential to drug enforcement. For young adults and teens, prevention is paramount. Experts suggest education programs that address the social aspects of drug use, not the familiar curriculum of the chemical nature of drugs. Decision making and coping skills curricula that is supplemented with self-esteem building and accurate information about peer behavior are essential to drug prevention for teens.

School-based drug use prevention programs have been an integral part of health education curricula and the U.S. anti-drug campaign for the past two decades. The most prevalent program in 1994 was D.A.R.E. (Drug Abuse Resistance Education). Since its inception in 1983, D.A.R.E. has been adopted by approximately 50 percent of local school districts nationwide.[48]

D.A.R.E.'s core curriculum, offered in the last grades of elementary school, focuses on teaching pupils the skills needed to recognize and resist social pressures to use drugs. It also provides information about drugs, teaches decision-making skills, builds self-esteem, and teaches how to choose healthy alternatives to drug use. Sadly, a study evaluating the effectiveness of the D.A.R.E. curriculum found that short-term effectiveness for reducing or preventing drug use behavior, alcohol, tobacco, and marijuana use is small and is less than that for interactive prevention programs.[49] It is generally found that curricula that moves from a less traditional teaching approach to a more student-centered, interactive approach may be more effective.

The DHHS created a new program for girls, *Girl Power*, a drug prevention program for nine- to fourteen-year-old girls. The message of this nontraditional drug prevention program is to teach confidence and promote self-esteem in girls at a time when previous studies have shown a loss of self-esteem in teen girls.

Violence

The United States has the highest rates of violence in the industrialized world.[50] Violence may range from bullying or verbal abuse to rape and homicide. The

Children's playing with guns often becomes a prelude to adolescent and young adult accidental death and homicide.

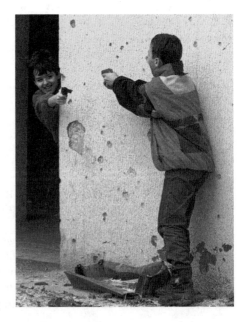

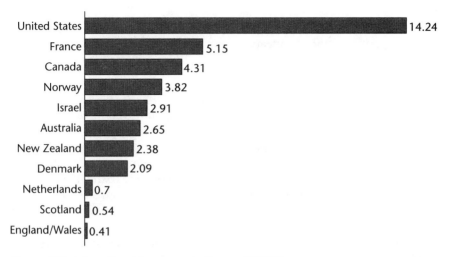

Figure 9.3 International handgun deaths per 100,000.

(*Source:* CDC, Bureau of Justice Statistics, 1999)

most common types of violence are those by acquaintances, followed by domestic violence, violence by strangers, and violence during robberies.[51] Violence exists in all age groups, in both genders and in every community. But some of the most prevalent and dangerous types of violent acts are committed by youth living in inner-city communities. "In many inner-city schools, not only do teachers practice fire drills, they also practice bullet drills."[52]

Adolescents aged twelve to nineteen have the highest victimization rates for crimes of violence and theft. Approximately one-third of these violent crimes involve a weapon, and approximately one-third of all robbery and assault victims sustain some sort of physical injury. Homicide rates are also highest among young adults and is the leading cause of death for both black males and females aged fifteen to twenty-four.[53] Access to weapons is a major contributing cause of accidental death from violent causes. Surveys show that guns are kept in 43 percent of American homes and that one-third of adolescents report that they could get a handgun if they wanted to.[54] The NASHS indicated that about 15 percent of adolescents carry a knife, 2 percent carry a gun, 10 percent carry another type of weapon, and 70 percent could get a gun if they wanted to. International handgun death rates are given in Figure 9.3.

Healthy People 2010 Objective: Reduce Weapon Carrying by Adolescents
on School Property

Target: 6 percent.

Baseline: 8.5 percent of students in grades 9 through 12 carried weapons on school property during the past thirty days in 1997.

Discussion: Which is the problem—students who carry weapons or a society that permits youth the means of acquiring weapons?

Gangs

There is no accepted, standard definition of a gang; however, the following criteria have been widely used in research: (1) formal organization structure, (2) identifiable leadership, (3) identified with a territory, (4) recurrent interaction, and (5) engaging in serious or violent behavior. Reports and estimates from responding agencies in 1995 indicate that there were more than 660,000 youth gang members and more than 23,000 gangs active in their jurisdictions during 1995.[55] The Department of Justice estimates there may be as many as 200,000 gang members in California alone.[56]

Gang membership is not well understood; however, some risk factors have been identified: [57]

1. *Racism:* When young people encounter both personal and institutional racism (i.e., systematic denial of privileges), the risks are increased. When groups of people are denied access to power, privileges, and resources, they will often form their own anti-establishment group.

2. *Poverty:* A sense of hopelessness can result from being unable to purchase wanted goods and services. Young people living in poverty may find it difficult to meet basic physical and psychological needs, which can lead to a lack of self-worth and pride. One way to earn cash is to join a gang involved in the drug trade.

3. *Lack of a support network.* Gang members often come from homes where they feel alienated or neglected. They may turn to gangs when their needs for love are not being met at home. Risks increase when the community fails to provide sufficient youth programs or alternatives to violence.

4. *Media influences.* Television, movies, radio, and music all have profound effects on youth development. Before youth have established their own value systems and are able to make moral judgments, the media promotes drugs, sex, and violence as an acceptable lifestyle.

Law enforcement surveys suggest that gang violence is increasing in more and more cities. The violence perpetrated by gangs is becoming more serious, with more injuries, and the use of more lethal weapons. About 6 percent of state prison inmates belonged to a gang prior to incarceration according to a 1991 Survey of Inmates in State Correctional Facilities. On the average, they had joined a gang at age fourteen.

Until the mid 1900s the majority of gangs in the United States were white. By the 1970s, about 80 percent of gang members were either black or Hispanic. In the 1990s, Asian gangs emerged. In 1991, twenty-seven cities reported female gangs with an estimated 7,205 female gang members. There is significant gang presence in public schools.[59] Thirty percent of students ages twelve

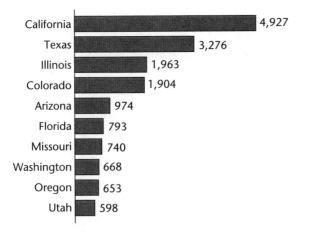

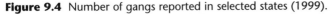

Figure 9.4 Number of gangs reported in selected states (1999).

(*Source:* Bureau of Justice Statistics. National Youth Gang Survey)

to nineteen reported the presence of street gangs in their school according to a 1996 survey. Number of gangs in selected states is given in Figure 9.4.

Prevention and intervention approaches generally have not been found to be effective, in part, because of inadequate evaluations of interventions. Intervention strategies have shifted from social intervention techniques to suppression strategies in the past two decades. Latest research suggest that opportunities provisions followed by community organization approaches may be the most effective deterrent and preventive measures in the future.[59] Gang violence is an immediate community health issue that is relatively new to health educators. It will require new training and understanding of these youth and their environments.

Suicide

Suicide among teens aged fifteen to twenty-four was the third leading cause of death in 1998, accounting for 15 percent of all suicides. More teenagers and young people die from suicide than from heart disease, cancer, AIDS, birth defects, strokes, pneumonia and influenza, and chronic lung disease *combined*. The 1990 objective was to reduce the rate of suicide among people fifteen to twenty-four to below 11 per 100,000. This objective was not met. In 1997, one in every twelve high school students reported having tried suicide, 27 percent had seriously contemplated it, and 2 percent were hurt during attempts, according to a CDC study of 12,000 high school students. Overall, youth suicide rates have been relatively stable since the baseline year of 1978. The risk for suicide among young people is greatest among young white males; however, from 1980 through 1995, suicide rates increased most rapidly among young black males. Although suicide among young children is a rare event, the dramatic increase in the rate among persons aged ten to fourteen years underscores the urgent need for intensifying efforts to prevent suicide among persons in this age group.

One-third of students in the NASHS study reported that they have seriously thought about committing suicide and 14 percent report having actually tried. The accessibility of firearms is a contributing factor to youth suicide. Among persons aged fifteen to nineteen years, firearm-related suicides accounted for 62 percent of the increase in the overall rate of suicide from 1980–1997. Every six hours, a youth aged ten to nineteen commits suicide with a gun.[60] The odds that potentially suicidal adolescents will kill themselves double when a handgun is kept in the home, since most teen suicides are impulsive, with little or no planning, and 70 percent of suicides occur in the victims' homes. The accessibility and ease in handling of a firearm accounts for unprecedented mortality among this age group due to handgun suicides.[61]

School Health

Each school day about 48 million youth in the United States attend almost 110,000 elementary and secondary schools for about six hours of classroom time. More than 95 percent of all youth aged five to seventeen years are enrolled in school. Schools are second only to homes among the primary places where children spend their time and thus are one of the significant places where children may be exposed to instruction regarding prevention of health risks.

School health programs are thought to be the most effective means of reducing deaths and promoting health among youth. Basic health services and health education should be a national goal for all children although Americans are far from providing this universal care for all children.

The comprehensive school health program has eight primary components. In 1990 those elements of school health education were identified:

1. a documented, planned, and sequential program of health education for students in kindergarten through grade 12

2. a curriculum that addresses and integrates education about a range of categorical health problems and issues at developmentally appropriate ages

3. activities to help young persons develop the skills they will need to avoid risky behaviors

4. instruction provided for a prescribed amount of time at each grade level

5. management and coordination in each school by an education professional trained to implement the program

6. instruction from teachers who have been trained to teach the subject

7. involvement of parents, health professionals, and other concerned community members

8. periodic evaluation, updating, and improvement[63]

See Chapter 17 for a complete discussion of comprehensive school health programs.

Healthy People 2010 Objective: Increase the Proportion of Schools that Provide Comprehensive School Health Education

Summary

The best measure of a nation's health is its infant mortality rate. The good news in the United States is that the infant mortality rate declined in the twentieth century and approached the Healthy People 2000 target. The bad news is that for blacks, the infant mortality rate is 2.5 times greater than for whites and is as high as the rate in some developing countries. Given all that we know about how to prevent infant mortality, increasing prenatal care, decreasing teen pregnancies, and providing better maternal care, there is little reason, other than neglect and perhaps racism, that black infant mortality is so high.

Whose responsibility is it to teach children and teens about diseases, hygiene, risk reduction, sexuality, and decision making? Most would agree that the ideal location would be the home and that the best teacher would be one's parents. However, if parents do not have the knowledge, skills, interest, or attention of their children to do this work, it must also be done somewhere by people trained to do the job. School health programs are a vital part of public health service and education. Growing problems such as HIV, new problems such as gangs, and exposed problems such as child sexual abuse, are requiring communities to learn skills and test new interventions. Making young people a part of the decision-making and intervention process will be an essential component of community action.

CYBERSITES RELATED TO CHAPTER 9

Children
  www.childrennow.org
  www.childadvocate.net
  www.childwelfare.com

QUESTIONS

1. What is the cost of infant morbidity or deprivation to society?
2. Why haven't mothers and infants received adequate attention in the United States?
3. How might racism affect our commitment to infants and children?
4. How can we teach young people about their health risks at a time when they feel invincible?
5. Should sexuality education, like alcohol/drug education, be required in the schools? At what age do schools begin sexuality education?

EXERCISES

1. See what prenatal/newborn health services are available in your community. Are they accessible to all? Are they affordable? Would you feel comfortable accessing them if the need arose?

2. Follow a junior or high school teen through a typical week of decision making about her or his health behaviors. What are the variables that impact decisions? What is the relative influence of parents, peers, religion, laws, developmental stage, fun and pleasure, and gender on these decisions?

3. If you are sexually active or have been sexually active, visit your private clinician or the public health testing service in your community and get an STD examination. If you are not yet sexually active, make a list of questions you will ask a new partner about her or his sexual history before you engage in sexual activity with this person. How and when will you approach these questions with a partner? How will you ensure your safety and health from STDs?

INTERNET INTERACTIVE ACTIVITY

CENSUS STATS

The Census Stats is a program that allows you to compare census data among counties within your state . The homepage for CensusStat is:

www.tier2.census.gov/dbappweb.htm

Example

Perhaps you want to know the number of children living in poverty in your state by county.

1. Go to CensusStat

tier2.census.gov/dbappweb.htm

2. Click on **USA Counties Data**

tier2.census.gov/usac/index.html

3. Select a state

North Carolina

4. Select a county

Alleghany County

5. Select a data set

Poverty

6. **submit**

7. Select

**Related children under 18 years old below poverty in 1989
Compare**

You have a table with comparative demographic data of persons in poverty in 1979 and 1989. You window looks something like this:

Persons for whom poverty status has been determined in 1979   9,477
Persons for whom poverty status has been determined in 1989   9,372
Persons below poverty level in 1979   1,857
Persons below poverty level in 1989   1,880

By scrolling through the data you now know the number of children under eighteen years old living in poverty in 1989 in Alleghany county—2,031.

You can click on the Table link and then select other counties from which to compare this variable or other vital statistics that interest you.

Exercise

1. Go to the Census Stat home page

   tier2.census.gov/dbappweb.htm

2. Click on **USA counties**

3. Select a state that you want to describe.

4. Obtain a general profile of your state by selecting this category from among possible categories of analysis.

5. By clicking between **Compare** and **Table,** and **categories available on the U.S. counties page,** build a general profile of your state as compared to three counties within your state. Describe your state and counties by building a table that uses ten demographic comparisons associated with children.

REFERENCES

1. www.who.org/whr/1998/factse.htm

2. WHO (1992). *Facts about WHO.* WHO. Geneva.

3. Ibid.

4. United Nations Children's Fund (1992). The State of the World's Children 1992.

5. www.health.gov/healthypeople/Document/HTML/Volume2/16MICH.htm#_Toc471971358

6. www.childstats.gov

7. Adamson, David (1990). *Defending the world.* London: Tauris and Co.

8. WHO, op. cit.

9. Life Expectancy Hits New High (2000). www.seniors.gov/articles/1001/life-expectancy

10. WHO, op. cit.

11. www.health.gov/healthypeople/Document/HTML/Volume2/16MICH.htm#_Toc471971358

12. Sternberg, Steve (1998). Teen-agers in turmoil. *USA Today*, October 5, p. A1.

13. U.S. Congress, Office of Technology Assessment (1988). Healthy children: Investing in the future. Washington, D.C. US Government Printing Office.

14. Kann, Laura, Warren, Charles, et al. (1995). Youth risk behavior surveillance—U.S., 1993. *Journal of School Health,* May, Vol. 65, No. 5, p. 163.

15. Snider, Mike (1992). U.S. children get a non-so-clean bill of health. *USA Today,* October 6, p. D6.

16. Healy, Michelle (1993). Kids build child safety into a home. *USA Today,* July 29, p. D4.

17. Kann, op. cit.

18. Ibid.

19. Ibid.

20. Ibid.

21. *Salt Lake Tribune* (1994). Child poverty. September 27, p. A2.

22. www.health.gov/healthypeople/Document/HTML/Volume2/ 16MICH.htm#_Toc471971358

23. Editorial (1994). *APHA Journal,* Vol. 84, No. 4 April p. 540.

24. www.health.gov/healthypeople/Document/HTML/Volume2/ 16MICH.htm#_Toc471971358

25. Ibid.

26. Ibid.

27. Laraque, Danielle (1994). The Central Harlem playground injury prevention project: A model for change. *AJPH.* October Vol. 84 (10), pp. 1691–1692.

28. Ibid.

29. NCPCA (1997). Child Abuse and Neglet Statistics. www.childabuse.org

30. Ibid.

31. Ibid.

32. resevoir.fhi.org/en/fp/fppubs/network

33. Ibid.

34. NCPCA, op. cit.

35. www.health.gov/healthypeople/Document/HTML/Volume2/16MICH.htm#_ Toc471971358

36. Ibid.

37. Ibid.

38. Brown, Robert. (1997). The pediatrician and the sexually active adolescent: Sexual activity. *Pediatric Clinics of North America* 44(12).

39. CDC (1993). 1993 Sexually Transmitted Diseases Treatment Guidelines. MMWR. September 24, 42(RR-14), Atlanta.

40. www.who.int/asd/figures/global_report.html

41. Heyman, R., & Killar, L. (1996). Teen talk. American Medical Association pamphlet.

42. Centers for Disease Control (CDC), Youth Risk Behavior Surveillance—United States, 1995. MMWR; 45(No. SS-4), 1–86, 1996.

43. Novello, Antonia C. (1992). Alcohol and kids: Its time for candor. *The Christian Science Monitor,* June 26., p. 19.

44. Ennett, Susan T. et. al. (1994). How effective is drug abuse resistance education? A meta-analysis of project DARE outcome evaluations. *AJPH,* September, Vol. 84 (9), p. 1394.

45. www.health.gov/healthypeople/Document/HTML/Volume2/16MICH.htm#_Toc471971358

46. Public Health Report Annual Supplement (1993). Measuring Use of Alcohol and Other Drugs Among Adolescents. USGPO. pp. 25–29.

47. Ennet, op. cit.

48. Ibid.

49. Howell, James C. (1994). Gangs. Office of Juvenile Justice and Delinquency Prevention. Fact Sheet #12, April.

50. Stayduhar, Katharine, & Sekhon, Linda (1998). Comprehensive plan to prevent adolescent injuries and viiolence: The role of clincians. *Physician Assistant* 22(3), pp. 83–89.

51. Shepherd, Jonathan. (1998). Tackling violence: Interagency procedures and injury surveillance are urgently needed. *British Medical Journal* 316(7135), pp. 879–881.

52. Winning the war against gangs (1996). Pamphlet.

53. Brown, op. cit.

54. Ibid.

55. National Youth Gang Center (1996). 1995 National Youth Gang Survey.

56. Nakamura, Raymond (1999). *Health and wellness: A multicultural perspective.* MA: Allyn & Bacon.

57. Glick, B. (1992). In New York: Governor's task force tackles growing juvenile gang problem. *Corrections Today,* 54, 92–97.

58. Winning the War Against Gangs, op. cit

59. Ibid.

60. National Center for Health Statistics (3/23/93).

61. Ibid.

62. Marx, E., Wooley, S.F., & Northrop, D. (eds.). *Health is academic: A guide to coordinated school health.* New York: Teachers College Press, 1998.

CHAPTER 10

Older Adults

Community Health in the 21st Century
The twenty-first century definitely will focus on the senior population—the
fastest growing portion of the population. There will be an emphasis on
chronic diseases such as arthritis and quality of life associated with a longer
lifespan. Hopefully, financial resources like Medicare and Social Security will
be viable and adequate to meet the demands of this very large population.

—Ann Hopkins, B.S. Health Education; Gerontology certificate,
Director of Health Promotion Services, YWCA

Chapter Objectives

The student will:

1. define gerontology and geriatrics.
2. discuss how life expectancy is increasing.
3. discuss Medicare and Medicaid in relation to long-term care.
4. list five characteristics of older adults.
5. discuss older adult health care priorities and how community health educators can intercede.
6. define elder abuse.
7. define and give one example of ageism.

Aging

Aging is the one life experience that is common to all human beings. There are similarities between the plight of children and that of older persons, but there are also important differences. In general, both populations are more likely to be influenced by their environment than to influence it.[1] Worldwide, between 1994 and 2030, people over sixty will triple in number, from half a billion to 1.4 billion.[2] Women in both developed and developing countries far outnumber aging men (Figure 10.1).

The population of those over sixty-five in the United States has more than tripled since 1900 to 35 million in 2000 and an estimated 70.2 million in 2030 as shown in Figure 10.2. We are in the midst of a longevity revolution that is enhanced by better public sanitation and personal hygiene, improved nutrition, and general medical progress.[3] The average age of the U.S. population has been increasing throughout this century. A 1997 longevity and retirement study

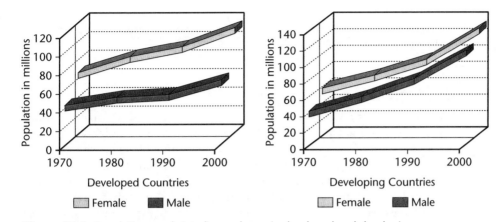

Figure 10.1 Population aged sixty-five and over in developed and developing countries by sex (1970 to 2000).

(*Source:* Office of Publications, WHO, 1992)

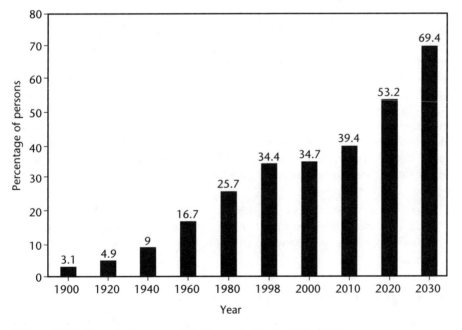

Figure 10.2 Percent of persons sixty-five and older in United States.

(*Source:* U.S. Census Bureau)

revealed that 41 percent of people now working feel it is at least somewhat likely that they will live to age eighty-five, 23 percent feel somewhat likely they will live to age ninety, and even 15 percent feel it is at least somewhat likely they will live to age ninety-five. America is on the brink of massive social change.[4]

Discussion: Why do older people often receive less respect as they grow older? Can this trend be reversed?

Life Expectancy

Life expectancy is an epidemiological concept that refers to the average duration of time that individuals of a given age can expect to live. Ability to survive the first year of life is a major variable in determining life expectancy for any cohort of people as discussed in Chapter 17. Life expectancy of a birth group of infants represents the average number of years that this cohort would live given the morbidity and mortality conditions of the times. Generally, females have a longer life expectancy than males, whites a longer life expectancy than people of color in the United States, and Midwesterners live longer than people in other geographical locations in the United States.

The United States has experienced an unprecedented gain of twenty-eight years in life expectancy from birth in this century alone. This figure is nearly equal to the total number of years added to life expectancy during the preceding 5,000 years of human history. From 1960 to 2000, life expectancy at age sixty-five was highest for white females, followed by black females, white males, and black males. In 1989, life expectancy at age eighty-five showed a crossover in that for each sex, life expectancy was higher for black than for white persons.[5] The average life expectancy at birth in 2000 in the United States for white men was 73.3 years and 79.6 years for white women compared to 64.9 years for black men and 73.9 years for black woman. Table 10.1 describes the life expectancy at birth according to gender by a variety of countries. Notice that Japan has the highest life expectancy for men and women, while the United States falls many countries lower on the table.

Discussion: What factors make life expectancy lower in the United States than in comparable countries? What community education programs might increase life expectancy in the United States?

The Demographics of Older Adults

Demographic trends are shifting toward an older population in the United States and this is sometimes referred to as "the graying of America." In 1998 there were 33 million people over the age of sixty-five. Between 1985 and 2020, the sixty-five and older population is expected to more than double. One in every five people will be an older adult. Not only will there be many older people in the twenty-first century, but the proportion of older women will increase. Women outlive men every place in the world where women no longer perform backbreaking physical labor and where adequate sanitation and reduced maternal mortality are present.

Table 10.1 Life expectancy at birth in some selected countries
2000–2005 and 2020–2025.

Country	2000–2005	2020–2025
World	63	70
MDC[1]	75	79
LDC[2]	62	69
Australia	79.2	81.0
China	71.2	75.5
France	79.0	81.5
Germany	78.8	81.0
Israel	79.2	81.6
Japan	81.5	84.9
Mexico	73.0	76.1
Russian Federation	66.0	72.0
United Kingdom	78.2	81.1
United States	77.5	80.7
Congo	51.6	60.9
Ethiopia	43.3	53.0
Mozambique	38.0	47.4
Nepal	59.8	68.9
Zimbabwe	42.9	56.3

[1]More developed countries.
[2]Less developed countries.

(*Source:* www.un.org/esa/population/wwp2000.at.pdf (2001))

Discussion: Since women outlive men, how should community health accommodate this demographic fact?

In the United States, women outlive men because of lower mortality from arteriosclerosis, lung cancer, chronic obstructive pulmonary disease, industrial accidents, suicide, and cirrhosis of the liver. For many older Americans, the so-called golden years are actually a very stressful time in search of affordable housing, health care, food, and leisure. Almost 20 percent of people over sixty-five years in the United States are considered poor or nearly poor. Figures 10.3 and 10.4 break down this figure by ethnicity, marital status, and gender. In 2000, the federal poverty level was $8,350 a year for one elderly person and $11,250 a year for an elderly couple. If you are a woman, black, Hispanic, or older than seventy-five years, your chances of being poor or nearly poor increase dramatically.[6] Thirty-four percent of older blacks, 22 percent of Hispanics, and 10 percent of whites live in poverty. The poorest of the poor elderly are black females, says Samuel Simmons, President of the National Caucus and Center on Black Aged.[7]

Poor older citizens spend nearly 20 percent of their limited incomes on out-of-pocket health care expenses often because they are not properly enrolled in

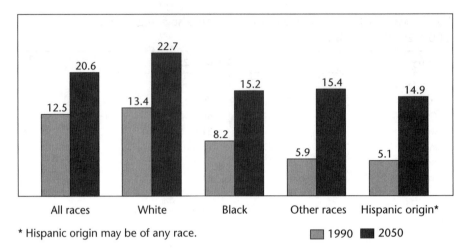

* Hispanic origin may be of any race.   ▢ 1990 ■ 2050

Figure 10.3 Percent of Americans living in poverty by race (1990 and 2050).

(*Source:* Older P{opulation of the United States. U.S. Census Bureau)

federal health programs such as Medicare and Medicaid which would fill health care gaps. People without savings must depend solely upon monthly Social Security payments that may be less than $400 a month. These poor will need to be plugged into food stamps, supplemental food programs, and Medicaid assistance to have an adequate quality of life.

Although the rate of poverty is lower for older Americans (12.9 percent) than the national rate, between 2.5 and 4.9 million suffer from hunger and food insecurity according to a national survey by the Urban Institute. Often people on fixed incomes must choose between buying food or medicines or paying a utility bill. Unfortunately, many seniors have incomes just above the poverty line which make them ineligible for food stamps or Supplemental Security Income. In 1993, nine out of ten low income seniors did not receive food stamps although they were hungry. Demographically, those most hungry are women, between sixty and sixty-four years old, Latino and have less than a high school education.

Older People of Color

The effects of institutionalized racism fall most heavily on black men, whose life expectancy is 7.4 years less than white men.[8] Older black citizens generally live in central cities with some of the worst housing and fewer social and health services than are available to more affluent, suburban older persons.

The distribution of older persons of color and whites in the United States is given in Figures 10.4 and 10. 5. The number of Hispanic elderly is expected to rise dramatically, from 5 percent of the total Hispanic population in 1980 to about seven times larger in 2030. In addition to lower life expectancy than whites, older Hispanics face poverty, poor housing, lack of medical care and education, and the turmoil of drastic changes in their traditional lifestyles. A

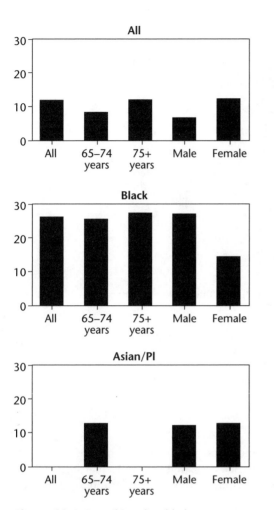
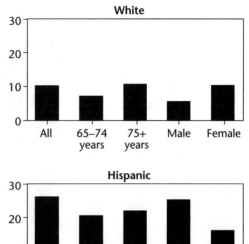
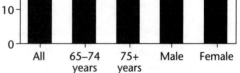

Figure 10.4 Describing the elderly poor: percentage in poverty by race, age, and gender (1998).

sense of personal privacy and pride make it difficult for older Hispanics to ask for and accept financial or medical aid through government programs.[9]

Of the 1.6 million Native Americans about 7 percent of the population is aged sixty-five and older. Over half live in rural areas, a far greater proportion than any other elderly subgroup. The Indian Health Service provides health care to most of these Native Americans, however, since they are among the poorest people in the United States, health care is seldom adequate to meet their tremendous needs.[10] One of the greatest hardships for these rural dwellers is their ability to even make it to a hospital or clinic, which may be miles and hours from their home.

Approximately 8 percent of Asian Pacific Islanders are over sixty-five years. About 90 percent of Asian Pacific Americans live in urban areas, usually connected to a rather strong family or extended family network. Health surveys

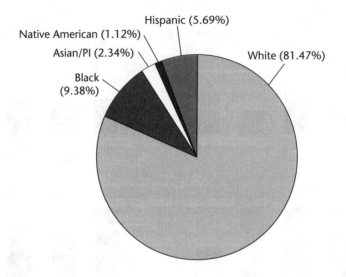

Figure 10.5 Racial diversity of people in the United States (1999).

(*Source:* U.S. Census Bureau)

have found that health issues vary by specific Asian ethnicity. Chinese Americans, for instance, tend to be quite poor, while Japanese Americans tend to be quite physically healthy and long-lived.[11]

Defining Aging

Biological aging refers to anatomical and psychological changes that occur over time in various systems of the body. Changes in molecular and cellular structures, tissue degradation, decreased immunity to disease, and lower metabolism are examples of biological aging.[12]

Social aging refers to the social habits and roles of an individual with respect to his or her culture.[13] The decrease in social interaction so often found in older people is partly the result of the withdrawal of society from the individual rather than the individual from society.[14]

Psychological aging is concerned with the interchanges between the person and the psychological or social environments. It is also concerned with an individual's adaptation to both the internal and external experiences of the world. The way aging is promoted through the media is extremely negative and is often internalized by older people.

Long-Term Health Care

In 1999, among those between the ages of sixty-five to seventy-four, only 1.5 percent were living in nursing homes. In total, among all people over sixty-five, only 4.3 percent are institutionalized. A surprise to many is that Medicare is not a major purchaser of nursing home care, but that Medicaid has the honors. Older patients who are chronically ill are discovering that unless they are eligible for Medicaid, their long-term health care costs, are not covered. Medicare pays only about 2 percent of all nursing facility costs although Medicare was the expected principal source of payment for 50 percent of the older population.[15] Medicare coverage for nursing facilities averages less than thirty days of care and that applies only to skilled nursing care. Medicare covers no long-term nursing facility or other residential care, and its home health care coverage is equally limited. The only comprehensive coverage of long-term care comes from Medicaid. This federal government program for low income people, administered by the states, pays for almost half the nation's total nursing facility costs and for much home care as well.

To be eligible for Medicaid, one has to deplete all of his or her financial resources first. The example was given of one woman who had to sell her graveplot to be eligible to enter terminal care facilities to die. It is alarming how many nursing home patients quickly end up in poverty by necessity. Nursing facility care averaged $3,500 per month in 1999. Most people exhaust their personal savings within six months of entering a residential care facility. One-third of disabled elderly who spend any time in a nursing home end up impoverished.[16]

The long-term care issue has been brought to national attention largely through the work of the American Association of Retired Persons' (AARP) campaign called Long-Term Care '88, as well as through a variety of other organizations. The late Congressman Claude Pepper's diligent efforts at achieving representation for older citizens, especially in relation to long-term care proved to be premature, but catalytic.

Characteristics of Older Adults

The demographic characteristics of men and women over sixty-five years from 1980 to 1998 are reported in Table 10.2. Of those women and men over sixty-five years, 80 percent are neither fully disabled nor institutionalized. The prevalence of disability in people over sixty-five has dropped in the past two decades.[17]

Although one cannot stereotype an older person, there are some characteristics and circumstances that tend to be rather common to this population:

1. Loss of status and an increased uncertainty about personal worth

2. Insecurity associated with feeling of inability to meet the demands of life

3. Apprehension about health

4. Difficulty in adjusting from a work routine to one of retirement

5. Inability to find avenues of service that will provide personal gratification

6. Difficulty in handling stresses created by social change

7. Limited incentive for social participation

Table 10.2 Characteristics of persons 65 years and over by gender.

Characteristic	Total				Male				Female			
	1980	1990	1995	1998	1980	1990	1995	1998	1980	1990	1995	1998
Total (million)	24.2	29.6	31.7	32.1	9.9	12.3	13.2	13.5	14.2	17.2	18.5	18.6
PERCENT DISTRIBUTION												
Marital status:												
Single	5.5	4.6	4.2	4.3	4.9	4.2	4.2	3.8	5.9	4.9	4.2	4.7
Married	55.4	56.1	56.9	56.6	78.0	76.5	77.0	75.1	39.5	41.4	42.5	42.9
Spouse present	53.6	54.1	54.7	54.2	76.1	74.2	74.5	72.6	37.9	39.7	10.6	40.7
Spouse absent	1.8	2.0	2.2	2.4	1.9	2.3	2.5	2.5	1.7	1.7	1.9	2.2
Widowed	35.7	34.2	33.2	32.5	13.5	14.2	13.5	14.9	51.2	48.6	47.3	45.2
Divorced	3.5	5.0	5.7	6.7	3.6	5.0	5.2	6.1	3.4	5.1	6.0	7.1
Family status:												
In families[1]	67.6	66.7	66.6	66.8	83.0	81.9	80.6	79.6	56.8	55.8	56.7	57.5
Nonfamily householders	31.2	31.9	32.4	31.9	15.7	16.6	18.4	18.4	42.0	42.8	42.4	41.7
Secondary individuals	1.2	1.4	1.0	1.3	1.3	1.5	1.0	2.0	1.1	1.4	0.9	0.7
Living arrangements:												
Living in household	99.8	99.7	99.9	100.0	99.9	99.9	100.0	100.0	99.7	99.5	99.9	100.0
Living alone	30.3	31.0	31.5	30.9	14.9	15.7	17.3	17.3	41.0	42.0	41.7	40.8
Spouse present	53.6	54.1	54.7	54.2	76.1	74.3	74.5	72.6	37.9	39.7	40.6	40.7
Living with someone else	15.9	14.6	13.7	14.9	8.9	9.9	8.1	10.0	20.8	17.8	17.6	18.4
Not in household[2]	0.2	0.3	0.1	-	0.1	0.1	-	-	0.3	0.5	0.1	-
Years of school completed:												
8 years or less	43.1	28.5	21.0	18.1	45.3	30.0	22.0	18.3	41.6	27.5	20.3	17.9
1 to 3 years of high school	16.2	16.1	[3]15.2	[3]14.9	15.5	15.7	[3]14.5	[3]14.1	16.7	16.4	[3]15.6	[3]15.4
4 years of high school	24.0	32.9	[4]33.8	[4]35.0	21.4	29.0	[4]29.2	[4]30.2	25.8	35.6	[4]37.1	[4]38.4
1 to 3 years of college	8.2	10.9	[5]17.1	[5]17.2	7.5	10.8	[5]17.1	[5]17.6	8.6	11.0	[5]17.0	[5]17.0
4 years or more of college	8.6	11.6	[6]13.0	[6]14.8	10.3	14.5	[6]17.2	[6]19.8	7.4	9.5	[6]9.9	[6]11.2
Labor force participation:[7]												
Employed	12.2	11.5	11.7	11.6	18.4	15.9	16.1	15.9	7.8	8.4	8.5	8.3
Unemployed	0.4	0.4	0.5	0.4	0.6	0.5	0.7	0.5	0.3	0.3	0.3	0.3
Not in labor force	87.5	88.1	87.9	88.1	81.0	83.6	83.2	83.5	91.9	91.3	91.2	91.4
Percent below poverty level[8]	15.2	11.4	11.7	10.5	11.1	7.8	7.2	7.0	17.9	13.9	14.9	13.1

- Represents zero. [1]Excludes those living in unrelated subfamilies. [2]In group quarters other than institutions. [3]Represents those who completed 9th to 12th grade, but have no high school diploma. [4]High school graduate. [5]Some college or associate degree. [6]Bachelor's or advanced degree. [7]Annual averages of monthly figures. *Source:* U.S. Bureau of Labor Statistics, *Employment and Earnings,* January issues. See footnote 2, Table 649. [8]Poverty status based on income in preceding year.

(*Source:* Except as noted, U.S. Census Bureau, *Current Population Reports,* P20-514, and earlier reports; P60-201; and unpublished data)

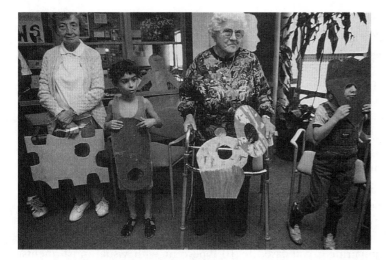

Long-term health care now includes integrating adult wisdom and experience with children's need for affection, respect, and interaction with others.

Normal aging also involves some physical manifestations that do not necessarily impair the efficiency of the body or lead to disease or death. They merely may bring about modification in an individual's lifestyle. As examples:

1. Skin: flaccid, dry, wrinkled; progressive hair loss or thinning; less sweat

2. Musculo-skeletal: limitations in mobility; stiffened joints, porous bones

3. Nervous system: slower reflexes; decrease in response to stimuli

4. Senses: hearing, taste, vision, touch, balance, and smell less acute

5. Respiratory: impairments with ventilation, diffusion, and circulation

6. Gastrointestinal: reduction in gastric motility; diminished peristalsis; hemorrhoids

7. Urinary: diminution of filtration rate; nighttime urination

8. Reproductive: ovulation terminates in women; sperm counts are reduced in men

9. Sexuality: response may be somewhat slower; vaginal drying; longer refractory period

10. Nutrition: slowed digestive processes; change in food habits

Among the noninstitutionalized older population, 70 percent rank their health as excellent or good although four out of five older adults have at least one chronic condition. Forty-eight percent have arthritis, 27 percent have heart conditions, 39 percent have hypertension, and 28 percent are hearing impaired. Only 10 percent cannot function independently. Functional independence means the ability to take care of ones feeding, toileting, and dressing. Even among the 10 percent who are not functionally independent, many of the disabilities experienced could be prevented by changes in lifestyle behaviors and habits. Across all age groups of the elderly and in both sexes, significantly greater numbers of white persons than black persons rate their health as excellent or very good, and significantly greater numbers of black than white rate their health as fair or poor.[18]

The 1979 Surgeon General Report on Aging suggested that new emphasis should be placed on "functional independence" instead of tertiary care. Four goals were: (1) the compression of mortality, (2) preventive gerontology, (3) successful aging, (4) redefining old age as over seventy-five years, and (5) extending healthspan.[19]

Health Priorities of Older People

Changes in our physical and mental abilities that occur as we age are often accentuated, such as the acuteness of our senses, cardiovascular health, mental agility, mobility, and memory. Perceptual impairments, especially hearing loss, increase with age. Thirty percent of persons over sixty-five years reported having hearing impairment compared to 10.1 percent with visual impairments. Hearing loss is more common among older men than older women. Vision and hearing are correctable and some blindness can be avoided through glaucoma testing. A major unresolved problem with hearing loss is the lack of adequate third-party insurance reimbursement. This is a critical reason why so many older people delay going for help with hearing problems. Medicare will reimburse for audiologic services, but will not pay for the hearing aid evaluation, consultation, or the hearing aid itself.

The four most common causes of visual impairment in people over sixty-five are macular degeneration, cataracts, glaucoma, and diabetic retinopathy. Most of these problems are avoidable either through prevention or early treatment, especially cataracts and glaucoma.[20]

Psychological illness that may be particular to older people are issues of loss and bereavement, although the AIDS epidemic has somewhat sensitized people to bereavement earlier than usually expected. Loss of meaningful employment, or lack of financial security, add to depression.

The Objectives for the Nation give highest priority to sensory deprivation control, although when surveyed, older people rank emotional needs much higher than physical needs. Among the common emotional reactions that older adults must anticipate and cope with are grief, guilt, loneliness, anxiety, depression, sense of impotence and helplessness, and rage.[21] These intrinsic, psychological reactions are often the result of concrete issues such as financial worries, sensory loss, disease, and disability, hospitalization and surgery, changes in body image, chronic pain, death and dying. Health programs must focus particularly on prevention of strokes, diabetes, sleep problems, depression, leg ulcers, arthritis, visual impairment, hearing impairment, and incontinence.[22] Simple moderate exercise and regular activity can reduce many unwanted conditions associated with aging. The most frequently occurring conditions per 100 people over sixty-five years in 2001 is shown in Figure 10.6.

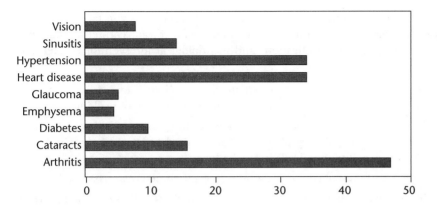

Figure 10.6 Percent of chronic health conditions of persons over 65 years (2001).

(*Source:* American Society of Consultant Pharmcists, 2001.
www.ascp.com/public/pr/fact/chronic.shtml)

Causes of Premature Death

Everyone dies, but the ways in which people grow old vary. The impact of societal change dramatically affects the aging process and how one ages. Therefore, using cohort studies to learn about aging is the preferred approach since these would account for social, political, and economic changes to a group. Cohort studies show differences in diet, exercise, standard of living, education, work history, medical care, sexuality, and experience with chronic and acute diseases.[23] The stresses of different cohorts affect the incidence and rates of premature and naturally caused death, and can better help community health educators adapt prevention programs accordingly.

Falls

The leading cause of accidental death among those over sixty-five is falls, which accounts for 56 percent of all deaths and has a rate of 56.7 per 100,000 among those over seventy-five years. Approximately 33 percent of adults aged sixty-five years or older fall each year, implicating environmental factors in one-third to one-half of their falls. In 1999, about 9,000 people over the age of sixty-five years died from fall-related injuries. Of all fall deaths, more than 60 percent involve people who are seventy-five years or older. Fall-related death rates are higher among men than women and differ by race. White men have the highest death rate, followed by white women, black men, and black women.[24]

A study of falls in the elderly found that 25 percent of falls occurred in the bedroom, 8 percent in the kitchen, and 22 percent in the dining room. Primary reasons for falls included: (1) trouble getting in and out of bed, (2) no grab bar for the toilet, (3) loose or wobbly grab bars, (4) difficulty with chairs and sofas, and (5) using furniture for support.[25]

Falls are caused by the interaction of a number of different factors. For this reason, fall prevention requires a combination of medical treatment, rehabilitation, environmental modification, and technological interventions. Interventions include:

- Physical conditioning and/or rehabilitation such as exercise to improve strength and endurance, physical therapy, gait training, or walking programs.
- Environmental assessments and modifications to improve mobility and safety (e.g., installing grab bars, adding raised toilet seats, lowering bed heights, installing handrails in the hallways).
- A review of prescribed medications to assess their potential risks and benefits.
- Technological devices (e.g., alarm systems that are activated when patients try to get out of bed or move unassisted, or protective hip pads).[26]

Primary Prevention   Primary prevention of fall-related injuries among older adults can be targeted to persons living independently in the community or residents of nursing homes. Research has established that effective fall intervention programs employ a multifaceted approach and incorporate both behavioral and environmental elements: exercises to improve strength and balance, environmental modifications, education about fall prevention, medication review and assessment to minimize side effects, and risk factor reduction.

Another unintentional injury associated with the risks associated with falls is pedestrian death. The elderly have the highest rate of all pedestrian deaths and injury in the United States. Only one in one hundred manages to cross the street in time allocated by crossing lights. Other hearing, balance, and vision impairments increase the risk of pedestrian injury for older Americans.

Suicide

One preventable cause of premature death among older people is suicide. Older Americans are disproportionately likely to commit suicide. Comprising only 13 percent of the U.S. population, individuals ages sixty-five and older account for 20 percent of all suicide deaths, with white males being particularly vulnerable. The highest rate is for white men ages eighty-five and older: 65.3 deaths per 100,000 persons in 1996 (the most recent year for which statistics are available), about six times the national U.S. rate of 10.8 per 100,000.

There is little increase in suicide mortality among widows, but there is a substantial increase among widowed men probably due to loss of spouse and lack of independent skills. Major depression, a significant predictor of suicide in elderly Americans, is a widely under-recognized and under-treated medical illness. According to one study, many older adults who commit suicide have visited their primary care physician very close to the time of the suicide: 20 percent on the same day, 40 percent within one week, and 70 percent within one month of the suicide.

Pneumonia and Influenza

According to Centers for Disease Control and Prevention, more than 40,000 older people in the United States die each year from pneumonia or influenza. With the aging of the U.S. population, increasing numbers of adults will be at risk for these major causes of illness and death. Persons with high-risk conditions (that is, heart disease, diabetes, and chronic respiratory disease) remain at increased risk for these diseases, as do persons living in institutional settings.

A new, once-in-a-lifetime vaccine for pneumonia is thought to be able to reduce the death rate from pneumonia by 50 percent. Vaccination against pneumococcal infections and influenza among persons aged sixty-five years and over has increased slightly for blacks and Hispanics although current levels of coverage among adults vary widely among age, risk, and racial and ethnic groups. For example, influenza vaccination rates for whites were 66 percent in 1997, whereas for blacks and Hispanics, rates were only 45 and 53 percent, respectively. In September 1997 the Department of Health and Human Services approved a plan to improve adult vaccination rates and reduce disparities among racial and ethnic groups. Better community health education to make clinicians and older Americans aware of this cost-effective vaccine is an important goal.

Healthy People 2010 Objective: Increase the Proportion of Adults Who Are Vaccinated Annually Against Influenza and Pneumococcal Disease

Increase in Adult Vaccinations	1997 Baseline	2010 Target
Noninstitutionalized adults aged 65 years and older		
Influenza vaccine	63	90
Pneumococcal vaccine	43	90

Alzheimer's Disease

During the last century there has been a change in the terminology used to describe the dementia condition now known as Alzheimer's disease. Some thought the condition was merely "senility," which was erroneously assumed to be inevitably associated with aging. Alois Alzheimer's first case (1906) was a fifty-one-year-old woman and because early-onset dementia was thought to be distinct from late onset, confusion over the proper diagnosis existed.

Whatever the diagnostic term, the epidemiologic figures are astounding. The National Institute on Aging (NIA) estimates that approximately 4 million persons (approximately 10.9 percent of the population over age sixty-five) have Alzheimer's disease. Diagnosis is usually determined through a patient's medical history and a physician's examination of the individual's cognitive functioning. Alzheimer's generally develops over an extended period of time with the duration of noticeable symptoms spanning four to eight years, and, in some instances, this illness may extend as long as twenty years or more. The disease usually begins between ages forty and ninety, with the greatest incidence occurring after age sixty-five. The cause of death is usually pneumonia or other health problems which may or may not be associated with the decline in functioning.[27]

More women than men suffer from this disease, probably a result of life expectancy for women compared to men. The rapidly aging population in this country, combined with the fact that our risk of getting dementia is increased by approximately 1 percent with each year after age sixty-five, suggests there may be as many as 7 to 9 million victims of Alzheimer's by the year 2025. That would mean an estimated increase in expenses from $50 billion to $200 billion in the next several decades.

Highly competitive and exciting research activity in Alzheimer's disease is in the forefront of aging research. Particularly critical has been the identification of a possible gene in familial Alzheimer's disease on the twenty-first chromosome, also the location of Down syndrome. Alzheimer's disease is now recognized as a multiple neurotransmitter deficiency disease, rather than a deficiency of a single neurotransmitter, such as acetylcholine. Unfortunately, there is still not a definitive diagnostic test, preventive treatment, or cure. However, better forms of care as well as better understanding of the underlying causation are developing.

Alcoholism

The literature suggests that about 10 to 15 percent of older people abuse alcohol. More than two million persons over sixty years are believed to suffer from alcoholism, and one-third of these become alcoholics only after becoming old. Those most at risk for alcohol abuse are males, especially elderly widowers.[28]

The National Institute on Aging reports that alcohol impairs older subjects in terms of reaction time and memory. It appears that older subjects not only were more severely impaired immediately after drinking, but also recovered slower. Chronic drinking contributes to poor nutrition, deterioration of the personality, memory loss, apathy, and premature death from cirrhosis, cardiovascular diseases, and cancer.

There are two types of problem drinkers—chronic and situational. Chronic abusers have been heavy drinkers for many years. Although many chronic abusers die by middle age, some live well into old age. Most older problem drinkers are in this group. Other people may develop a drinking problem late in life, often because of "situational" factors such as retirement, lowered income, failing health, loneliness, or the death of friends or loved ones. At first, having a drink brings relief, but later it can turn into a problem. Drinking status of men and women over sixty-five years is given in Table 10.3.

Elder Abuse

Federal definitions of elder abuse, neglect, and exploitation appeared for the first time in the 1987 Amendments to the Older Americans Act. Since the

Table 10.3 Drinking status (in percents) of men and women by selected demographics (1990).

Characteristic	65 years and older			
	Abstainer	Former	Current	Heavier Drinker
Men	21	23	56	15
Women	57	12	31	6

(*Source:* National Health Inventory Survey)

Table 10.4 Types of substantiated elder maltreatment.

Maltreatment	Number of Reports	Percentages
Neglect	34,525	48.7
Emotional/psychological abuse	25,142	35.4
Financial/material exploitation	21,427	30.2
Physical abuse	18,144	25.6
Abandonment	2,560	3.6
Sexual abuse	219	0.3
Other	994	1.4
Total incidents	70,942	

(*Source:* Department of Health and Human Services. Administration on Aging. National Elder Abuse Incidence Study, (1998)

recognition of elder abuse as a community health issue, prevention programs have begun in all fifty states.

There are several types of abuse specific to the elderly. First are physical abuses. These include mental health mistreatment, bodily impairment, and bodily assaults. Second is psychological abuse, which includes humiliation and harassment. Third is sociological abuse, which is manifested in deprivation of living conditions. The fourth abuse is legal abuse, which encompasses material and personal exploitation and theft.[29] Sadly, most abuse takes place within the home or family circle, perpetrated by relatives, acquaintances, home-service workers, or in institutions where the elderly reside.[30]

The National Elder Abuse Incidence Study (NEAIS) and data collected by Adult Protective Services (APS)[31] are reported in Table 10.4. The best national estimate is that a total of 449,924 elderly persons, aged sixty and over, experienced abuse and/or neglect in domestic settings in 1996. Of this total, 70,942 (16 percent) were reported to and substantiated by APS agencies, but the remaining 378,982 (84 percent) were not reported to APS.[32]

Specifically, negligence, a violation of another due to carelessness, can occur from the outside as well as from self-neglect, which may be the result of decreased mental and physical abilities. All types of abuse add up to violations of human rights. Some basic rights that every older person should have are the right to choose, the right to privacy, the right to independence, the right to a decent quality of life, and the right to protection.[33]

Legislation for elder abuse has only recently been improved. In 1965 the Older Americans Act was passed, but protection for the abused was not directly mentioned in this act. It wasn't until 1981 that the Select Committee on Aging of the House of Representatives issued a report titled, "Elder Abuse: An Examination of a Hidden Problem." In 1984 the Family Violence Prevention and Treatment Act was passed by Congress. This Act provided grants to states to combat abuse and it encouraged research in finding occurrences of elder abuse.[34]

In 1990, the Nursing Home Reform Amendment passed, providing civil and criminal actions that could be taken at an institutional level to prevent abuse. One law that most states currently have on their books is mandatory reporting of suspected abuse. Reporting is often made through human services or law enforcement groups rather than health departments so much of the necessary health care for victims is not met.

Studying Aging

Preparing for this universal experience should be the job of each individual and every community. A great challenge to health is to distinguish between attributes of aging as opposed to those of disease.

Gerontology is the academic study of the natural aging process with its pathologies in biological, social, and psychological terms. **Geriatrics** is concerned with the care of older men and women. The first White House Conference on Aging, in 1961, laid the groundwork for the establishment of the National Institute on Aging. In addition, there are now fifteen organized geriatrics programs in medical schools.

Community Health Interventions

With health care costs and the number of older Americans rising, health promotion and disease prevention programs should be a priority for everyone who

---

BOX 10.1 *Recent Statistics on the Elderly in America*

- 35,808 people were over 100 years old.
- 80 percent were white; women outnumbered men 2 to 1.
- Half resided alone or with family members.
- 90 percent had incomes under $5,000 a year.

- 603 people over the age of 60 were HIV positive.
- Only 3 percent of United States companies had policies that assist employees who care for an elderly relative.[35]

works for, and with, the aging. Chronic conditions, disabilities, and life-threatening illnesses frequently can be prevented or controlled, often through relatively inexpensive programs that save millions in health care costs and, most importantly, enable older people to remain active and independent members of their families and communities. Community health educators need to begin their work with the aged by creating new health information and educational materials that are specific to this population. All public and private health efforts should be directed toward preventive clinical services.

Since the objective of health education is to change lifestyles and behavior, it is important to understand attitudes and beliefs of many older people that may facilitate or obstruct this objective. For instance, over one-third of older people smoke. They are also less likely to be influenced by advice about healthy diet and they feel more fatalistic about their health problems, considering them to be part of the natural process of aging.[36]

There are periods in the lives of older people that lend themselves to community health education advice: retirement, bereavement, discharge from a hospital, and initial stages of disability. Most older persons have at least one chronic condition and many have multiple conditions. The most frequently occurring conditions per one hundred elderly in 2000 were: arthritis (forty-nine), hypertension (forty), heart disease (thirty-one), hearing impairments (twenty-eight), orthopedic impairments (eighteen), cataracts (sixteen), sinusitis (fifteen), and diabetes (thirteen) (Figure 10.6).

Health education is particularly helpful in reducing strokes, diabetes, sleep problems, depression, leg ulcers, arthritis, visual impairment, hearing impairment, and incontinence (problems previously mentioned). Additionally, those topics highlighted in this chapter will be other areas of focus into the twenty-first century.

More and more evidence is available that indicates that exercise and activity may be one of the best preventive behaviors available to seniors. Stamina, muscle strength, suppleness, and skill can be regained in old age with moderate exercise. Prevention of diabetes, stroke, cardiovascular problems, mental alertness, osteoporosis, decreased lung function, agility, and sexuality are all affected by moderate exercise.

Weight training is equally helpful. Researchers have found that the elderly, even those in their mid-nineties, can greatly increase their overall muscle, ligament, and tendon strength as well as bone density. These improve an older person's balance and ability to walk, resulting in maximum independence and a decreased incidence of falls. Weight training may also help to lower cholesterol levels and does not have an adverse effect on blood pressure or heart function, as previously thought.[37]

Nutrition programs and education also are essential to good health and independence. Home-delivered and congregate meals, which must consist of one-third of the daily Recommended Dietary Allowances can be provided through schools, churches, and activity centers. Nutrition programs offer meals and related services to some 3.2 million older Americans each year; however, there is still a need to expand good nutrition activities since an estimated 4 million older Americans suffer from food deprivation—the inability to afford, prepare, or gain access to food.

Another serious problem for older people that community health professionals can help with is the possibility of **iatrogenic disease** caused by the misuse of prescribed medication. The frequency of major side effects from drugs increases steadily with age. Studies have shown that the level of prescribing is age related, with a steep rise in those over seventy-five years old; 58 percent have been reported as having received a prescription within the previous 4 weeks.[38]

Ageism

Adaptation to aging is impeded by the stigmatized status that accrues to older people in our culture. The discrimination and devaluation of older people is called **ageism**. Ageism is diseaselike in and of itself and is exhibited by those who will someday become its victim. Ageism is evident in mandatory retirement of people who are able and wish to continue working. It is evident in the ageist jokes, cartoons, and media representation of older people. Ageism pervades our ability to look at older people as sexual, sensual, and in need of intimacy. Ageism is as insidious as racism, sexism, and homophobia and requires public health consciousness.

Age discrimination can be obvious, such as a business hiring a pretty, inexperienced young woman instead of an older woman with a strong background in similar jobs. But it's the subtler forms of age discrimination that may have the most powerful effect on cutting short the productive years of Americans— the law partner who is moved to a smaller office when he or she passes sixty, the fifty-year-old professional who knows hard work won't bring any more promotions, the vacancy filled by a younger staff member before older workers even know about it, and the new boss who makes life so miserable for the sixty-year-old secretary he inherits that she quits.[39]

Learning to cope with a stigmatized identity that does not allow for older peoples' needs for sexuality, intimacy, independence, intellectual stimulation, and physical activity is an important step to positive, healthy, self-acceptance in a society that is less accepting. Better than coping, however, might be to become politically active around these issues and challenge stereotypes and discrimination head on, legally or through public activism.

In addition to age stigma, it should be remembered that approximately 1.75 million older persons are gay or lesbian. These older people need to be accorded the same respect, privacy, and human rights as heterosexuals. This means that the problems associated with nursing homes and hospitals for all older people, such as privacy, dignity, role loss, sexuality, and friendship networks should be extended to gay and lesbian people and their partners as they would be for heterosexual people and their partners.

Summary

Older people are gaining in political clout due to their numbers, and are asking for and receiving the perks of power. Unfortunately, the delicate balance of the health and quality of life of the young and the health and quality of life of aging becomes precarious when one group has voice and the other has not. Anticipating old age by promoting good health at younger ages and instilling a respect among young people for the contributions and choices older adults make is an important health initiative. Other initiatives include social programming and physical activities for older adults.

CYBERSITES RELATED TO CHAPTER 10

Aging

    www.seniornet.com

    www.asaging.org

QUESTIONS

1. How does one prepare for aging as a young adult?

2. What health programming exists in your community for older adults? Is it affordable and accessible?

3. Define "old."

4. How does society determine when a person should retire? How can this transition be made in a positive way?

5. What are signs of ageism in your community?

6. What personal behaviors and beliefs do you have about older adults that are probably ageist?

EXERCISE

Interview a grandparent or close older friend. Discuss how he or she looks at him or herself in terms of physical, emotional, sexual, spiritual, and social health. What life lessons does this person have to share? What misconceptions changed as a result of this discussion?

INTERNET INTERACTIVE ACTIVITY

HEALTH AND AGING CHARTBOOK FROM HEALTH, UNITED STATES, 2001.

The *Health and Aging Chartbook* from Health, United States, 2001, describes the health of older Americans. The chartbook is divided into sections on population, health status, and health care access and utilization. The data presented are from nationally representative health surveys or vital statistics and cover the population sixty-five years of age and over.

    This report can be viewed only with Adobe Acrobat 5.0 or newer. You will need to download a copy of Acrobat 5.0. *Acrobat® Reader™* which is free and freely distributable software that lets you view and print Adobe *Portable Document Format* (PDF) files.

adobe.com/prodindex/acrobat/readstep.html

Example

1. Go to the access page for the Health and Aging Chartbook

   www.cdc.gov/nchs/products/pubs/pubd/hus/hus.htm

2. Click on the **View/download** PDF

3. You will now be in Acrobat Reader. On the left of your page is the Table of Contents for the chartbook. Clicking on any item in the Table of Contents will take you to that page in the chartbook. You can also work through the chartbook page by page by clicking on the arrow icon at the bottom of the page or using the scroller on the right side of the page.

4. Click on **Trend Tables** (page 16) and review the most recent trends in size of the population, living arrangements, life expectancy, chronic conditions, visual and hearing impairments, and nursing home residency. You can peruse the chartbook by moving through these pages.

Exercise

1. Go to the homepage for the **Health and Aging Chartbook from Health, United States, 2001**.

2. Using the data available in the chartbook describe the health status of older Americans by giving one example of a table or a figure (these will need to be copied using your print command) from the chartbook that describes the following aspects of both men and women over the age of sixty-five.

   life expectancy

   selected leading causes of death for men and woman

   osteoporosis in women

   physical conditions for both genders

   care access and utilization

   unmet needs

   health risk factors

   chronic conditions

3. Go to **Vital and Health Statistics Data from State Health Departments in the USA** homepage

   depts.washington.edu/~hsic/phealth/state/state-vs.html

4. On this page, find your state health department and click on its link.

5. Based on the data available through your state health department, how does the older population in your state compare to the national data you found using the chartbook?

REFERENCES

1. Riley, Matilda White (1994). Changing lives and changing social structures: Common concerns of social science and public health. *APHA Journal*, p. 1215.

2. Shapiro, Joseph (1994). Gray boomers. *US News and World Report*, October 10, p. 14.

3. Butler, Robert N. (1991). *Aging and mental health*. N.Y.: Macmillan Publishing.

4. www.aoa.dhhs.gov/may98/agewell.html

5. CDC (1992). Highlights from health data on older Americans: United States, 1992. DHHS, National Center for Health Statistics, Series 3, No. 27.

6. Douglas, Maria (1992). "Golden years often tarnished." Knight Ridder News Service, *The Oregonian*, June 25, p. A10.

7. Ibid.

8. Butler, op. cit.

9. Ibid.

10. Ibid.

11. Ibid.

12. Wantz, Molly S. (1991). *The aging process: A health perspective*. Winthrop Publishers, Inc.

13. Rosenthal, Evelyn R. (1991). *Women, aging and agism*. N.Y.: Harrison Park Press.

14. Young, Stephen. (1993). Against aging. *New Scientist*, April 17, V. 138.

15. CDC (1999). *The aging chartbook*. www.cdc.gov/nchs/data/pdf.

16. Ibid.

17. Ibid.

18. Ibid.

19. Somers, Anne R. (1990). "Improving the elderly 'healthspan' and postponing 'old age'." In *The Nation's Health* by Philip Lee, pp. 389–394.

20. Butler, op. cit.

21. Ibid.

22. Somers, op. cit

23. Riley, op. cit..

24. www.cdc.gov/ncipc/factsheets/falls.htm

25. Northridge, Mary E. (1995). Home hazards and falls in the elderly. *American Journal of Public Health*, Vol. 85, No. 4., April, p. 509.

26. www.cdc.gov/ncipc/factsheets/falls.htm

27. www.aoa.dhhs.gov/may98/agewell.html

28. Butler, op. cit.

29. Pritchard, Jacki. (1992). *The abuse of elderly people, a handbook for professionals*. London: Jessica Kingsley Publishers.

30. Butler, op. cit.

31. www.aoa.gov/abuse/report/GFindings.htm#p15

32. Ibid.

33. Pritchard, op. cit.

34. Meagher, M. Steven (1993). Legal and legislative dimensions. Taken from *Adult protective services, research and practice*. Bryand Byers and James Hendricks, editors. Illinois: Charles C. Thomas Publishers.

35. Ehrlich, Phyllis, & Anetzberger, Georgia (1991). Survey of public health departments on procedures for reporting elder abuse. *Public Health Reports, 106*(2), March/April, 151–154.

36. Jones, Dee (1991). Health maintenance for frail elderly. In *Oxford textbook of public health*. New York: Oxford University Press.

37. www.aoa.dhhs.gov/factsheets/health.html

38. Jones, op cit.

39. www.aoa.dhhs.gov/factsheets/ageism.html

CHAPTER 11

Ethnically Diverse People:

PEOPLE OF COLOR, IMMIGRANTS, AND MIGRANT FARMWORKERS

Community Health in the 21st Century
Asian Americans are at high risk for HIV/AIDS because of their reluctance to discuss sexuality. Breast cancer is also increasing because of Asian women's modesty and reluctance to have preventive BSE and other cancer prevention tests.

—Yung-Chih Fang, M.S., Health Education HIV/AIDS Education Program Coordinator for the Asian Association of Utah

Chapter Objectives

The student will:

1. list the five primary health concerns for African Americans, Hispanic Americans, Asian Americans, Pacific Islander Americans, immigrants, refugees, and migrant farmworkers.

2. discuss how a community health educator can improve his or her cultural sensitivity.

3. explain how culturally unique Hispanic American populations may differ in their health needs.

4. describe how social, political, economic, and religious differences impact the health of diverse people.

Defining Ethnic Diversity

"The United States is one of the most diverse countries in the world. There is no other place in the world where so many different people live and work together."[1] Unfortunately, this diversity is not celebrated and valued in a manner that would enhance the health and quality of life of these diverse people. The health status of the ethnic/racial, non-white, and socially diverse groups in the United States is influenced by past racial inequities and present institutional and personal prejudice in education, employment, housing, politics, and health care systems. The result is greater morbidity, higher rates of mortality, and

Table 11.1 Ethnicity and disease: Disorders associated with genetic factors.

Ethnicity	High Frequency	Low Frequency
Ashkenazi Jews	Tay-Sachs Kaposi's sarcoma	Cervical cancer
African American	Sickle cell anemia Hypertension	Skin cancer Osteoporosis
Mediterrean/Chinese	β -Thalassemia	
Southeast Asian	α-Thalassemia	
American Indian	Diabetes	
Japanese	Gastric cancer	Breast Cancer

(*Source:* Adapted from McKusick, Victor, 1973, & Simpson, Joe, 1992)

lower life expectancy for non-Anglo members of our communities. Personal fears and hesitancy in accessing health care, and institutional barriers to accessing health care are felt by people of color, people with disabilities, people of diverse sexual orientations, older Americans, and sometimes adolescent Americans. The result is a greater need for community health education that reaches out to minority populations and invites them in.

Race is a social category. In the same way that gender has come to be separate from biological sex, so too can biological race be distinguished from social definitions of race. Since race to a large extent is constructed socially, racial definitions often change from society to society. This is evident in Wagley's (1965) example of a man who traveled from Puerto Rico to Mexico to the United States, changing his race from white to mulatto (mixed) to Negro. Defining race varies from nation to nation as illustrated in South Africa where Japanese are "honorary" whites, in Nazi Germany where Jews were a race, and in Great Britain where East Indians and South Americans are black.[2]

It has become politically correct to refer to all people, other than self-identified Anglo, as "people of color." This semantic distinction is no solution to the health care problem of distinguishing among differences and utilizing culturally appropriate models for care. Table 11.1 demonstrates the unique genetic predispositions of some ethnic groups and their relationship to health. Familiarity with ethnically related illnesses contributes to better preventive health education. The term "people of color" does, however, give non-Anglo people a common political "family" from which to derive power statistically. As it is politically correct to refer to childbearing aged females as "women," it is also correct to refer to the many combinations of blacks, Hispanics, Asians, Native Americans, Pacific Islanders, and others, as people of color. The term "third-world" people or "third-world" countries suggests that on a numerical hierarchy, white people might be "first world," ergo, better. The shift from "third-world people" to "developing" when referring to economic status or people of color is less white, Eurocentric, and less classist.

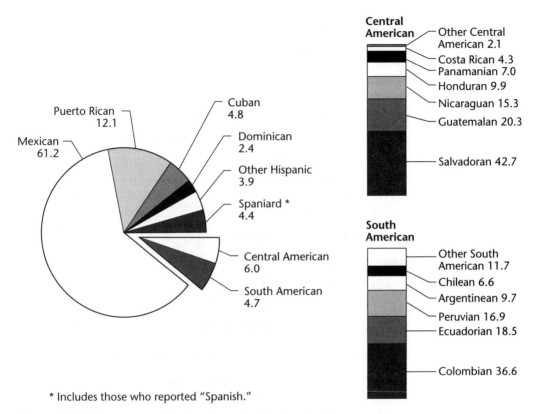

Figure 11.1 Hispanic population by place of origin (percent).

(*Source:* U.S. Census Bureau)

Empirical data about health status also are not politically correct and could be more helpful only if they were actually able to differentiate more specifically among geocultural populations as suggested in Figure 11.1. It is not enough to just say that a person is Hispanic or Asian American. There are discrete cultural variations that influence health care and prevention.

Over the next decade, the composition of the nation will become more racially and ethnically diverse, thereby increasing the need for effective prevention programs tailored to specific community needs. Poverty, lack of adequate access to quality health services, lack of culturally and linguistically competent health services, and lack of preventive health care also are underlying factors that must be addressed. The Centers for Disease Control (CDC) has studied local health departments and reports the percent of those health departments that provide culturally and linguistically appropriate services in Figure 11.2.

Discussion: Why would a community health educator want to know about the diversity of his or her community when planning prevention programs?

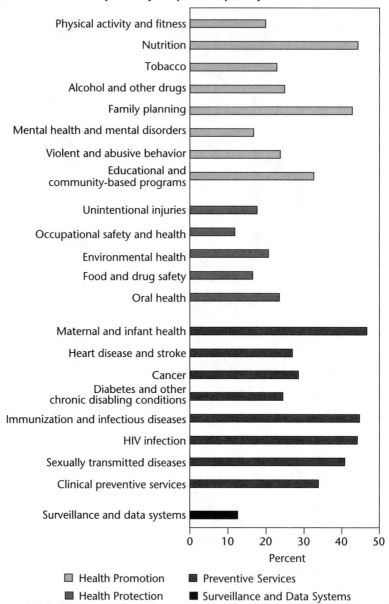

Services by Healthy People 2000 priority areas

Figure 11.2 Culturally appropriate health services in local health departments in the United States (1997).

(*Source:* Healthy People 2010)

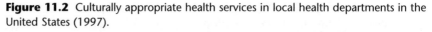

Discussion: Given the great diversity in America, should we be a melting pot or a stew?

The tendency to statistically and demographically identify as "other" for all His-panics in census and trend data is confusing and inappropriate for health care planning. Fully 40 percent of all Hispanics in the country indicated their race as "Other" in the 1980 Census, 4 percent identified as black, and 55.6 percent identified as white. Less than 2 percent of non-Hispanics identified as "Other."[3] If only these simplified data are used in place of culturally and ethnically spe-cific data, behavior change programs and intervention programs are at risk for failure because of their potential lack of cultural sensitivity. It was not until the 1990 census that Hispanics were able to identify as such, not having to choose among white, black, or Other as racial categories. The Census category, His-panic, however, still fails to differentiate among the unique cultural differences of Hispanics as it is a word invented by the U.S. government.

Another attempt at letting citizens better define their racial and ethnic her-itage was attempted in the 2000 Census. Regrettably, even with many racial variations from which to choose, the push to politicize race for financial gain and the complexity of multiracial backgrounds still made the 2000 Census inac-curate and controversial. Many people of Spanish origin refer to themselves by terms other than Hispanic, such as Latino/Latina or Chicano/Chicana; however, the term *Hispanic* will be used in this chapter to represent this ethnically diverse population.

Hispanic Americans

The year 2000 Census counted 32 million persons of Hispanic origin in the United States (12 percent of the total population). Figure 11.3 shows the pro-portion of racial diversity in 1999 and projected in 2050. (Complete data from the 2000 Census were not available for the printing of this edition of this book.) About 350,000 Hispanic immigrants come to the United States every year. By 2050 the population is projected to be 96 million, or 25 percent of the popula-tion. Thus, Hispanics now comprise the largest minority population in the United States.

Hispanics as an ethnic group are younger than the U.S. population with a median age of twenty-six. One-third of all Hispanics are children under eight-een years ,and 40 percent live in poverty. This is 2.5 times the rate of poverty among white children. Eighty-eight percent live in metropolitan areas.[4] Thirty-nine percent of Hispanics less than sixty-five years (7.2 million) have no health insurance. Inability to obtain health insurance for Hispanics occurs because many work for small businesses, are self-employed, or work in low-skill jobs that do not offer insurance.

Table 11.2 gives the number of live births in 1990 and in 1998 for all races. Table 11.3 reports the birth rates for Hispanics. Crude mortality rates show no overall gaps between Hispanics and non-Hispanics; however, incidence of unin-tentional injuries, homicide, chronic liver disease, cirrhosis, and AIDS rank higher for Hispanics (Table 11.4 on page 298). Since cardiovascular diseases and cancer rates are actually lower for Hispanics than non-Hispanics, this may be a

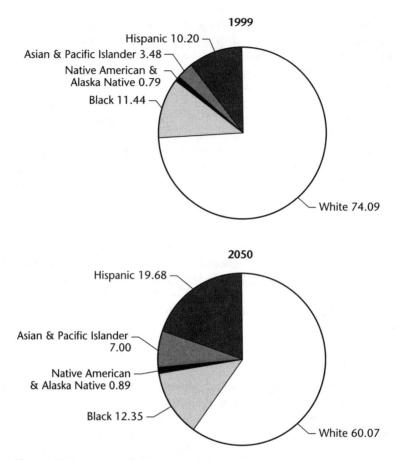

Figure 11.3 Percent of ethnicity in U.S. population 1999 and 2050.

(*Source:* U.S. Census Bureau)

reason why demographers have a tendency to report Hispanics among white vital statistics. Two exceptions are stomach cancer, which is twice as high in Hispanic children as it is in white children, and cervical cancer among Hispanic women, who are the highest of any minority group except Vietnamese women.

Hispanics are disproportionately affected by the HIV/AIDS epidemic. In 1999 there were 49.9 AIDS cases per 100,000 Hispanics compared to 29.9 cases for the total population. In part, as a result of the AIDS epidemic and Hispanic HIV rates, in 1996 the Department of Health and Human Services announced the "Hispanic Agenda for Action" initiative to ensure that the workforce and programs are more reflective of and sensitive to Hispanics in our population.

Barriers to obtaining health care include few Hispanic physicians, lack of English language, 39 percent without health insurance, and family cohesion that emphasizes family over individual needs. In 1998 the National Health Interview Survey was translated into Spanish to improve the collection of health information about Spanish-speaking Americans.

Table 11.2 Live births by race of mother (1999).

Race and Hispanic Origin	Number of Births (1,000)	
	1990	1998
Total	4,158	3,942
White	3,290	3,119
Black	684	610
American Indian, Eskimo, Aleut	39	40
Asian and Pacific Islander	142	173
Filipino	26	31
Chinese	23	28
Japanese	9	9
Hawaiian	6	6
Hispanic origin	595	735
Mexican	386	516
Puerto Rican	59	57
Cuban	11	13
Central and South American	83	98
Other and unknown Hispanic	56	50

[4,158 represents 4,158,000. Represents registered births. Excludes births to nonresidents of the United States. Data are based on Hispanic origin of mother and race of mother. Hispanic origin data are available from only forty-eight states and the District of Columbia in 1990]

(*Source:* U.S. Center for Health Statistics; *Vital Statistics of the United States,* annual; *National Vital Statistics Report (NVSR)* (formerly *Monthly Vital Statistics Report*); and unpublished data)

Table 11.3 Crude birth rates, by age for Hispanic mothers (1980–1997).

Race of Mother, Hispanic Origin of Mother, and Year	Crude Birth Rate	Fertility Rate	Age of Mother									
			10–14 Years	15–19 years			20–24 Years	25–29 Years	30–34 Years	35–39 Years	40–44 Years	45–49 Years
				Total	15–17 Years	18–19 Years						
Hispanic mothers												
1980	23.5	95.4	1.7	82.2	52.1	126.9	156.4	132.1	83.2	39.9	10.6	0.7
1990	26.7	107.7	2.4	100.3	65.9	147.7	181.0	153.0	98.3	45.3	10.9	0.7
1991	26.7	108.1	2.4	106.7	70.6	158.5	186.3	152.8	96.1	44.9	10.7	0.6
1992	26.5	108.6	2.6	107.1	71.4	159.7	190.6	154.4	96.8	45.6	10.9	0.6
1993	26.0	106.9	2.7	106.8	71.7	159.1	188.3	154.0	96.4	44.7	10.6	0.6
1994	25.5	105.6	2.7	107.7	74.0	158.0	188.2	153.2	95.4	44.3	10.7	0.6
1995	25.2	105.0	2.7	106.7	72.9	157.9	188.5	153.8	95.9	44.9	10.8	0.6
1996	24.8	104.9	2.6	101.8	69.0	151.1	189.5	161.0	98.1	45.1	10.8	0.6
1997	24.2	102.8	2.3	97.4	66.3	144.3	184.2	161.7	97.9	45.0	10.8	0.6

(*Source:* National Vital Statistics System)

Table 11.4 Death rates for ten leading causes of disease for Hispanics, both sexes (1998).

Rank	Cause of Death (Based on the Ninth Revision, International Classification of Diseases, 1975), Hispanic Origin, Race for Non-Hispanic Population, Sex, and Age	Number	Rate per 100,000
	Hispanic, both sexes, all ages		
...	All causes	98,406	325.3
1	Diseases of heart	24,596	81.3
2	Malignant neoplasms, including neoplasms of lymphatic and hematopoietic tissues	19,528	64.6
3	Accidents and adverse effects	8,248	27.3
...	Motor vehicle accidents	4,339	14.3
...	All other accidents and adverse effects	3,909	12.9
4	Cerebrovascular diseases	5,587	18.5
5	Diabetes mellitus	4,741	15.7
6	Pneumonia and influenza	3,277	10.8
7	Homicide and legal intervention	2,978	9.8
8	Chronic liver disease and cirrhosis	2,845	9.4
9	Chronic obstructive pulmonary diseases and allied conditions	2,528	8.4
10	Certain conditions originating in the perinatal period	1,987	6.6
...	All other causes (Residual)	22,091	73.0

(*Sources:* Centers for Disease Control. National Center for Health Statistics)

Despite poverty, poor access to medical care, and a lack of health insurance, Hispanics surprisingly are less likely than whites to die of most of the major chronic illnesses. A study reported in *The Journal of the American Medical Association* (JAMA) found that with the exception of diabetes, liver disease, and homicide, Hispanics' morbidity and mortality was significantly better for all forms of cancer, heart disease, and pulmonary disorders.[5] Former Surgeon General Antonia Novello theorized that Latino culture, which frowns on drinking and smoking and promotes strong family networks, helps keep the population healthy in spite of socioeconomic disadvantages.[6]

While "Hispanic" or "Latino" has become a convenient way to refer to Americans of Central or South American heritage, the term masks a variety of ethnic, racial, national, and cultural backgrounds. There are distinctive cultures that build an Hispanic community in the United States that may be best defined by the country of origin, such as Puerto Rico, Mexico, Cuba, Nicaragua, or the countries of South America.

Puerto Ricans

Puerto Ricans are one of the major Hispanic subgroups in the United States. They represented 12 percent of the Hispanic population in the United States in 1995. In 1990, half of Puerto Ricans in the United States lived in Bronx County, New York (pop. 1,196,000, 49 percent Hispanic) or elsewhere in New York City.

Table 11.5 Infant deaths by race of mother (1988–1997).

Race and Hispanic Origin	1988	1989	1990	1991	1995	1996	1997
Total	9.6	9.5	8.9	8.6	7.6	7.3	7.2
White, non-Hispanic	8.0	7.8	7.2	7.0	6.3	6.0	6.0
Black, non-Hispanic	18.1	18.0	16.9	16.6	14.7	14.2	13.7
Hispanic	8.3	8.1	7.5	7.1	6.3	6.1	6.0
Mexican American	7.9	7.7	7.2	6.9	6.0	5.8	5.8
Puerto Rican	11.6	11.7	9.9	9.7	8.9	8.6	7.9
Cuban	7.2	6.2	7.2	5.2	5.3	5.1	5.5
Central and South American	7.2	7.4	6.8	5.9	5.5	5.0	5.5
Other and unknown Hispanic	9.1	8.4	8.0	8.2	7.4	7.7	6.2
Asian/Pacific Islander	6.8	7.4	6.6	5.8	5.3	5.2	5.0
Chinese	5.5	6.4	4.3	4.6	3.8	3.2	3.1
Japanese	7.0	6.0	5.5	4.2	5.3	4.2	5.3
Filipino	6.9	8.0	6.0	5.1	5.6	5.8	5.8
Other Asian/Pacific Islander	7.0	7.3	7.4	6.3	5.5	5.7	5.0
Native American/Alaska Native	12.7	13.4	13.1	11.3	9.0	10.0	8.7

(Infant deaths per 1,000 live births)

(*Source:* U.S. Census Bureau)

While, like many Hispanics, they speak Spanish, they have a cultural heritage that is distinct from Cubans, South Americans, and Mexicans.

In general, the socioeconomic data on Puerto Ricans paint pictures that are distressing. More Puerto Ricans live outside New York City (NYC) than in the city; however, data about Puerto Ricans are drawn primarily from NYC since it has the most dense concentration of Puerto Ricans in the United States. Therefore, those looking at these data should be aware that they may not represent Puerto Ricans who live in California, Florida, or Texas.

In 1995 there were 2.6 million Puerto Ricans in the United States and 3.3 million in Puerto Rico. On the whole, Puerto Ricans are quite young with the median age 23.7 when compared to whites (approximately thirty-two years) and blacks (approximately twenty-eight years). Table 11.5 shows an infant mortality rate in 1997 of 7.9 per 1,000, as compared to all mothers (see Table 7.3), which may be the consequence of the reality that overall, approximately 30 percent of Puerto Rican families live below the poverty line and that the mean household income is approximately $13,000.

A serious concern for health planners is that half of Puerto Rican families have only a single female head of household. Most live at the poverty level maintaining a feminization of poverty pattern among Puerto Ricans.[7] Puerto Rican teens have the highest birth rate of all Hispanic populations, 20.5 per 1,000.

Mexican Americans

In the United States, 61 percent of the Hispanic population in 1995 was of Mexican origin, Los Angeles being the population center for Mexican Americans. Of the 8.7 million Mexican Americans, 64 percent speak Spanish as their first language. Mexicans often differentiate politically as "Chicano," a term created by Caesar Chavez as part of the United Farmworkers activism of the 1960s. Mexican Americans who may be less activist may call themselves Latinos, choosing not to associate with a political label.

The Mexican American birth rate is 29.6 per 1,000 and is the highest among the American Hispanic groups. The infant mortality rate in 1996 of 5.8 per 1,000 was lower than the U.S. rate of 7.2.

Cuban Americans

Of all the Hispanic groups, Cubans, who were 5 percent of the Hispanic population in 1995, have been the most conspicuous and successful. Cuban American infant mortality is the lowest of all Hispanic groups at 5.5 per 1,000. The majority of Cuban Americans are in two age categories, the ages of forty to fifty-four, and fifteen to twenty-four. Over half the country's Cuban Americans live in the Miami area, where they make up 70 percent of Hispanics.

Native Americans

The Indian Health Service (IHS), a component of the U.S. Public Health Service (PHS), provides health related services to about one million of the eligible 2.5 million Native Americans and Alaska Natives. The most current, but not necessarily accurate data about the health status of U.S. indigenous people comes from the IHS.[8] For a variety of reasons, many Native people are not considered eligible for tribal membership and are not considered in the data. An individual is eligible for IHS care if "he or she is regarded as an Indian by the community in which he or she lives as evidenced by such factors as tribal membership, enrollment, residence on tax-exempt land, ownership of restricted property, active participation in tribal affairs, or other relevant factors in keeping with general Bureau of Indian Affairs practice in the jurisdiction."

Native Americans are not one homogeneous group, but diverse nations with differences in spiritual and cultural practices. They can be differentiated in terms of their language, spirituality, geography, economic structure, and political structures. The 1990 Census identified 278 reservations and 209 Alaska Native villages and counted 1.9 million Native Americans (8 percent of the population), Eskimos, and Aleuts living throughout the United States both on and off reservations. The four largest tribes are Cherokee (308,132), Navajo (219,198) Chippewa (103,826), and Sioux (103,255). Two-thirds of the tribes have fewer than 1,000 tribal members.[9]

Unemployment rates are high. Fifty percent of Native Americans are unemployed and a considerable number are under-employed. The median income for Native American families was $21,750 in 1990 compared to the U.S. median of $35,225. In 1990, 23.7 percent lived below the poverty line compared to the U.S. total of 10.4 percent. The median age was 22.9 years compared with the U.S. median age of 32. This makes 45 percent of Native Americans less than twenty years old. Only 37 percent of all Native American men in the United States reach sixty-five years.

Native Americans remain the poorest and the most disadvantaged of all racial or ethnic groups in the United States, as shown by death rates from a wide range of diseases (Figure 11.4). When compared to national averages, Native Americans have the highest rate of alcoholism (438 percent greater), tuberculosis (400 percent greater), diabetes (155 percent greater), accidents (131 percent greater), homicide (57 percent greater), pneumonia and influenza (32 percent greater), syphilis (300 percent greater), and suicide (27 percent greater). It is thought by many that alcoholism is the number-one health problem facing Native Americans and contributes to many of the other health problems suffered by native populations. According to senate hearings, mortality from alcohol-related causes among Native Americans was twenty-two times higher than the national average, and alcohol abuse is associated with four of the top ten causes of death for Native Americans, including accidents, cirrhosis of the liver, homicides, and suicides. Native Americans die from tuberculosis at six times the rate of other races. Their suicide rate is twice the national average.

Although there has been an improvement in crude mortality rate, the infant mortality rate of 8.7 per 1,000 was 1.1 times the U.S. rate for all races combined. Most infant deaths have been attributed to sudden infant death syndrome (SIDS). The cause of SIDS is unknown, but it has been reported among low birth weight infants born to women who smoke. The percentage of low birth weight babies among Native Americans is 6.1, which is actually similar to the total U.S. percentage of 6.9.

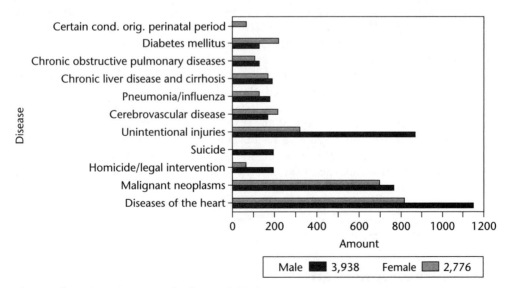

Figure 11.4 Native American death rates (1997).

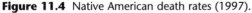

(*Source:* CDC, NCHS: Vital Statistics of the U.S., Vol. 2, PHS, Washington, D.C.)

On average, mortality rates due to cardiovascular diseases and cancer were lower than those for all U.S. races combined; however, the accidental death rate (172.6 per 1,000) is 3.4 times that of the United States. The diabetes rate of 29.1 is 2.8 times higher than the national rate, and death due to suicide (17.5/100,000) exceeded the U.S. rate by a ratio of 1.7.

Among children, infant diarrhea due to unsanitary drinking water and polluted ground water contribute to high infant mortality. Otitis media, an inner ear infection, is found among 75 percent of Native American children. This condition causes permanent hearing impairment if not treated early.

The systematic sterilization of Native American women has been a government policy that has only recently been addressed and challenged by health activists. It is one more of many indignities toward our Native populations.[10]

There is very little information on the health status of Native Americans living in urban areas, although they constitute about 54 percent of their total population. Also, the overall mortality rates do not necessarily show the reservation specific rates that may be grossly higher than overall rates.

Poverty is probably the primary indicator of poor health among Native populations. With the loss of original tribal lands, the loss of mineral and water rights, the broken treaties, and what some think may be racial genocide of native populations, it is little wonder that death is so high among them.

The good news is that the health of Native Americans has improved on many measures over the past fifteen years. Even so, in almost every IHS service area, health status is far behind that of the rest of the U.S. populations. There is considerable risk for death by accidents, suicide, homicide, and other "social" causes. Motor vehicles are included in nearly half of all accidental injuries, and the rate of such accidents among Native Americans is higher than that of any other group.[11] The treatment of Native populations in our country as well as the treatment of Native populations in other colonial nations is an embarrassment and an outrage.

It would not surprise the community health educator to find that stress related problems are high among Native peoples. The mores and cultural patterns of non-Native populations imposed upon Native Americans have disrupted their traditional way of life. A sense of powerlessness and hopelessness has often been observed as a result; however, Native Americans continue to draw upon traditional sources of strength to cope with these stressors. Traditional strengths include the family, the tribe, and the land itself.[12] These should not be discounted when suggesting health promotion and prevention programs. Traditional health practices of indigenous people include ceremonies, herbs, and steam baths or sweat lodges. Health practices are commonly intertwined with spiritual beliefs.[13]

African Americans

The term "African American" has replaced the term "black" among many demographers, social scientists, political activists, and other persons of African descent having U.S. citizenship. This term, however, does not reflect the wide variety of people of color whose genetic heritage is Negro, but whose cultural background may be Caribbean, South American, or even European instead of African. Similarly to Hispanics, black Americans reflect great diversity and cultural heritage, even though the greatest number have their historical beginnings in the Americas as captive African slaves.

Racial inequity and ethnic invisibility are often demonstrated by excluding the populations of Native Americans, Asians, and Hispanics from demographic and epidemiological comparison, and comparing only blacks and whites on a variety of conditions as reflected in much of the vital statistic data for the nation.

> **Discussion:** Why are so many health data given only by the demographic characteristics of white and black? Where are the rest of the data?

In his book, *Two Nations,* Andrew Hacker gives examples of the problems of racism in the United States, as demonstrated by the black/white comparison:

1. In the United States, 44.8 percent of black children live in poverty compared with 15.9 percent of white children;

2. 63.7 percent of black children are born out of wedlock, compared with 14.9 percent of whites;

3. Black women have 635 abortions compared to 274 per 1,000 for white women; and

4. One out of every five black males spends part of his life behind bars.

In 2000, there were 35.5 million African Americans in the United States with 81 percent living in metropolitan areas. The poverty rate was 28.2 percent compared to the U.S. total of 10.4 percent. Infant mortality was 13.7 per 1,000

BOX 11.1 *Black and White Children in America*

Compared to white children, black children are:

Twice as likely to:
- die in the first year of life
- be born prematurely
- suffer low birth weight
- have mothers who receive late or no prenatal care
- see a parent die
- live in substandard housing

Three times as likely to:
- be poor
- have their mothers die in childbirth

- live in a female headed family
- be placed in an educable mentally retarded class
- die of known child abuse

Four times as likely to:
- be murdered before one year of age or as a teenager
- be incarcerated between fifteen and nineteen years of age.[16]

BOX 11.2 *The African American Health Crises*

Heart Disease—27 percent greater in black men than white men; 55 percent higher in black women than white women.

Diabetes—one in every ten African Americans has diabetes; 55 percent more likely than whites to have diabetes. This is especially true in older African American women.

Lupus—over 500,000 individuals have lupus in the United States. Nine out of ten of these are women from the ages of fifteen to forty-five. Sixty percent of these individuals are black.

Infertility—1.5 times more than whites.

AIDS—African Americans and Latinos together total 21 percent of the population, but account for 46 percent of the U.S. AIDS cases so far.

Hypertension—high blood pressure is twice as common in blacks as in whites, affecting one in three African Americans.

Infant Mortality—twice as likely as white children to die before their first birthday.

Cancer—10 percent more often than the general population. Once acquired, the mortality rate is 20 to 40 percent higher.

Addiction—drug abuse-related issues account for 39 percent of the emergency room visits nationally. Seventy to seventy-five percent of the nation's 2 to 2.5 million heroin addicts are black.

(*Source:* www.africanamericanhealth.com/physical.htm)

compared to the nation's rate of 7.2; probably reflecting the low birth weight difference of 13 percent compared to 6.9 percent. Maternal mortality (16.5 per 1,000) was more than twice the national rate (7.2 per 1,000).

Black longevity has increased, but a 50 percent difference remains in adjusted death rates for blacks and whites. If blacks had the same death rates as whites, 59,000 black deaths a year would not occur.[14]

A 1985 Children's Defense Fund (CDF) study, *Black and White Children in America: Key Facts*,[15] found that black children have been sliding backward. Black children today are more likely to be born into poverty, lack early prenatal care, have a single mother or unemployed parent, be unemployed as teenagers, and not go to college after high school graduation.

Despite Medicaid, 22 percent of blacks are without any medical insurance coverage. Further, the rate of increase of black physicians is declining in part due to the reduction in federal funding of higher education.

Blacks have more undetected diseases than whites. Older blacks suffer from more functional limitations than older whites, a situation of "accelerated" or unequal aging associated with poverty and the inequities of education and employment.

Morbidity is particularly high for cardiovascular illness associated with high blood pressure, which is epidemic among blacks. Cervical cancer among black women is also higher than the general population.

Being black puts a male twice as likely to die from stroke, have 2.2 times higher mortality from diabetes, have 3.2 times higher mortality from kidney disease, and six times more likely to be murdered as his white counterparts.

BOX 11.3 *The Black Church as a Participant in Community Health Interventions*[17]

Historically, African Americans have mistrusted traditional medical practices since institutional racism has excluded blacks from total participation in medical systems. Consequently, this and other reasons have led to longer durations between visits to health care facilities and delays in diagnosis and treatment. To counteract this resistance, the black church seems to be an ideal resource for promoting health care and health access to members of the black community, because the church is community based. Information including voter registration, pre-school immunization programs, job hunting, soup kitchens, AIDS education, hypertension programs, cancer screening, and aging services are often available through black churches. Research shows that health behaviors change for the better when they are influenced directly by the church.

Effective health promotion programs in black churches should consider:

a. Explicit and implicit organization guidelines that address the philosophies of both the health providers and the black church should not be in conflict.

b. The organization should have pre-existing reinforcement contingencies for rewarding its members.

c. The organization should be able to influence entire families to meet on a large scale.

d. The health provider should have an understanding of the relationship between the black community and the black church.

e. Church deacons and ministers should be involved.

f. Non-African American health providers should be understanding of black Americans' spiritual differences from their own.

Like Native Americans, poor housing and sanitation for many poor black families is a major threat to health due to crowding and infestation. Job and housing conditions also expose black families more often than whites to certain cancer risks, such as lead.

A specific health risk for African Americans and some ethnic groups from countries around the Mediterranean Sea is **sickle cell anemia,** a chronic blood disease characterized by the presence of sickle or crescent-shaped blood cells that cannot adequately carry hemoglobin. There are about 50,000 persons with sickle cell anemia in the United States and 3 million carriers of the cell trait, or 10 percent of the black population of the United States. It is a genetically transmitted disease that can be readily diagnosed with a simple and inexpensive blood test that could easily be part of community health fairs. The condition develops at the time of conception but signs and symptoms do not appear until the infant is stricken with an upper respiratory infection or tonsillitis, which may be accompanied by severe debilitation. It is estimated that one in every 500 black children born in the United States has sickle cell anemia. Death occurs in many of its victims by the age of twenty; the rest die by age forty.

Clinically, sickle hemoglobin cells differ from normal cells by only two amino acids, have a shortened life span, and are unable to transport oxygen as normal hemoglobin cells do. Distorted, sickle-shaped cells that cannot pass easily through small blood vessels block vessels and prevent oxygen from reaching body tissues. When this happens, painful sickle cell symptoms occur. Other symptoms include impaired growth and development, jaundice, kidney problems, and a dangerous susceptibility to infection. There is no cure, but testing for the genetic trait can improve reproductive counseling and early treatment among infected newborns.

Kinship and family ties are extremely important for African Americans. The church is a powerful source of emotional strength and is becoming a very important resource for community health education programs. Support for drug and alcohol prevention, AIDS prevention, and teen pregnancy prevention programs have been found among African American clergy and churches.[18]

Asian Americans and Pacific Islanders

Data from the 2000 Census shows that almost 11 million Asian and Pacific Islanders (AAPIs) have the greatest percentage of growth (107.8 percent) of all racial/ethnic groups in the United States. They constitute 4.1 percent of the population but will double to 6.6 percent by the year 2025. The largest immigration of Asians is among Chinese (24 percent), followed by Filipinos (20 percent) (Figures 11.5 and 11.6). Total growth of the Asian population in the United States increased from 3.5 million to 11 million persons between 1980 and 2000. In 1998, 60.7 percent of Asian American and Pacific Islanders were foreign-born, 61 percent from the Philippines, Korea, and China.

Leading causes of death for Asian Americans and Pacific Islanders are given in Figure 11.7. Heart diseases, cancer, and cardiovascular diseases are the primary causes of death in these populations—as in the population as a whole. Smoking is a major preventable behavior implicated in these high rates. Among Asian men, the smoking rate has decreased from 55 percent to 24 percent in the past ten years; however, female smokers (10 percent) are "closeted" and underreported.[19]

Two infectious diseases that have followed immigrant Asian and Pacific Islander subgroups to this country are tuberculosis and hepatitis B. Among Southeast Asian Americans, the tuberculosis rate (45.9 per 100,000) is five times the national average, and the rate of hepatitis B carriers is six times the national average.[20] Hepatitis rates are particularly high among those over forty-five years. The overall carrier rate in the United States is estimated to be .3 percent of the population.[21] Tuberculosis is still the leading cause of death in some Asian countries and has become a serious health problem in some Asian communities in large American cities. Among Southeast Asian immigrants, the incidence is 40 times higher than the incidence rate for the rest of the population. Refugee transit camps now screen pregnant women and vaccinate infants of those who are carriers of hepatitis B and all children under age six.[22]

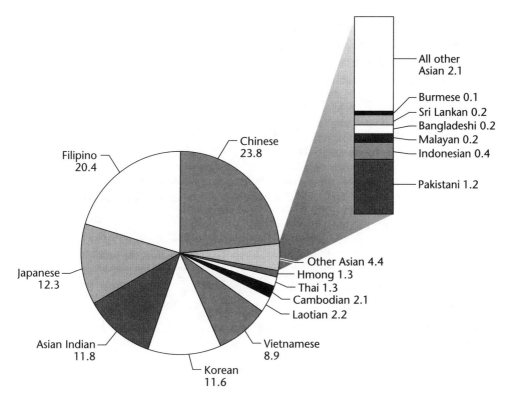

Figure 11.5 Asian population by place of origin (in percent).

(*Source:* U.S. Census Bureau)

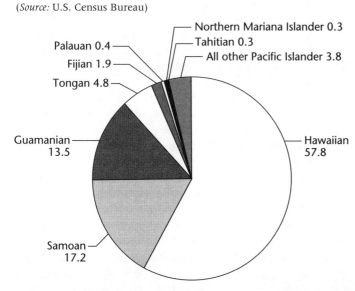

Figure 11.6 Pacific Island population by place of origin (in percent).

(*Source:* U.S. Census Bureau)

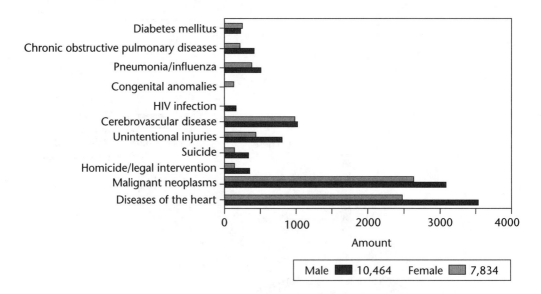

Figure 11.7 Leading causes of death for Asians and Pacific Islanders (1991).

(*Source:* CDC, NCHS: Vital Statistics of the U.S., Vol. 2, PHS, Washington D.C.)

Southeast Asian Americans are also at high risk for thalassemia, hemoglo-binopathies, hypertension, parasitism, and anemia. In 2000, AIDS cases had increased 71 percent since 1995 among refugees from Southeast Asia.

In general, 50 percent of Asian refugees have one or more parasites, six times the national average for hepatitis B, and 40 percent of refugees are positive for tuberculosis. Among specific Southeast Asian populations, Laotians have the highest rate of parasitism, Cambodians the poorest overall health, and Vietnamese the highest rate of positive tuberculosis—five times the national average. Of those residing in America, 66 percent of Laotians, 50 percent of Cambodians, and 35 percent of Vietnamese live in poverty. These people cannot afford health insurance or often do not know how to access health care for the economically disadvantaged. AAPIs are second only to Hispanic Americans in numbers of people who are uninsured. Some 36 percent of AAPIs under age sixty-five had no health insurance as compared of 16 percent of the U.S. population under sixty-five.[23] It is estimated that two million Asian Americans and Pacific Islanders lack health insurance, with Korean Americans the most likely to be uninsured.

As Pacific Islanders move from their tropical homeland to temperate and western communities in the United States, their health problems change from acute issues such as infant mortality, maternal mortality, and communicable diseases to more chronic conditions such as hypertension and diabetes. The increase in diabetes can be directly related to a change in diet from root vegetables such as taro, yams, and sweet potatoes to canned meat and canned fish. The consumption of sugar and salt increases enormously and alcohol use increases as well.

Table 11.6 Immigrants admitted as permanent residents by country of birth, 1981–1996.

Country of Birth	1981–90, Total	1991–94, Total	1995	1996	Country of Birth	1981–90, Total	1991–94, Total	1995	1996
Total	**1,013,620**	**504,893**	**114,664**	**128,565**	China[3]	7,928	3,431	803	845
					Hong Kong	1,916	440	48	47
Europe[1]	**155,512**	**213,840**	**46,998**	**51,977**	Iran	46,773	17,669	1,245	1,212
Albania	353	2,545	314	154	Iraq	7,540	6,814	3,848	3,802
Bulgaria	1,197	1,314	105	100	Laos	142,964	28,182	3,364	2,155
Czechoslovakia	8,204	1,138	38	25	Philippines	3,403	695	80	80
Hungary	4,942	1,163	28	40	Syria	2,145	497	258	208
Poland	33,889	6,782	245	183	Thailand	30,259	14,451	2,932	1,940
Romania	29,798	14,100	592	447	Turkey	1,896	360	58	42
Soviet Union, former[2]	72,306	181,711	40,120	42,356	Vietnam	324,453	111,265	28,595	29,700
Armenia	(NA)	(NA)	214	182	**North America**[1]	**121,840**	**67,409**	**16,265**	**28,070**
Azerbaijan	(NA)	(NA)	1,594	1,446	Cuba	113,367	41,473	12,355	22,542
Belarus	(NA)	(NA)	3,421	3,480	El Salvador	1,383	3,078	283	262
Moldova	(NA)	(NA)	1,597	1,415	Guatemala	(NA)	806	158	234
Russia	(NA)	(NA)	8,176	9,745	Nicaragua	5,590	19,759	727	766
Ukraine	(NA)	(NA)	14,937	16,636	**South America**	**1,976**	**1,606**	**497**	**922**
Uzbekistan	(NA)	(NA)	3,258	4,144	**Africa**[1]	**22,149**	**21,233**	**7,527**	**5,464**
Yugoslavia	324	707	4,744	7,820	Ethiopia	18,542	13,062	1,802	985
Asia	**712,092**	**200,735**	**43,314**	**42,076**	Sudan	(NA)	1,398	935	1,089
Afghanistan	22,946	8,080	616	369	Other	51	70	63	56
Cambodia	114,064	5,610	268	210					

NA Not available. [1]Includes other countries, not shown separately. [2]Includes other republics and unknown republics, not shown separately. [3]Includes Taiwan.

(*Source:* U.S. Immigration and Naturalization Service, *Statistical Yearbook,* annual; and releases.)

Peoples of Guam and Tonga rely heavily on traditional community healers that are still referred to as "witch doctors." There are long-held traditional beliefs in evil spirits call "taotaomona" in Guam.[24]

Immigrants

Immigrants made up more than one-third of the nation's growth in the 1980s. We are a nation of immigrants.[25] One of the controversies regarding recent immigrants as well as undocumented laborers is their utilization of health and social services. The use of such programs depends basically on: (1) the legal status of the immigrant, (2) the societal mores and traditions in the immigrant's country of origin, (3) the amount of knowledge about such programs available to the individual, and (4) the degree of need. In general, most legal immigrants do not take advantage of health and social programs available to them and consequently are among some of the primary groups at greatest risk for infection of communicable diseases, infant morbidity and mortality, maternal morbidity and mortality, and stress-related syndromes. Extended families and traditional healers compensate somewhat for lack of government assistance, but better education would probably mean better health status. The number of immigrants by location of origin is given in Table 11.6.

Table 11.7 Refugees and asylum-seekers worldwide (1999).

Region	Refugees	Asylum-Seekers	Returnees	IDPs and Others of Concern	Total
1. Great Lakes	869,100	15,730	477,300	736,700	2,098,830
2. East and Horn of Africa	1,122,640	7,030	193,420	51,600	1,374,690
3. West and Central Africa	877,960	15,060	532,410	865,600	2,291,030
4. Southern Africa	195,100	22,960	75,940	0	294,000
5. North Africa	199,760	370	17,700	70	217,900
6. The Middle East	207,410	18,240	22,500	166,500	414,650
7. South-West Asia	3,133,800	170	193,700	343,700	3,671,370
8. Central Asia	42,200	5,390	42,820	20	90,430
9. South Asia	333,930	100	40,210	717,600	1,091,840
10. East Asia and the Pacific	573,800	7,090	16,140	39,100	636,130
11. Eastern Europe	666,400	28,350	110	2,145,800	2,840,660
12. South-Eastern Europe	595,000	6,000	285,400	1,374,020	2,260,420
13. Central Europe and the Baltic States	93,580	14,230	0	15,800	123,610
14. Western Europe and Turkey	1,847,050	532,340	1,800	265,000	2,646,190
15. North America and the Caribbean	661,630	645,630	0	0	1,307,260
16. Central America	56,030	0	7,830	20,000	83,860
17. South America	16,320	330	30	800,000	816,680
Total	11,491,710	1,319,020	1,907,310	7,541,510	22,259,550

(*Source:* U.S. Committee for Refugees. World Refugee Survey)

Refugees

Refugees are immigrants who arrive in America, or other countries, from war-torn countries, economically depressed nations, and religiously intolerant societies. Statistics on refugees and other uprooted people are often inexact and controversial. One country's refugee is another's illegal alien. Today's internally displaced person may be tomorrow's refugee. As such, government tallies cannot always be trusted to give full and unbiased accounts of refugee movements.[27] Table 11.7 reports the number of refugees worldwide as of 1999.

The United Nations estimates there are at least 100 million international migrants living outside the countries in which they were born, or about 2 percent of the world's population. An estimated 18 million are refugees—fleeing political strife and warfare—while 20 million are fleeing other violence or environmental destruction, including drought.[28]

Refugees come to America with "the shirt on their back" and little else. The greatest number of refugees has come from Southeast Asia with a new increase from Central America and the Caribbean. Instead of finding shelter, employment, and opportunity, many have been incarcerated in internment camps where only minimal living conditions are maintained in crowded, stressful, dirty compounds. Among these "homeless" are people with tuberculosis, psychological illnesses, anger, hunger, and other physical and social traumas. Few refugees have been inoculated for common communicable diseases and they bring new, exotic parasitic and fungal conditions that challenge the medical community. Among refugees there are elevated crude death rates and perinatal and childhood mortality rates.

Table 11.8 Regional refugee ceilings and admissions (1999–2000).

	1999 Ceilings	1999 Admissions	2000 Ceilings
Africa	12,000	13,038	18,000
East Asia	9,000	10,204	8,000
Eastern Europe	38,000	38,654	27,000
USSR/Former USSR	23,000	16,922	20,000
Latin America	3,000	2,110	3,000
Near East and South Asia	4,000	4,078	8,000
Unallocated Reserve		2,000	6,000
Total	91,000	85,006	90,000

(*Source:* U.S. Department of State, Bureau of Population, Refugees, and Migration. Tabulated by the U.S. Committee for Refugees)

The number of refugees worldwide in 1999 was approximately 11.5 million.[29] The number of refugees allowed into the United States is based upon the region from which they come. These ceilings are given in Table 11. 8.

Refugee mental health providers and resettlement workers are increasingly aware that refugees and survivors of torture need greater, earlier access to culturally appropriate mental health services to help them deal with both the trauma from which they fled and the challenge of adjusting to life in the United States. Several refugee mental health programs in the United States are addressing some refugees' psychological needs on the local level. But there has been little coherent, nationwide coordination of refugee mental health services with other refugee services, and virtually no mental health outreach services to refugees and victims of torture. Consequently, the needs of newly arrived refugees and asylees are often misunderstood, and some receive no mental health services at all. Psychological support for asylum-seekers and survivors of torture who do not arrive under an organized resettlement program is particularly tenuous. Asylum-seekers face legal uncertainty and lack access to the social services afforded to resettled refugees, factors that compound problems associated with their lack of psychological support.[30]

Migrant Farmworkers

The distinction between refugees and economic migrants is often blurred, since political turmoil and economic collapse often go hand in hand. Internationally in 1991, of the non-refugee migrants, 35 million were in Africa, up to 15 million in Western Europe, 15 million in North America, and 15 million in Asia and the Middle East.[31]

Food would not get to our table if it were not for the 5 million migrant and seasonal farmworkers in the United States. Although not all migrant farmworkers are people of color, 80 percent are ethnic minorities representing black, southeast Asian, and Hispanic as well as white men, women, and children day-haul laborers who are transported daily to and from farms; male migrant Puerto Rican, Haitian, black, and Jamaican workers living in labor camps; Mexican American migrant families living in towns and camps; and year-round local res-

Five million migrant and seasonal farmworkers bring fruits and vegetables to the tables of 230 million in the United States. Most of these workers do not have health insurance despite their high-risk profession.

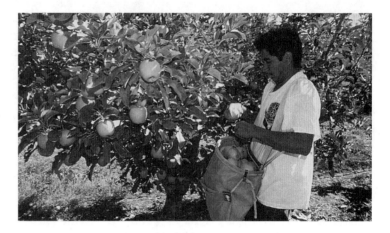

idents who do farm work during the agricultural season. Seventy percent of migrant farmworkers are foreign born. Eighty percent are male, and most adult farmworkers are married and have children. The average annual income for the migrant seasonal farmworker is approximately $6,000 a year and this seldom includes the benefits of health insurance, social security payments, or living allowances.[32] Since they are continually moving, they do not live in a specific location long enough to qualify for federal Medicaid insurance. Today growers have a surplus of workers and they have little incentive to make life better for their hired harvesters.

The Census reports approximately 5 million migrant and seasonal workers and their families in the United States who are at risk for a variety of occupational hazards and ailments worsened by limited or nonexistent health care services. Occupational health studies of agricultural workers generally exclude migrant and seasonal farmworkers because of their necessary migrant work patterns, illegal status, and their return to their country of origin when work is no longer available. As a result, it is difficult, if not impossible, to find any accurate figures about the health status of this population.

Migrant farmworkers have a developing-world health status, although they live and work in one of the richest nations on earth. Unsanitary working and housing conditions make farmworkers vulnerable to health conditions no longer considered to be threats to the general public. Poverty; frequent mobility; low literacy; language, cultural, and logistic barriers impede farmworkers' access to social services and cost-effective primary health care. Economic pressure makes farmworkers reluctant to miss work when it is available. In addition, they are not protected by sick leave and risk losing their jobs if they miss a day of work. These circumstances cause farmworkers to postpone seeking health care unless their condition becomes so severe that they cannot work. At this point, many farmworkers must rely on expensive emergency room care for their health care needs.[33] Migrant health centers provide accessible care for farmworkers, but existing centers have the capacity to serve fewer than 20 percent of the nation's farmworkers.

BOX 11.4 *Major Health Problems of Migrants*

Accidental injury and death	Stress
Pesticide exposure	Chronic diarreah
Neuropsychological disorders	Hypertension
Poor nutrition	Alcohol and drug use
TB and other respiratory diseases	Violence
Parasitic infestation	HIV/AIDS
Congenital disorders	Diabetes
Oral health	Infant mortality

"When the man who feeds the world by toiling in the fields is himself deprived of the basic rights of feeding, sheltering and caring for his own family, the whole community is sick."—Cesar Chavez

Although accurate health data for migrant families and individuals are not available, some facts are well documented. The migrant worker faces "a harvest of illness, injury, and death" from pesticide poisonings, parasitic infections, machinery accidents, tuberculosis, and AIDS.[34] Many live and work under the conditions of poor sanitation and nutrition. Many families live in substandard, overcrowded housing, if they have housing at all. Men, women, and children perform backbreaking, often dangerous work using poorly designed equipment, for which they are paid meagerly and rarely insured. Farmworkers are exposed to pesticide contamination and parasitic infection rates comparable to rates in developing countries.

Farmworker housing is often substandard or nonexistent. Over the last decade much housing has been demolished and not replaced. Farmworkers must move frequently to seek employment. If labor camp housing is not available, they are often unable to find or afford housing. As a result, many farmworkers must camp in the open or sleep in their vehicles. Even among those with housing, 35.2 percent of farmworker housing lacked inside running water in eight major agricultural labor states (California, Florida, Texas, Washington, Colorado, Michigan, New York, and Ohio).[35]

The infant mortality rate for migrants is 125 percent higher than the national average. Birth injuries increase the rates of cerebral palsy and mental retardation. Life expectancy for a migrant farmworker is forty-nine years compared to the national average of seventy-five years. In 1998, 48 of every 100,000 agricultural workers died of work-related unintentional injuries, compared to the national industrial average of nine workers per 100,000.

The rate of parasitic infection among migrants is estimated to be eleven to fifty-nine times higher than that of the general U.S. population, and the incidence of malnutrition is higher than among any other population in the country. Lack of toilets, hand-washing facilities, poor drinking water at the worksite, and crowded dormitory living increase the rates of infectious diseases, diarrhea, pneumonia, influenza, and tuberculosis (which is twenty-five times the national average).

Migrant farmworkers suffer as much as twenty times the rate of diarrhea among the urban poor. The death rates for farmworkers from influenza and pneumonia have been reported to be as much as 20 percent and 200 percent higher, respectively, than the national average. Rates of heart disease, diabetes, hepatitis, and cirrhosis of the liver are higher among this population than national rates.[36]

Women workers must urinate more frequently during pregnancy, but due to the lack of toilets in the fields, urine retention is common. This promotes chronic urinary tract infections which have been associated with an increased rate of hypertension, toxemia, and anemia. Delay in seeking health care is not uncommon. Ultimately, both maternal and fetal survival are put at risk.

Although no accurate figures exist, there is an indication that psychiatric disorders and family dysfunction are high among migrant farmworkers due to the frequency of moving and the loss of ties with nuclear families in countries of origin.

Because the ability to work is based on the perceived health status of a farmworker by her or his employer, migrant workers are often unwilling to admit that they might be ill, and frequently they do not seek health care despite serious health concerns. Barriers to adequate health care also include lack of financial resources and the inability to effectively communicate health care needs when caregivers do not speak the language of the worker.

Often the health care provider has a lack of sensitivity to the needs of culturally diverse patients, assuming that the client's lifestyle and beliefs are those of the majority white middle class. Lack of understanding about cultural medical tradition such as healing rituals, homeopathic medicines, and traditional healers make routine health care incomprehensible and culturally contraindicated.

Another barrier found in the health care system is institutional inflexibility in caring for patients who lack the resources to pay. Rigid institutional standards that prevent negotiation in treatment plans and demeaning quality of care to poor patients aggravate an already overwhelming health care barrier. Some migrant workers are not citizens and are often denied access to affordable and subsidized health care.

Lack of transportation from the fields or labor camps to health care facilities, limited health clinic hours due to shortage of funding and staff resources, major cutbacks in critically important health and social services, and lack of money to pay for basic health care services are primary barriers to health care.

The Healthy People 2000 objectives for migrant workers included: (1) reducing alcohol and drug abuse, (2) improving nutrition, (3) improving mental health, (3) reducing environmental hazards, (4) improving occupational safety, (5) preventing injuries, (6) reducing violent and abusive behavior, and (7) preventing and controlling HIV infection. These objectives are still important and necessary for 2010.

Disparities in Minority Health Education

A compelling disparity of most minority groups in the United States is socio-economic status. Poverty and near poverty appear as underlying elements of many health problems for groups that are also often targets of racism. Economic and educational disadvantages of many peoples are aggravated by behavioral and environmental risk factors specific to populations and locations. The role of health education is not only to address individual risks, but to raise public awareness about the global nature of preventive health behaviors.[37]

Cultural Sensitivity

Delivery of health services requires the humane and culturally sensitive under-standing of all people both in and out of the United States. Effective prevention programs in diverse communities must be tailored to community needs and take into consideration factors concerning individuals, such as disability status, sexual orientation, and gender appropriateness, which also play a significant role in determining health outcomes, behaviors, use patterns, and attitudes across age, racial, and ethnic groups.

The differences in disease patterns among whites and people of color are striking, but these differences are cultural, and/or environmental, and more often based upon socioeconomic factors, not racial factors. There are no diseases that are genetically related to any particular racial group; even sickle cell ane-mia, a disease common to African Americans, is seen in non-black people. Fac-tors such as housing conditions, employment or lack thereof, urban over-crowding, discrimination, dietary habits, alcohol, smoking, and the lack of awareness or availability of health care are all alterable conditions that can be addressed for all people.[38]

The art of healing has been practiced by traditional healers in virtually all cultures. Given the diversity of cultures that can now be found in almost any country, particularly our own, sensitivity to the myriad of beliefs about health and illness must be melded with nonethnocentric and nonracist community health education. Native Americans are going to seek out and depend upon their tribal healers (medicine men and women); Asians upon their practition-ers (hakims and vaids); South and Central Americans may want to work with traditional healers (curanderos).

It is also important to be sensitive to gender issues associated with health care and ethnicity. For instance, Arab and Asian women who are recently from their country of origin are not used to being touched by a male doctor; nor is an Asian man accustomed to being touched by a female doctor.

Language barriers between clinicians and clients are often significant among intercultural health care. Because of the plethora of indigenous lan-guages and dialects among refugees and immigrants, every attempt should be made to find bilingual translators. In 1992, a California migrant worker was released, after over a year in a mental hospital, when it was discovered his "schizophrenia" was actually the inability of any health care clinician to speak his Mexican dialect.

What some might think of as alternative therapies, are actually not "alternative" and are efficacious to those who practice them. Homeopathy, food therapy, herbal therapy, massage therapy, yoga, and even magic may be important parts of many people's health care and may work for traditional or clinical illness. The key to successful community and personal health education is finding a way to integrate traditional and contemporary methods in a sensitive, noncondescending manner that builds confidence among traditional people and their caregivers.

A caveat is the potential for misusing someone's culture in evaluating and educating clients of different backgrounds. Cultures do not exist in a vacuum. They are always part of a particular context, made up of and influenced by historical, geographical, economic, social, and political elements. People may act or think in a particular way, not because of their race or culture, but because they are rich or poor, employed or unemployed, able or disabled, powerful or powerless. Community health should avoid reducing all aspects of an individual or a group's life down to its culture, while ignoring class factors. Perhaps the best "worst" example is the way demographic data are reduced to white, black, and other. Many Hispanics are quite "white" and many are quite "black." Pacific Islanders do not share the cultural beliefs of Asians. Native Americans of different tribes have unique characteristics. Puerto Rican Hispanics can be differentiated from Cubans, Mexicans, and Spaniards. Gay men whether black, Hispanic, Asian, or white should be evaluated in their unique framework, and not just as "gay men" as if all were nonethnic. Lumping people into colors is actually racist and often leads to spurious information. It also promotes stereotyping and the loss of the richness of diversity.

Healthy People 2010 Objective: Increase the Proportion of Local Health Departments with Community Health Promotion and Disease Prevention Programs for Racial and Ethnic Minority Populations

Selected Local Health Department Community Health Promotion and Disease Prevention Programs That Are Culturally and Linguistically Competent	1996–97 Baseline	2010 Target
	Percent	Percent
Cancer	30	50
Educational programs	33	50
Environmental health	22	50
Family planning	42	50
Heart disease and stroke	28	50
HIV	45	50
Immunizations and infectious diseases	48	50
Maternal, infant (and child) health	47	50
Mental health (and mental disorders)	18	50
Nutrition and overweight	44	50
Occupational safety and health	13	50
Oral health	25	50
Physical activity and fitness	21	50

Summary

Oppression is a health risk to people of color. In fact, being a person of color may be hazardous to your health in our society. While modifiable lifestyle factors are the primary risks, underlying poor health among minority people is a legacy of economic deprivation and social oppression.

African Americans still suffer the greatest health risks, morbidity, and mortality, overall, than all other people of color. There are, however, specific health risks associated with each ethnicity that can be addressed by community health education. People of color should not be lumped into the category other and addressed by health care providers as one group.

CYBERSITES RELATED TO CHAPTER 11

African Americans
 www.africanamericanhealth.com

Native Americans
 www.codetalk.fed.us
 www.aaip.com

Hispanics
 www.hispanichealth.org
 latino.si.edu

Asian Americans
 www.baylor.edu/~charles_kemp/asian_health.html
 Usenet: soc.culture.asian.american

QUESTIONS

1. What are the health implications of being a racial minority in the United States today?

2. What are the implications for the collection of health data and the implementation of health programs when we are or are not politically correct in our use of language?

3. Select a specific minority group from those discussed in this chapter and discuss how a politically aware community health professional can improve the quality of life and the health status, while reducing the health risks of this group.

EXERCISES

1. Imagine yourself as the director of a community health conference on AIDS and the risks to minority populations. Prepare for this conference by thinking about who your keynote, plenary, and workshop speakers would be. How would they represent your diverse cultural populations? What workshop titles would appeal to what cultural groups? What areas of sensitivity would need to be anticipated in bringing diverse peoples together?

Assuming you are not a person of color, how does this impact your role as director of the conference and representative of the health community?

2. An interesting experiment has been conducted to measure racial preferences among blacks and whites. You can take assess your own racial attitudes by going to buster.cs.yale.edu/implicit/. Read the introduction and then click on **Measure Your Implicit Attitudes** and follow the links to **Take the Race IAT**.

INTERNET INERACTIVE ACTIVITY

THE MEDICALLY UNDERSERVED DATABASES: BUREAU OF PRIMARY HEALTH CARE, HEALTH RESOURCES, AND SERVICES ADMINISTRATION

The Bureau of Primary Health Care is primarily responsible for serving the medically underserved. An essential program for the medically underserved is the Community Health Center Program, which provides primary and preventive health care services in medically-underserved areas throughout the United States and its territories.

The bureau has a number of databases from which the community health educator can access data regarding medically underserved. Its homepage for the databases is:

bphc.hrsa.gov/bphc/

Example

The community health educator is interested in the characteristics of Alabama's medically underserved population.

1. Go to the database homepage

bphc.hrsa.gov/bphc/

2. Click on **Databases** and then an **HRSA State Profiles**

3. Click on **State Profiles** and then select **Alabama for Fiscal Year 1998**.

4. The profile tells us

the % of population by minority status
% over 65 years
% under 18 year
number of migrant workers
number of seasonal farmworkers
% below poverty
number on Medicaid
number of uninsured
health status including low birth weight
number of counties designated as medically underserved
number of people without a primary care physician
% using Community Health Centers by race, age, gender, economic status

Exercise

The community health educator wants to know how her or his state compares with another state in the same geographical region regarding numbers and characteristics of the medically underserved.

1. Go to the databases for the **Bureau of Primary Health Care**

   bphc.hrsa.gov/bphc/

2. Build a table that compares the demographic characteristics, services provided, and money spent on the medically underserved in your state and the comparative state.

3. How does your state compare to the national data?

4. Use the **Medically Underserved Areas/Medically Underserved Populations** to enhance your description of the needs and services provided by your state to the underserved.

   bphc.hrsa.gov/databases/mua/search.cfm

5. Go to Health Professional Shortage Areas (HPSAs)

   bphc.hrsa.gov/databases/hpsa/hpsa.cfm

6. Use the **Data Search Form** to access the counties in your state that have medical, mental, and dental personnel shortages.

7. Go back to county profiles and describe the demographic characteristics of those counties that have the greatest professional shortages. What are the greatest health concerns in those counties?

REFERENCES

1. Nakamura, Raymond (1999). *Health and wellness: A multicultural perspective.* MA: Allyn & Bacon.

2. Rodriquez, Clara E. (1989). *Puerto Ricans born in the USA.* Boston: Unwin Hyman.

3. Ibid.

4. Acosta-Belen, Edna, & Sjostrom, Barbara (1988). *The Hispanic experience in the United States.* New York: Praeger.

5. *Salt Lake Tribune* (1993). Study Says Latinos Less Likely to Suffer from Most Diseases. November 24, p. A4.

6. *Salt Lake Tribune*, op. cit.

7. Acosta-Belen, op. cit.

8. Trujillo, Michael (1997). "Indian Health Service Home Page," www.tucson.ihs.gov

9. A look at American Indian life (1994). *Salt Lake Tribune*, April 25.

10. Stiffarm, L. A., & Lane, P. (1992). The demography of native North America: A quest of American Indian survival. In M. A. Jaimes (ed.), *The state of Native America* (pp. 23–54). Boston: South End Press.

11. AAHE (1994). Cultural awareness and sensitivity. Guidelines for Health Educators. Virginia.

12. Acosta-Belen, op. cit.

13. Olson, op. cit.

14. Lee, Philip R., & Estes, Carroll L. (1990). *The Nation's Health,* 3rd ed. Boston: Jones & Bartlett.

15. Edelman, Marian (1985). *Black and white children in America: Key facts.* Children's Defense Fund. Washington, DC.

16. Edelman, Marian (1992). *Families in peril.* Children's Defense Fund, Washington, DC.

17. Scandrett, Alfonso (1994). The black church as a participant in community health interventions. *Journal of Health Education* May/June, Vol. 25, No. 3.

18. AAHE, op. cit.

19. McAvoy, Brian, & Donaldson, Liam (1990). *Health care for Asians.* London: Oxford University Press.

20. O'Hare, A. (1990). A new look at Asian Americans. *American Demographics,* October.

21. DHHS (1992). *Healthy People 2000. Full report with commentary.* Boston: Jones & Bartlett.

22. DHHS (1997). Healthy People 2000. Progress Review: Asian and Pacific Islanders. Washington, DC.

23. Ibid.

24. Lequette, Cely (1994). Personal interview, SLC, Utah.

25. Vobejda, Barbara (1990). U.S. growth in the 1980s fueled by immigrants. In *Earth's eleventh hour*, William O. Dwyer (1995). Boston: Allyn & Bacon.

26. Nakamua, op. cit.

27. www.refugees.org/world/statistics/wrs99_tableindex.htm

28. Robinson, Eugene (1993). Worldwide migration nears crisis. In *Earth's eleventh hour*, William O. Dwyer (1995). Boston: Allyn & Bacon.

29. www.unhcr.ch/

30. www.refugees.org/world/statistics/wrs99_tableindex.htm, op. cit

31. Robinson, op. cit.

32. USHHS (1990). Migrant and seasonal farmworker health objectives for the year 2000. Office Migrant Health.

33. www.ncfh.org/aboutfws/facts.htm#services

34. Dixon, Jennifer (1992). Panel report: Migrant farm workers still abused. *Salt Lake Tribune.* November 1, 1992, p. A22.

35. www.ncfh.org/aboutfws/facts.htm#services, op. cit.

36. Ibid.

37. USHHS, op. cit.

38. AAHE, op. cit.

CHAPTER 12

Emerging Communities of the 21st Century

Community Health in the 21st Century
"The time has come for Americans to acknowledge the reality of diversity—
this includes sexual orientation and the contributions of, needs of and
inequalities suffered by lesbians, gay men, bisexuals, and other sexually
diverse people. The 21st century will include more open participation by
gay men and lesbian health professionals, and the identification of health
risks unique to their constituents."

—Ben Barr, M.S.W., Former Director, Utah AIDS Foundation

Primary prevention by changing individual's behaviors that contribute
to many occupational injuries, especially spinal cord injuries.

—Frederick I. White, Ed.D., Manager,
Disabilities Prevention Program

Chapter Objectives

The student will:

1. list the three primary health risks for lesbians.

2. list the three primary health risks for gay men.

3. explain why homophobia is a social illness.

4. describe ways community health professionals can make the differently abled feel more integrated into their communities.

5. explain how "isms" come from a similar basis and impact victims in similar ways.

Lesbians, Gay Men, and Bisexual Communities

A minority population that until now has been ignored in public health texts is the lesbian, gay, and bisexual communities of our nation. In fact, there were no Healthy People 2000 objectives for these special populations although other special populations were identified and targeted. There are, however, specific community health risks that are presently being met by many communities and community health professionals, and these populations are discussed in many objectives for Healthy People 2010, although the Gay and Lesbian Medical Association believes "it completely ignores the specific health needs of the lesbian, gay, bisexual, and transgendered community."[1]

The plural, communities, is used because, like any group, there are more differences than there are similarities among people of different sexual orientations, and the combination of these differences define the whole. Neither lesbians, gay men, nor bisexuals are homogeneous or easily defined outside familiar and exaggerated stereotypes. Common myths and their corrections about lesbians and gay men are discussed in Box 12.1. It is the responsibility of health professionals to know and be sensitive to these communities in the same way that an appropriate understanding of native cultures or immigrant or African American cultures is essential to the planning and implementation of health education programs. While AIDS may seem like the only impetus for coming to consciousness about gay men, some other very important issues face gay men, bisexuals, and lesbians in ways that nonhomophobic professionals can address.

Health professionals should be aware that there are three components to gender identity relative to a given society. The first is *core gender identity*, which describes a person's innermost concept of oneself as male or female.[2] For the majority of people on the planet one is either male or female. There are, however, a small minority within any culture who ultimately are defined as transsexuals, those whose physical gender manifestation does not match the internal concept of self as male or female.

The second category is *gender role*, which is the set of roles prescribed for females and males by one's culture, society, generation, or other external factors. These are culturally defined and vary across the planet.[3] People emigrating from other countries often must modify traditional gender roles to assimilate into their newly adopted country.

The third category is *sexual orientation*. This is a continuum of erotosexual attraction that varies from person to person.[4] As Alfred Kinsey discovered in the early 1950s, society cannot be dichotomized as heterosexual and homosexual. There is tremendous variation between those parameters that may change throughout one's life. In general, however, most people, by late teens or early adulthood, have a personal sense of their primary sexual orientation as heterosexual, homosexual, or bisexual. While the term sexual preference has been used commonly in the past to denote primary sexual and emotional attraction, since the Stonewall riots in 1969, the official beginning of the gay liberation movement, sexual orientation has replaced sexual preference since it does not suggest a choice in one's orientation. Research from the National Institutes of Health and other research since 1990 is strongly suggesting that sexual attraction is not a choice but a physiologically defined characteristic, much like left-handedness, hair color, or musical ability. Given the great diversity even among homosexuals and heterosexuals, the cause of one's sexual orientation is probably a combination of biological, social, cultural, and environmental factors.

Gay men and lesbians are, perhaps, the most understudied groups in the United States. Little is known about their health status, their economic status,

BOX 12.1 Myths and Facts about Homosexuality

There are numerous misconceptions about being gay or lesbian. They nevertheless continue to circulate, adding to the fires of the prejudice. These misconceptions include:

Misconception No. 1: Men and women are gay or lesbian because they can't get a heterosexual partner. This belief is reflected in such remarks about lesbians as "All she needs is a good lay" (implying a man). Similar remarks about men include "He just needs to meet the right woman." Research indicates that lesbians and gay men have about as much heterosexual high school dating experience as their peers. Furthermore, the majority of lesbians had sexual experiences with men; many of those experiences were pleasurable (Bell et al., 1987).

Misconception No. 2: Lesbian and gay men "recruit" heterosexuals to become gay. People are not recruited or seduced into being gay anymore than they are recruited into being heterosexual. Most gay men and lesbians have their first gay experience with a peer, either a friend or an acquaintance. They report having had homosexual feelings prior to their first experience (Bell et al., 1981).

Misconception No. 3: Gay men are child molesters. This is a collary to the misconception above. The overwhelmingly majority of child molesters are heterosexual males who molest girls; these men include fathers, stepfathers, uncles, and brothers. A large percentage of men who molest boys identify themselves as heterosexual (Arndt, 1991).

Misconception No. 4: Homosexuality can be caught. Homosexuality is not the flu. Some parents express fear about having their children taught by homosexual teachers. They fear their children will model themselves after the teacher or be seduced by him or her. But a child's sexual orientation is well established by the time he or she enters school, and a teacher would not have an impact on that child's orientation (Marmor, 1980).

Misconception 5: Gay men and lesbians could change if they wanted. There is no evidence that gay men and lesbians can change their sexual orientation. The belief that they should reflects assumptions that homosexuality is abnormal or sinful. Most psychotherapy with gay men and lesbians who are unhappy about their sexual orientation aims at helping them adjust to it.

Misconception No. 6: Homosexuality is condemned by the Bible. The Bible condemned same-sex sexual activities between men, not homosexuality. Some biblical scholars believe that the rejection of same-sex sexual activities was based on historical factors including the lack of the concept of sexual orientation, the explorative and abusive nature of much same-sex activity in ancient times, the belief that the purpose of sex procreation, and purity or holiness concerns that such acts were impure (there were similar concerns about sexual intercourse with a menstruating woman). There is increasing debate among religious groups as to whether same-sex relationships are inherently sinful.

their political preferences, or their demographic trends. They are not represented in clinical trials, even those markedly directed toward AIDS. They are not considered as an independent variable in most health research. The result is a lack of sufficient information upon which to create health education programs and promote behavior change or health promotion.

While bisexuals, transsexuals, and other diversities of sexual orientation and lifestyles exist within any community, this chapter will focus on lesbians and gay men. Unfortunately, there has not been enough public health research or social research conducted on other sexually diverse people to introduce the reader to accurate community health information regarding these other populations at this time. The authors encourage community health professionals to get to know each community's diverse populations and learn from the professional interaction with these populations what their needs and risks may be.

> **Discussion:** What are the demographic characteristics of your GLTB communities? What are the specific health needs of your GLTB communities?

Because of the nature of **homophobia**—the irrational fear toward lesbians and gay people—and **homohatred**—the hostile and violent behavior against lesbians and gay people in our population—an accurate assessment of the vital statistics of gay men and lesbians cannot be made with assurance. Justifiable fear and threats of loss of job, children, housing, health insurance, social status, and biological family support systems keep many gay men and lesbians from freely and accurately identifying themselves for demographic analysis or health status study. It is estimated that most surveys about homosexuality reflect at the most only 5 percent of the so-called "out" population, and these persons represent typically urban, middle class, white males. However, the initiation of lesbian and gay professional caucuses in the American Public Health Association, the American Medical Association and other health professional groups, as well as lesbian and gay health organizations are recent sources of identification of the community health issues of these populations, if not solutions to many problems.

Another prejudice that prevents an accurate look at different sexual lifestyles and the assimilation of diversity into American life is **heterosexism.** Heterosexism is "the system by which heterosexuality is assumed to be the only acceptable and viable life option. Often heterosexism is quite subtle or indirect and may not even be apparent."[5]

The issue of same sex marriage or even the promotion of marriage as an established requirement for a healthy adult leads to grave psychosocial problems among young gay men and lesbians, those who by law have a characteristic that does not permit marriage, or those who do not wish to marry.[6]

Heterosexism forces lesbians, gay men, and bisexuals to struggle constantly against their own invisibility and makes it much more difficult for them to integrate a positive sexual identity. This situation is not unlike African Americans and Asians who only see white faces in all forms of media or when beauty is defined by a Caucasian norm.[7]

Lesbians and Gay Men

The gay and lesbian communities share the same social and community health problems as any contemporary community. Proportionately high incidences of partner abuse, child abuse, alcoholism, drug dependency, mental illness, and issues of aging exist in gay and lesbian communities. What is poorly recognized and studied is that at least one-fourth of homeless teens are gay and that suicide is higher among gay teens than their non-gay peers. Whereas one in ten heterosexual teens attempts suicide, two to three of every ten gay teens attempt suicide.[8] Gay people are often diagnosed as mentally ill because of their lifestyle, not due to the stresses associated with social discrimination, internalized homophobia, isolation, and loss that causes depression and anxiety.

Any community's attempts at legalizing discrimination and encouraging bigotry against the lesbian and gay men's populations takes tremendous emotional energy to face privately and publicly. The stress and constant threat of violence and hatred adds another dimension of interpersonal and community stress on gay men and lesbians. Gay bashing, the physical violence against people presumed to be nonheterosexual, is an everyday occurrence in our country. It is usually perpetrated by very misinformed, poorly socialized, hate-filled teenaged or young adult males. It leaves the carnage of death, disability, terror, paranoia, and post-traumatic violence syndromes that make this issue an important public health and health education issue for schools and communities.

Table 12.1 describes the actual types of hate crimes reported to the FBI by states in 1997. Figure 12.1 shows the status of hate crime legislation by state in 1999. Without hate crime legislation that includes sexual orientation, it is difficult to fully protect gay men and lesbians under the law.

Discussion: What laws protect the rights of lesbians and gay men in your community? Should there be more laws or fewer?

Substance Abuse

A study of 455 lesbians (42 percent) and gay men (58 percent)[9] found similar illicit and licit drug use for different age groups. However, inhalant use was greater among gay men and cigarette use was more prevalent among lesbians. Lesbians had a 20 percent higher cigarette use rate than among U.S. women in general. The least prevalent drugs used were crack and heroin. Marijuana, inhalants, and club drugs were the most popular illicit drugs used by gay men. The following paragraph gives the reader some of the comparisons between gay men and lesbians, and heterosexual populations.

Among all adults aged twenty-six to thirty-four, 73.7 percent of men and 55.2 percent of women have used alcohol in the past month. Comparative figures for gay men and lesbians were 81.3 percent and 66.7 percent. Among all adults aged thirty-five+, 28.6 percent of men and 22 percent of women reported smoking cigarettes in the past month, compared with 47.8 percent for gay and bisexual men and 38.1 percent for lesbians.[10] The association with smoking among gay men suggests a general tendency to be less health conscious, to be influenced by class and gay socialization patterns, and to be affected by the AIDS epidemic.

Table 12.1 Number of hate crime incidents, offenses, victims, and known offenders by bias motivation, 1997.

	Incident	Offenses	Victims[1]	Known Offenders[2]
Total	8,049	9,861	10,255	8,474
Single-Bias Incidents				
Race	**4,710**	**5,898**	**6,084**	**5,444**
Anti-White	993	1,267	1,293	1,520
Anti-Black	3,120	3,838	3,951	3,301
Anti-American Indian/Alaska Native	36	44	46	45
Anti-Asian/Pacific Islander	347	437	466	351
Anti-Multiracial Group	214	312	328	227
Religion	**1,385**	**1,483**	**1,586**	**792**
Anti-Jewish	1,087	1,159	1,247	598
Anti-Catholic	31	32	32	16
Anti-Protestant	53	59	61	19
Anti-Islamic	28	31	32	22
Anti-Other Religious Group	159	173	184	120
Anti-Multireligious Group	24	26	27	11
Anti-Aethiest/Agnosticism	3	3	3	6
Sexual Orientation	**1,102**	**1,375**	**1,401**	**1,315**
Anti-Male Homosexual	760	912	927	1,032
Anti-Female Homosexual	188	229	236	158
Anti-Homosexual	133	210	214	103
Anti-Heterosexual	12	14	14	14
Anti-Bisexual	9	10	10	8
Ethnicity/National Origin	**836**	**1,083**	**1,132**	**906**
Anti-Hispanic	491	636	649	614
Anti-Other Ethnicity/National Origin	345	447	483	292
Disability	**12**	**12**	**12**	**14**
Anti-Physical	9	9	9	11
Anti-Mental	3	3	3	3

[1]The term "victim" may refer to a person, business, institution, or a society as a whole.

[2]The term "known offender" does not imply that the identity of the suspect is known, but only that an attribute of the suspect is identified that distinguishes him/her from an unknown offender.

(*Source:* FBI statistics)

As noted earlier, social stresses may be the enhancing variable in the significantly greater use of alcohol and tobacco among gay men and lesbians; however, since little research has been done among these populations, the complete picture is not known. Clearly, these are immediate community health prevention priorities among those who do work with the gay and lesbian communities.[11]

The AIDS epidemic has created a whole new dimension of health care consciousness around the advocacy role of health care workers to speak for those who have no voice in our system, whether they be children, non–English-speaking immigrants, the disabled, or lesbians and gay men.

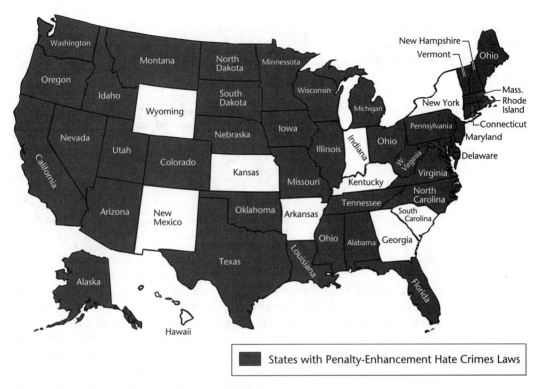

Figure 12.1 States with hate crimes laws (1999).

(*Source:* Human Rights Coalition)

Health Services

Another universal issue for gay men and lesbians, much like that of different cultures, is finding health care practitioners who "speak their language," are culturally sensitive, are willing to listen and learn, and are ethical in their relationship with clients. One study reported that 71.3 percent of health care workers said their quality of care for gay men was poor to fair and 68 percent said they were unaware of health and social resources for gay men.[12]

Defining "Family" in Our Society

Perhaps an issue for our society is to redefine "the family." For gay people the family is their life partner and the significant friends and lovers who create a support network when traditional support systems such as biological family, church, and state have failed. Where domestic partners are not acknowledged by law or convention, many partners are denied access to their life partner during life-threatening or even everyday decision making that married heterosexuals would have privilege to without question. Lack of legal and conventional understanding of the diversity of "the family" has left couples of many years without the right or invitation to participate in decisions around surgery, life

Lesbians and gay men have redefined "family" by creating new, inclusive relationships that promote community support. Since the Stonewall Riot in June 1968, Pride Day has been celebrated throughout the United States to raise awareness and community pride.

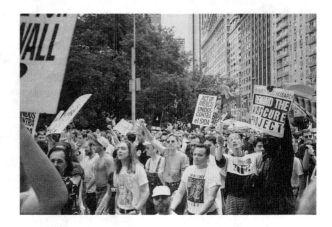

support, burial, or grief. Some business leaders such as Levi Strauss, Lotus Development Corp., Montefiore Medical Center in New York, and Ben and Jerry's Ice Cream have recognized these inequities and have included domestic partners as part of "family" health care benefits. A study at Lotus Software showed that including gay family partners did not increase cost of health care to the companies, and in fact, improved personnel relations and company working conditions. The employee pays an additional premium, the same whether it's a gay or straight employee. The fear of the cost of AIDS has not materialized as a cost issue. Compare the $50,000 or $60,000 cost with a heart or liver transplant or cancer treatment and the difference is significantly less.

In 1992, a lesbian city social worker took time off to care for her seriously ill domestic partner. Her request for sick leave was denied because her partner was not legally her spouse. This issue is not unique. It has been a problem for domestic partners as well as heterosexual couples who live out of wedlock or for adult children of an ill parent who are all denied sick leave because the illness is not in their "immediate, legal family." Congress has passed a family leave act that will give more flexibility to those who need time off to care for sick loved ones, but defining "family" and "loved ones" still leaves gay and lesbian couples without due process. In the case of the Denver social worker an appeal to the courts found in her favor and ruled she was entitled to three days of sick pay. This is the beginning of setting a precedent for other alternative family constellations. Recently, a Minneapolis Civil Rights Commission panel voted to require the city and the library board to stop refusing to provide health care benefits to a library employee's woman partner. This trend is occurring throughout the United States.

It is estimated that about twenty private employers, including the American Psychological Association, are known to offer spousal benefits to domestic partners, although no comprehensive list exists. Some companies, like U.S. West Communications offers parental leave to employees regardless of their sexual orientation or marital status. Other benefits include child care, bereavement leave, and life insurance.

Lesbian Issues

The term "lesbian" is used in different ways by public and mental health professionals, and its definition has long been a source of debate among women who self-identify as women who love women. Though most health professionals use the term lesbian to describe women who engage in sexual activities exclusively with women, the definition is actually much broader.[13] Adrienne Rich, poet and philosopher, described a lesbian continuum that includes women who are women identified but do not have sexual relationships with women, bisexuals who may have male and female lovers throughout their lives, and those who self-identify as sexually attracted only to women. On the definition continuum there are diverse relationships, behaviors, emotions, attachments, affections, political beliefs, and family constellations. There are also women who love women who are uncomfortable using the label lesbian to define their wide variety of life experiences, because the term lesbian has been used by heterosexuals in such a pejorative way. Many women who love women may find the term "gay" or "women identified" more descriptive. In this chapter, the term lesbian refers to women whose primary sexual and emotional interaction is associated with the love of another woman, or of those who think of themselves as part of a lesbian community. The most important issue for community health is to assist women of many persuasions to have access to sensitive, nonjudgmental health care, and participation in drug trials and health education that is specific to the unique nature of women's diversity.[14]

Because lesbians are female, the major health problems of women strike lesbians proportionately. There is some evidence, however, that two conditions may be disproportionately represented: (1) breast cancer and (2) immune deficiency disorders. Also, some problems such as alcoholism and drug abuse may seem accentuated due to clustering of women in these populations. It is estimated that one-third of lesbians have a problem with alcohol or substance abuse, five to seven times greater than heterosexual women.[15] A national study of 1,925 lesbians in fifty states found that 33 percent reported regular use of alcohol and 6 percent drank alcohol daily. Alcohol dependency was higher among older lesbians. Alcoholism is more prevalent among lesbians because of the importance of gay bars as "safe," confidential social centers, the alienation and isolation lesbians experience in society, and the lack of treatment agencies responsive to the lesbian client.[16] Excessive alcohol use among women correlates with higher rates of cirrhosis, accidents, suicide, depression, hypertension, menstrual and reproductive problems, malnutrition, colon and stomach cancer, and gastrointestinal hemorrhage.[17]

Gynecologically, lesbians report less endometriosis, few sexually transmitted diseases, and much lower incidence of cervical neoplasia. Vaginal infections of all types occur similarly for lesbians and other women, though less chronically. It is estimated that 25 to 50 percent of lesbians will or have been pregnant.[18] A study by Conway found that 80 percent of lesbian clients at one clinic had practiced heterosexual intercourse and, therefore, were at risk for cervical abnormalities.[19] Nulliparity, low parity, and delayed childbearing all may be associated with increased risk of breast, ovarian, and endometrial cancers. Strategies favored by some lesbians for achieving conception (unprotected sex with known donor, a stranger, or insemination with untested semen) pose risks for transmission of sexually transmitted diseases and HIV.[20]

Unfortunately, many lesbians delay preventive gynecological health care because of the issues associated with "coming out" to a practitioner. Lesbians report encountering clinical providers' embarrassment, fear, ostracism, refusal to treat, cool detachment, shock, voyeuristic curiosity, insults, rough physical handling, and breaches of confidentiality when they have disclosed their sexual orientation.[21] Although 81 percent of women surveyed in the national study were between the ages of twenty-five and forty-four, only 50 percent reported having obtained a Pap smear within the last year and 5 percent had never obtained one.[22] Lesbians were less likely than bisexual women to report a history of cystitis and vaginal and sexually transmitted diseases, however, because sexual practices among lesbians may include both oral-genital and genital-genital contact, they may be at risk for transmitting genital herpes, hepatitis A, and HIV.[23]

Breast Cancer   There is really no longitudinal research that addresses the concerns among lesbians regarding their risk of breast cancer. Among the known risk factors for breast cancer is not giving birth. On the whole, lesbians are less likely to have given birth and may be at somewhat higher risk than women in general. What may not be a statistically significant difference is that this risk (this has yet to be studied) may be potentiated by less preventive screening. The National Lesbian Survey found that 21 percent performed monthly breast exams, as opposed to 50 percent of single women and 63 percent of married women responding in the National Health Interview Survey in 1985.[24] A 1998 retrospective study among 1,109 heterosexual women and lesbians being seen at the Lyon-Martin Clinic in Oakland, California found no significant differences between the two groups on risk factors such as a family history of breast cancer, current or past alcohol use, or in ever having had a mammogram. In addition, there was no significant difference in the prevalence of breast cancer between the two groups—five cases were identified in the lesbians, three in the heterosexual women. The researchers recommended further, longitudinal research.[25]

Lesbians are less likely to seek health care that may routinely screen for breast cancer in heterosexually active lifestyles. The result is often later diagnosis with poorer prognosis for breast cancer among diagnosed lesbians. A major concern of the National Lesbian and Gay Health Conference has been the lack of national interest in breast cancer (and other women's health issues) which puts lesbians in double jeopardy.

Chronic Fatigue Syndrome (CFS)   A condition of prolonged and overwhelming fatigue, achy joints, loss of memory, weight loss, and other chronic conditions was first described by physicians in Incline Village, Lake Tahoe, Nevada, in the early 1980s. The numbers suggested an epidemic among women in this community. Nationally, the physician's concerns aroused little suspicion and in the 1980s this growing collection of signs and symptoms were most frequently diagnosed among white, upper middle-class professions. It was thought to be caused by stress and the 1980s emphasis on self, money, promotion, and prestige and was dubbed "Yuppie Flu." As the yuppies lost ground, the disease did not, and today more and more immune system-related diseases are being diagnosed among not just white middle-class professionals, but among all members of the population.

Lesbians, in particular, have been outspoken about the incidence among their friends, lovers, and "community." It is not thought that CFS is specific to lesbians, but yuppies had the financial means to get treatment and thus become visible. People of color, lesbians, and others who find it difficult to access health care, were much less able to afford or seek treatment for CFS, and therefore, were not found to be at risk until much later.

Lesbians, who have fought on the front lines of the AIDS epidemic, have taken health care among themselves seriously and are beginning to make their health needs visible to the medical profession. Breast cancer and CFS have been the two conditions that have most frequently been identified when lesbian health professionals have shared their data. It is recommended that lesbians be included as a cohort in research that might identify etiology and treatment of CFS.

HIV/AIDS In the early days of the AIDS epidemic, lesbians were sarcastically called "the chosen people" since the disease was thought to be a problem for those having sex with men. This attempt at humor has given many lesbians a false sense of security that they cannot become infected. The stereotype was that lesbians did not have sex with men. The CDC has chosen to define a lesbian as a woman who has reported "sex relations exclusively with females since 1977." According to the CDC, as of 1990 there were 143 cases of AIDS among lesbians. Since the CDC definition of lesbian is completely out of touch with the reality of the wide variety of sexual behaviors in any woman's life, including a lesbian's, the incidence reported is thought to be grossly underestimated. Underreporting may also be the result of secrecy that lesbians and bisexuals may maintain when dealing with the health care profession. Lesbians are as diverse as all humanity. Some have had sexual intercourse with men prior to exclusive relationships with women, many define themselves as bisexual and enjoy sex with men and women, and some are married to men and have women lovers on the side. Perhaps even more hidden is the reality that some lesbians are sex workers and are exposed to HIV and other risks of being a sex worker such as violence, infections, and stress. Although only five cases of woman to woman transmission have been documented worldwide, it is also possible for women to expose other women to HIV through unsafe sexual practices such as among those who practice unsafe sadomasochistic sexual practices.[26]

As are exclusively heterosexual women, lesbians may be injection drug abusers, may be transfused, receive an organ transplant, be raped, or otherwise exposed to infected blood through occupational hazards. From June 1980 through September 1989, seventy-nine women with AIDS reported only having female-to-female sexual relationships. Most of these women were injection drug users.[27] A study in a community clinic in New York City found that among HIV infected women, thirty-one cases were lesbian. When asked to state their risk factors the results included sixteen injection drug users, seven prior sexual contact with men, five prostitutes, two female-to-female transmission, and one contaminated transfusion recipient.[28] The point of this analysis is that lesbians have been omitted from public health information written specifically for them and many still live with the misconception that they are not at risk because they are lesbian.

Birthing   Many lesbians are choosing to become mothers. For lesbians, the health care hurdles involve working with sperm banks, obstetricians or midwives, prenatal education givers, maternity and baby stores, and friends and family who may lack the knowledge, sensitivity, or social poise to make this a special, joyous choice. There are still many professionals who refuse to permit lesbians access to the system, which means lesbians must "pass" or go around the system, often putting themselves and their baby at risk.

Gay Men's Issues

Sexual labels to define identity are a common means of talking about and understanding the diversity of sexual orientations. A common word to mean heterosexual is *straight,* and a common term for homosexual is *gay.* Although gay is often used to talk about all people who do not define themselves as heterosexual, it is more generally being used to describe men who find emotional and physical attraction primarily toward other men. When men are referred to as gay, community health professionals should remember that there is a vast continuum of diverse lifestyles that may include gay. Some men may be or have previously been married to women, dating women as well as men, exclusively involved with men, or making a living selling sex to other men.

In general, the CDC refers to the population described above as men who have sex with men (MSM). Different lifestyle choices require different health considerations and risk reduction programs. Since MSM have some unique health risks they should be considered as part of this population whether or not they self-identify as gay.

Mental Health   Research among gay men shows some health trends that should be considered in working for the gay community. For instance, gay men score slightly higher than heterosexual men on the Hopkins Depression Symptoms checklist. Episodes of depression related to AIDS anxiety was reported in one study at 40.1 percent of gay men.

Substance Abuse   Studies suggest that 30 percent of gay men are chemically dependent compared to 10 to 12 percent of non-gay men. Depression and chemical dependency seem to be triggered not so much by one's sexual orientation as by the stress associated with being "different" in a homophobic society. The pressure to remain "closeted" and invisible, to "pass" and to play roles to maintain one's job or social standing creates tremendous anxiety and stress, as it does for other minority populations. Twelve-step programs that do not target gay recovering alcoholics do not adequately deal with the unique issues associated with being homosexual in a heterosexist society, so many gay twelve-step programs have begun across the country. One of the noted national recovery programs for gays and lesbians is The Pride Institute, which provides private counseling by gay therapists, twelve-step programs for gay people, gay-friendly residential inpatient programs, and support groups for positive reinforcement regarding alternative lifestyles.

Communicable Diseases   At higher rates among gay men than non-gay men are HIV infection, gonorrhea, and hepatitis A and B. Fifty percent of gay men had experienced at least one STD in the past according to a study in San Francisco. Before the education and acceptance of safer sex practices by gay men, the conditions mentioned were serious and common health concerns of gay men. The nature of some sexual behaviors, namely anal penetration and multiple anonymous sexual partners, made chronic STD infections the norm. Chronic STDs, over time, appear to have led to penicillin-resistant strains of many bacteria, as well as depressed immune systems that left many gay men at very high risk for HIV infection.

There are many enteric diseases for which gay men may be at risk. The most common means of transmission of enteric pathogens is through fecal–oral routes. Two common enteric bacterial infections are caused by *Shigella* and *Campylobacter jejuni* bacteria. Common parasitic infections include those caused by *Entamoeba histoytica* and *Giardia lamblia*. Also, approximately 80 percent of gay men test positive for Cytomegalovirus (CMV) antibodies, and hepatitis B is a common viral infection passed through fecal–oral transmission.[29]

Hepatitis A, B, and C   High rates of hepatitis A, B, and C are found among MSM. Unprotected sex and use of illicit intravenous or intranasal drugs increase the risk for developing hepatitis. Occupational exposure to infected blood, tattooing, body piercing or sharing razors or toothbrushes can lead to hepatitis infection. Despite the fact that safe, effective vaccination exists for both hepatitis A and B, most men who have sex with men have not chosen immunization to protect themselves and others against these sometimes fatal diseases. According to a recent four-city survey, only one-third of the MSM respondents have been immunized against hepatitis B.

Even fewer, less than a fourth of those interviewed, have been immunized against hepatitis A. A survey of 250 men in New York, Los Angeles, Chicago, and San Francisco reveals other troubling data. For example, 62 percent incorrectly believed that condoms would prevent transmission of hepatitis A. More than 50 percent did not know that MSM are at a significantly higher risk than the rest of the population. Most problematic, however, was that while vaccination rates were directly proportional to the degree of openness a patient has about his sexuality, not all of the MSM is these heavily gay areas were "out" to their doctors.[30]

HIV/AIDS   Older gay adolescents, gay men, and racial and ethnic minorities are disproportionately represented among those infected with HIV. Although the AIDS epidemic seems to have stabilized among gay men in some areas of the country, there is evidence of a future second wave in that group, especially among those who are now gay teens who do not know anyone infected with HIV. There are, however, many clinical differences in health risks between adolescent teens and adult gay males and females. Gay teens usually are much less able than their non-gay peers to discuss sexually related health issues with providers. Less than ten percent of pediatricians surveyed said that they provided comprehensive care to teenage patients on the issues of sexuality, substance abuse, body image or mental health, let alone health care specific to gay teens.[31]

Fathering   Some gay men also have an interest in being fathers through adoption and require the sensitivity and help of a social system that often sees single fatherhood, especially among gay men (even if partnered) as socially deviant despite lack of any evidence to support such a conclusion. Gay men who are fathers become active in all the childhood school, health, religious, and social institutions in which their children participate. Remembering to include partners at social events and to not be heterosexually presumptuous may help to make gay parenting less stressful for communities.

Gay and Lesbian Youth   Gay and lesbian youth face numerous issues that might be addressed through public health and school health interventions. Because society has created a mythology about gays and lesbians, young people are quick to believe the myths about nonheterosexuals without looking at the data available. As a result, nonheterosexual youth face or expect widespread violence, discrimination, humiliation, and threats. The result of such fear and stress includes the following risks:

1. Loss of self-esteem. Eighty-six percent of high school students said they would be very upset if classmates called them gay or lesbian. Nearly two-thirds of high school counselors express negative attitudes and feelings about homosexuality and homosexual persons.

2. Sexually transmitted diseases. Homosexual and bisexual male teens were found to have a greater number of sexual partners than heterosexual teens. Forty-five percent of gay teens reported a past history of STDs.

3. Violence. One survey found 45 percent of males and 20 percent of females having experienced verbal or physical assaults in secondary school because they were perceived to be gay or lesbian.

4. Drop-out rate. Twenty-eight percent of gay and lesbian youth drop out of high school.

5. Suicide. Gay youth account for approximately one-third of all youth suicides. Suicide is the leading cause of death among gay and lesbian youth.

6. Homelessness. Gay youth comprise about 25 percent of all youth living on the street. Twenty-six percent of gays and lesbians are forced to leave home because of conflicts over their sexual orientation.

7. Substance abuse. Gay youth report more use of drugs, alcohol, and tobacco than their heterosexual peers.

8. Sexual abuse. Approximately 15 percent of gay youth report being victims of sexual abuse.

9. Eating disorders. Male gay youth are more likely to be underweight than heterosexual youth. They have a higher risk of binge eating, using laxatives, and obsessions with thoughts of food.

Differently Abled People

People with disabilities form 7 to 10 percent of the world's population. At least 2 percent of a nation's population is in need of rehabilitation services at any one point in time.[32] In 1999, the most common disabilities in the United States were: (1) arthritis/rheumatism (27 percent), (2) back/spinal injury (21 percent), (3) heart problems (17 percent), (4) respiratory problems (10 percent), (5) other (25 percent).[33] Table 12.2 describes the rate of reported chronic diseases—

BOX 12.2 The Americans with Disabilities Act

There are four titles to the ADA. Some examples of the regulations within each title are given below.

Title I—Employment

- Employers may not discriminate against an individual with a disability in hiring or promotion if the person is otherwise qualified for the job.
- Employers can ask about one's ability to perform a job, but cannot inquire if someone has a disability or subject a person to tests that tend to screen out people with disabilities.
- Employers will need to provide "reasonable accommodation" to individuals with disabilities. This includes steps such as job restructuring and modification of equipment.
- Employers do not need to provide accommodations that impose an "undue hardship" on business operations.

Title II—Transportation

- New buses ordered on or after August 26, 1990, must be accessible to individuals with disabilities.
- Transit authorities must provide comparable paratransit or other special transportation services to individuals with disabilities who cannot use fixed-route bus services, unless an undue burden would result.
- New bus stations must be accessible

Title III—Public Acommodations

- Public accommodations such as restaurants, hotels, theaters, doctors' offices, pharmacies, retail stores, museums, libraries, parks, private schools, and day care centers may not discriminate on the basis of disability. Private clubs and religious organizations are exempt.
- Auxiliary aids and services must be provided to individuals with vision or hearing impairments or other individuals with disabilities, unless an undue burden would result.
- Physical barriers in existing facilities must be removed if removal is readily achievable.

Title IV—Telecommunications

- Companies offering telephone service to the general public must offer telephone relay services to individuals who use telecommunications devices for the deaf (TDDs) or similar devices.

Table 12.2 Chronic conditions per 1,000 by sex (1996).

Type of Chronic Condition	Male	Female	Type of Chronic Condition	Male	Female
Selected skin and musculoskeletal conditions			**Selected digestive conditions**		
Arthritis	411.2	534.5	Ulcer	30.0	30.3
Gout, including gouty arthritis	46.4	19.5	Hernia of abdominal cavity	53.3	44.9
Intervertebral disc disorders	37.4	28.4	Gastritis or duodenitis	17.9	34.6
Bone spur or tendinitis, unspecified	12.0	19.5	Frequent indigestion	20.3	43.0
			Enteritis or colitis	7.1	10.7
Disorders of bone or cartilage	8.9	38.6	Spastic colon	10.7	17.0
Trouble with bunions	17.0	25.6	Diverticula of intestines	22.8	55.6
Bursitis, unclassified	25.7	46.8	Frequent constipation	21.3	42.8
Sebaceous skin cyst	3.1	1.1	**Selected circulatory conditions**		
Trouble with acne	—	—	Rheumatic fever with or without heart disease	17.7	7.7
Psoriasis	28.2	5.4			
Dermatitis	32.6	19.8	Heart disease	311.3	238.0
Trouble with dry (itching) skin, unclassified	50.9	47.4	Ischemic heart disease	184.8	109.1
			Heart rhythm disorders	69.7	68.7
Trouble with ingrown nails	40.7	35.5	Tachycardia or rapid heart	28.2	32.7
Trouble with corn and calluses	26.7	31.8	Heart murmurs	23.9	16.5
Impairments			Other and unspecified heart rhythm disorders	17.4	19.5
Visual impairment	103.8	70.0			
Color blindness	40.2	3.4	Other selected diseases of heart, excluding hypertension	56.8	60.1
Cataracts	140.1	194.3			
Glaucoma	54.1	60.4	High blood pressure (hypertension)	298.0	410.8
Hearing impairment	386.8	243.2	Cerebrovascular disease	93.8	44.4
Tinnitus	117.4	66.1	Hardening of the arteries	45.8	32.1
Speech impairment	15.2	9.2	Varicose venis of lower extremities	46.2	102.9
Absence of extremities (excludes tips of fingers or toes only)	26.6	14.3	Hemorrhoids	40.4	76.3
Paralysis of extremities, complete or partial	20.8	17.5	**Selected respiratory conditions**		
			Chronic bronchitis	48.8	74.1
			Asthma	37.5	51.3
Deformity or orthopedic impairment	156.5	158.4	Hay fever or allergic rhinitis without asthma	45.7	83.6
Back	50.1	82.1	Chronic sinusitis	109.6	122.5
Upper extremities	43.4	21.8	Deviated nasal septum	10.7	3.0
Lower extremities	69.9	74.5	Chronic disease of tonsils or adenoids	—	1.4
			Emphysema	33.2	31.9

(*Sources:* Centers for Disease Control. National Center for Health Statistics)

conditions for men and women—who had specific disabling limitations. Figure 12.2 shows the percentage of those with specific disabilities.

Discussion: What infrastructures in your community should be changed to make your community accessible?

On July 26, 1990, the landmark **Americans With Disabilities Act (ADA)** was enacted in the United States. This legislation was originally proposed by the National Council on Disability, an independent federal agency that

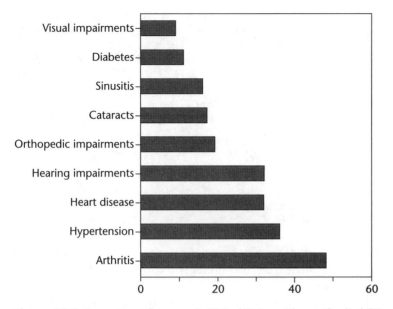

Figure 12.2 Percentage of persons in United States with specific disabilities.

(*Sources:* Centers for Disease Control. National Center for Health Statistics)

reviews and makes recommendations concerning federal laws, programs, and policies affecting individuals with disabilities.[34] The ADA was codified in Public Law 101–336. The purpose of the Act is:

1. To provide a clear and comprehensive national mandate for the elimination of discrimination against individuals with disabilities.

2. To provide a clear, strong, consistent, enforceable standard addressing discrimination against individuals with disability.

3. To ensure that the federal government plays a central role in enforcing standards.

4. To invoke the sweep of congressional authority … in order to address the major areas of discrimination faced day-to-day by people with disabilities.[35]

It is believed that there are about 43 million Americans with one or more physical or mental disabilities. In 1998, 12.4 percent of public school children had a disability. This number is increasing as the population grows older. Historically, society has tended to isolate and segregate individuals with disability, and despite some improvements, such forms of discrimination against individuals with disabilities continues to be a serious and pervasive social and community health problem.

Discrimination against individuals with disabilities persists in such critical areas as employment, housing, public accommodations, education, transportation, communications, recreation, institutionalization, health services, voting, and access to public services. Unlike individuals who have experienced discrimination on the basis of race, color, gender, national origin, religion or age,

It is hard to know if "disabled" is an appropriate term when referring to those who accomplish great feats with, and in spite of, apparent barriers.

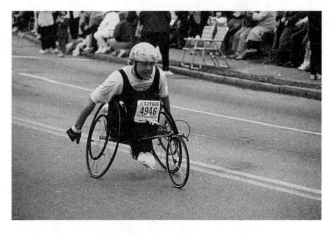

individuals who have experienced discrimination on the basis of disability, like lesbians and gay men, often have had no legal recourse to redress such discrimination and inequities.

Not only should community health educators work as advocates for the differently abled, there should be a concerted effort in public health locations to meet the physical and logistical needs of those with disabilities. Individuals with disabilities continually encounter various forms of discrimination, including intentional exclusions, the discriminatory effects of architectural, transportation and communication barriers, overprotective rules and policies, failure to make modifications to existing facilities and practices, exclusionary qualification standards and criteria, segregation and relegation to lesser services, programs, activities, benefits, jobs, and other opportunities. The CDC supports such measures through the Disabilities Prevention Program. The two main goals of the DPP are (1) to reduce the incidence and severity of primary and secondary disabilities and (2) promote the independence and productivity of people with disabilities and to further the integration of people with disabilities into the community.

The World Health Organization has developed a classification for disability that is given in Table 12.3. WHO defined impairment as any deviation from the norm in physical terms. It recommends that impairment should be used to include both abnormalities and malfunctions. Thus, an impairment is "any loss or abnormality of psychological, physiological, or anatomical structure or function." Disability occurs when an impairment results in a reduction of what would be regarded as normal activity for the affected individual. A person with a disability cannot perform as well as his or her peer group. A handicap is a disadvantage for a given individual, resulting from an impairment or a disability that limits or prevents the fulfillment of a role that is normal for that individual. The distribution of persons with special needs worldwide is shown in Figure 12.3.

Ableism

Ableism is the systematic, institutionalized, oppression of, and discrimination against people with disabilities. Ableism supports the belief that non-disabled

Table 12.3 World Health Organization disability classifications.

Impairments: anomaly, defect or loss of body part or defect in function system	Handicaps: the value attached to an individual's situation or experience when it departs from the norm
1. Intellectual	
2. Psychological	1. Orientation
3. Language	2. Physical independence
4. Aural	3. Mobility
5. Ocular	4. Occupational
6. Visceral	5. Social integration
7. Skeletal	6. Economic self-sufficiency
8. Disfiguring	
9. Generalized, sensory, other	

Disabilities: excesses or deficiencies of customarily expected activity, performance or behavior

1. Behavior
2. Communication
3. Personal care
4. Locomotor
5. Body disposition
6. Dexterity
7. Situational
8. Particular skills

(*Source:* deKleinjn-deVrankkrijken (1995). The International Classification of Impairment and Disability Handicaps. *Disability and Rehabilitation.* Vol. 17, No. 314)

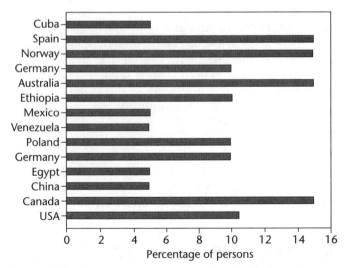

Figure 12.3 Proportion of persons worldwide with special needs.

(*Source:* MacKay, Judith. 1993. *State of Health Atlas.* Copyright Swanston Publishing Limited.
New York: London, Simon and Schuster)

people are superior to, more capable than, and have a higher quality of life than people with disabilities. Community health professionals need to make a conscious decision to interrupt these beliefs and challenge and change oppressive, ableist practices. Listed below are some helpful ways to combat ableism:

1. Have printed materials in braille, on audiotape, or in large print.

2. Do not touch a person with disability's wheelchair in an intimate fashion when you are not intending intimacy.

3. Do not use the word "blind" to connote ignorance, stupidity, or fear such as in "blind rage."

4. Do not pull a child away from a person with a visible disability or prevent the children asking the person with a disability questions.

5. Do not assume that a person with a disability needs or wants your help.

6. Do not see a person with a disability as completely nonsexual.

Summary

American society will always have to be conscious of and sensitive to the needs, talents, rights, health risks, and protection of minorities in our population. Probably the most meaningful step for lesbians and gay men will be their individual and collective effort to become visible in a society that blatantly denies them equal rights with other citizens. For example, at the 1992 Republican Presidential Convention, Patrick Buchanan was adamant in his histrionic denunciation of gays and lesbians and was outspokenly opposed to equal access under the law. Given the actual number of gay men and women in this country and on the planet, there is a need for courage to confront bigotry, by all citizens who love freedom and celebrate diversity.

No short-term panaceas exist for the problems of obtaining quality health care for lesbians and gay men. There is a wide gulf of misunderstanding, ignorance, and prejudice between health practitioners in the traditional medical establishments and those gay people who need medical services. The rights of persons who are differently abled took many years to finally find recourse through the Americas With Disabilities Act. Hopefully, gay men and lesbians will soon find similar public consciousness.

Acknowledging that the health care issues of people who are differently abled are not significantly different from able-bodied people, and pursuing a health care policy of equal access to health care for all people, will begin to address this problem. More importantly is a change in the homophobia and ableism that exists parallel with racism and sexism to an appreciation of differences among all people.

CYBERSITES RELATED TO CHAPTER 12

Gay, Lesbian, and Bisexual Resources
   www.gayhealth.com
   www.glma.org/policy/hp2010/

Americans With Disabilities Act
   www.usdoj.gov/crt/ada
   www.adata.org

QUESTIONS

1. How and why do the health care problems of the gay and lesbian community differ from the non-gay community?

2. What might be the best definition of "family" in the 1990s?

3. Why should the community health educator know the provisions of the ADA law?

EXERCISES

1. Interview a gay man about his fears, concerns, joys, life choices, and health care in the "age of AIDS." Find out about this man's childhood and adulthood. What are his life goals, his political beliefs, his hobbies, and his spiritual pursuits? Who does he call his family?

2. Teach yourself empathy by simulating a disability for a day or two. Try being visually impaired, hearing impaired, illiterate, paralyzed, disfigured, or severely arthritic. What are the community and social barriers you encounter? What would your community need to do to fully implement the ADA to meet your abilities and disabilities?

INTERNET INTERACTIVE ACTIVITY

GAY/BISEXUAL MALE YOUTH SUICIDE PROBLEMS:
THE 1999 OREGON YRBSS RESULTS

Data about gay youth and suicide are relatively new. The most extensive and comprehensive resources on gay and bisexual male suicide problems available on the web at this time may be at :

   www.virtualcity.com/youthsuicide/news/oregon-youth-suicide.htm

From this page the community health educator may link to a number of web sites that contain information about gay youth suicide.

One set of data is based on the CDC Youth Risk Behavior Surveillance Survey and reports the results of Gay Youth Risks in Oregon:

   www.virtualcity.com/youthsuicide/gbsuicide3.htm#oregon97

Exercise

1. Go to the homepage for the **Oregon Youth Risk Behavior Survey Results for Gay/Bisexual Male Suicide Problems**

   www.virtualcity.com/youthsuicide/gbsuicide3.htm#oregon97

2. Go through the results of tables provided by the state of Oregon on this web site and, based on the data available, describe the relationship between harassment based on one's sexual orientation and the risk of suicide.

3. Review the articles found at the **Youth Suicide Problems, Gay/Bisexual Male homepage**

   www.virtualcity.com/youthsuicide/

4. Go to www.virtualcity.com/youthsuicide/gbsuicide3.htm

5. Through the links on this page compare the CDC/Oregon youth suicide data with the YRBSS results from other states that addressed issues of homosexuality. Minnesota 1987; Massachusetts 1993, 1995, 1997; Vermont 1995, 1997, 1999; Washington 1995; Wisconsin 1997; Oregon, 1997, 1999; San Francisco, 1997; and Connecticut 1997.

6. Based on the data provided through these states, what are common risks and characteristics of gay male youth?

REFERENCES

1. www.glma.org/media/newsreleases/index.html. Gay Docs Outraged at Exclusion of Gay and Lesbian Health Issues in Federal Health Plan.

2. Blumenfeld, Warren J., & Raymond, D. (1988). *Looking at gay and lesbian life.* Boston: Beacon Press.

3. Ibid.

4. Ibid.

5. Ibid.

6. De Leeuw, Evelyne (1995). Marriage for all? No challenge for the 1990's. *Health Promotion International*, Vol. 10, no. 2, p. 163.

7. Blumenfeld, op. cit.

8. Dempsey, Cleta L. (1994). Health and social issues of gay, lesbian and bisexual adolescents. *Families in Society: The Journal of Contemporary Human Services.* No. 3(75), pp. 160–167.

9. Skinner, William F. (1994). The prevalence and demographic predictors of illicit and licit drug use among lesbians and gay men. *APHA Journal*, August, vol. 84. No. 8, p. 1307.

10. Stall, Ronald (1999). Cigarette smoking among gay and bisexual men. *APHA Journal*, December, Vol. 89, No. 12, p. 1875.

11. Skinner, op. cit.

12. Baker, Judith A. (1993). Is homophobia hazardous to lesbian and gay health? *American Journal of Health Promotion*, No. 4 (7), pp. 255–256.

13. Rich, Adrienne (1980). Compulsory heterosexuality and lesbian existence. *Signs 5*, No. 4, summer.

14. Adamson, David (1990). *Defending the world.* London: Tauris and Co.

15. Denenberg, Risa (1995). Report on lesbian health. *Women's Health Issues*, Vol. 5, No. 2, Summer, p. 91.

16. Smith, Mindy, & Heaton, Caryl (1990). Health concerns of lesbians. *Physician Assistant*, January, pp. 81–92.

17. Denenberg, op. cit.

18. Hidalgo, Hilda, & Peterson, Travis (1985). *Lesbian and gay issues*. Maryland: National Association of Social Workers.

19. Conway, Mollie, & Humphries, Evelyn (1994). Bernhard clinic meeting need in lesbian sexual health care. *Nursing Times*, No. 32 (90), pp. 40–41.

20. Stevens, Patricia E. (1994). Protective strategies of lesbian clients in health care environments. *Research in Nursing and Health*, No. 3(17), pp. 217–227.

21. Ibid.

22. Trippet, Susan E., & Bain, Joyce (1990). Preliminary study of lesbian health concerns. *Health Values*, No. 6(14), pp. 30–36.

23. Hidalgo, op. Cit.

24. Denenberg, op. cit.

25. Roberts, Stephanie (1998). Differences in risk factors for breast cancer: Lesbian and heterosexual women. *Journal of the Gay and Lesbian Medical Association*, Sept.

26. Cole, Rebecca, & Cooper, Sally (1991). Lesbian exclusion from HIV/AIDS education. *SIECUS Report*. Dec. 1990/Jan. 1991, p. 18.

27. Buehler, J.W. (1990). Epidemiology of reported cases of AIDS in lesbians, U.S. 1980–1989. *American Journal of Public Health*, No. 80 (11), pp. 1380–1381.

28. Ribble (1989). HIV infection in lesbians. International Conference for AIDS 1989. June 4–9. Abstract No. WAP 10.

29. Ibid.

30. www.glma.org/media/newsreleases/index.html. Gay Docs Outraged at Exclusion of Gay and Lesbian Health Issues in Federal Health Plan.

31 Anderson, Martin M., & Morris, Robert (1993). HIV and adolescents. *Pediatric Annals*, July 22(7), pp. 436–446.

32. WHO (1993). Facts about WHO.

33. Stang, Patti, & Ward, Sam (1995). Americans with disabilities. USA Snapshots. *USA Today*, August 28, p. A1.

34. Federal Register (1991). July 26, Vol. 56, No. 44.

35. Perritt, Henry (1993). *Americans with Disabilities Act handbook*. Vol. 2. New York: Wiley Law Publications.

CHAPTER 13

Issues in Women's Health

Community Health in the 21st Century
"Everytime we take a few steps forward in terms of women's reproductive rights, people in positions of power manage to push us back a few more steps. The primary issue for women today and in the future will be the control of their own bodies and their own decision making. Once women control their own bodies, they can begin to have control over their economic, political, and social life."

—Laurel Ingham, BS., Health Education,
Health Educator, Women for Choice

Chapter Objectives

The student will:

1. state the purpose of the Women's Health Equity Act.

2. explain why it has been difficult to get women's health issues on the political agenda.

3. list five health concerns specific to women.

4. contrast the issues of women in developing countries with those in developed countries.

Health Concerns of Women

It is time to put women's health needs on the public health agenda, not in the narrow context of maternal and child health, nor in the restrictive sense of reproductive health, but in the broad context of what is commonly called women's status and empowerment.[1] In the area of research, women have long been excluded in clinical study populations. In a long-term study of coronary heart disease risk factors, the multiple risk factor intervention trials included 15,000 men and no women. The Physician's Health Study demonstrated the value of aspirin as a preventive therapy for coronary disease in a study of 22,071 men and no women. A 1990 study of the correlation between coffee-drinking and heart disease included no women in its study population of 45,589. The extrapolation from data of this type has long been questioned but the practice of excluding women continues.[2] Community health can redress such omissions by looking at women as a specific at-risk population, and thus prepare prevention programs with the variety of women's races, cultures, ages, and life experiences in mind.

Today, women's health research must include such diverse areas as cardiovascular and cerebrovascular diseases, hormone therapy, osteoporosis, mental health, substance abuse, obesity, diabetes, AIDS, and the role of women in clinical trials and health education research. In 1990, Representatives Olympia Snowe and Pat Schroeder introduced the Women's Health Equity Act (WHI). It contained twenty separate provisions dealing with women's health, most of which had been neglected or underrepresented in previous research. This bill was defeated in 1990 and 1991. It was not until 1993 that the bill was finally passed into law as part of the National Institutes of Health (NIH) Revitalization Amendments. The WHI is a fourteen-year, $625 million program that supports biomedical research with the goal of preventing heart disease, cancer, and osteoporosis among women.[3] In addition to a substantial list of activities, this legislation requires the inclusion of women and minorities as research subjects unless inappropriate.[4]

Former President Bush vetoed the NIH Reauthorization Act in the spring of 1992 which would have increased funding for the 22-bill Women's Equity Act. He vetoed the package for women because he opposed an aspect of the act that would lift an administration ban on the use of fetal tissue in medical research. The Clinton administration signed the NIH Act into law in June 1993.

This legislation, and pressure from many consumer groups, particularly women with breast cancer, and the National Women's Health Network, have prompted the NIH to make a commitment to include women in clinical trials. The NIH established an Office of Research on Women's Health whose underlying job is to address past neglect to women's health issues. Since about 1990, information has come forward from a General Accounting Office study showing that women have been excluded from medical research trials and that women's diseases have been given a low priority in research funding. Encouraging is the news that more women are entering the medical profession and many are involved in public health. In 1992, both the Surgeon General of the United States, Dr. Antonia C. Novello, and the director of the NIH, Dr. Bernadine Healy, were women. President Clinton nominated an African American woman, Joycelyn Elders as Surgeon General, and appointed the first woman to serve as Secretary of the Department of Health and Human Services, Donna Shalala.

Overall, women report a greater incidence than men of chronic conditions that may not be life-threatening, but certainly affect day-to-day quality of life. Chronic conditions were greater for women in all categories but visual and hearing impairments, hernias, and paralysis. Except for injuries in the under age forty-five category, women's complaints of acute conditions are 20 percent to 30 percent more than men's in all categories (see Table 12.2). Despite this greater morbidity, men's mortality rates are higher for all leading causes of death except diabetes.[5] National research initiatives have yet to look at these gender discrepancies in such a way that women become a focal point for the

---

BOX 13.1 Milestones for the Inclusion of Women in Clinical Trials

- **1985**—The Public Health Service Task Force on Women''s Health Issues stated that the lack of research on women's health had compromised quality of information and care for women.
- **1986**—The National Institutes of Health adopted a policy requiring the inclusion of women in clinical trials.
- **1990**—The Society for the Advancement of Women's Health Research was founded to bring national attention to the problem of the exclusion of women from clinical trials and the need for greater federal funding for diseases and conditions prevalent in, and unique to, women.
- **1990**—A General Accounting Office report revealed that women were still being excluded. The Physician's Health or "Aspirin" Study, designed to examine the impact of taking aspirin on cardiovascular disease, was one of many large studies revealed to be excluding women.
- **1990**—The NIH Reauthorization Act of 1990, with input from the Society, cre-

ated the Office of Research on Women's Health, to direct an NIH focus to women's health issues.
- **1990**—The Congressional Caucus for Women's Issues introduced the Women's Health Equity Act which called for (among other things) inclusion of women and minorities in clinical trials; establishment of research centers on osteoporosis, contraception, and infertility; and expansion of existing studies to examine how less typically "female" conditions such as AIDS, lung cancer, and cardiovascular disease impact women differently from men.
- **1993**—The NIH Revitalization Act of 1993 mandates development of guidelines on the inclusion of women and minorities in clinical trials.
- **1993**—The FDA rescinded earlier guidelines recommending restrictions on the participation of women with child-bearing potential and left the determination of risks and benefits of their inclusion to patients, investigation sponsors, and institutional review boards.

(*Source:* Society for Women's Health Research)

---

research in terms of biology, psychological variables, behavior, use of the health care system, or the combined effects of factors.

In 1991 a major study showed that doctors were treating women with heart disease, kidney disease, and lung cancer less aggressively than men with the same illnesses.[6] Further, since women had not been part of the research on cause or treatment of these and other diseases, treatment designed for men's physiology, weight, metabolism, and endocrine systems was being used without thought about the implications to women.

The report published by the Council on Ethical and Judicial Affairs of the AMA (American Medical Association) revealed that women were far less likely than men to receive kidney transplants or a diagnostic test for lung cancer. The Council cited evidence suggesting that "physicians are more likely to attribute women's health complaints to emotional rather than physical causes," and that additionally, doctors might consider men's role in society "greater than women's."[7] Mortality rates for the leading causes of death among women in the United States in 1999 are given in Table 13.1.

Table 13.1 Leading causes of death for women by race (1999).

Cause of Death	White Rate	Black Rate	Hispanic Rate
All causes	897.8	742.8	288.0
Diseases of the heart	289.8	224.2	78.3
Malignant neoplasm	220.4	160.5	61.4
Cerebrovascular disease	75.7	58.0	19.6
COPD	44.1	16.5	7.8
Pneumonia/Influenza	37.8	22.1	10.6
Accidents	25.4	22.9	8.3
Diabetes	14.5	37.5	17.2
Alzheimer's disease		23.9	
Nephritis	9.5	12.9	5.5
Septicemia	9.1	13.3	
HIV		13.7	

(*Sources:* Centers for Disease Control. National Center for Health Statistics)

Primary morbidity and mortality rates for illnesses and conditions such as breast cancer, osteoporosis, infertility, silicone breast implants, STDs, and birth control have long been ignored by a health care system that has been controlled by men. Research in AIDS has not included women in the drug trials, and lesbians as a group have not been studied as a possible at-risk group.

Feminist analysis sees women's health risks as a reflection of men's relative dominance of women, the change in economic dynamics for some women in labor and production, and the changing conditions of reproduction. Economic disparity between men and women is probably the most important contributing factor to the difference in health status for all people. In 1998 the median income for women was $24,393 and $39,414 for men.[8] Black and Hispanic women made considerably less. In 2000 women still made only 75 cents for every dollar made by men.

Women's health activists are now holding the medical and political communities accountable and making equality in health research and care the women's rights cause of the next decade. Wendy Wasserman, legislative aide for U.S. Representative Patricia Schroeder of Colorado said, "The same women who fought for abortion rights are now fighting for money for breast cancer research and menopause research."

The World Looks at Women's Health

In September 1994, 180 nations met at the Cairo Conference on World Population and Development. Although this was a controversial conference since it addressed issues such as abortion, contraception, and condom use, ultimately a plan was written upon which participants could agree. The plan addressed the primary source of, and the victims of poor worldwide family planning, the social/political/economic status of women. The plan:

- Calls on countries to meet the needs of about 120 million women who want to use birth control but do not have access to it. It calls for comprehensive health care for women and says there should be freedom of choice in matters of birth control, health care services, and decisions about family planning.

- Promotes sex equality and calls for global primary school education by 2015. (Two-thirds of the world's 960 million illiterate people are female.)
- Urges countries to eliminate violence against women, prohibit female genital mutilation, infanticide, and prenatal sex selection.
- Recognizes unsafe abortion as a worldwide problem that should be addressed.
- Makes the plan's provisions subject to national sovereignty, local custom, and cultural religious beliefs.[9]

The Primary Health Issues of Women Worldwide

Breast Cancer

Despite many political and economic differences among women of the world, women's anatomy creates a sisterhood around a number of universal women's health concern. Certainly, breast cancer is a fear for most women, especially as economic development increases, communicable diseases are controlled, and nutrition improves. Demographic variables related to risk are given in Table 13.2.

The incidence rate and death rate of breast cancer are increasing in the United States. Breast cancer fatality rates for women are given in Figure 13.1. Thanks to consumer pressure and the visibility of women in positions of responsibility in Washington, DC, breast cancer received $135 million in research funding for the 1998–1999 fiscal year. An additional $1.8 million was allocated to the Stamp Out Breast Cancer Act of 1999. The past two decades have seen unprecedented advances in understanding of what makes breast cancer grow; in particular, the central roles of hormones such as estrogen and progesterone, and their signaling pathways; and of important genes involved in the genesis and progression of breast cancers such as HER-2/neu, p53, PTEN, BRCA-1, and BRCA-2. Research during this period has been focused on in-depth analysis of these known modulators of breast cancer biology, which has led to important tools for clinical care.

In addition to increased funding, a seventeen-state study released in 1992 by the CDC showed that more women are having mammograms, the x-ray detection procedure thought to reduce the risk of dying from breast cancer by 20 to 30 percent. Despite this important preventive test, many insurance companies in the United States refuse to cover routine mammograms as part of their policies, preventing particularly low-income women from benefitting from this procedure. Disparity among women of color, poor women, and white middle class women for routine mammograms screening is indicated in Table 13.3.

Discussion: Why is mammography not economically feasible for so many women?

Table 13.2 Major factors affecting breast cancer risk.

Variable	Risk
Demographic	
age	Over age 40
race	Decreased in Asian Women
social status	Increased with high SES
Genetic	
positive family history	Increased if first degree
Reproductive	
early menarche	Increased
single	Increased after age 50
first pregnancy	Increased over age 30
oophorectomy	Decreased if before age 40
Pre-existing	
Breast cancer	Increased if proliferative
X-irradiation	Increased if excess exposure in adolescence
Nutrition	
high fat, protein	Increased
low selenium	Increased

(*Source:* American Cancer Association)

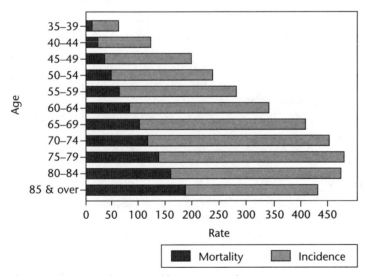

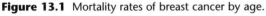

Figure 13.1 Mortality rates of breast cancer by age.

(*Source:* National Cancer Institute)

In 1993, the *American Journal of Public Health* identified several occupational groups as being at increased risk of dying from breast cancer. Those at greatest risk were white and black women executives, including administrators and managers, professionals, and administrative support workers including clerical workers (Table 13.4).

Table 13.3 Percent of women who have had clinical breast exams and Year 2000 target.

Clinical Breast Exam & Mammogram:	1987 Baseline	2000 Target	Percent Increase
Ever Received—			
Hispanic women aged 40 and older	20%	80%	All
Low-income women aged 40 and older			a
(annual family income <$10,000)	22%	80%	b
Women aged 40 and older with less			c
than high school education	23%	80%	d
Women aged 70 and older	25%	80%	e
Black women aged 40 and older	28%	80%	0 100 200 300
Received Within Preceding 2 Years—			
Hispanic women aged 50 and older	18%	60%	All
Low-income women aged 50 and older			a
(annual family income <$10,000)	15%	60%	b
Women aged 50 and older with less			c
than high school education	16%	60%	d
Women aged 70 and older	18%	60%	e
Black women aged 50 and older	19%	60%	0 100 200 300

Baseline data source: National Health Interview Survey, CDC.

(*Source:* U.S. Dept. of HHS. PHS, *Healthy People, 2000: National Health Promotion and Disease Prevention Objectives, Full Report.* DHHS Pub. No. 91-5212 (Washington, DC. USGPO, 1991))

Table 13.4 Breast cancer in white and black women by occupation.
(PMR = proportionate mortality ratio)

Occupational Group	Number of Breast Cancer Deaths		PMR	
	White	Black	White	Black
Executive/administration	2,816	143	109	139
Professional	6,001	560	129	150
Technicians and support	753	106	84	107
Sales	3,231	135	99	134
Clerical	8,502	424	113	133
Service	3,960	1,517	74	83
Housewives	26,690	1,852	91	85

(*Source:* From the *American Journal of Public Health.* Copyright © 1993 by the American Public Health Association. Reprinted with permission)

Black women are more likely to die of breast (31.4 per 100,000) and colon and rectum cancer (20.0 per 100,000) than are women of any other racial and ethnic group. White and black women have the highest mortality rates of lung

BOX 13.2 New Cancers in Women in 2000 and Five-Year Survival Rates

Type	Number	Survival Rate (%)
Breast	178,700	85
Lung	80,100	14
Colon/Rectal	67,000	60
Uterus	36,100	69
Ovary	25,400	46
Non-Hodgkin's	24,300	51
Melanoma	17,300	88
Bladder	14,900	81
Pancreas	14,900	4
Cervix	13,700	69

(*Source:* American Cancer Society)

and bronchus cancer followed by Native American, Asian/Pacific Islander, and Hispanic women.[10]

Black women also had increased risk if they worked in sales and precision production occupations. Occupations with the lowest proportionate mortality ratios for both black and white women included service, farming, transportation, and labor. This study found that no established predisposing workplace exposure explained these increases; however, the delay in childbearing among professional, working women may be a factor that will need to be assessed further.[11]

The best prevention for breast cancer appears to be regular breast self-examination and clinical exams, reduction of fat intake, and awareness of hereditary and workplace risk. Mammographies after age forty are recommended for low-risk women and an earlier baseline mammography is recommended for high-risk women. Research is needed to determine if there are other factors that put women at risk for breast cancer.

Healthy People 2010 Objective: Increase the Proportion of Women Aged Forty Years and Older Who Have Received a Mammogram Within the Preceding Two Years.

Target: 70 percent.

Baseline: 68 percent of women aged 40 years and older received a mammogram within the preceding 2 years in 1998 (preliminary data, age adjusted to the year 2000 standard population).

Osteoporosis

Bone integrity is maintained by a balance between bone formation and bone resorption. This process is at its height during the early years of life, peaks at age thirty to thirty-five, and from then on bone loss exceeds bone gain. The ultimate

Table 13.5 Risk factors for osteoporosis.

Constitutional	Nutritional
Ethnic (white or Asian)	Low calcium intake
Small boned	Gastric or bowel resection
Lean	Malabsorption
Inactive	Anorexia nervosa
Positive family history	Alcohol abuse
Endocrine	Other factors
Hypogonadism	Nulliparity
Hyperthyroidism	Long-term anticonvulsants
Hyperparathyroidism	Smoking
Hypercotisolaemia	
Hypopituitarism	

development of osteoporosis is determined both by peak bone mass achieved at the end of the accretion phase and by the rate of net bone loss. The risk factors for osteoporosis are given in Table 13.5. There is some evidence that calcium loss can be aggravated by several alcoholic drinks a day, smoking, eating too much protein, and consuming too much phosphorus.

Half of all women over the age of forty-five and 90 percent of all women over the age of seventy-five suffer from osteoporosis, a post-menopausal disorder in which bones become increasingly brittle resulting in falls and serious, life-threatening breaks. Each year 260,000 women suffer hip fractures as a result of osteoporosis. Hormone replacement therapy (HRT) has been the medical practitioner's therapy of choice and is commonly prescribed without even a word of caution. HRT is prescribed although its long-term effects are still unknown and the risk of breast and endometrial cancer increases with estrogen use. The NIH is launching a fourteen-year, large-scale, federal study, The Women's Health Initiative, which will study how factors such as nutrition and hormone therapy affect women over fifty.

In 1995, a study comparing 40,000 postmenopausal women followed for six years compared women who had used hormonal replacement (HRT) with those who had never used hormone replacement. Results showed that fracture incidence was substantially reduced with hormone replacement therapy, as has been thought. Other results showed increased incidence of endometrial cancer, breast cancer (though not statistically significant), lower incidence of colon cancer, and substantial reduction of cardiovascular deaths with HRT.[12]

Reproductive Cancer

There were an estimated 12,800 cases of invasive cervical cancer, with an estimated 4,600 cervical cancer deaths in 2000. Mortality rates have also declined sharply over the past several decades. Incidence rates have decreased steadily over the past several decades. From 1992 to1996, the incidence rate in black women (11.2 per 100,000) was higher than the rate in white women (7.3 per

Table 13.6 Percent of women who have had a Pap test and Year 2000 target.

Pap Test:	Special Population Targets		
	1987 Baseline	2000 Target	Percent Increase
Ever Received—			
Hispanic women aged 18 and older	75%	95%	All
Women aged 70 and older	76%	95%	a
Women aged 18 and older with less than high school education	79%	95%	b, c
Low income women aged 18 and older (annual family income <$10,000)	80%	95%	d

Received Within Preceding 3 Years—			
Hispanic women aged 18 and older	66%	80%	All
Women aged 70 and older	44%	70%	a
Women aged 18 and older with less than high school education	58%	75%	b, c
Low income women aged 18 and older (annual family income <$10,000)	64%	80%	d

Baseline data source: National Health Interview Survey, CDC.

(*Source:* U.S. Dept. of HHS. PHS, *Healthy People, 2000: National Health Promotion and Disease Prevention Objectives,* Full Report. DHHS Pub. No. 91-5212. Washington, DC: USGPO, 1991)

100,000). As Pap screening has become more prevalent, carcinoma in situ of the cervix occurs more frequently than invasive cancer.[13]

Healthy People 2010 Objective: Increase the Proportion of Women Who Receive a Pap Test.

	1998 Baseline (%)	2010 Target (%)
Women aged 18 years and older who have ever received a Pap test	92	97
Women aged 18 years and older who received a Pap test within the preceding 3 years.	79	90

It is well known that the Pap test is the most important diagnostic tool for early treatment of cervical cancer. Yet, only 75 percent of women get a Pap test (Table 13.6).

Ovarian cancer, one of the most deadly forms of malignancy and one about which little is known, is finally beginning to get the proper research funding it deserves. There were an estimated 23,100 new cases of ovarian cancer and

14,000 deaths in the United States in 2000. It accounts for 4 percent of all cancers among women and ranks second among gynecologic cancers. Ovarian cancer causes more deaths than any other cancer of the female reproductive system. During 1992 to 2000, ovarian cancer incidence rates were significantly declining, probably due to more community health attention to early detection and more frequent visits to clinicians by older women.

Fertility and Birth Control

The World Health Organization reported in 1992 in "Reproductive Health, a Key to a Brighter Future" that without fertility regulation, women's rights are mere words. A woman who has no control over her fertility cannot complete her education, cannot maintain gainful employment ... and has very few real choices open to her." (Figure 13.2 shows the relationship between education and childhood mortality in developing countries.) The report said that 381 million people used contraception in developing countries between 1985 and 1990 with the greatest increase in east Asia. In 1992, between 6.5 million to 10 million Chinese women were sterilized by the governments one-child family planning policy.[14] However, despite some increase in contraception use, International Planned Parenthood reports that more than 500 million women worldwide lack access to reliable contraception. In the United States there are more than 600,000 unintended pregnancies each year among fifteen- to nine-

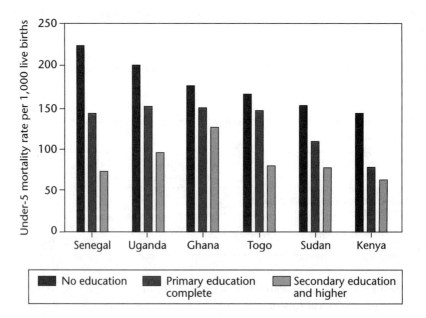

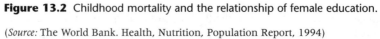

Figure 13.2 Childhood mortality and the relationship of female education.

(*Source:* The World Bank. Health, Nutrition, Population Report, 1994)

Table 13.7 Contraceptive use by women 15–44 years.

		Age		
Contraceptive Status and Method	**All Women**	**15–24 Years**	**25–34 Years**	**35–44 Years**
All women (1,000)	60,201	18,002	20,758	21,440
Sterile	29.7	2.6	25.0	57.0
Surgically sterile	27.9	1.8	23.6	54.0
Noncontraceptively sterile	3.1	0.1	1.2	7.4
Contraceptively sterile	24.8	1.7	22.4	46.6
Nonsurgically sterile	1.7	0.7	1.3	2.8
Pregnant, postpartum	4.6	5.9	6.9	1.3
Seeking pregnancy	4.0	2.1	6.2	3.5
Other nonusers	22.3	44.4	13.3	12.6
Never had intercourse	10.9	30.8	3.4	1.4
No intercourse in last month	6.2	7.0	5.3	6.5
Had intercourse in last month	5.2	6.6	4.6	4.7
Nonsurgical contraceptors	39.7	45.0	49.1	26.1
Pill	17.3	23.1	23.7	6.3
IUD	0.5	0.1	0.6	0.8
Diaphragm	1.2	0.2	1.2	2.0
Condom	13.1	13.9	15.0	10.7
Periodic abstinence	1.5	0.5	1.8	2.0
Natural family planning	0.2	—	0.3	0.3
Withdrawl	2.0	1.6	2.3	1.9
Other methods	3.9	5.6	4.2	2.1

(*Source:* U.S. National Center for Health Statistics, *Advance Data from Vital and Health Statistics,* No. 182)

teen-year-olds. More than half end in abortion. Worldwide, about 150,000 unwanted pregnancies end every day in abortion. Contraception use in the United States is described in Table 13.7.

Substance Use and Fertility

Fertility is affected by a mother's use of illegal and legal drugs during pregnancy. It is suggested that 1 million of the 4 million babies born each year in the United States may be exposed to some legal or illegal drug. A study conducted by the National Institute on Drug Abuse of 2,613 women who gave birth in 1992 found that:

- 5.5 percent used an illegal drug, mostly marijuana or cocaine
- 18.8 percent used alcohol
- 20.4 percent smoked cigarettes
- Illegal drug use was most common in blacks—11.3 percent reported it as did 4.4 percent of whites and 4.5 percent of Hispanic mothers

- Alcohol use was most common among whites—22.7 percent reported it as did 15.8 percent of blacks and 8.7 percent of Hispanic mothers

- Among women who both smoked and drank, 20 percent also used marijuana and 9.5 percent used cocaine[15]

Substance abuse during pregnancy affects a fetus in different ways. Heavy alcohol exposure can lead to mental retardation and abnormal physical development.[16] Smokers have more miscarriages and stillbirths. Their babies are lighter, shorter, and have a higher risk of SIDS. Cocaine is linked with lower birth weight, smaller head size, and developmental delays. Marijuana may be linked with lower birth weight.[17]

Family Planning

Funding for family planning programs dropped significantly throughout the 1980s, due in part to the strong lobby of conservative, anti-abortion groups. Birth control options have remained generally unchanged since the 1960s, when oral contraception came on the market. Norplant, implanted progesterone capsules, and injected Depo Provera are the only significant new choices in the last three decades.

WHO suggests that access to contraception is a major necessity for women's health in the world today. Increased contraception has helped women in developing countries reduce the fertility rate from 6.1 per 1,000 in 1965–1970 to 3.9 per 1,000 from 1985–1990.

The United States government provided $425 million for international family planning programs in 2001. Both Bush administrations, however, gave no money to two family planning programs—International Planned Parenthood Federation and the United Nations Populations Fund—because these organizations provide information on abortion. Abortion services became a defining criterion for international aid during both Bush administrations. The World Health Organization reported that 381 million people used contraception in developing

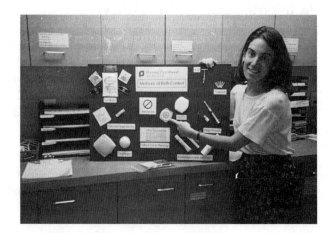

Community health educators take an active role in providing family planning information at the nation's Planned Parenthoods.

BOX 13.3 *Worldwide Contraception Rates*

Female sterilization	26%
Vasectomy	19%
Oral contraception	15%

(*Source:* Alan Guttmacher Institute, 2000)

---

countries in 1985–1990, up from only 31 million in 1960–1985. Female sterilization is still the most widespread form of contraception, accounting for 21 percent of all methods used, followed by male sterilization with 19 percent.

Breast Implants

Over 150,000 women a year receive silicone breast implants and 80 percent are for cosmetic reasons. In 1991, the safety of silicone-gel breast implants was questioned as many women developed immune disorders, severe neurological impairment, and acute pain, perhaps associated with silicone leakage. Consumer outrage led to the discovery that the Dow Chemical Company, the primary maker of silicone implants, may have kept negative safety research from the FDA and thus from women. In 1992, the FDA ruled that more testing was required and put a moratorium on cosmetic silicone implants. Results of further research, reported in 1999, have not substantiated the claims that silicone implants impair women's immune system.

Sexually Transmitted Diseases

Worldwide, an estimated 333 million curable STDs occur annually. Each year an estimated 15 million new STD infections occur in the United States, and nearly 4 million teenagers and college-age students are infected with an STD. Infected persons should, but often do not, seek medical care because as many as 85 percent of women and up to 50 percent of men with chlamydia have no symptoms. Women are at higher risk than men for most STDs, and young women are more susceptible to certain STDs than are older women. The higher risk is partly because the cervix of adolescent females is covered with cells that are especially susceptible to STDs, such as chlamydia.

Women suffer more frequent and more serious STD complications than men. Among the most serious STD complications are pelvic inflammatory disease, ectopic pregnancy, infertility, and chronic pelvic pain. Women are biologically more susceptible to infection when exposed to a sexually transmitted agent. Often, STDs are transmitted more easily from a man to a woman. Acute STDs (and even some complications) often are very mild or are completely asymptomatic in women. STDs are more difficult to diagnose in women due to the physiology and anatomy of the female reproductive tract. This combination of increased susceptibility and "silent" infection frequently can result in women being unaware of an STD, which results in delayed diagnosis and treatment.[18]

STDs in pregnant women can cause serious health problems or death to the fetus or newborn. Sexually transmitted organisms in the mother can cross the placenta to the fetus or newborn, resulting in congenital infection, or these organisms can reach the newborn during delivery, resulting in perinatal infections. Regardless of the route of infection, these organisms can permanently damage the brain, spinal cord, eyes, auditory nerves, or immune system. Even when the organisms do not reach the fetus or newborn directly, they can significantly complicate the pregnancy by causing spontaneous abortion, stillbirth, premature rupture of the membranes, or preterm delivery. For example, women with bacterial vaginosis are 40 percent more likely to deliver a preterm, low birth weight infant than are mothers without this condition.[19]

Chlamydia   *Chlamydia trachomatis* has the properties of both a bacterium and a virus. It affects the urinary tract and reproductive organs of both women and men. Chlamydia is responsible for hundreds of thousands of cases of pelvic inflammatory disease (PID), a leading cause of infertility and ectopic pregnancy. The infertility rate of women ages twenty to twenty-nine tripled between 1975 and 1992. Chlamydia testing is still not routinely done during gynecological examinations of sexually active women by private physicians outside of community-based clinics like Planned Parenthood.

Healthy People 2010 Objective: Reduce the Proportion of Adolescents and Young Adults with *Chlamydia trachomatis* Infections

Reduction in *Chlamydia trachomatis* infections	1997 Baseline (%)	2010 Target (%)
Females aged 15 to 24 years attending family planning clinics	5.0	3.0
Females aged 15 to 24 years attending STD clinics	12.2	3.0

Chancroid   Chancroid is a painful ulceration of the genital area caused by *Hemophilus ducreyi*. In developing countries very little demographic information is available about sexually transmitted diseases, although tropical infections, particularly chancroid, are among the most common of genital ulcerations. Women may carry the bacteria but are generally asymptomatic for chancroid.

Gonorrhea   Although the rates vary among countries, the trend over the last thirty years has been an increase in gonorrhea with a recent stabilization of the rate. In developed countries the figures tend to be more complete although many patients are treated by private physicians who do not report cases to public officials. In the United States the highest rate in females is found among those fifteen to nineteen years at 1451 per 100,000 in 1999. Figure 13.3 shows the rates of gonorrhea according to race and ethnicity.

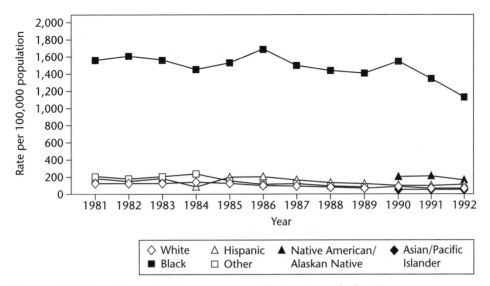

Figure 13.3 Rates of gonorrhea in women according to race and ethnicity.

(*Source:* CDC, Sexually transmitted disease surveillance, 1992. Atlanta. In The women's health data book, p. 38)

Healthy People 2010 Objective: Reduce Gonorrhea

Target: 19 new cases per 100,000 population.

Baseline: 123 new cases of gonorrhea per 100,000 population in 1997.

Gonorrhea is a primary cause of pelvic inflammatory disease (PID) in women and urethritis among men. Of 850,000 reported PID cases, 20–80 percent can be attributed to gonorrhea. PID is a growing concern to women because of its potential to cause infertility. Diagnosis of PID is often delayed because signs and symptoms resemble common menstrual discomfort that is often misdiagnosed until the pain is severe enough to warrant invasive diagnosis. By this time, infertility has often occurred.

Herpes Simplex (Genital Herpes) Genital herpes is a viral disease that tends to recur periodically and for which there is no cure. Herpes virus is transmitted by intimate contact between mucous membrane surfaces. There are two types of herpes simplex virus, type I (fever blisters or cold sores) and type 2 (genital herpes).[20] In the United States genital herpes is not a reportable disease, so no uniform or universal data are collected. It has been estimated that the prevalence of genital herpes is approximately 45 million cases in the United States and the CDC estimates there are between 200,000 and 500,000 new cases each year in the United States.

Industrialized countries such as Scandinavia report similar incidence. A survey in Sweden found that herpes could be isolated from 8.4 percent of the cervices of all females attending studied STD clinics. Genital herpes (simplex II) is thought to be associated about 10 percent of the time with cervical cancer.[21]

Neonatally transmitted herpes simplex is reported in about 5 per 10,000 births. Seventy percent of babies born with herpes-related central nervous system damage will die and 60 percent of those babies who survive will be neurologically impaired.

Randomized trials show that systemic acyclovir provides partial control of the symptoms and signs of herpes episodes when used to treat first clinical episodes. However, acyclovir neither eradicates latent virus nor affects subsequent risk, frequency, or severity of recurrences after the drug is discontinued.[22]

Human Papillomavirus (HPV)   HPV until recently was known as genital warts. It is estimated there are nearly one million consultations a year in the United States for HPV infection. HPV is usually asymptomatic; however, secondary infection and ulceration can occur with abrasion. It is implicated in about 70 percent of cervical cancer cases.

A 1992 *JAMA* article reported that of sexually active women, 30 percent were infected with HPV. It appears that HPV infection in combination with a low folic acid (B vitamin) level increases a woman's risk for cervical cancer. There are 13,000 new cervical cancer cases each year in America, with 5,000 related deaths. HPV is probably the greatest risk factor for cervical cancer and mortality.

The treatment, locally applied podophyllum resin is only about 60 percent effective while cryotherapy or electrocautery therapy are somewhat effective in eliminating symptoms.[23]

Syphilis   In the United States there has been a disturbing increase in the number of cases of infectious syphilis. Syphilis is a highly contagious disease caused by the Treponema pallidum, a delicate organism that is microscopic and resembles a corkscrew in shape. The disease may be acquired or congenital. The spirochete enters the body through the skin or mucous membrane during sexual or close body contact. Congenital syphilis is transmitted to the fetus in the infected mother through the placental barrier. In 1992 there were 120,000 cases in the United States. Part of the increase is considered to be the reallocation of resources away from traditional STD programs to AIDS. The lesson from this, and one equally applied in developing countries, is that the control of HIV and AIDS will only come through good STD programs and revitalized global leadership.

Encouraging is the decline in rates of congenital syphilis in developed countries due to early diagnosis and control of syphilis in pregnant women. Infant mortality due to congenital syphilis is negligible in the United States, which meets the 1990 national objective of 1.5 cases per 100,000 children under one year. Unfortunately, congenital syphilis still represents a major health problem in many developing countries.

Table 13.8 Women and AIDS internationally (1997).

Region	Number of Women Infected with HIV (in 1,000s)	Percent of HIV-Infected Adults Who Are Women
Sub-Saharan Africa	9,915	50
Caribbean	99	33
South and Southeast Asia	1,478	25
Eastern Europe and Central Asia	36	25
North Africa and Middle East	41	20
Western Europe	105	20
North America	170	20
South and Central America	244	19
East Asia and Pacific	48	11
Australia and New Zealand	0.0	5
TOTAL	**12,137**	**41**

(*Source:* AIDS Epidemic Update. UNAIDS, Dec. 2000)

> *Healthy People 2010 Objective:* Eliminate Sustained Domestic Transmission of Primary and Secondary Syphilis
>
> *Target:* 0.2 case per 100,000 population.
>
> *Baseline:* 3.2 cases per 100,000 population in 1997.

HIV Women are the fastest growing group of those infected with HIV (14 percent of all reported cases), the virus that causes AIDS, yet almost no research has been done on women and AIDS. Young heterosexual women, especially minority women, are increasingly acquiring HIV infection and developing AIDS. In 1998, 41 percent of reported AIDS cases in persons aged thirteen to twenty-four years occurred in young women, and more than four of every five AIDS cases reported in women occurred in minority women (mostly African American or Hispanic). The U.S. spread of HIV infection through heterosexual transmission closely parallels other STD epidemics.[24]

Compelling worldwide evidence indicates that the presence of other STDs increases the likelihood of both transmitting and acquiring HIV infection. Prospective epidemiological studies from four continents, including North America, have repeatedly demonstrated that when other STDs are present, HIV transmission is at least two to five times higher than when other STDs are not present. Biological studies demonstrate that when other STDs are present, an individual's susceptibility to HIV infection is increased, and the likelihood of a dually infected person (having HIV infection and another STD) infecting other people with HIV is increased. Conversely, effective STD treatment can slow the spread of HIV at the individual and community levels. Worldwide AIDS cases for 1997 are given in Table 13.8. Worldwide, 3,000 women are infected daily with HIV, primarily through heterosexual transmission.

The Centers for Disease Control and Prevention 1992 list of what opportunistic infections may indicate HIV infection excluded women's experience.

Chronic vaginal yeast infections, genital warts (HPV), and chronic pelvic inflammatory disease are beginning to become more commonly recognized as presenting signs of HIV infection, but clinicians did not universally have this information from the CDC. With the change in the AIDS definition in 1993, chronic vaginal yeast infections were added as an opportunistic infection.

The Menstrual Cycle

Virtually no research has been conducted at the federal level on the menstrual cycle. In 1992 the Office of Technology Assessment published a study that outlined the need for more research on menopause and hormone therapy. A longitudinal study of fifty years' worth of menstrual histories (The Tremin Trust), located at the University of Utah School of Nursing, has been plagued by funding problems since no agency thinks this extraordinary data bank is worth studying.

Abortion

To many women, safe and legal abortion is the fundamental issue of their health care. Of the 50 million induced abortions worldwide, it is estimated that approximately 200,000 women die annually, mostly in developing countries, from unsafe, illegal abortions. Many others are permanently injured and mortally wounded. The need and demand has always outweighed the restrictions and difficulty in obtaining safe, legal, medical abortions, and the result is often death. Estimated abortion rates per 100,000 women in countries where abortion is legal and illegal are reported in Table 13.9. Worldwide rates are shown in Figure 13.4.

Discussion: Using only health factors as criteria, what are the pros and cons of legal abortion in developed versus developing countries?

BOX 13.4 Global Estimated Risk of Death from Unsafe Abortion (WHO)

	Unsafe Abortions	Number of Deaths	Risk
World Total	30 million	70,000	1 in 300
MDC	2.5 million	600	1 in 3,700
LDC	20 million	69,000	1 in 250
Africa	3.5 million	23,000	1 in 150
Asia	9.2 million	40,000	1 in 250
Europe	260,000	100	1 in 2,600
Latin America	4.2 million	6,000	1 in 800
Oceania	2600	<100	1 in 400
USSR (former)	2.1 million	500	1 in 3,900

Table 13.9 International abortion frequencies and rates.

Country (Year)	Abortions	Rate per 1,000
Australia (1988)	63,000	16.2
Bulgaria (1987)	119,900	64.7
Canada (1987)	63,600	10.2
China (1987)	10,349,500	31.4
Cuba (1988)	155,300	58.0
England (1987)	156,200	14.2
Netherlands (1986)	18,300	5.3
United States	1,588,600	28.0
* France (1987)	161,000	13.3
* German Fed. Rep (1986)	92,200	7.0
* India (1987)	588,400	3.0
* Israel (1987)	15,500	16.2
* Romania (1983)	421,400	90.9
* Soviet Union (1987)	6,818,000	54.9
** Brazil (1980)		150
** Mexico (1980)		113
** Peru (1980)		33

*Incomplete statistics

**Estimated illegal abortions

(*Source:* Henshaw, Stanley K. (1990). Induced abortion: A world review, 1990. *Family Planning Perspectives, 22*[2], March/April)

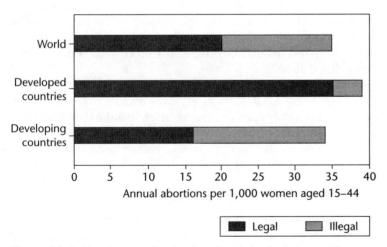

Figure 13.4 Abortion rates by developed and developing countries.

(*Source:* Alan Guttmacher Institute, 2000)

The CDC began abortion surveillance in 1969. In the United States, abortion rates remain fairly stable (about 1.3 million a year throughout the 1990s), although access has diminished because of restrictions by the previous presidential administrations on public funding, abortion counseling (the gag rule), and parental notification. Although the majority of surveyed voters appear to want legal abortion, many favor access limitation. On July 1, 1992 the Supreme Court upheld *Roe* v. *Wade,* allowing for safe legal abortions in the first trimester, but also upheld Pennsylvania's right to restrict abortions as long as restrictions pose "no undue hardship" on women seeking legal abortions. Despite rulings by the Supreme Court in 1995 that gave women unrestricted access to women's clinics, violence against clinics continues (Table 13.10). Between 1977 and the end of 1994, 1,712 bombings, arsons, blockades, episodes of vandalism, stalkings, assaults, and other acts of violence took place at clinics throughout the country.[25] The Clinton administration eliminated the gag rule in 1993 and now allows the constitutional right of women to seek a safe legal abortion. In 1994, the Freedom of Access to Clinic Entrances Act (FACE) was signed into law. FACE prohibits the use of force, threats of force, physical obstruction, and property damage intended to interfere with those obtaining or providing reproductive health services. It does not apply to peaceful praying, picketing, or communication by anti-choice demonstrators.[26] Despite this, in 1997 30 percent of abortion clinics reported some type of violence.

Abortion is a class issue. Women of low economic means are not able to receive federal or state funding for abortion as part of their health care assistance. The legislation that restricts funding is called the Hyde Amendment and has passed Congress without much opposition until 1993, when those representing economically disadvantaged women pressed a more sympathetic Congress to lift this restriction. However, until the Hyde Amendment is lifted, the right to choose under *Roe* v. *Wade* is only allowed to women of economic means. Further, if Roe were overturned, it is a fact that abortions will continue to be performed and that those with less money will have less safe abortions and greater risk of death than economically privileged women who will be able to secure safer, even illegal abortions.

The greatest potential threat to those seeking an abortion in the future could come from a growing medical trend of fewer doctors trained to do an abortion. A radical and certainly risky alternative, **menstrual extraction** (self-abortion), has been proposed by some women activists, but virtually all women hope that this alternative to safe, legal abortion does not become a necessity. Today, abortion has seen a liberalizing trend internationally.

RU-486

Import restrictions have prevented distribution of RU-486, an abortion-inducing pill that may be helpful in treating illness, including breast cancer and endometriosis, because of the strong, vocal anti-abortion lobby. On July 4, 1992 the first arrest of the illegal importation of RU-486 was made in New York as a pregnant woman returned from France with this banned drug. On October 7, 1992 a Scottish researcher announced in the *New England Journal of Medicine* that RU-486 is 100 percent effective as birth control and has virtually no side effects. In May 1994, the FDA allowed for the limited use and testing of RU-486 in the United States. It was approved for general use in September 2000.

Table 13.10 Violence against abortion clinics (1994).

Violence	1992	1993	1994	Total 1977–1994
Murder	0	1	4	5
Attempted murder	0	1	8	9
Bombing	1	1	3	40
Arson	16	5	9	92
Attempted bomb	13	7	4	68
Invasion	26	24	2	347
Vandalism	116	113	42	585
Assault & battery	9	9	7	95
Death threats	8	78	59	225
Kidnaping	0	0	0	2
Burglary	5	3	3	34
Stalking	0	188	22	210
Total	194	434	159	1,712
Disruption				
Hate mail/calls	469	628	381	1,833
Bomb threats	112	22	14	311
Picketing	2,898	2,979	1,407	7,763
Total	3,379	2,929	1,802	9,912
Clinic Blockades				
# of incidents	83	66	25	634
# arrests	2,580	1,236	217	33,661

(*Source:* The National Abortion Federation, Washington, DC: Reprinted with permission.)

Maternal Morbidity

Pregnancy, delivery, and the first year of life—despite all progress—is a period in which there are numerous problems for the mother. During pregnancy some women develop elevated blood pressure. Data from 1980 indicate that a small proportion of women develop eclampsia, which increases the chance of severe bleeding (5 percent), threatened abortion (8–10 percent), and premature delivery (8–10 percent). During pregnancy Caesarean sections have increased with a certain number of sequelae. Other anomalies include placenta previa (1 percent) and hemorrhage requiring transfusion (2–3 percent).

A more common problem in the past ten years has been the increase in ectopic or tubal pregnancy. The rate of ectopic pregnancies has increased from one in every 250 normal pregnancies to one in every seventy.[27] This appears to be associated with an increase in sexually transmitted diseases among women which leads to pelvic inflammatory disease (PID) and blocked fallopian tubes. Death from ectopic pregnancy is ten times greater than from childbirth and fifty times greater than from a legal abortion.

In 1998, 281 maternal deaths were reported, the major causes of which were hemorrhage, ectopic pregnancy, pregnancy-induced hypertension, embolism, infection, and other complications of pregnancy and childbirth. U.S. rates are

Table 13.11 Maternal death rates for selected causes by race (1998).

Cause of Death (Based on the Ninth Revision, International Classification of Diseases, 1975)	Number				Rate			
			All Other				All Other	
	All Races	White	Total	Black	All Races	White	Total	Black
Complication of pregnancy, childbirth, and the puerperium	281	158	123	104	7.1	5.1	14.9	17.1
Pregnancy with abortive outcome	32	15	17	14	0.8	*	*	*
Ectopic pregnancy	19	7	12	9	*	*	*	*
Spontaneous abortion	2	2	–	–	*	*	*	*
Legally induced abortion	6	3	3	3	*	*	*	*
Illegally induced abortion	–	–	–	–	*	*	*	*
Other pregnancy with abortive outcome	5	3	2	2	*	*	*	*
Direct obstetric causes	229	129	100	85	5.8	4.1	12.2	13.9
Hemorrhage of pregnancy and childbirth	24	16	8	5	0.6	*	*	*
Toxemia of pregnancy	47	23	24	22	1.2	0.7	2.9	3.6
Obstructed labor	–	–	–	–	*	*	*	*
Complications of the puerperium	99	60	39	35	2.5	1.9	4.7	5.7
Major puerperal infections	6	4	2	2	*	*	*	*
Venous complications in pregnancy and the puerperium	3	3	–	–	*	*	*	*
Obstetrical pulmonary embolism	43	32	11	9	1.1	1.0	*	*
Other and unspecified complications of the puerperium, not elsewhere classified	46	21	25	23	1.2	0.7	3.0	3.8
All other complications of the puerperium	1	–	1	1	*	*	*	*
Other direct obstetric causes	59	30	29	23	1.5	1.0	3.5	3.8
Indirect obstetric causes	20	14	6	5	0.5	*	*	*
Delivery in a completely normal case	–	–	–	–	*	*	*	*

*Figure does not meet standards of reliability or precision.
–Quantity zero.

(*Source:* Vital Statistics of the United States)

given in Table 13.11. The overall maternal mortality rate has fluctuated between approximately 7 and 8 per 100,000 live births since 1987 when it was 6.6 per 100,000 live births. Moreover, the gap between African Americans and whites remains, with the maternal mortality rate among African Americans 3.5 times that of whites in 1996. The rates among African Americans have been at least three to four times higher than those of whites since 1940. The rate among African Americans also has not declined; it still fluctuates between about 18 and 22 per 100,000 live births.[28]

Perhaps one of the factors in maternal mortality is the inaccessibility of private physicians. The rising cost of malpractice insurance, coupled with the increase in maternal risks, and the unrealistic expectation that all outcomes should be perfect have made many clinicians leave the practice or limit their practice to healthy women. More than $2 billion is spent each year in the United States on medical professional liability insurance. That is $500 million more than what is spent annually to salvage an estimated 165,000 low birth weight newborns. The growing crisis in malpractice suits and medical liability insurance is actually cutting women off from choices in practitioners and services.[29] Only "good girl" patients, those at very low risk, are often even considered by health care providers. This gate-keeping method prevents reproducing women, half the world's more than 3.5 billion women, from speaking out against the system that they rely on but that has the power to exempt them.

> **Healthy People 2010 Objective:** Reduce Maternal Deaths
>
> *Target:* 3.3 maternal deaths per 100,000 live births.
>
> *Baseline:* 8.4 maternal deaths per 100,000 live births in 1997.

The primary causes of maternal mortality worldwide, but declining in developed countries, are hemorrhage, infection, and toxemia. An unnecessary increase in caesarean section births has increased the risk of mortality from anesthetic complications. Safe, legal abortions have also been an important contributor to a decrease in maternal mortality. Life expectancies for women for selected countries are given in Figure 13.5. Data indicate that 20 to 40 percent of all deaths among women aged fifteen to forty-nine are from pregnancy-related causes in most developing countries as opposed to less than 1 percent in the United States and most of Europe.[30]

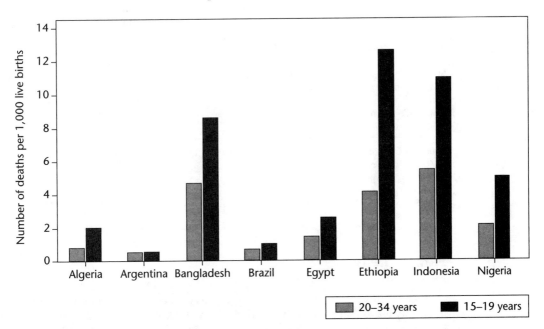

Figure 13.5 Maternal mortality in selected countries (1980s).

(*Source:* Women, health, and development. Progress report, World Health Assembly, Geneva, WHO, 1991)

Table 13.12   Maternity leave benefits among selected countries.

Country or Area	Number of Weeks of Maternity Leave	Percentage of Wages in Covered Period
Australia	6 (B) + 6 (A)	100
Austria	8 (B) + 8 (A)	ave. earnings
Belgium	7 (B) + 8(A)	82
Bulgaria	120 days	100
Canada (Federal)	17	57 for 15 wks
Denmark	4 (B) + 14 (A)	(variable)
Finland	105 days	80
France	6 (B) + 10 (A)	84
Germany	6 (B) + 8 (A)	100
Greece	15	100
Hungary	24	100
Iceland	1 (B) + 1 (A) mos	(variable)
Ireland	14	70
Israel	12	75
Italy	2 (B) + 3 (A) mos	80
Japan	14	60
Liechtenstein	8 (A)	80
Luxembourg	6 (B) + 8 (A)	100
Malta	13	100
Netherlands	16	100
New Zealand	14	unpaid
Norway	12 (B) + 6 (A)	100
Poland	16	100
Portugal	90 days	100
Romania	112 days	(variable)
Russian Federation	140 days	100
Spain	16	75
Sweden	6 (B) + 6 (A)	90
Switzerland	8 (A)	100
Turkey	6 (B) + 6 (A)	two-thirds
United Kingdom	14	90
United States (Federal)	12	unpaid

(*Source:* ECA Windham, 1999. www.relojournal.com/june1999/benefits.htm)

Discussion: What makes birthing so risky for women in developing countries?

Family Leave

Of the Fortune 500 companies, 44 percent provide for paternity leave, which averages eighteen days. Sixty percent of these major U.S. companies provide maternity leave that averages fifty-six days. In 1992, President Bush vetoed family leave legislation for U.S. businesses and federal government. The election of Bill Clinton in 1992 opened the door to the government's finally signing a family leave bill in 1993. Worldwide maternity leave benefits are given in Table 13.12.

Violence

The abuse of women has escalated in the last decade. During each year women were the victims of more than 4.5 million violent crimes, including approximately 500,000 rapes or other sexual assaults. In 29 percent of the violent crimes against women by lone offenders the perpetrators were intimates—husbands, former husbands, boyfriends, or former boyfriends. In the United States, women are more likely to be injured, raped, or killed by a current or former male partner than by all other types of assailants combined. During the same period, 1979 to 1990, only 4 percent of the crimes against men were committed by women partners or family members. Women today, are protected by the Violence Against Women Act of 1994.

Internationally, one of the horrendous forms of culturally sanctioned violence is genital mutilation of young girls and women. The World Health Organization reports that a sexual inequity exists in most parts of the world, as evidenced by the fact that 100 million women, mainly in East and West Africa and the Middle East, have suffered genital mutilation. Mutilation occurs with the complete removal of the clitoris through often unsterile, brutal cutting, and infibulation, the sewing together of the labia majora to prevent penetration. The primary reason for this violence is to keep women in sexual servitude by making them visibly virgin at marriage and then to prevent sexual enjoyment due to the scarring and mutilation of the genital organs. Table 13.13 reports violence trends against women worldwide in the mid-1980s.

Globally, physical, sexual, and psychological violence occurs in the family, including battering, sexual abuse of female children in the household, dowry-related violence, marital rape, female genital mutilation, and other traditional practices harmful to women. Non-spousal violence and violence related to exploitation occur within the general community, including rape, sexual harassment and intimidation at work, in educational institutions, and elsewhere. There are still parts of the world where trafficking in women and forced prostitution are part of life. Beginning before birth with sex-selective abortions, and at birth when female babies may be killed by parents who are desperate for a son, violence continues to have a profound effect on women throughout their lives. As young children, girls may be given less food and health care than their brothers. Female children are much more likely than their brothers to be raped or sexually assaulted by family members and by strangers. The genitalia of infant and young girls may be operated on, without anesthetic, for a variety of cultural reasons. If an unmarried woman is raped she may be forced to marry her attacker, or she may end up in prison for committing a criminal act. If she becomes pregnant before she is married, she may be beaten, ostracized, or murdered by family members, even if the pregnancy is the result of a rape.

After marriage, the greatest risk of violence continues to be in women's own homes, where they may be attacked, raped, or killed by their husbands. If they become more vulnerable, through pregnancy, old age, mental illness, or disability, women are even more likely to be attacked. If women find themselves far

Table 13.13   Violence against women in selected countries.

	Domestic Violence	Incest	Homicide in Family	Sexual Assault and Rape	Sexual Harassment
Developed regions					
Australia	x		x		
Austria	x		x		
Belgium	x	x		x	x
Canada	x		x	x	x
Finland	x	x		x	x
France				x	
Germany	x	x	x		x
Greece	x		x	x	
Italy		x		x	
New Zealand	x		x		
Poland	x				
Portugal				x	
Spain					x
United Kingdom	x			x	x
United States	x	x	x	x	x
Africa					
Kenya	x		x		
Nigeria	x				
Uganda	x				
Latin America and Caribbean					
Argentina	x				
Brazil	x			x	
Chile	x	x	x		
Colombia	x	x		x	
Dominican Republic			x		
Ecuador	x				
Jamaica	x	x		x	
Peru	x				
Puerto Rico	x		x		
Trinidad and Tobago	x	x		x	
Venezuela				x	
Asia and Pacific					
Bangladesh	x		x		
China			x		
India	x		x	x	x
Israel	x				
Kuwait	x				
Malaysia	x			x	
Philippines				x	
Thailand	x		x		

(*Source:* Reproduced, by permission of WHO, from: *Women's health: Across age and frontier.* Geneva: World Health Organization, 1992)

from home, or imprisoned or isolated in any way, they are more likely to be attacked. In times of armed conflict and war, assaults escalate, including those committed against women by friendly and hostile forces alike, and by their own husbands.[31] The U.N. estimates that one-fourth of women worldwide are physically battered. In India, 6,200 dowry deaths were reported in 1998.

You can take a sexual abuse survey and determine your own risk for violence at www.dviworld.org/

Discussion: How can health education programs help to stop the vicious cycles of violence that are passed on from one generation to another?

Quantifying acts of violence is difficult: Information gathering systems break down during conflict, victims may be reluctant to report being raped, and figures can be manipulated for political ends. Nevertheless, something of the nature and the scale of the problem of gender-based and sexual violence during conflict and displacement is illustrated by the following reports and statistics:

- In Bosnia-Herzegovina, aside from the unreported cases, the number of raped women was estimated (1993) to be 20,000 to 50,000.

- In 1971 the number of raped women in Bangladesh was estimated at 200,000.

- According to cautious estimates, 110,000 women were raped in the Berlin area after World War II. Less conservative estimates cite the number as 900,000 raped and abused women.

- In 1985, 3 percent of Vietnamese boat women between the ages of eleven and forty were reported to have been abducted and/or raped at sea.

- A randomly chosen sample of twenty Ethiopian refugees who had fled forced relocation and ethnic persecution in Ethiopia were interviewed in a refugee camp in Somalia in 1986: Seventeen knew someone in their village, and three knew someone in their family, who had been raped by the Ethiopian militia.

- Among 210,000 mostly Somali refugees living in Kenya, 192 cases of sexual abuse were documented. One hundred eighty-seven of the victims were women, four were children, one was a man.[32]

War

The violence of war is a dramatic public health issue. It impacts all aspects of one's life and health. For women, war is particularly impactful because women and children are the primary victims of war. War destroys health care systems, creates shortages of food and medical supplies, and results in poor obstetrical care. During war sexually transmitted diseases increase as a result of rape, torture, and lack of condoms. HIV infection is now a complication of wartime sexuality. Adding to the horrors of war, more than 100 million antipersonnel land mines are scattered throughout the world. They pose a particular danger to women who perform much of the agricultural work in the world.[33]

Summary

Women's health issues have long been ignored as funded research interests by the U.S. government. As women have taken seats in the senate, as governors, and as heads of major health organizations, the research needs of woman have seen new opportunities and funding. With new research into breast cancer, menopause, reproduction methodology, and domestic violence will come reductions in morbidity and mortality rates and greater opportunities for prevention and health promotion among women.

CYBERSITES RELATED TO CHAPTER 13

Maternal/Child Health
>   www.nmch.org
>   www.mchb.hrsa.gov
>   www.mchpolicy.org

Women's Issues
>   www.wwwomen.com/category/health1.html
>   dir.yahoo.com/Health/Women_s_Health

QUESTIONS

1. Why are women, despite being greater in number, a "minority"?
2. What fundamental changes must be made at federal, state, and local levels to improve the health of women?
3. If women had control of public health, what would be the significant changes?

EXERCISE

Imagine yourself a woman in a developing country. Select the country and describe your physical, emotional, intellectual, sexual, mental, and spiritual health. What could be done by community health professionals to improve your situation?

INTERNET INTERACTIVE ACTIVITY

BEHAVIORAL RISK FACTOR SURVEILLANCE SYSTEM

The Behavioral Risk Factor Surveillance System (BRFSS) survey was developed by the Centers for Disease Control (CDC). BRFSS utilizes a standardized questionnaire to collect information on self-reported health habits and risk factors that contribute to the development of chronic diseases. The survey is conducted over the telephone using groups of randomly selected telephone numbers. Specially trained staff complete the interviews and record responses. The homepage for seeking results is:

www2.cdc.gov/nccdphp/brfss/index.asp

Example

1. Go to the homepage for the Behavioral Risk Factor Surveillance System

   www2.cdc.gov/nccdphp/brfss/index.asp

2. Fill in the categories

   Nationwide
   1998
   Health Status

3. Click

   Go

4. You can now click on each survey question or category and get the results of the nationwide health status. For instance, for the question How is your general health?, you should get a page that looks something like this:

Nationwide - 1998
Health Status

How is your general health?

	Excellent	Very good	Good	Fair	Poor
Median	23.6	33.6	27.9	9.8	3.3
# States	52	52	52	52	52

# of States includes District of Columbia and Puerto Rico
See notes for data users.

You now know that for fifty-two states and territories reporting, 23.6 percent felt they had excellent health, 33.6 percent had very good heath, and 3.3 percent had poor health.

Exercise

The community health educator wants to know the status of women's health in her or his state.

1. Go to the Behavioral Risk Factor Surveillance System

   www2.cdc.gov/nccdphp/brfss/index.asp

2. Select your state, the most recent year, and women's health. Then click Go.

3. Describe the status of women's health in your state grouped by Race and then by Age.

4. After you have analyzed the data, describe ten target populations that may need community health intervention based on the survey data.

REFERENCES

1. Turshen, Meredeth. (1989). *The politics of public health.* N.J.: Rutgers University Press.

2. thomas.loc.gov/cgi-bin/query/z?r102:E27FE1-48:

3. Davis, Karen (1995). Editorial: The federal budget and women's health. *AJPH*, August *85*(8), p. 1051.

4. Nickman, Nancy A. (1993). Gender equity issues in clinical research. *Journal of Pharmacy Practice*, Vol. VI, No. 5 (October), pp. 202–210.

5. Ibid.

6. American Medical Association Council on Ethical and Judicial Affairs: Gender disparities in clinical decision making. *JAMA* 266:559–562, 1991.

7. Turnquist, Kristi. (1992). Body of evidence. *The Sunday Oregonian*, July 5, p. L1.

8. U.S. Census Bureau, Current population reports, P-60, #206.

9. Hale, Ellen (1994). Population plan wins OK from 180 nations. *USA Today*. September 22, p.c.

10. www.health.gov/healthypeople/Document/HTML/Volume2/ 16MICH.htm#_Toc471971359

11. Rubin, C.H. et. al (1993). Occupation as a risk identifier for breast cancer. *American Journal of Public Health.* September, Vol. 83: No. 9, p. 1311.

12. Folsom, Aaron R., Mink, Pamela, et al. (1995). Hormonal replacement therapy and morbidity and mortality in a prospective study of postmenopausal women. *AJPH*, August *85*(8), p. 1128.

13. www.cancer.org/statistics/cff2000

14. Sun, Lena H. (1993). China lowers birthrate at levels in West. In *Earth's eleventh hour* by William O. Dwyer. Boston: Allyn and Bacon.

15. Painter, Kim (1994). Gauging use of drugs, alcohol in pregnancy. *USA Today*, September 13, p. D1.

16. Rogers, Estelle H. (1995). Reproductive rights update, ACLU, NY.

17. Painter, op. cit.

18. Goldenberg, R.L., Andrews, W.W., et al. (1997). Sexually transmitted diseases and adverse outcomes of pregnancy. *Clinics in Perinatology* 24(1): 23–41.

19. www.health.gov/healthypeople/Document/HTML/Volume2/ 25STDs.htm#_Toc470354135

20. McGoldrick, Kathryn E. (1986). *Women in society: Making a difference.* New York: Todd & Honeywell.

21. Boston Women's Health Collective. (1992). *The new our bodies ourselves.* New York: Simon and Schuster.

22. Boston Women's Health Collective, op. cit.

23. Turnquist, op. cit.

24. CDC. HIV/AIDS Surveillance Report. (1998); 10(No.2). Altanta, GA.

25. Rogers, op. cit.

26. Ibid.

27. Green, Lawrence W. (1990). *Community health*. St. Louis: Times Mirror/Mosby.

28. www.health.gov/healthypeople/Document/HTML/Volume2/ 25STDs.htm#_Toc470354135

29. McGoldrick, op. cit.

30. Brown, Lester R. (1992). *State of the world 1992*. New York: W.W. Norton.

31. www.who.int/eha/pvi/infokit/women.htm

32. Ibid.

33. Levy, Barry S., Sidel, Victor W. (1997). *War and public health*. New York: Oxford University Press.

Section IV

Community Health Priorities and Issues for the 21st Century

At any given time, there are any number of specific community health issues that may arise for individuals, among groups, or within the environment. This text has chosen four health priorities, beyond the ten leading causes of death, which seem to have increased in importance in the 1990s, and appear to be important for the twenty-first century. Chapter 14 introduces the reader to the growing concern among community health educators for the spread of communicable diseases and the emergence of super pathogens that are not easily treated.

Virtually all adults will be part of the work force sometime in their adulthood. Chapter 15 discusses the complex nature of occupational health problems within the working community.

The social stresses of a complex, hi-tech, fractured society appear to be increasing despite many intervention programs that begin in elementary school. Chapter 16 describes the personal and social illnesses associated with alcohol and drug abuse and interpersonal violence.

Chapter 17 talks about the importance of school health in the twenty-first century. If young people can be made aware of their health risks and the threats to the environment, and if they can modify their behaviors and become good decision makers, community health will have its challenges greatly reduced in the future.

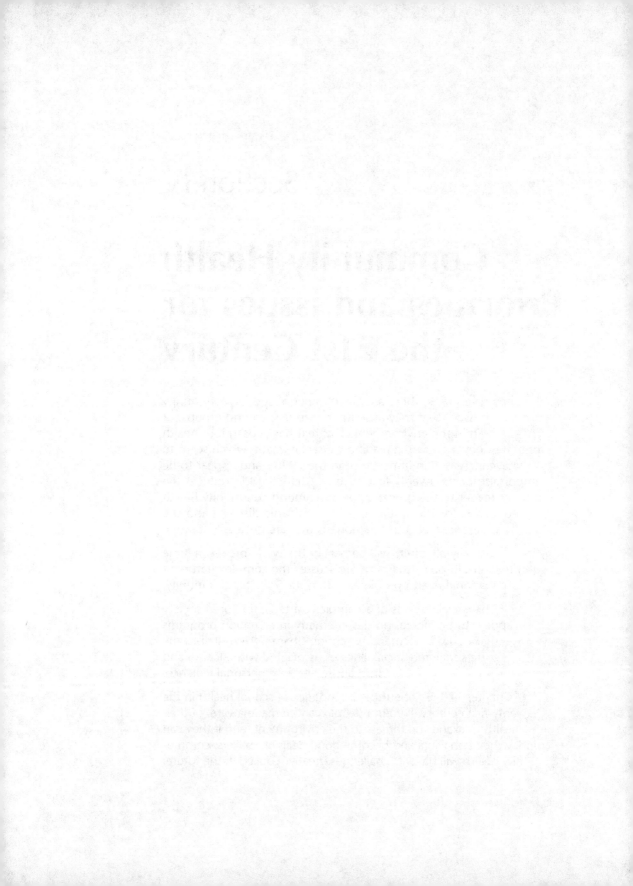

CHAPTER 14

Communicable Diseases

Community Health in the 21st Century
Infectious diseases are increasing. Hopefully there will be emphasis on
preventive and early intervention health services rather than treatment.
There is new emphasis on maternal and child care—this is the basis for the
future of the next generation.

—Nan Streeter, R.N.; M.S. Reproductive Health, Division
of Family Health Services

Chapter Objectives

The student will:

1. differentiate among respiratory, alvine, vector-borne, and open lesion diseases.

2. list the five pathogens.

3. know what diseases are prevented by immunization.

4. explain the difference among active, passive, acquired, natural, and herd immunity.

5. describe the risk for the spread of disease during the incubation period of an illness.

6. suggest prevention methods for the spread of communicable diseases.

7. give six reasons why new diseases are emerging.

Communicable Diseases in Contemporary Society

Improved sanitation, routine immunizations, diverse pharmaceuticals, and epidemiological principles have decreased the threat of communicable disease, making it no longer one of the major killers in the United States. In less developed countries, communicable diseases still pose the greatest threat to life and are the major emphasis of the World Health Organization. Worldwide, more than one-third of all deaths are caused by infectious, communicable diseases. The number of deaths in 1999, worldwide, associated with selected infectious diseases is given in Figure 14.1.

The first discussion of contagion found in literature was in the sixteenth century *de Contagione*. Not much more was found until the ninteenth century. Paleopathologists, however, have traced diseases back 500 million years. They have discovered bacteria, trauma, parasites, arthritis, and "cave gout."

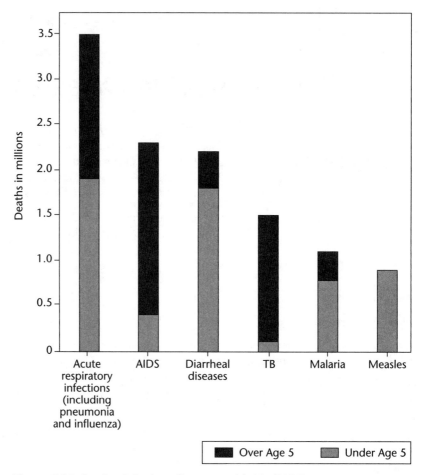

Figure 14.1 Leading infectious diseases worldwide (1999).

(*Source:* World Health Organization)

In the United States many communicable diseases are reportable, meaning each new case must be reported to the Centers for Disease Control and Prevention within forty-eight hours. Table 14.1 lists the reportable diseases and their incidence. Diseases that are reportable are those that are communicable and can develop into epidemics without proper control, vaccination, or treatment.

The pathogens that cause disease are bacteria, viruses, parasites, helminths (worms), and fungi. These pathogens are transmitted by a variety of pathway systems including: (1) respiratory, (2) alvine discharge, (3) vector-borne, and (4) open lesion pathways.

The human body is the greatest reservoir of potentially pathogenic organisms. The skin, intestines, and body fluids harbor innumerable organisms that given a change in host, agent, or environment can become pathogenic to the host or to others. Some organisms can be transmitted to others indirectly through airborne droplets of saliva, through water or food, or via a vector.

Table 14.1 Selected reportable diseases in the United States (1998).

Name	Total	Name	Total
AIDS	46,521	Malaria	1,611
Botulism, total	116	Measles (rubeola)	100
Chlamydia	604,420	Meningococcal disease	2,725
Cryptosporidiosis	3,793	Mumps	666
Escherichia coli O157:H7	3,161	Pertussis (whooping cough)	7,405
Gonorrhea	355,642	Rabies, human	1
Haemophilus influenzae	1,194	Rubella (German measles)	364
Hepatitis A	23,294	Salmonellosis	43,901
Hepatitis B	10,258	Syphilis, total all stages	37,540
Hepatitis, C/non-A non-B	3,518	Toxic-shock syndrome	138
Legionellosis	1,355	Tuberculosis	18,851
Lyme disease	16,801	Varicella (chickenpox)	82,727

(*Sources:* Centers for Disease Control. MMWR Weekly Report)

Other organisms require direct contact, usually through intimate contact (not necessarily sexual) with another human or animal for transmission. Vectors, water, milk, food, air, **fomites** (inanimate objects such as clothing, doorknobs, drinking fountains, and toys), and soil are common means of transmission of disease. Intermediate animal hosts are required for completion of the life cycle of many animal parasites.

Respiratory Diseases

The respiratory system consists of a tubular air passageway from the external environment to the lungs. Bacteria and viruses, entering with inspired air, can set up various sites of infection along the respiratory tract. Diseases of the nose and throat are called upper respiratory diseases. Those of the trachea, bronchi, and lungs are lower respiratory diseases. The common cold is a respiratory disease that is within everyone's experience.[1]

Respiratory diseases follow a characteristic cycle of incubation, prodrome, fastigium, defervescence, and convalescence (Figure 14.2). The most common U.S. acute respiratory diseases are influenza, pneumonia, streptococcal sore throat, and chickenpox. All young children worldwide have from four to eight

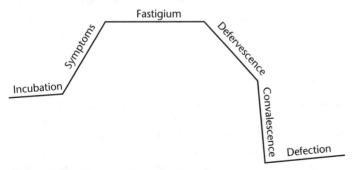

Figure 14.2 Progress of a respiratory disease.

episodes of respiratory infections per year. Many of these episodes are self-limiting infections of the upper respiratory tract. However, the incidence of acute lower respiratory infections, in particular pneumonia, is very high in developing countries. Four million children die every year due to these infections.[2]

The Respiratory Disease Cycle

There are 5 stages to the respiratory disease cycle:

Incubation is that time from exposure to a pathogen to the first signs and symptoms. During the incubation period, the organisms are reproducing and triggering the immune system to develop antibodies. Incubation periods may vary from two days for the common cold to ten or more years for HIV. During incubation, many diseases are communicable through carriers. The legendary Typhoid Mary was a New York cook in the early 1900s who carried the typhoid bacillus in her system without any signs or symptoms of having the disease. She spread the disease through droplets from her saliva into food as she cooked. HIV positive persons are a contemporary example of carriers throughout incubation, although they may have no idea they are infected.

Prodrome begins with the first symptoms. People with herpes simplex I or cold sores know the prodrome time as that sense of annoyance around the lip that suggests that within the next twenty-four hours a blister will appear. Some diseases are communicable during the prodrome period.

Fastigium is when the disease is at its worst. These are a few days after you start feeling ill, when you are bedridden with fever, aches, discharge, nausea, headache, and other symptoms. Usually you are very contagious in this stage.

Defervescence indicates the disease is declining in severity, although you may relapse.

Convalescence is a high-risk time for others, because a patient will feel well enough to go about his or her activities; however, spreading the infection may still be quite possible.

Alvine Discharge Diseases

Alvine discharge diseases are passed through the alimentary canal, from mouth to anus. These diseases include cholera, hepatitis, dysentery, and salmonellosis, and usually occur as a result of poor sanitation or contaminated food, water, or milk.

Vector-Borne Diseases

Vector-borne diseases are a group of diseases closely correlated with environmental conditions that require an insect vector for transmission. The most common vector-borne diseases are given in Table 14.2. Throughout history, biting flies have been indirectly responsible for a large proportion of human illnesses and deaths. Fleas are the vectors of bubonic plague, murine typhus,

Table 14.2   Some major vector-borne and zoonotic diseases of humans.

Disease	Mode	Animals Usually Involved	Vector	Distribution
Yellow fever	V	Monkeys, marsupials	*Aedes* mosquitoes	Africa Cen. & S. America
Viral encephalitis	V	Rodents, birds, horses, monkeys	Mosquitoes or ticks	Many types; temperate and tropical areas
Dengue	V	Humans	*Aedes* mosquitoes	Pacific, S.E. Asia, Caribbean, S. America
Rabies	D	Dogs, wild mammals		Cosmopolitan
Influenza	D, I	Swine, birds		Cosmopolitan
Typhus	V	Rodents	Lice	Africa, Asia, Cen. & S. America, Balkans
Murine typhus	V	Rodents	Fleas	Cosmopolitan
Scrub typhus	V	Rodents	Mites	Asia, S. Asia, N. Australia
Q fever	D, I	Cattle, sheep, goats, birds		Cosmopolitan
Spotted fevers	V	Rodents, other mammals	Ticks	Several types; Australia, N. & S. America, Africa, India
Psittacosis	D, I	Birds		Cosmopolitan
Anthrax	D, I	Cattle, goats, horses, swine		E. Mediterranean, Asia, Caribbean, Latin America
Brucellosis	D, I, M	Cattle, goats, sheep, swine		Cosmopolitan
Plague	D, V, I	Rodents	Fleas	Widespread
Lyme disease	V	Deer, rodents	Ticks	N. America, Europe
Relapsing fever	V	Rodents	Ticks or lice	Asia, Africa, Mid-East, S. America, Europe
Tuberculosis	D, M	Humans, cattle, goats, cats, dogs, swine		Cosmopolitan
Leishmaniasis	V	Dogs, wild animals	Sand flies	Asia, India, Africa, Cen. & S. America
Malaria	V	Humans	*Anopheles* mosquitoes	Mainly in tropics
Chagas disease	V	Small mammals, dogs	Triatomid bugs	Cen. & S. America
Sleeping sickness	V	Large mammals, cattle	Tsetse flies	Tropical Africa
Filariasis	V	Primates, cats, dogs	Mosquitoes	Widespread in tropics
Trichinosis	E	Swine, bear		Widespread in temperate areas
Hydatid disease	E	Sheep, dogs		E. Mediterranean, New Zealand, S. America, Europe, California
Tapeworms	E	Cattle, swine, dogs		Cosmopolitan
Schistosomiasis	V	Humans, cattle, rodents, swine, primates	Snails	Asia, Africa, Mid-East, Caribbean, S. America

Abbreviation
D Direct   M Milk
E Eating (ingestion)   V Vector-borne
I Inhalation

(*Source:* Herman Koren, 1991. *Handbook of environmental health and safety,* Vol. 1. Chelsea, MI: Lewis Publishers. Used with permission.)

tapeworms, salmonellosis, and tularemia. Other common vector-borne diseases include malaria and yellow fever passed by a mosquito, tularemia passed by a flea, and encephalitis passed by a fly.

Lyme disease (LD) is a growing vector-borne disease most specific to the Northeast and upper Midwestern portions of the United States. LD is now the most common arthropod-borne illness in the United States. In 1998 there were 12,801 cases with 90 percent found in the geographic northeast of the United States, which includes ten states.

Lyme disease was first noted in 1977, when investigators linked arthritis-like symptoms in children from Lyme, Connecticut, to a corkscrew-shaped bacterium. In the late 1990s a vaccine was developed that provided limited protections against LD, but most prevention comes from physical precautions when in wooded areas. Lyme disease is spread by deer ticks that feed off rodents in their early stages and then hunt for larger supplies of blood, such as deer, domestic animals, or humans.

Open Lesion Diseases

Open lesion diseases include the sexually transmitted diseases that are passed through open sores in the genitalia, through abrasions in the vagina, or through the cervix or meatus (portal of entry or exit) of the penis. They also include diseases that require direct contact with an open lesion or through a portal of entry in the skin such as with HIV infection through infected needles. These diseases include tuberculosis, anthrax, scarlet fever, and leprosy.

Zoonoses

Zoonoses are conditions in which humans are accidentally infected with a disease that ordinarily would be an animal disease. An example is jungle yellow fever. Yellow fever spreads from infected monkeys by mosquitoes who carry this infected blood to other monkeys and sometimes humans. Another example is viral encephalitis, which is transmitted by mosquitoes to humans, although the normal hosts would be wild birds.

BOX 14.1 *Prevention for Lyme Disease*

- **Wear enclosed shoes and light-colored clothing** with a tight weave to spot ticks easily.
- **Scan clothes and any exposed skin frequently** for ticks while outdoors.
- **Stay on cleared, well-traveled trails.**
- **Use insect repellant containing DEET (diethyl-meta-toluamide)** on skin or clothes if you intend to go off-trail or into overgrown areas.

- **Avoid sitting directly on the ground or on stone walls** (havens for ticks and their hosts).
- **Keep long hair tied back,** especially when gardening.
- **Do a final, full-body tick-check at the end of the day** (also check children and pets).

Nosocomial Diseases

The measures used to increase or prolong life, such as radiation, chemotherapy, and organ transplants, often alter the body defenses and predispose patients to infections from organisms from which they would be resistant under normal conditions. These pathologies, acquired in a hospital, are called **nosocomial infections.** The most common agents of nosocomial bacterial infections are gram-negative *Escherichia coli, Pseudomonas aeruginosa,* and species of Enterobacter, Proteus, and Providencia. Of the gram-positive bacteria, *Staphylococcus aureus* and teterococcal group B streptococci are most frequently reported.

Nosocomial infections occur worldwide and are recognized as a major cause of morbidity and mortality, particularly in the developed world. These infections occur among hospital patients and staff when a patient is the reservoir and inadequate sterilization or prevention takes place. In the United States, the infection rates of hospital discharges is thought to be about 10 percent.

A variety of clinical presentations occur as a result of bacterial nosocomial infections, but the great majority involve urinary tract infection (42 percent), surgical wound infection (24 percent), and lower respiratory tract infection (10 percent).

Microorganisms That Cause Communicable Diseases

Bacterial Infections

Bacteria are the greatest single cause of disease. Bacteria are the lowest form of life, and have the highest power of reproduction.[3] Bacteria are of particular interest to the community health educator, because they are generally quite preventable through proper sanitation or immunization.

Following is a brief review of the common bacterial infections in industrialized countries, the frequency of occurrence, duration of morbidity, and general impact on the health economy.[4] Since many viral and bacterial diseases are not reportable by law, any numbers given below are generally underestimates of actual incidence of these infections.

Campylobacter enteritis, from the bacteria of the genus *Campylobacter,* is distributed worldwide. In the United States, 2 to 3 million cases a year occur primarily among infants and young adults. In developing countries the disease occurs almost exclusively among young children. Prevention rests on thorough cooking and proper preparation of foods derived from animal sources, particularly poultry.

Chlamydia trachomatis is a spherical bacterium found worldwide and may be sexually transmitted through genito-urinary infections in men and women. The CDC estimates there are about 4 million cases a year, a rate that is two to three times that of gonorrhea. Women may be completely asymptomatic in over 60 percent of all cases. Untreated chlamydia infection accounts for the greatest cause of infertility due to pelvic inflammatory disease and resultant scar tissue. Chlamydia also contributes to ectopic pregnancy and complications in newborns.[5]

Gonorrhea is sexually transmitted among men and women, heterosexual or homosexual. Men are symptomatic in approximately 50 percent of the cases, while women are asymptomatic in approximately 80 percent of the cases. When symptoms do appear, they include inflammation of the urethra, epididymis, cervix, fallopian tubes, conjunctivitis of the eyes in newborns, and late stage arthritis and endocarditis in older adults. Gonorrhea is reportable.

Haemophilus influenzae causes two important groups of clinical disease particular to infants and children—invasive diseases (meningitis, epiglottitis, or sepsis) and otitis media (inflammation of the inner ear), the most common childhood disease among Native Americans.

Escherichia coli can cause several types of gastrointestinal illness. Some evidence suggest that *E. coli* is the third most common bacterial cause of diarrhea in some regions of the United States, behind salmonella (35,000 cases a year) and campylobacter.

Pneumococcal infection is a streptococcus infection most often seen in lobar pneumonia and otitis media.

Pneumococcus bacteria cause hundreds of thousands of cases of pneumonia nationwide each year. The bacteria are responsible for about half the 24 million annual U.S. office visits to pediatricians for treatment of earaches. A new concern to community health is that many strains of pneumococcus have become penicillin resistant. Researchers know that such resistant bacteria can cover the globe in a matter of years. It also means that there may not an effective treatment for many common bacterial diseases that are seen today. Before 1980 only a few scattered cases of penicillin-resistant strains were known. Now they are common worldwide.[6]

Salmonella causes different clinical syndromes including gastroenteritis, enteric fever, and typhoid fever. The most common form of salmonellosis is acute gastroenteritis. Over 2 million cases of salmonellosis are estimated to occur in the United States each year. While most are not reported, there were 48,000 reported cases in 1998. The principal reservoirs are animals, including poultry, livestock, and pets.

Staphylococcal infection is an ubiquitous bacterium normally present on the skin and in the gastrointestinal tracts. Infections usually occur sporadically but can occur in small epidemics. **Toxic shock syndrome** is a potentially fatal condition whose etiology is staphylococcus.

Streptococcal pyogenes comprise more than seventy serologically distinct types. Most of these strains can produce upper respiratory tract infection and subsequent rheumatic fever. Streptococci cause a variety of acute clinical diseases including tonsillitis, skin infections such as impetigo, and pyoderma. Type B Strep diseases are transmitted by close, intimate contact with infected persons.

Type A streptococci require proper preparation and storage of food, particularly milk and eggs. Food handlers with skin lesions or respiratory illness should be excluded from work.

Syphilis is a worldwide disease with a higher frequency in urban and highly populated areas. There were 6,657 reported cases in the United States in 1998, representing approximately 50 percent of the true incidence. Syphilis is transmitted through direct contact with infectious exudates of the primary or secondary lesions. Sexual intercourse is the most common means of transmission.

Tuberculosis (TB) is a chronic infectious disease caused by two varieties of mycobacteria, *M. tuberculosis* and *M. bovis*. TB has infected humans since the neolithic era sometimes in epidemic numbers. After a thirty-year decline, tuberculosis has re-emerged as a serious public health problem worldwide. It is one of the leading infectious disease in the world, infecting 1.7 billion people and killing more than 1.5 million people a year (Figure 14.1). The World Health Organization says about 8 million new cases occur each year.

In the United States, there were 18,361 cases in 1998.[7] Several large cities, including New York City (19.1 per 100,000), Atlanta (8.9 per 100,000), Los Angeles (14.9 per 100,000), and Miami (13.4 per 100,000), have experienced outbreaks in hospitals and among high-risk populations. New York City is thought to be a "living laboratory of TB" with the highest number of TB cases in the country.[8] In 1998, New York City had 1,558 cases, as compared to 544 cases in Los Angeles, 424 in Houston, and 473 in Chicago.[9] It is estimated that 20 percent of cases go unreported. In 1999, 24.5 percent of TB cases were white, 31.9 percent were black, 19.7 percent were Asian, 22.4 percent were Hispanic, and 1.4 percent were Native American (Figure 14.3).

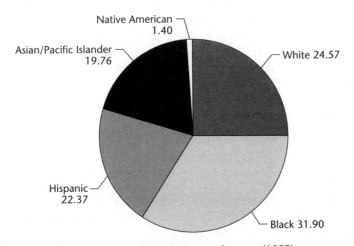

Figure 14.3 United States tuberculosis cases by race (1999).

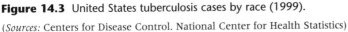

(*Sources:* Centers for Disease Control. National Center for Health Statistics)

Healthy People 2010 Objective: Reduce Tuberculosis

Target: 1.0 new case per 100,000 population.

Baseline: 6.8 new cases of tuberculosis per 100,000 population in 1998.

There is an important difference between infection with TB and active TB diseases. With infection, the TB bacteria are in the person's body, their skin test is positive, their chest x-ray is normal and the person is NOT contagious. When a person has active TB disease, the bacteria is in the body, skin test is positive, chest x-ray is abnormal, sputum is usually positive, and some of the symptoms include cough, fever, weight loss, and night sweats. This person is contagious prior to treatment.

TB is especially prevalent in economically disadvantaged neighborhoods where there is substandard housing, crowding, and inadequate health services. Cities overcrowded with the homeless, the poor, the mentally impaired, and people who are on drugs, imprisoned or HIV positive are pockets of TB infection risk. This may make reaching these target objectives difficult at the present time.

The Three Fs of Tuberculosis
Feces, Fingers, Flies

Among the greatest concerns is what health officials call multi-drug resistant TB, which affects about 9 percent of U.S. patients. Many of these cases develop when a person with regular TB fails to complete the prescribed treatment, which means taking two or more drug regimens for six to twelve months. As patients begin to feel well, they discontinue the full course of treatment, allowing the bacteria to mutate into a strain that is impervious to the first drug regimen. The new strain will be far more difficult to treat medically and may cost the patient up to $200,000.[10] The case fatality rate of drug resistant TB is 40–60 percent. The highest priority for TB control is to ensure that persons with the disease complete curative therapy. If treatment is not continued for a sufficient length of time, such persons often become ill and contagious again. Completion of therapy is essential to prevent transmission of the disease as well as to prevent outbreaks and the development and spread of drug-resistant TB.

Cholera is an acute, diarrhea illness caused by infection of the intestine with the bacterium Vibro cholerae. Cholera is usually transmitted through contaminated water or water life such as shellfish. The infection is often mild, but sometimes it can be severe. Cholera produces a profuse yet painless diarrhea, then vomiting, muscle cramps, and death from dehydration in a matter of hours. Treatment consists of oral rehydration of almost five gallons electrolyte-enriched water.

In January 1991, epidemic cholera appeared in Peru and Ecuador. This epidemic, which killed over 3,000 people, was an example of a phenomenon that is becoming increasingly common throughout developing countries. According to the United Nations Environment Programme, "four of every five common diseases in developing countries are caused either by dirty water or lack of sanitation, and water-borne diseases cause an average of twenty-five thousand deaths a day in the Third World."[11] There were six reported cholera cases in the United States in 1990 and twelve in 1991 when the Peruvian epidemic spread north.

Vibrio cholerae, the deadliest of all infectious diseases, appears to have mutated into a new deadly strain that may ignite the eighth cholera pandemic since 1817. Although the pandemic will probably be most contained in developing countries, 14 million Americans travel abroad yearly, and the only protection against this bacteria is clean food and uncontaminated water.

Plague is caused by a small, gram-negative, extremely virulent organism, Bacillus pestis (*Pasteurella pestis*). During the Middle Ages the Black Death came the nearest to exterminating the human race when it killed 25 million people in Europe. The bacillus enters the body through the skin by means of the bite of a flea that carries the infection to humans. Plague is primarily a disease of rats. When a rat dies of the disease, the infected fleas leave it and go in search of a new warm-blooded host. A patient with plague is not infective unless fleas carry the infection from him or her to others.[12]

Viral Infections

Changes in the environment, human mobility, living patterns, and the naive belief that humans had conquered viral epidemics have brought public health to the twenty-first century with a renewed challenge of preventing new and previously unknown viral epidemics. The Ebola virus epidemic in Zaire in 1995 was probably only a warning to the planet.

Viruses are RNA or DNA enclosed in a protein coat that require a host to reproduce. They are intracellular parasites whose transmission is the most hazardous part of the infectious cycle because of the damage they do to host cells. The steps in viral infection include:

BOX 14.2 Antibiotics and the Plague

Surat, India, a few hours north of Bombay, has long been known as the "filthiest city" in India. It was here that the September 1994 plague epidemic in India began. Within two weeks, fifty-five people had died, 600 more were infected, and a fourth of the population of 400,000 had fled. The exodus spread the disease to numerous other towns in India. Although antibiotics will cure plague, they cannot prevent it. Many healthy residents thinking differently, began taking massive amounts of tetracycline, which actually weakened their immune systems and put them at greater risk for infection.[13]

1. Virus attaches to a cell, penetrates, and begins uncoating.
2. Messenger RNA synthesizes genomic nucleic acid synthesis.
3. Maturation and assembly of virion, which is released from the cell. Because of the cell damage, viruses are difficult to cultivate.

Among the RNA viruses of significance to humans are the *Picarnaviridae* and the *Paramyxoviridae*. The Picarnaviridae include the enterovirus that causes polio and the rhinovirus that is found in humans and cattle. They also include cardiovirus, which causes encephalomyocarditis and aphthovirus, which is also known as hoof and mouth disease. The Paramyxoviridae cause mumps and parainfluenza 1–4, measles and canine distemper, and pneumovirus which causes respiratory virus.

Among the DNA viruses are the *Papovaviridae*, which causes human papilloma virus and perhaps cancers; *Poxviridae*, which is the etiology of smallpox and cowpox; and *Herpesviridae*, which is responsible for herpes simplex, herpes zoster, Epstein Barr virus, and cytomegalovirus.

Reported cases of some viral infections for 1998 are given below:

Measles (Rubeola)	100
German Measles (Rubella)	364
Chickenpox (Varicella)	82,455
Herpes Simplex II	app. 500,000
Hepatitis C	3,528
Hepatitis A	23,229
AIDS	46,521

Hepatitis

There has been an alarming increase in the incidence of viral hepatitis in the United States. **Hepatitis A** accounts for 40 percent of reported cases of hepatitis cases in a community. Children in day care, travelers, and those who live in unsanitary conditions are often at risk for hepatitis A from fecal contaminated food (such as raw shellfish) and water. Person-to-person spread is more likely to occur in settings where there is close contact between client and caregiver (such as in a day care center), from food handlers, or in a hospital. The time between exposure to the virus and symptoms is four to six weeks and this virus is most contagious during the first week of symptoms. Infection hampers liver function and can cause flu-like symptoms and jaundice. About 24,000 United States cases were reported in 1998. Today there is a new hepatitis A vaccine that is the most recent FDA approved vaccine in use.

The 1998 incidence was up to 30,000 new hepatitis B cases and 3,816 new **hepatitis C** infections. The recent hepatitis B (HB) vaccine may reduce this incidence in the next decade; however, only 60 percent of the source of infection can be identified and a large proportion of these high-risk groups cannot be identified before they are at risk of acquiring infections so they might receive the vaccine. The pool of carriers in the United States is also increasing, with 12,000 to 20,000 new individuals entering the pool each year.

Healthy People 2010 Objectives: Reduce Hepatitis A and B

Target for Hepatitis A: 4.5 new cases per 100,000 population.

Reduction in Hepatitis B	1997 Baseline (%)	2010 Target (%)
Rate per 100,000		
Adults		
19 to 24 years	24.0	2.4
25 to 39 years	20.2	5.1
40 years and older	15.0	3.8

Public health experts do not agree on who needs to be tested for hepatitis B and C infections. The CDC does not encourage universal testing because the treatment for symptom-free infected persons is problematic and the test for hepatitis C is not as precise as the CDC would want. The CDC does recommend testing pregnant women for hepatitis B, since they can pass the disease on to the fetus. Hepatitis D and hepatitis E also exist in the United States, however, they do not infect many people.

Hepatitis C Hepatitis C virus (HCV) infection is the most common bloodborne infection in the United States. Based on data from the CDC Sentinel Counties Study of Viral Hepatitis, it is estimated that as many as 180,000 new HCV infections occurred each year during the 1980s. Since 1989, the annual number of new infections has declined by 80 percent. However, in 1996, data from the third National Health and Nutrition Examination Survey, conducted from 1988 through 1994, indicated that approximately 4 million Americans (1.8 percent) are infected with HCV. Many of these chronically infected persons might not be aware of their infection or be clinically ill, because symptoms of hepatitis C-related chronic liver disease might not develop for ten to twenty years after infection. However, such persons can infect others and are at risk for chronic liver disease or other HCV-related chronic diseases. Cirrhosis develops in 10–20 percent of persons with HCV-related chronic hepatitis during the first two decades after infection, and 8,000–12,000 persons die from HCV-related chronic liver disease each year.[14]

Healthy People 2010 Objective: Reduce Hepatitis C

Target: 1 new case per 100,000 population.

Baseline: 2.4 new cases of hepatitis C per 100,000 population in selected counties in 1996.

Yellow Fever

The environmental reasons for vector-borne diseases are fairly well understood except for yellow fever. The virus is found only in the western hemisphere and

Africa. There is no evidence that yellow fever has even become established in the Asian tropics, even though many Asian mosquitoes are perfectly good vectors in the laboratory. Yellow fever struck repeatedly in the United States during the eighteenth and nineteenth centuries. The most recent epidemic struck New Orleans in 1905.

In 1904 when the United States took over the Canal Zone, this part of Panama was probably the most fever-ridden location on earth. The Panama Canal is probably the most compelling example of the price paid by countries due to vector disease. After eight years of effort, 300 million dollars and almost 20,000 deaths from malaria and yellow fever, the Compagnie Universelle du Canal Interoceanique de Panama went bankrupt and abandoned its efforts to build the canal. By 1905, more than 4,000 men were employed in mosquito extermination alone.

Parasites

Parasites are members of the animal kingdom that have acquired the power of living in the body of another animal known as the host. One of the most remarkable features of the parasite's life cycle is that the eggs produced in the body of a host do not develop in the same animal. They are transferred to a new reservoir by a vector. Disease-producing parasites belong to two groups, protozoa and worms. The worms are divided into roundworms, tapeworms, and flukes.[15]

Protozoa

Protozoa are single-cell animals that are parasitic and free-living. Protozoa are a serious problem in developing countries, but they exist in the United States as well. They are commonly found in fecally contaminated food and water and are carried by arthropod vectors. Common protozoa include:

1. Trypanosoma carried by the tsetse fly
2. Leishmania carried by sand flies
3. Plasmodium carried by anopheles mosquitos
4. Toxoplasma gondii carried in rat feces
5. Pneumocystis carini carried in human intestine
6. Trichomonads transmitted through sexual intercourse or close sexual contact
7. Giardia carried in contaminated water
8. Ectamoeba histolytica found in food and water[16]
9. Cryptosporidium found in food and water

Toxoplasmosis

Toxoplasmosis is a parasitic disease found throughout the world. It is caused by a single-celled organism called *Toxoplasma gondii.* Although up to 50 percent of the U.S. adult population has been infected with the parasite, most people show no signs or symptoms. However, pregnant women who acquire the infection may suffer stillbirth or birth babies with neurologic problems or blindness. In immune-deficiency patients, the illness can be fatal.

The primary sources of infection are cat feces and raw or poorly cooked meat. Emptying kitty-litter boxes and handling raw meat without washing hands immediately afterward are two of the most common ways people become infected. Although only 10 percent of adults will have symptoms, they include fluctuating low fever, swollen glands, muscle aches, rash, headache, and sore throat.

Malaria

Another good example of a vector-borne disease, caused by a protozoan, is malaria, spread by the water-breeding Anopheles mosquito. More than half the world's population live in malaria-prone regions in about 100 countries in tropical and subtropical regions.

Malarial parasites now infect an estimated 270 million people every year, killing more people than HIV. Its prevalence is approximately 500 million people worldwide. There is no cure. Malaria control has been tried by various methods (Figure 14.4), with marginal success. In 1955, WHO declared that the disease would soon be eradicated. Forty-five years later, in 2000, this was still only a wish. The safe, cheap drugs that used to provide effective protection against

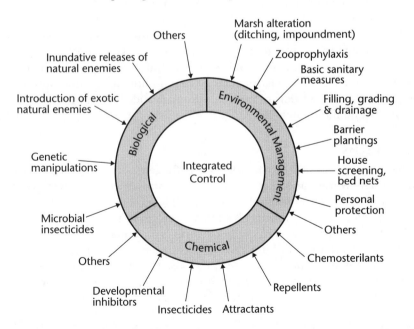

Figure 14.4 Components of mosquito, thus malaria control.

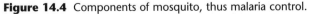

(*Source:* Reproduced, by permission of WHO, from *Manual on environmental management for mosquito control.* Geneva, World Health Organization, 1982, WHO Offset Publication #66)

malaria are no longer dependable in many parts of the world, since the parasite responsible for the severe form of the disease, known as ***Plasmodium falciparum***, is developing resistance to drugs. The mosquitos that transmit the parasite to humans are also developing resistance to pesticides in many parts of the world.[17]

Forty percent of the world's population, some 2.2 billion persons in over ninety different countries, live in areas threatened by malaria. The greatest number of cases is in Africa, and malaria is endemic in tropical Asia and Latin America.[18] One-tenth of all infant mortality in Africa, where rates are typically 150 deaths per 1,000 live births, is due to malaria. An average of four people in the United States discover they have malaria each day. Malaria is often cited as the most important communicable disease in the world.

Malaria was controlled before 1970 by spraying breeding areas with DDT, dieldrin, and other pesticides. Because of repeated spraying, most of the malaria-carrying species of **Anopheles** mosquito have become genetically resistant to most of the insecticides used. Today, in some parts of the world, progress against the disease is at a standstill, and in some areas the situation is worsening.[19]

The WHO estimates that only 3 percent of the money spent worldwide each year on biomedical research is devoted to malaria and other tropical diseases, even though more people suffer and die worldwide from these diseases than from all others combined. Early diagnosis and prompt treatment are fundamental to malaria control. Vector control includes environmental management to reduce or eliminate mosquito breeding sites.

Attempts at malaria eradication have, unfortunately, failed. Effective implementation of the WHO Global Malaria Control Strategy depends upon: (1) sustained political commitment from all sectors of government; (2) integration of malaria control into health systems, and coordination with relevant non-health sectors; (3) full partnership of communities in malaria control activities; and (4) mobilization of adequate human and financial resources, both nationally and internationally.[20]

Helminths

Helminths are parasitic worms that are pathogenic. They include flatworms such as tapeworms and flukes; and roundworms such as pinworms. Most helminths are found in tropical areas of the planet, infecting about 1.5 billion children and adults worldwide. They are a problem in the southern part of the United States in particular, where hookworm is a common problem.

Helminths can live in humans for years or decades producing eggs or larvae. They migrate through viscera via the vascular or intestinal systems. Their greatest threat to human life is the severe anemia or diarrhea they can produce as they use human nutrients, reproduce, to make produce toxins.

Fungi

Fungi, including yeasts and molds, are plants, although they are higher on the scale of life than bacteria. They lack chlorophyll, and they cannot manufacture their own food, so they are either saprophytes or parasites, living on and at the expense of other plants, animals, and people. Fungi are omnipresent in the air, so they can be generally troublesome. They require high humidity, warmth, and a free supply of oxygen.

Fungal infections known as the mycoses or mycotic diseases damage tissue through hypersensitivity to the proteins of the fungi. They can cause superficial infections and systemic infections. Common fungal infections include candida albicans or candidiasis, which causes vaginal yeast infections; histoplasmosis, which has had a reemergence since the AIDS epidemic; and dermatomycoses or ringworm, a contagious disease often seen in children. Prevention of these fungal infections includes maintaining an environment that is dry and not exposed to fungi. Treatment is usually penicillin and sulfa drugs.

Emerging New Diseases

One of the greatest concerns to community health and to the global community is the emergence of "new diseases." Actually, diseases that seem to appear overnight and spread at epidemic rates are usually not new, but previously contained, previously preventable, or previously geographically isolated pathogens that have evolved, mutated, spread, survived, and manifested themselves under new conditions. Among those recognized at the end of the twentieth century are: HIV, hantavirus, dengue hemorrhagic fever, Ebola virus, human papilloma virus, peptic ulcer virus, Creutzfeldt-Jacob disease, and herpes virus (Table 14.3).

The question raised most often by the public is, Why are these new diseases emerging? The answer lies in multiple causes, but in general it may be attributed to a twenty-first century global community, not nineteenth or early twentieth century definable communities. Almost all local problems now have global implications. The following factors have greatly increased the demand for disease surveillance and vigilance and certainly for prevention where possible:

1. Human demographic movement and change
2. Technological and industrial changes
3. Economic development and changes in land use
4. Travel and commerce
5. Adaptation, antimicrobial resistance, and mutation by organisms in the environment
6. Changes in climate and ecology
7. A breakdown and loss of commitment toward public health measures
8. Inadequate public health infrastructures and surveillance

Box 14.3 Hot Viruses

"A hot virus from the rain forest lives within a 24-hour plane flight from every city on earth. All of the earth's cities are connected by a web of airline routes. Once a virus hits the network, it can shoot anywhere in a day—"

Richard Preston, author of *The Hot Zone*

Table 14.3 Newly identified infectious diseases and pathogens.

Virus	Year	Virus	Year
Nipah virus	1999	Hepatitis E	1988
H5N1 (avian flu)	1997	Human herpesvirus 6	
nvCJD	1996	HIV	1983
Australian bat lyssavirus		*Escherichia coli* O157:H7	1982
HHV8 (Kaposi sarcoma virus)	1995	Lyme borreliosis	
Sabia virus	1994	HTLV-2 virus	
Hendra virus		Human T-lymphotropic virus	1980
Hantavirus pulmonary syndrome	1993	*Campylobacter jejuni*	1977
(Sin Nombre virus)		*Cryptosporidium parvum*	1976
Vibro cholerae O139	1992	Legionnaires' disease	
Guanarito virus	1991	Ebola	
Hepatitis C	1989		

(*Source:* WHO Fact Sheet, No. 97, 1998)

Anthrax

Anthrax is an acute infectious disease caused by a spore-forming bacterium called bacillus anthracis. Until 2001, it was a rarely occurring disease and was generally aquired following contact with anthrax-infected animals or anthrax-contaminated animal products. Anthrax has become a public health concern because of its use as a biological warfare agent in the twenty-first century. In humans, three types of anthrax infections can occur based on the route of exposure: cutaneous (skin exposure), inhalational (inhalation exposure), and gastrointestinal (ingestion exposure). Symptoms are dependent on the route of exposure. Those most often associated with skin infections are itching, boils, and formation of a black scab. Symptoms most often associated with inhalation infections are fever, chest pain, and difficulty breathing. Symptoms most often associated with ingestion infections are nausea, vomiting, and diarrhea. Direct person-to-person spread of anthrax is extremely unlikely, if it occurs at all.[21]

Exposure Through Criminal/Terrorist Acts Unsuspecting citizens and workers whose jobs would not ordinarily involve anthrax exposure (e.g., occupations that do not involve animals, animal hides, or fibers) have been exposed through acts of terrorism. Conventional thinking was that terrorists were likely to target places where large populations could be found such as large buildings, sporting events, or mass transit systems.[22] However, after the World Trade Center tragedy in 2001, anthrax terrorism was perpetrated by mailing anthrax spores to smaller targets which ultimately expanded the range of people exposed as a result of handling anthrax tainted envelopes. As an emergent new public health crisis, health initiatives are primarily directed toward job and personal safety through education that stresses awareness and vigilance. Public health will also begin preparations for other forms of biological warfare such as smallpox and botulism contamination.

Health Care Workers Health Care personnel working in occupational settings, such as hospitals, clinics, and laboratories, are susceptible to anthrax exposures from contaminated patients as well as clothing and/or equipment. Exposures can come from activities such as treating or decontaminating contaminated patients.[23]

Preventing Communicable Diseases: Immunization

Immunizing Against Infection

The decrease in incidence of infectious diseases is the most significant public health achievement of the past 100 years. Notwithstanding the progress made, infectious diseases remain important causes of illness and death in the United States. Many of these could be prevented through proper and universal immunization.

The beginning of immunization has been incorrectly cited as the day in 1796 when British physician, Edward Jenner, vaccinated his own young son against smallpox. He had noticed that milkmaids who caught a similar disease, cowpox, during the course or their work, were somehow protected against the more deadly human disease, smallpox. He reasoned correctly that if he injected material from the scab of a woman with cowpox into the bloodstream of volunteers, he could protect them against smallpox. His work was in fact preceded by the work of Mary Wortley Montagu who introduced inoculation against smallpox to Britain after she had seen it practiced in Turkey in 1716–1718. She used material from a smallpox scab but, because the disease was more serious than cowpox, the inoculation sometimes proved fatal.[24] This beginning in the science of immunization has probably been one of the most significant moments in human history.

Immunity

When a host has no specific resistance to a pathogen, the host is susceptible and may be converted to immunity status by a variety of mechanisms. Complete resistance to a pathogen is termed immunity and is specific for each infection. Immunity is the body's ability to produce antibodies, blood chemicals that kill, paralyze, agglutinize or engulf antigens, pathogenic organisms. There are different types of immunity.

Active acquired immunity occurs when a person's own immune system produces the necessary and specific antibodies to a particular antigen. After a person has had an infectious disease, such as measles, the flu, or even a cold, the body has an active immunity that prevents any further contagion (infection) by that specific antigen.

Active immunity can also occur by fooling the body into thinking it is exposed to a pathogen by inoculating the body through vaccination before any onset of a disease. Immunization of children or adults is the introduction of small amounts or attenuated amounts of antigen into the system to trigger the permanent production of antibodies.

Table 14.4 History of vaccine development since 1720 (approximate).

Year	Vaccine	Year	Vaccine	Year	Vaccine
1720	Smallpox	1945	Pertussis	1968	Rubella
1885	Rabies	1948	Yellow Fever	1970	Meningococcus
1918	Typhoid		Influenza	1974	Pneumococcus
1925	Tuberculosis	1952	Polio (Salk)	1978	Hepatitis B
	Diphtheria	1955	Polio (Sabin)	1985	H. Influenza b
1935	Tetanus	1960	Measles	1994	Hepatitis A
1941	Cholera	1965	Mumps		

(*Source:* Bennett, John V., 1991. Biological applications and interventions in public health, in *Oxford textbook of public health*. Vol. 3, p. 71. Used by permission of Oxford Press, London)

Table 14.5 Vaccination levels among children aged 19–35 months (1998).

Vaccine	Rate (percent)
Diphtheria-tetanus-pertussis (DtaP)	84
Haemophilus influenzae type b (Hib)	93
3 doses hepatis B vaccine (hep B)	87
Measles-mumps-rubella (MMR)	92
3 doses polio vaccine	91
1 dose varicella vaccine	43

(*Source:* Centers for Disease Control)

Passive immunity occurs when antibodies are produced in some other individual or animal and then "borrowed" by means of injecting them into the infected person's bloodstream. The duration of passive immunity activity is relatively short and is used when a susceptible person has been exposed to a disease and there is not enough time for the body to produce its own active immunity.

Acquired passive immunity are those antibodies that a newborn baby inherits from her or his mother as blood is diffused through the placenta into the fetus' bloodstream. It lasts approximately six months; however, it does not protect an infant from all pathogens during this time. This passive immunity can be extended if a baby is breastfed through the milk of the nursing mother.

Natural immunity is the genetic immunity one species may possess to a particular disease to which some other species is at risk or susceptible. For example, dogs can get distemper whereas humans exposed to this antigen do not become infected. Domestic animals are immune to human diseases such as measles.

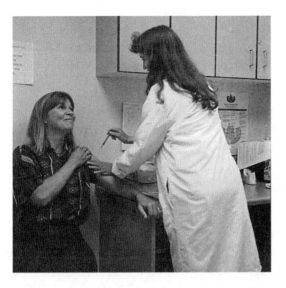

When a measles outbreak occurs, even adults must sometimes return for vaccination.

Vaccinating for Immunity

Over one dozen vaccines are used with some frequency in developed countries as a result of vaccine development since 1720 (Table 14.4). Eight of these vaccines are routinely used in U.S. childhood immunization programs—diphtheria, pertussis, tetanus, polio, measles, mumps, *Haemophilus influenza*, Hepatitis B, and rubella, but the percentage immunized varies by race, location, and economic status.

In recent decades the incidence of these eight diseases has fallen by over 99 percent, and vaccine coverage rates at school entry exceed 98 percent. Among the 2 percent of all unvaccinated adolescents in the United States, 40 percent live in the American inner-city populations. The percent of immunized children 19–35 months old in 1998 with Healthy People 2010 targets is given in Table 14.5.

Although immunization is usually required for public school admission, many states make exceptions. For instance, in Utah there are three exemptions:

1. Medical: A signed letter from a physician stating why a child should not be immunized;

2. Religious: A signed letter from a parent saying that immunizations are against one's religion;

3. Personal: A signed letter from a health worker and a parent expressing a personal reason for no immunization.

With these exemptions in even one state, it becomes clear that trying to immunize all children is very difficult.

In 1974, the World Health Assembly created the Expanded Programme on Immunization (EPI) to address a significant world problem. Less than 5 percent of the world's children are vaccinated for six preventable diseases: diphtheria, measles, pertussis, poliomyelitis, tetanus, and tuberculosis. When the EPI was formed, a goal of "Immunization for all by 1990" was set. Although the goal

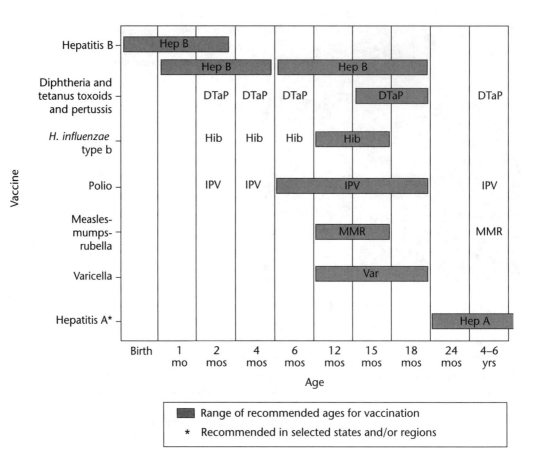

Figure 14.5 Recommended childhood immunization schedule.

(*Sources:* Centers for Disease Control. National Center for Health Statistics)

was not reached by 1990, great improvements were made. The use of vaccines has soared, and today over 60 percent of the world's children received the last of the three-dose series of either the polio or DPT vaccine. This translates into 1 to 2 million lives saved per year from the ravages of the six EPI identified diseases that killed 5 million children a year prior to vaccination. The recommended schedule for immunizing children is shown in Figure 14.5.

Sadly, 46 million infants are not yet fully immunized in the world today. Approximately 2.4 million children died of vaccine-preventable diseases in 1998, and of these close to 2 million died from measles alone; one every 15 seconds.[25]

Although there are about twenty vaccines in use for prevention of bacterial and viral infections (Table 14.6), a notable problem is the lack of useful vaccines for parasites that contribute to morbidity and mortality in developing countries. Parasites are a major cause of intestinal infections that cause severe diarrhea and dehydration throughout developing countries.

Table 14.6 Conventional human viral vaccines in use or in trial.

Current Vaccines		Vaccines Under Trial	
Agent	**Type**	**Agent**	**Type**
BCG	live, attenuated	M. leprae	inactivated
V. cholerae	inactivated	V. cholarae	subunit/whole organism
S. typhi	inactivated	V. cholarae	live, attenuated
S. pertussis	inactivated	S. typhi(Ty 21a)	live, attenuated
S. pneumaniae	cap. polysaccharide	S. typhi	live, attenuated
(pneumococcus)		(aro A mutant)	
H. influenzae,type B	cap. polysaccharide	S. typhi	Vi capsular polysaccharide
Cl. tetani (tetanus)	toxoid	B. pertussis	subunit(s)
C. diphthenae (diphtheria)		H. influenzae,	polyccharide/diptheria
Vaccinia	live, attenuated	type b	toxoid conjugate
Polio (OPV)	live, attenuated	Varicella-zoster	live, attenuated
Polio (IPV)	inactivated	Cytomegalo	live, attenuated
Measles	live, attenuated	Hepatitis A	inactivated
Adeno	live		live, attenuated
Yellow fever	live, attenuated	Influenza	
Mumps	live, attenuated	(ca-variant)	live, attenuated
Influenza	inactivated	(human-avian	live
Influenza	subunit	reassortant)	
Hepatitis B	subunit	Dengue	live, attenuated
Japanese B encephalitis	inactivated	Rota (Rhesus monkey)	live
Rabies	inactivated	(human)	live, attenuated
		Parainfluenza	live
		Type 3 (bovine)	
		Japanese B encephalitis	live, attenuated

(*Source:* Bennett, John V., 1991. Biological applications and interventions in Public Health. Vol. 3, p. 71. Used by per mission of Oxford Press, London)

The benefit/cost ratio of immunization programs provides one of the strongest returns of any health activity. For example, while the United States spent over $150 million per year in the 1960s to keep smallpox out of the United States through vaccination, a $30 million investment in global smallpox eradication now provides the United States with annual savings five times our total investment. United States investment exceeded our annual dues to the World Health Organization.[26]

Preventable Childhood Diseases

Pertussis

Pertussis, also known as whooping cough, is a potentially fatal childhood disease that can be prevented with the five-shot childhood DTP immunization series. There are presently about 4,500 pertussis cases a year in the United States and 50 million cases worldwide. Internationally, over 600,000 deaths from pertussis occur each year. A minority of those DPT immunized children may suffer lethargy, persistent crying, high fever, and loss of consciousness, with the traditional DTP series. The incidence of pertussis has declined from at least 100 per 100,000 cases per year from 1930–1945 to 1 per 100,000 during 1973–1985. There are now several thousand cases per year because of lack of vaccination.

Signs and Symptoms   The most characteristic symptom of pertussis is a wet cough that comes in paroxysms and is often preceded by a feeling of apprehension or anxiety and tightness in the chest. The disease usually lasts for a least six weeks regardless of treatments. Complications of pertussis may include cerebral hemorrhage, convulsions and brain damage, pneumonia, emphysema, or collapsed lung.[27] Antibiotics may help reduce the period of contagion. Pertussis immune globulin (an immune system booster) may help shorten the illness and prevent complications and death in children under two years of age.

Diphtheria

Diphtheria is an acute bacterial infection characterized by a sore throat and development of a membrane that may cover the throat. Complications of diphtheria include: (1) myocarditis, which can lead to heart failure, and (2) transitory paralysis of the limbs, muscles of respiration, or muscles of the throat or eye. Diphtheria is fatal in 10 to 15 percent of cases. The incubation period is two to four days.

Between 1900 and 1920 the mortality rate from diphtheria declined by 50 percent. This preceded the immunization era. By the 1960s the number of cases declined to 200 per 1,000 per year. In the 1980s there were zero to five cases per year. In 1990, there were only four reported diphtheria cases; however, after the collapse of the former Soviet Union, the situation changed dramatically. Epidemics broke out in Russia and Ukraine and spread throughout the region. In 1994, 47,802 cases and 1,742 deaths were recorded. WHO predicted that between 150,000 and 200,000 new cases will occur in the region in the next decade.[28]

Tetanus

Since 1976, there has been a decline in tetanus cases with less than 100 cases of tetanus per year in the United States. The majority of cases are people over fifty years old, and tetanus is now recognized as primarily a disease of older adults in the United States. It is recommended that all adults receive a tetanus booster every ten years. In 1985–1986 only five percent of tetanus cases were people less than twenty years old. Worldwide, however, tetanus kills 780,000 newborn babies a year.

Tetanus is caused by the introduction of the tetanus bacillus into an open wound, and is found in the soil and the intestinal tracts of farm animals. Incubation for tetanus varies from one day to three weeks. Treatment is drastic and includes muscle relaxants, sedatives, antibiotics, immune globulin, and antitoxins. Feeding is usually through a stomach tube and an artificial airway may be required.

> ## BOX 14.4 The DTP Controversy
>
> Among a variety of childhood immunizations, probably the most controversial is the DTP vaccination. DTP is a combination vaccination for diphtheria, tetanus, and pertussis. This vaccination is controversial to many parents because of the possible side effects of the pertussis part of the vaccine, which may include brain damage. A comprehensive DTP study, specifically looking at pertussis, was conducted at UCLA in 1978–1979. Children who received the DTP vaccine were compared to those who received the DT vaccine. The UCLA study data show that 50 percent of those vaccinated with DTP developed fever, 34 percent irritability, 35 percent had crying episodes, and 40 percent had localized inflammation. Excessive sleepiness was reported in 31 percent of DTP compared to 14 percent of DT controls. A similar 1983 study found significant difference in seizure occurrence when 134,000 children received DTP, compared to 133,000 DT recipients. Both studies have been criticized for threats to validity. The estimated risk of occurrence of persistent neurological damage one year later was 1:170,000.
>
> The results of the largest study of its kind ever done about the effects of pertussis vaccine was reported in the *Journal of the American Medical Association* in January 1994. This federally financed study of 218,000 children up to twenty-four months old, studied for one year, found that the vaccine does not lead to increased risk of serious neurological illness. Some have thought DTP is associated with SIDS. Reviewing seven major studies, the American Academy of Pediatrics Task Force on Pertussis concluded there is no convincing evidence for a causative role for DTP immunization in SIDS.

Measles

In the United States, only one child in every 1,000 is likely to have clinical measles. Of those infected with measles, 50 percent are among those five to nineteen years old, and 24 percent were over twenty years. The risk of measles in preschool-age African American and Hispanic children was eight to ten times higher than that of white children. There is a possibility, with universal immunization, that measles could be eradicated from the United States.

The major barrier to better worldwide measles control, especially in Africa, is the difficulty of immunizing children at an age early enough to prevent natural measles. Current vaccines, given as the measles-mumps-rubella (MMR) vaccine at age twelve to eighteen months, provide good protection in the absence of maternal antibodies. However, the presence of maternal antibodies provides variable risk rates before nine months of age. In many areas of the world, children are at risk of natural measles by five to six months of age.[29]

The WHO estimates that 1.1 million deaths associated with measles occur each year worldwide. If the measles vaccination program were terminated there would be massive epidemics worldwide.

Polio

The introduction of inactivated polio vaccine in 1955 led to a rapid decrease in poliomyelitis incidence. When the oral polio vaccine was introduced, the reduction was dramatic, and the United States is now considered to be free of wild polio virus. There were, however, seven reported cases of polio in 1990; all were vaccine associated.

In developing countries where polio is endemic, WHO believes polio can be eliminated in the twenty-first century. The Pan American Health Organization launched a program in 1986 to eliminate polio from the western hemisphere by the end of 1990. In May 1988, the WHO set a similar target of eradication of polio for the entire planet for the year 2000, which was met for the Western Hemisphere.

Two good vaccines, inactivated and oral, exist for the prevention of polio, yet both vaccines have limitations. The oral vaccine is easily administered, is widely used in countries that have become polio free, and has the advantage of immunity spread from those directly immunized to others not immunized. It has the disadvantage of poor results in tropical areas, thought to be due to the interference of other intestinal viruses. Inactivated vaccines have been recently improved and under field conditions in Geneva have been shown to provide 89 percent efficacy with two doses. An advantage of inactivated vaccine is that it can be combined with DPT. The disadvantage is that the inactivated vaccine is more expensive than oral vaccine, and if combined with DTP, is not given until six weeks of age.[30]

An interesting and sad development is that many people who suffered polio in the 1940s and 1950s are now experiencing a recurrence of debilitating symptoms called post-polio syndrome. Science is not sure why this is occurring, however, people who have had polio should be aware of this possibility and seek medical care.

Mumps

Mumps is an RNA virus acquired by the respiratory route that infects the salivary glands and sometimes the ovaries, testes, and pancreas. After an incubation period of two to three weeks, the disease starts with malaise and fever and is usually followed by painful swelling of the parotid glands.[31]

Rubella (German Measles)

Rubella virus is also a small RNA virus transmitted via the respiratory system. It causes a mild disease characterized by a light rash, low-grade fever, and lymphadenopathy. The importance of rubella is that it is a major cause of congenital heart defects, cataracts, mental retardation, or deafness in the infant when acquired by the mother in the first trimester of pregnancy.[32]

Mumps and rubella vaccines are now included with the measles vaccine (MMR), the combination reaching over 98 percent of children by school entry. For rubella, one child in 10,000 will get the natural disease, thus decreasing the risk of disease in pregnant women who may be exposed to the virus while interacting with an infected child.

There is a belief among some that mumps and rubella can be wiped from the planet within ten years if a global effort is initiated. Since mumps and

> ### *BOX 14.5 Smallpox*
>
> On October 26, 1977 in the town of Merka, Somalia, the last case of naturally occurring smallpox was reported. The eradication of smallpox, eighteen decades after Jenner's discovery of a vaccine, culminated the most extensive global health initiative that had ever and probably ever will be attempted. In one decade, from 1966–1976, the world-wide record of over 130,000 reported cases annually (and millions of unreported cases) dwindled to zero.[33]

rubella are less infectious than measles, and since they can be joined with the measles vaccine at almost no additional cost, it is logical for the world to consider giving MMR vaccine everyplace where the world is now giving only measles vaccine, according to the World Health Organization.

Unfortunately, the WHO task force concluded that five other disease are *not* now candidates for global eradication: hepatitis B, neonatal tetanus, diphtheria, pertussis, and yellow fever.

Haemophilus Influenzae **Type B**

Since 1985 children have been vaccinated against *Haemophilus influenzae* type B (Hib), the most common cause of bacterial meningitis and other severe infections in the extremely young. Hib can cause meningitis, encephalitis, retardation, and other severe, potentially deadly conditions. It is now recommended that Hib vaccines be given at the same time as the DPT shot, in the other arm. A new study of children in the United States shows the vaccine has produced a huge benefit, preventing illness and by extension, saving lives and preventing mental retardation and hearing loss, two potential aftereffects of Hib infections.

The number of Hib infections among babies has plummeted since 1985, with Hib-caused hospitalizations falling from 151 per 100,000 children to 6 per 100,000. This reduction corresponds with a reduction in related Hib infections from 12,000 meningitis cases annually to only 1,200 in 1998.

Pneumococcal Pneumonia

Each year up to 60,000 adults, most sixty-five years and older, die of preventable infectious diseases (influenza, pneumococcal infection, and hepatitis B). The recent development of the pneumococcal vaccine can prevent up to 60 percent of serious pneumococcal infections. This vaccine is a once-in-a-lifetime shot that prevents the most common type of deadly pneumonia.

Summary

The eradication of smallpox gave the world hope that other organisms that cause disease might also be eradicated. Unfortunately, this has not been the case. Microorganisms have the same need and ability to survive as humans and animals. As they are attacked by pesticides and pharmaceuticals, they evolve through mutation or resistance to more virulent or complex forms.

Further, our global society is so transient and mobile that isolating disease is very difficult and sometimes impossible due to long incubation periods, carriers, poor and inadequate reporting, and the myriad of social problems in the world that contribute to disease.

Fortunately, for those of us in the United States, communicable diseases, with the exception of perhaps STDs, are not a major threat at this time, giving us the opportunity to study and prevent chronic diseases. However, "ever vigilant" should be our motto.

It is too bad that a controversy has arisen about the use of childhood immunization, because vaccination has been one of the most effective community health initiatives in all of history. Immunization has saved more lives and changed the course of human events in ways that will never be completely appreciated. The role of community health education now is to resell the value of immunization to those who are afraid and to the governmental agencies that will need to allocate resources and energy to a renewed effort of public immunization.

Cybersites Related to Chapter 14

Disease Prevention
   www.cdc.gov/nccdphp
   www.cdc.gov/ncidod
   www.cdc.gov/niosh/homepage.html
   www.cdc.gov/ncipc
   www.who.int

Questions

1. Select one communicable disease. How would the world go about eradicating this disease?

2. What are the major communicable diseases of your community and what is being done by your community to eliminate or reduce their incidence?

3. Should the federal government finance a public child immunization program? Why? Why not?

4. What are the factors that make the United States at risk for another measles epidemic? How at risk is your university or college for a measles epidemic?

5. What are the pros and cons of immunizing a child with DPT?

Exercises

1. Become familiar with the TB prevention program in your community. Through interviews, visits, and media, determine what personal, governmental, and community action is being taken. How do each of the following populations interpret and respond to TB—school systems, prisons, local health departments, immigrants, politicians, and parents?

2. Go through your health history, and if you have children, go through their history and document when all immunizations were given. If any boosters need to be given, make arrangements to do so.

INTERNET INTERACTIVE ACTIVITY

NATIONAL NOTIFIABLE DISEASES SURVEILLANCE SYSTEM

The National Electronic Telecommunications System for Surveillance (NETSS) is a computerized public health surveillance system that provides weekly data on cases of nationally notifiable diseases. The information and description page for NETSS is:

www.cdc.gov/eod/hissb/act_int.htm

The Centers for Disease Control and Prevention (CDC) acts as a common agent for the states and territories in the collection and reporting of nationally notifiable diseases. Reports of the occurrences of nationally notifiable diseases are transmitted to CDC each week from the fifty states, two cities, and five territories through the National Electronic Telecommunications System for Surveillance. Provisional data are published weekly in the *Morbidity and Mortality Weekly Report;* final data are published each year in the annual *Summary of Notifiable Diseases, United States.* The timeliness of the provisional weekly reports provides information that CDC and state or local epidemiologists use to detect and more effectively interrupt outbreaks. Also, reporting provides the timely information needed to measure and demonstrate the impact of changed immunization laws or a new therapeutic modality. The finalized annual data also provide information on reported disease incidence, which is necessary for the study of epidemiologic trends and the development of disease prevention policies. Different reportable diseases will be featured periodically on the *Social Statistics Briefing Room.*

Example

The community health educator would like to know the summary of reported cases, by month, United States, 1998.

1. Go to the CDC homepage for the summary of notifiable diseases in the United States:

www2.cdc.gov/mmwr/summary.html

2. Click on **View This Issue**

3. Scroll through this document and note the outbreaks of various diseases by month, state, region, age group, and ethnicity.

Exercise

The community heath educator wants to know what disease outbreaks were most prevalent during winter months of the most recent year. The educator also wants to know how her or his state compares with the states that border the state in terms of the incidence of influenza, gonorrhea, lyme disease, toxic shock, hepatitis A, B, and C, and mumps.

1. Go to the most recent **Summary of Notifiable Diseases, United States.**

2. Build a table that will answer the question above regarding most prevalent diseases during the winter months.

3. Build a table that compares the diseases above by your state and the bordering states.

4. Based on the available data:

   What is the trend for measles?

   Where is lyme disease most prevalent?

   Who has the highest rates of gonorrhea by race?

   What is the most common cause of botulism?

   In what states has cholera been reported? Why do you think this is?

   What is the age group most at risk for pertussis?

   What is the difference between TB for U.S. and foreign-born persons?

   What is the most common STD?

   Do we still have leprosy in the United States? Where? How many cases a year?

REFERENCES

1. Mulvihill, Mary Lou (1991). *Human diseases, a systemic approach*, 3rd ed. Norwalk: Appleton & Lange.

2. Ibid.

3. Boyd, William (1971). *An introduction to the study of disease*, 6th ed. Philadelphia: Lea and Febiger.

4. Gregg, Michael, & Parsonnet, Julie (1991). The principles of an epidemic field investigation. In *Oxford textbook of public health*, Vol. II, pp. 400–415. New York: Oxford University Press.

5. Hansfield, H. Hunter (1993). *Chlamydia in the '90's*. New Jersey: Roche Molecular Systems.

6. *Salt Lake Tribune* (1994). Antibiotics losing their punch in bacteria fight. February 20, p. A7.

7. www.who.int/infectious-disease-report/pages/graph3.html

8. Manning, Anita (1992). Tuberculosis makes a menacing comeback. *USA Today*, November 17, 1992. p. 4D.

9. www.who.int/infectious-disease-report/pages/graph3.html

10. Manning, op. cit.

11. Gore, Al. (1992). *The earth in balance*. New York: Houghton McMillan.

12. Boyd, William (1971). *An introduction to the study of disease.*, 6th ed. Philadelphia: Lea & Febiger.

13. Blank, Jonah (1994). Bombay's rat patrol takes on the plague. *US News and World Report*, October 10, p. 14.

14. www.cdc.gov/epo/mmwr/preview/mmwrhtml/00056071.htm#00003632.htm

15. Mulvihill, op. cit.

16. Ibid.

17. WHO (1992). *Facts about WHO*. Geneva: WHO.

18. Ibid.

19. Ibid.

20. Bryan, Jenny (1988). *Health and science*. New York: Hampstead Press.

21. http://www.osha.gov/bioterrorism/anthraxfactsheet.html (2001). OSHA Fact Sheet and References on Worker Health and Safety for Anthrax Exposure.

22. Ibid.

23. Ibid.

24. Manning, Anita (1995). Many young adults at risk for measles. *USA Today*, August 11, p. D1.

25. Bennett, op. cit.

26. Ibid.

27. Neustaedter, Randall (1990). *The immunization decision*. Berkeley, CA: North Atlantic Books.

28. *Public Health Reports* (1995). Diptheria epidemic becomes international heath emergency. Sept/Oct, Vol. 110, p. 514.

29. Cody, C. Baraff, L. J., et al. (1981). Nature and rates of adverse reactions associated with DTP and DT immunization in infants and children. *Pediatrics, 68,* 650–660.

30. Bennett, op. cit.

31. Kent, Thomas H., & Hart, Michael (1993). *Introduction to human disease*, 3rd ed. Norwalk, Conn: Appleton-Century-Crofts.

32. Ibid.

33. Bennett, op. cit.

CHAPTER 15

Occupational Health

Community Health in the 21st Century
(1) Continuing efforts in reducing cumulative trauma disorders, ergonomic
awareness and reducing risks associated with back injuries. (2) Training in
regard to bloodborne pathogens and prevention through inoculation. (3) Cor-
porate support for health/physical fitness via worksite health promotion
which includes: spa discount memberships, health needs assessments,
seminars, walking tracks, and wellness resources.

—James C. Bergseng, B.S. Community Health Education
Project Safety Engineer

Chapter Objectives

The student will:

1. list, in order, the ten major occupational health conditions.

2. describe the role of OSHA in preventing occupational injuries.

3. suggest prevention measures that can be taken in industry, agriculture, and business to reduce occupational injuries and deaths.

4. explain the purpose of HAZCOM and the responsibilities of employers and employees under this law.

Health Risks of Working People

On March 25, 1911, 146 people, most of them women, burned to death because the doors of Triangle Shirtwaist Company were locked. The Manhattan factory, where low-wage piecework was done, locked the doors as a preventive measure against even a momentary lull in productivity. Unbelievably, a similar incident occurred in 1993, when the fire doors to a poultry processing factory in North Carolina were sealed shut to prevent workers from exiting. When a fire broke out in the poultry processing factory, many people, almost exclusively women, were killed.

Today, preventive measures in the workplace mean saving people's lives and reducing their risk. Unfortunately, without government oversight and health and safety legislation, workplaces often remain dangerous environments, much like workplaces of the past. For instance, over 22,000 garment factories in this country, hiring mostly immigrant women, remain dangerous, demanding, low-paying, unventilated, fire hazards with little, if any, safety inspection, correction, or oversight. Additionally, in New York City, locked exits is the second most common safety violation.[1]

Over 117 million U.S. citizens spend about one-third of their time daily either at work or in transit between home and work. The role of community health education in the workplace is to protect the worker through a safe and risk-free environment. Early efforts to promote health in the workplace have come from unions that have demanded healthy environments and health benefits for their membership. In the past few decades, the federal government has stepped in to assure health and safety for workers who do not have the representation of unions.

A total of 5.9 million injuries and illnesses were reported in private industry workplaces during 1998, resulting in a rate of 6.7 cases per 100 equivalent full-time workers.[2] The National Institute for Occupational Safety and Health (NIOSH) estimates that each year in the United States about 100,000 people die from occupational illnesses, and about 2 million suffer disabling injuries on the job. This means that each day an average of 137 persons die from work-related diseases, and an additional seventeen die from injuries on the job. Although the legal responsibility for the health and safety of workers lies with businesses and management, inadequate and negligent health and safety promotion in the workplace affects the families and communities of workers and makes occupational health a public health concern. Preventing occupational injuries has become a major focus and responsibility of employees, employers, unions, and government-regulating agencies.

Two-thirds of workers in the world today have working conditions below the minimum standards set by the International Labour Organisation. Worldwide, there are 33 million occupational injuries per year with about 145,000 deaths. Although global data are not carefully collected, it is known that workers in many countries still suffer from occupational hazards that resemble those found among American workers.[3]

The diseases caused in and by the workplace span a broad range of human illnesses and traumas as shown on Table 15.1. There were about 392,000 newly reported cases of occupational illnesses in private industry in 1998. Manufacturing accounted for three-fifths of these cases. Disorders associated with repeated trauma, such as carpal tunnel syndrome and noise-induced hearing loss, were the dominant type of illness reported, making up 65 percent of the 392,000 total illness cases.[4] Other morbidity on the job include: lung cancer and mesothelioma in asbestos workers, cancer of the bladder in dye workers, leukemia in workers exposed to benzene, chronic bronchitis in workers exposed to dusts, heart disease among workers exposed to carbon monoxide, disorders of the nervous system among workers using solvents, kidney failure

Table 15.1   Occupations and their risks.

Type of Work	Common Hazards	Health Effects
Household workers: over 859,000	Cleaning substances (drain and oven cleaners, bleach, aerosol sprays, waxes), pesticides	Irritation or burns of skin, eyes or lungs, allergies
	Lifting, falls, infections from children, electric shock, noise	Muscle soreness, slipped disc, torn ligaments, bursitis
Clerical workers: over 14.7 million	Stress, video display terminals (VDTs)	Headache, heart disease, eyestrain, neck and back pain
	Poor air quality and ventilation, toxic substances from photocopy, duplicators, corrections fluids	Nausea, colds, respiratory problems, eye, nose and throat irritation
		Cardiovascular disease
	Noise	Anxiety, hearing damage
	Poor lighting and chair design	Varicose veins, neck and back pain, eyestrain
Hospital workers: 3.7 million	Infections	Infection from patients, utensils, specimens
	Lifting and falls	Back strain, slipped disc, torn ligaments
	Radiation	Tissue damage, genetic changes from x-rays and chemical hazards
	Chemical hazards (sterilizing gases, anesthetic gases, drugs)	Skin and respiratory irritation, liver, kidney, nervous system damage, cancer, reproductive problems
	Stress, electric shock	Headaches, heart disease, gastrointestinal problems
Retail salespersons: 4.1 million	Standing lifting, stress	Leg pain, varicose veins, back and shoulder pain, headaches, irritability, high blood pressure
	Safety hazards (blocked aisles, exits; poorly designed equipment)	Accidents
	Poor ventilation	Colds, respiratory problems, eye, nose and throat irritation
	Infection	Communicable diseases
Artists: 115,000	Solvents	Dizziness, dermatitis, damage to liver, kidneys, nervous system
	Paints, solder	Damage to kidneys, liver, lungs, reproductive system, from heavy metals
	Clays, glazes, welding fumes, fumes from firing	Lung damage
	Poor equipment maintenance; poor ventilation	Accidents, fire
Health care lab workers: 240,000	Handling biological specimens or animals	Infection
Lab technicians and related support staff: 1,872,000	Toxic chemicals, including carcinogens	Organ damage, changes in genetic material, reproductive problems, cancer
	Radiation in specimens, radioisotopes, machinery using radiation	Tissue changes or genetic changes, reproductive problems

Table 15.1   *(Continued)*

Type of Work	Common Hazards	Health Effects
Textile, apparel and furnishings machine operators (includes sewers and stitchers): 949,000	Chemicals (fabric treatment, dyes, cleaning solvents)	Skin and lung irritation, damage to liver, kidney and nervous system, dermatitis
	Synthetic fiber and cotton dust	Asthma, respiratory disease
	Noise	Hearing loss
	Vibration	Wrist and hand inflammation
	Heat, cold, poor ventilation	Heat stress, colds
	Unsafe equipment	Accidents, electric shock
	Lifting, standing, sitting	Back and shoulder strain, varicose veins
	Stress	High blood pressure, headaches, anxiety
Electrical and electronic technicians: 47,600	Solvents	Dermatitis, dizziness, damage to nervous system and organs such as liver
	Acids	Skin burns and irritation
	Sitting and standing, fine work under microscope, repetitive work	Back and shoulder pain, varicose veins, headaches
	Stress	Heart disease, gastrointestinal problems
	Solder fumes, poor ventilation	Eye, nose and throat irritation, lung disease
Meat wrappers: number unknown	Lifting	Shoulder and back strain
	Standing	Low back pain, varicose veins
	Repetitive motion	Swelling and inflammation of the hands
	Plastic wrap fumes	Asthma, eye, nose and throat irritation, nausea, flulike symptoms
	Cold, cuts, slips, falls	Numbness, circulation problems
Hairdressers and beauticians: 672,000	Standing	Low back pain and varicose veins
	Chemicals (hair sprays and dyes, aerosol sprays, cosmetics and other preparations)	Lung disease, reproductive effects, cancer, allergies, skin irritation
Laundry and dry cleaners: 269,000	Laundry: soaps, bleaches, acids	Irritation or burns on hands, irritation of eyes, nose or throat
	Dry cleaning: solvents	Dermatitis, dizziness, damage to nervous system or liver
	Both: lifting	Back injuries, strains, hernias
	Heat	Heart disease
	Contamination	Exposure to whatever chemicals or biologicals are used

(*Source: The new our bodies, ourselves.* Boston Women's Health Collective, Simon and Schuster, 1992. Reprinted with permission)

in lead workers, infertility in men and women using lead and certain pesticides, and traumatic musculoskeletal injuries.[5] Table 15.2 is a rather interesting list of specific diseases and disabilities associated with their industry or occupation.

New occupational diseases, such as the repetitive trauma of carpal tunnel syndrome, are occurring as a result of new technology that uses repeated

Table 15.2   Occupationally related unnecessary disease, disability, and death.

Condition	Industry/Occupation	Agent
Pulmonary tuberculosis (O)	Physicians, medical personnel	*Mycobacterium tuberculosis*
Silicotuberculosis	Quarrymen, sandblasters, silica processors, mining, metal foundries, ceramic industry	$SiO2$.—*Mycobacterium tuberculosis*
Plague (O)	Farmers, ranchers, hunters, field geologists	*Yersinia pestis*
Tularemia (O)	Hunters, fur handlers, sheep industry workers, cooks, veterinarians, ranchers	*Francisella tularensis*
Anthrax (O)	Shepherds, farmers, butchers, handlers of imported hides or fibers, veterinarians, veterinarian pathologists, weavers	*Bacillus anthracis*
Brucellosis (O)	Farmers, shepherds, veterinarians, laboratory workers, slaughterhouse workers	*Brucella abortus, suis*
Tetanus (O)	Farmers, ranchers	*Clostridium tetani*
Rubella (O)	Medical personnel, intensive care personnel	Rubella virus
Hepatitis A (O)	Day care center staff, orphanage staff, mental retardation institution staff, medical personnel	Hepatitis A virus
Hepatitis B (O)	Nurses and aides, orphanage and mental institution staff, medical personnel	Hepatitis B virus
Non-A, non-B hepatitis (O)	As above from hepatitis A and B	Unknown
Rabies (O)	Veterinarians, animal and game wardens, laboratory researchers, farmers, ranchers, trappers	Rabies virus
Ornithosis (O)	Bird breeders, pet shop staff, poultry producers, veterinarians, zoo employees	*Chlamydia psittaci*
Hemangiosarcoma of the liver	Vinyl chloride polymerization industry, vintners	Vinyl chloride monomer Arsenical pesticides
Malignant neoplasm of nasal cavities (O)	Woodworkers, cabinet-makers, furniture makers Radium chemists and processors Chromium producers, users Nickel smelting and refining	Hardwood dusts Radium Chromates Nickel
Malignant neoplasm of larynx (O)	Asbestos industries and utilizers	Asbestos
Malignant neoplasm of trachea, bronchus, and lung (O)	Asbestos industries and utilizers Topside coke oven workers Uranium and fluorspar miners Chromium producers, users Nickel smelters, processors, users Smelters Mustard gas formulators Ion exchange resin makers, chemists	Asbestos Coke oven emissions Radon daughters Chromates Nickel Arsenic Mustard gas Bis (chloromethyl) ether, chloromethyl methyl ether
Mesothelioma	Asbestos industries and utilizers	Asbestos
Malignant neoplasm of bone (O)	Radium chemists and processors	Radium
Malignant neoplasm of scrotum	Automatic lathe operators, metal workers Coke oven workers, petroleum refiners, tar distillers	Mineral/cutting oils Soots and tars, tar distillates
Malignant neoplasm of bladder	Rubber and dye workers	Benzidine, naphthylamine, auramine, magenta amino-biphenyl, 4-nitrophenyl

Table 15.2   (*Continued*)

Condition	Industry/Occupation	Agent
Malignant neoplasm of kidney and other urinary organs (O)	Coke oven workers	Coke oven emissions
Lymphoid leukemia, acute (O)	Rubber industry Radiologists	Unknown Ionizing radiation
Myeloid leukemia, acute (O)	Occupations with exposure to benzene Radiologists	Benzene Ionizing radiation
Erythroleukemia (O)	Occupations with exposure to benzene	Benzene
Hemolytic anemia, nonautoimmune (O)	Whitewashing and leather industry Electrolytic processes, arsenical ore smelting Plastics industry Dye, celluloid, resin industry	Copper sulphate Arsine Trimellitic anhydride Naphthalene
Aplastic anemia (O)	Explosives manufacture Occupations with exposure to benzene Radiologists, radium chemists	TNT Benzene Ionizing radiation
Agranulocytosis or neutropenia (O)	Occupations with exposure to benzene Explosives and pesticide industries Pesticides, pigments, pharmaceuticals	Benzene Phosphorus Inorganic arsenic
Methemoglobinemia (O)	Explosives and dye industries	Aromatic amino and nitro compounds
Toxic encephalitis (O)	Battery, smelter, and foundry workers	Lead
Inflammatory and toxic neuropathy (O)	Pesticides, pigments, pharmaceuticals Furniture refinishers, degreasing operations Plastic-coated-fabric workers Explosives industry Rayon manufacturing Plastics, hydraulics, coke industries Battery, smelter, and foundry workers Dentists, chloralkali workers Chloralkali plants, fungicide makers, battery makers Plastic industry, paper manufacturing	Arsenic and arsenic compounds Hexane Methyl *n*-butyl ketone TNT CS2 Tri-*o*-cresyl phosphate Inorganic lead Inorganic mercury Organic mercury
Cataract (O)	Microwave and radar technicians Explosives industries Radiologists Blacksmiths, glass blowers, bakers Moth repellent formulators, fumigators Explosives, dye, herbicide and pesticide industries	Microwaves TNT Ionizing radiation Infrared radiation Naphthalene Dinitrophenol, dinitro-*o*-cresol
Noise effects on inner ear (O)	Exposure	Excessive noise
Raynaud's phenomenon (secondary) (O)	Lumberjacks, chain sawyers, grinders, chippers Vinyl chloride polymerization industry	Whole-body or segmental vibration Vinyl chloride monomer
Extrinsic allergic alveolitis	Farmer's lung, baggassosis, bird fancier's lung, malt worker's lung, mushroom worker's lung, maple bark disease, miller's lung	Various agents
Extrinsic asthma (O)	Jewelry, alloy and catalyst makers Polyurethane, adhesive, paint workers Alloy, catalyst, refinery workers Solderers Plastic, dye, insecticide makers	Platinum Isocyanates Chromium and cobalt Aluminum soldering flux Phthalic anhydride

(*Continued*)

Table 15.2   Occupationally related unnecessary disease, disability, and death. *(Continued)*

Condition	Industry/Occupation	Agent
Extrinsic asthma (O) *(continued)*	Foam workers, latex makers, biologists	Formaldehyde
	Printing industry	Gum arabic
	Nickel platers	$NiSO_4$
	Bakers	Flour
	Plastics industry	Trimellitic anhydride
	Woodworkers, furniture makers	Red cedar and other wood dusts
	Detergent formulators	*Bacillus*-derived exoenzymes
Coalworkers pneumocconiosis	Coal miners	Coal dust
Asbestosis	Asbestos industries and utilizers	Asbestos
Silicosis	Quarrymen, sandblasters, silica processors, mining, metal, and ceramic industries	Silica
Talcosis	Talc processors	Talc
Chronic beryllium disease of the lung	Beryllium alloy workers, ceramic and cathode ray tube makers, nuclear reactor workers	Beryllium
Byssinosis	Cotton industry workers	Cotton, flax, hemp, and cotton-synthetic dusts
Acute bronchitis, pneumonitis, and pulmonary edema due to fumes and vapors (O)	Refrigeration, fertilizer, oil refining	Ammonia
	Alkali and bleach industries	Chlorine
	Silo filters, arc welders, nitric acid industry	Nitrogen oxides
	Paper and refrigeration industries, oil refining	Sulphur dioxide
	Cadmium smelters, processors	Cadmium
	Plastics industry	Trimellitic anhydride
Toxic hepatitis (O)	Solvent utilizers, dry cleaners, plastics industry	Carbon tetrachloride, chloroform, tetrachloroethane, trichloroethylene
	Explosives and dye industries	Phosphorus, TNT
	Fire and waterproofing additive formulators	Chloronaphthalenes
	Plastics formulators	Methylenedianiline
	Fumigators, gasoline, fire extinguisher formulators	Ethylene dibromide
	Disinfectant, fumigant, synthetic resin formulators	Cresol
Acute or chronic renal failure (O)	Battery makers, plumbers, solderers	Inorganic lead
	Electrolytic processes, arsenical ore smelting	Arsine
	Battery makers, jewellers, dentists	Inorganic mercury
	Fluorocarbon formulators, fire extinguisher makers	Carbon tetrachloride
	Antifreeze manufacture	Ethylene glycol
Infertility, male (O)	Formulators	Kepone
	DBCP producers, formulators, and applicators	Dibromochloropropane
Contact and allergic dermatitis (O)	Leather tanning, poultry dressing plants, fish packing, adhesives and sealant industry, boat building and repair	Irritants (e.g., cutting oils, solvents, acids, alkalis), allergens

(Source: Landrigan, P. J. & Baker, D. B., 1991. In *Oxford textbook of public health,* 2nd ed. Vol 3, pp. 456–457. By permission of the Oxford University Press)

motions of computer work or mass production technology. This was 60 percent of the year's job-related injuries and illnesses and was seen most often among keyboard operators and production line workers. In 2000, NIOSH announced broad rules effected in 2001 that protect 100 million workers from repetitive stress injuries. See Table 15.3.

Table 15.3 Number and percent of non-fatal occupational injuries involving repetitive motion (1997).

Occupation	Repetitive Motion		Repetitive Typing or Keyentry		Repetitive Use of Tools		Repetitive Placing, Grasping, or Moving Objects, Except Tools	
	Number	Percent	Number	Percent	Number	Percent	Number	Percent
All occupations	75,188	100.0	11,160	100.0	10,471	100.0	24,621	100.0
Assemblers	6,874	9.1	—	—	1,541	14.7	2,846	11.6
Laborers, nonconstruction	3,464	4.6	—	—	495	4.7	1,548	6.3
Textile sewing machine operators	2,049	2.7	—	—	80	0.8	1,100	4.5
Truck drivers	1,614	2.1	—	—	169	1.6	561	2.3
Cashiers	1,546	2.1	187	1.7	98	0.9	503	2.0
Packaging and filling machine operators	1,473	2.0	—	—	66	0.6	824	3.3
Secretaries	1,464	1.9	1,096	9.8	54	0.5	46	0.2
Welders and cutters	1,315	1.7	—	—	451	4.3	409	1.7
Machine operators, not specified	1,268	1.7	—	—	164	1.6	584	2.4
Electrical and electronic equipment assemblers	1,221	1.6	—	—	286	2.7	455	1.8
Data-entry keyers	1,177	1.6	1,015	9.1	57	0.5	—	—
Janitors and cleaners	944	1.3	—	—	209	2.0	375	1.5
Hand packers and packagers	943	1.3	—	—	—	—	686	2.8
Cooks	882	1.2	—	—	153	1.5	270	1.1
Stock handlers and baggers	868	1.2	—	—	—	—	429	1.7
Production inspectors, checkers, and examiners	820	1.1	—	—	78	0.7	434	1.8
General office clerks	817	1.1	507	4.5	—	—	74	0.3
Construction laborers	775	1.0	—	—	355	3.4	149	0.6

(*Source:* Occupational Safety & Health Administration, Department of Labor Statistics)

Occupational Risks

The full range of occupational risks is unknown; however, the list seems to be endless given the types of occupations and the types of jobs that put people at risk as noted in Table 15.2. For example, 8 to 10 million workers have been or are currently exposed to asbestos. Half a million workers have been exposed to cotton dust. Five percent of coal miners develop pneumoconiosis (black lung disease), and 1 million workers are exposed to silica in mines, foundries, blasting, stone, and glass industries. There are high rates of leukemia among shoemakers, rubber tire workers, and glue workers who use benzene-based compounds. High bladder cancer rates are found among dye workers, and neurological damage occurs among industrial painters and pesticide manufacturers. Multiple myeloma is found among petroleum workers, pancreatic and rectal cancer among thorium refinery workers, and sterility, melanoma, leukemia, and Hodgkin's disease are found to be high among farmworkers.[7] It is estimated that 7.7 million workers are exposed full time to one or more neurotoxic agents such as chlorinated hydrocarbons and other acrylamides.

Repetitive motion injuries like carpal tunnel syndrome are occurring more frequently as more workers use computers or mass production technology.

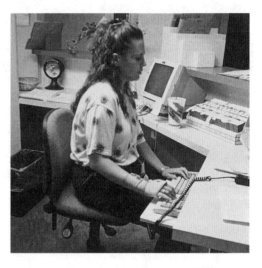

BOX 15.1 *Common Occupational Environmental Hazards and Resulting Health Problems*[6]

1. Temperature—heatstroke, burns, heat rashes, frostbite, hypothermia, trench-foot
2. Illumination—fatigue, accidents, burns
3. Vibration—neuritis, decalcification of the carpal and metacarpal bones, muscle atrophy, Raynaud's syndrome (dead fingers)
4. Ergonomics—back pain, headaches, nervousness, aching muscles, depression
5. Noise—hearing loss, fatigue, insomnia, psychological disorders, ulcers
6. Electromagnetic radiation—cell damage, genetic damage, nausea, fatigue, blood and intestinal disorders, hair loss, CNS damage, lung cancer, skin cancer, and leukemia
7. Dusts, fumes, gases, mists and aerosols—respiratory distress

---

White-collar and service sector workers are also at risk. Carpal tunnel syndrome, as noted above, is one of the leading occupational diseases affecting video display terminal workers. Modern office buildings with sealed windows are often the environment for sick building syndrome. Sick building syndrome is caused by chemical irritants in carpets, paint, glues, and cleaners. Back pain from poorly designed office furniture causes as much chronic illness as any chemical exposure. Sometimes only estimates are possible because of the long latency period for many chronic diseases associated with the workplace. Many workers are exposed to a variety of agents in different environments and locations over many years making epidemiological analysis difficult and statistical rates difficult to calculate.[8] The National Research Council believes these data are seriously underreported. It is acknowledged that occupationally related deaths exceed the reported incidence by a factor of five and that job injuries are

Table 15. 4 National occupational research agenda priorities.

Category	NORA Priority Research Areas
Disease and injury	Allergic and irritant dermatitis
	Asthma and chronic obstructive
	Pulmonary disease
	Fertility and pregnancy abnormalities
	Hearing loss
	Infectious diseases
	Low-back disorders
	Musculoskeletal disorders of the upper extremities
	Traumatic injuries
Work environment and workforce	Emerging technologies
	Indoor environment
	Mixed exposures
	Organization of work
	Special populations at risk
Research tools and approaches	Cancer research methods
	Control technology and personnel
	Protective equipment
	Exposure assessment methods
	Health services research
	Intervention effectiveness research
	Risk assessment methods
	Social and economic consequences of workplace illness and injury
	Surveillance research methods

(*Source:* National Occupational Research Agenda. National Institute for Occupational Safety & Health)

ten times more frequent than officially reported. The error factor of occupationally related diseases is unknown but probably exceeds 100.[9]

The National Occupational Research Agenda (NORA), developed by the National Institute for Occupational Safety and Health (NIOSH) in partnership with more than 500 outside organizations and individuals, was released in April 1996 as a framework to guide occupational safety and health research into the twenty-first century. The NORA process resulted in a consensus on the top twenty-one research priorities for occupational safety and health (see Table 15.4).

Occupational Death

Among job-related mortality figures, a study among workers from 1990 to 1999 found that the numbers and rates of fatal injuries from 1990 through 1999 remained relatively stable, over 5,000 deaths per year and about 4.3 deaths per 100,000 workers. Motor vehicle-related fatalities at work, the leading cause of death for U.S. workers since 1980, accounted for 23 percent of deaths during the sixteen-year period. Workplace homicides became the second leading cause

Table 15.5 Fatal occupational injuries by event or exposure (1998).

Event or Exposure	Number	Event or Exposure	Number
Total	6,026	Assaults and violent acts	960
		Homicides	709
Transportation incidents	2,630	Shooting	569
Highway	1,431	Stabbing	61
Collision between vehicles, mobile equipment	701	Other, including bombing	79
		Self-inflicted injuries	223
Moving in same direction	118		
Moving in opposite directions, oncoming	271	Contact with objects and equipment	941
Moving in intersection	142	Struck by object	517
Vehicle struck stationary object or equipment	306	Struck by falling object	317
		Struck by flying object	58
Noncollision	373	Caught in or compressed by equipment or objects	266
Jackknifed or overturned—no collision	300		
Nonhighway (farm, industrial premises)	384	Caught in running equipment or machinery	129
Overturned	216	Caught in or crushed in collapsing materials	140
Aircraft	223	Falls	702
Worker struck by a vehicle	413	Fall to lower level	623
Water vehicle	112	Fall from ladder	111
Railway	60	Fall from roof	156

(*Source:* Occupational Safety & Health Administration, Department of Labor Statistics)

of death in 1990, surpassing machine-related deaths, which is the third leading cause of occupational deaths. An average of twenty workers die each week as a result of workplace homicides in the United States. Highway-related incidents were the leading cause of job-related fatalities among men; homicides were the leading cause of fatal injuries among women workers.[10]

Although the rankings of individual industry divisions have varied across the years, the largest number of traumatic occupational deaths consistently are found in construction, transportation and public utilities, and manufacturing. Industries with the highest traumatic occupational fatality rates per 100,000 workers are mining, agriculture, forestry and fishing, and construction.[11]

Motor Vehicle Deaths

Highway crashes continued as the leading cause of on-the-job fatalities during 1998, accounting for 24 percent of the fatal work injury total. (See Table 15.5.) This figure is mainly from an increase in the number of workers killed in highway crashes between oncoming vehicles. Slightly over two-fifths of the 1,431 victims of job-related highway fatalities were employed as truck drivers. The number of workers fatally struck by vehicles rose to 413 in 1998, an increase of 13 percent from their 1997 total and the highest number in the seven-year period that fatality census data has been compiled. In contrast to job-related fatalities, total highway and pedestrian fatalities dropped in 1998 from 1997, according to preliminary figures from the United States.

Table 15.6 Workplace homicides for selected industries (1994–1998).

Industry	1994	1995	1996	1997	1998
Total homicides	1,080	1,036	927	860	709
Retail trade	530	422	437	395	286
Grocery stores	196	152	146	141	95
Eating and drinking places	135	121	135	109	69
Gasoline service stations	41	36	23	34	24
Taxicab	87	68	50	74	48
Detective and armored car services	49	27	29	21	18
Police protection	65	61	45	61	50

(*Sources:* Centers for Disease Control. National Institute for Occupational Safety & Health)

Table 15.7 Major fatal events in construction (1997–1998).

Event	1997 Number	1998 Number	1998 Percent
Total construction fatalities (private sector)	1,107	1,171	100
Falls	377	383	33
From roofs	129	123	11
From scaffolds	63	84	7
From ladders	63	54	5
From building girders or other structural steel	38	29	3
Electrocutions	140	171	15
Highway crashes	125	147	13
Worker struck by vehicle	86	103	9
Struck by falling objects	65	67	6
Trench cave-ins	26	36	3
Collapsing structures	28	28	2

(*Sources:* Centers for Disease Control. National Institute for Occupational Safety & Health)

Homicides

The second leading cause of on-the-job deaths, workplace homicides, fell to its lowest level in the past seven years in 1998. A total of 709 workers died as a result of job-related homicide. Robbery continued to be the primary motive of job-related homicides in retail trade when a motive could be ascertained from the source documents. As Table 15.6 shows, outside of security work, taxicab drivers are at high risk for homicide on the job.

Other Occupational Fatalities

In 1998, deaths resulting from on-the-job falls totaled 702, nearly the same as the worker homicide total (Table 15.7). Modest increases in falls from roofs and scaffolds resulted in seven-year highs for these two totals. Most of the worker deaths resulting from falls from roofs and scaffolds occurred in the construction industry, which accounts for about half the fatal workplace falls each year. Electrocutions accounted for 6 percent of the fatal injuries. Contact with overhead power lines accounted for about half the deaths from electrocution.

Healthy People 2010 Objective: Reduce Deaths from Work-Related Injuries

Reduction in Deaths from Work-Related Injuries

	1998 Baseline (%)	2010 Target (%)
Deaths per 100,000 Workers Aged 16 Years and Older		
All industry	4.5	3.2
Mining	23.6	16.5
Construction	14.6	10.2
Transportation	11.8	8.3
Agriculture, forestry, and fishing	24.1	16.9

Occupational Morbidity

Occupational illness can affect virtually every organ system of the body although compensation for injury or loss does not cover all cases (Figure 15.1). The National Institute for Occupational Safety and Health (NIOSH) has developed a rank-order list of the ten most important categories of occupational illness. The rank order is:

1. lung disease
2. musculoskeletal injuries
3. cancers other than lung
4. traumatic injuries
5. reproductive disorders
6. cardiovascular disease
7. neurotoxic disorders
8. noise-induced loss of hearing
9. dermatological conditions and
10. psychological disorders

Lung Disease

Major categories of lung disease include the dust diseases of the lung or pneumoconioses, lung cancer, occupational asthma, industrial bronchitis, and other irritants and infections. It is hard to determine accurately the total prevalence of these diseases because for many conditions, such as asbestos-related lung cancer, it may take twenty-five years or more for the symptoms to appear. Lung disease is a major killer of the population and is aggravated in the workplace with smoking in and off the job.

Dusts can be classified as inert, irritating, combustible, and toxic. Inert dusts are present in paper and fiber manufacturing. They are found in miners,

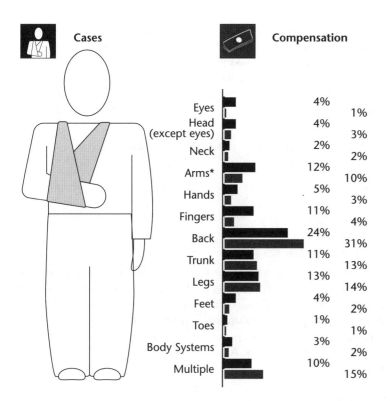

Cases   Compensation

	Cases	Compensation
Eyes	4%	1%
Head (except eyes)	4%	3%
Neck	2%	2%
Arms*	12%	10%
Hands	5%	3%
Fingers	11%	4%
Back	24%	31%
Trunk	11%	13%
Legs	13%	14%
Feet	4%	2%
Toes	1%	1%
Body Systems	3%	2%
Multiple	10%	15%

*Includes multiple or NEC extremity injuries amounting to less than 2 percent of the total cases and compensation.

Figure 15.1 Percent distribution of on-the-job injuries and compensation by part of body.

(*Source:* National Safety Council. *Accident Facts,* 1994, Itasca, IL: Author)

BOX 15.2 Occupational Injuries in a Typical Year

- 40 workers are killed in trench cave-ins
- 30 workers die from carbon monoxide poisoning—often vehicle mechanics
- 22 workers die from heatstroke—often farmers and laborers
- 17 workers are fatally crushed by forklifts
- 16 flaggers are struck and killed by vehicles

- 15 workers are killed by lightning
- 13 workers are killed by accidental discharge of a firearm
- 12 farmworkers are killed when gored or trampled by bulls
- 12 workers are electrocuted when cranes contact overhead power lines
- 10 workers are killed by exploding tires, typically when inflating the tire

(*Source:* U.S. Department of Labor, Bureau of Labor Statistics)

grinders, and sand and gravel pit workers. Air quality surveillance attempts to prevent dust-related injury by requiring that dusts be kept to minimum levels by using exhaust systems or water soaking.

Asbestos, which has now been regulated, is the primary cause of mesothelioma, a type of lung cancer. Fiberglass has yet to be regulated, although the filaments of fiberglass that may get in the lungs causes similar lung irritation.

Healthy People 2010 Objecive: Reduce Dust-Related Deaths

Target: 1,900 deaths.

Baseline: 2,928 pneumoconiosis deaths among persons aged 15 years and older in 1997.

Musculoskeletal Injuries

Musculoskeletal injuries are generally caused by strains, overuse, repetitive motion trauma, or trauma to moving parts of the human body. These injuries include back, arm, leg strains and pain, immobility, or broken bones. Musculoskeletal injuries are the principal cause of disability of people in their working years, afflicting over 20 million persons. They account for one-third of annual worker's compensation claims. Almost half of all workers are affected at some time during their working life.

Occupational Cancer

Because of the long latency between cancer-causing exposure and symptoms, this occupational morbidity can only be estimated. At even the lowest estimate, 17,000 cancer deaths in the United States each year are attributable to workplace exposure (Figure 15.2).

BOX 15.3 Occupationally-Related, Disabling, Unintentional Injuries by Affected Body Area

Disabling work injuries in the entire national totaled approximately 3,200,000 in 1993. Of these, about 9,100 were fatal.

Injuries to the back occurred most frequently, followed by leg injuries, arm, trunk, and thumb and finger injuries, according to state labor department reports.

Eyes	130,000
Head (except eyes)	130,000
Neck	60,000

Arms	380,000
Hands	160,000
Fingers	350,000
Back	770,000
Trunk	350,000
Legs	420,000
Feet	130,000
Toes	30,000
Body systems	100,000
Multiple	320,000

(*Source:* National Safety Council. *Accident facts*, 1994, Itasca, IL: Author)

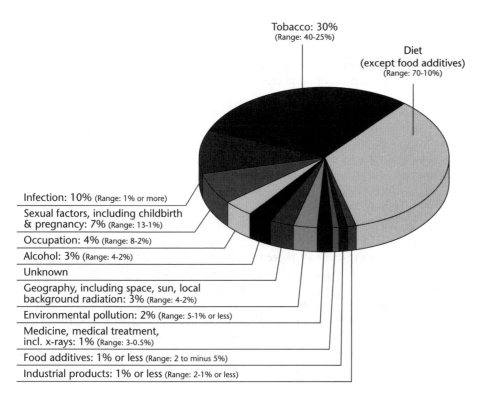

Tobacco: 30%
(Range: 40-25%)

Diet
(except food additives)
(Range: 70-10%)

Infection: 10% (Range: 1% or more)

Sexual factors, including childbirth
& pregnancy: 7% (Range: 13-1%)

Occupation: 4% (Range: 8-2%)

Alcohol: 3% (Range: 4-2%)

Unknown

Geography, including space, sun, local
background radiation: 3% (Range: 4-2%)

Environmental pollution: 2% (Range: 5-1% or less)

Medicine, medical treatment,
incl. x-rays: 1% (Range: 3-0.5%)

Food additives: 1% or less (Range: 2 to minus 5%)

Industrial products: 1% or less (Range: 2-1% or less)

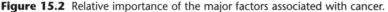

Figure 15.2 Relative importance of the major factors associated with cancer.

(*Source:* Benarde, Melvin A. *Our precarious habitat.* Copyright © 1990 John Wiley & Sons, Inc. Reprinted by permission of John Wiley and Sons, Inc.)

Occupational Trauma

Annually, at least 10 million persons in the United States suffer traumatic injuries at work. These injuries include amputations, fractures, lacerations, eye loss, acute poisoning, and burns as shown on Box 15.3. In 1995, NIOSH reported 5,314 occupational fatalities in the United States. The major causes of work-related trauma deaths in the United States were highway motor vehicle incidents (34 percent), falls (13 percent), industrial vehicle incidents (11 percent), blows other than by vehicles (8 percent), and electrocution (7 percent).

Reproductive Disorders

Most knowledge about reproductive toxicity comes from laboratory studies; however, infertility due to loss of spermatogenesis among male farmworkers is well documented. Additionally, reproductive anomalies are common to the partners and the children of farmworkers. Laundering clothing that has been exposed to pesticides causes the pesticides to enter the systems of all family members.

A 1980s government study found PCB pesticide in every human sperm sample tested. Environmental toxins can disrupt the production of male hormones in the testes, causing loss of sex drive and impotence. Men exposed to lead have decreased fertility and malformed sperm. Higher rates of birth defects are showing up among the children of Vietnam veterans exposed to Agent Orange, an herbicide contaminated with dioxin that was used for deforestation in Vietnam.

Among women exposed to occupational toxins, damage may be direct to the ovaries, resulting in early menopause, ovarian disease, and ova mutation. There may also be an increase in spontaneous abortion and birth defects. Fetal development during the first three months is particularly at risk. Finally, certain toxins concentrate in human breast milk, to be passed on to newborns. According to an EPA study, 99 percent of all American women have enough PCB in their breast milk to show up in tests.

A recent study among 418 California female dental assistants found that those exposed to high levels of unventilated nitrous oxide for five hours or more a week were only 40 percent as likely to become pregnant when trying as compared to unexposed women. Previous studies have identified nitrous oxide as a toxin, but this was one of the first studies to implicate the chemical to decreased fertility. At least fifty chemicals have been shown to produce impairment of reproductive functions in animals. Paternal exposure before conception may reduce fertility and produce unsuccessful fertilization or abnormal fetus development. Maternal exposure after conception may result in fetal death and structural and functional abnormalities in newborns.[12]

Noise-Related Health Problems

As sound passes through the fluid-filled inner ear, it moves tiny projections called microvilli on the surfaces of millions of sensory cells suspended in the fluid. The motion sets off chemical reactions in sensory cells that produce electrical impulses. These impulses are entered through the auditory nerve to the brain, where the incoming signal is analyzed and interpreted as sound.[13] Even common everyday sounds have the ability to cause damage to the sensory cells (Table 15.8).

With normal hearing, you can hear sounds with frequencies ranging from 16 to 20,000 cycles per second (20,000 Hertz or Hz). When certain frequencies become prolonged, permanent loss in ability to hear with potential deafness can occur.

According to the Environmental Protection Agency, nearly half of all citizens, mostly urban residents, are regularly exposed in their neighborhood and in their jobs to noise pollution—any unwanted, disturbing, or harmful sound that impairs or interferes with hearing, causes stress, hampers concentration and work efficiency, or causes accidents. Every day, one of every ten people lives, works, or plays around noise of sufficient duration and intensity to cause some permanent loss of hearing. Over 60 million people are significantly disrupted by noise pollution from cars, trucks, buses, jackhammers, construction equipment, motorcycles, power lawnmowers, vacuum cleaners, sirens, and unwanted loud noise. Table 15.8 describes the effects of some common sounds.

Table 15.8 Common noises and their typical consequences.

Source	Sound Pressure (dbA)	Effect from Prolonged Exposure
Jet takeoff (25 meters away)	150	Eardrum rupture
Air-raid siren	140	
Jet takeoff (100 meters away), earphones at loud level	130	
Live rock music, chain saw, boom stereo systems in cars	120	Human pain threshold Maximum vocal level
Steel mill, riveting, automobile horn at 1 meter, "boom box" stereo held close to ear	110	
Subway, outboard motor, power lawn mower, motorcycle at 8 meters, farm tractor, printing plant, jackhammer, garbage truck	100	
City traffic, diesel truck, food blender	90	Hearing damage (8 hours), speech interference
Garbage disposal, clothes washer, average factory freight train at 15 meters, dishwasher, alarm clock	80	Possible hearing damage
Freeway traffic at 15 meters, vacuum cleaner, noisy office or party, TV audio	70	Annoying
Air conditioner	60	Intrusive
Quiet suburb (daytime), conversation in living room	40	Quiet
Library, soft background music	30	
Quiet rural area (nighttime)	30	
Broadcasting studio	20	Very quiet

(*Source:* Miller, G. Tyler, 1992. *Living in the environment,* 7th ed. © Belmont: Wadsworth Publishing Company, p. 235. Reprinted with permission.)

The 2010 national objective was to reduce the prevalence of occupational noise-induced hearing loss. There are no national data to measure this objective, however, meeting this goal depended on three sources:

1. Continued improvements in engineering should lower noise levels.

2. Major shifts in technologies that will yield lower levels.

3. Widespread education and training for employees.

Internationally, noise pollution may be much worse since there are few if any regulations that control for noise in developing countries. In downtown Cairo, the noise levels are ten times the limit set by United States health and safety standards.[14] However, when compared to the former Soviet Union, Scandinavian countries, and many western European countries, the United States lags behind. Europeans have developed quieter jackhammers, pile drivers, and air compressors that do not cost much more than earlier, noisy models. Most European countries also require that small sheds and tents be used to muffle construction. The United States trails in development because of industry pressure against establishing stricter workplace noise standards.

Industry has convinced government to cut, dramatically, the EPA's budget for noise pollution, which has resulted in lax enforcement of noise control laws.[15] Federal laws require U.S. employers to use engineering or other controls to adhere to certain noise standards, but only to the extent feasible. Compliance and enforcement are lax because the law does not specify what is or is not feasible.[16]

Occupational Skin Disorders (OSDs)

In 1997 occupational skin diseases or disorders (OSDs) constituted 13.5 percent of all occupational illnesses, or 57,900 reported cases in the U.S. workforce. It is estimated that there are approximately 1 to 1.6 million unreported dermatological injuries each year in the United States.

Strategies for the prevention of OSDs include identifying allergens and irritants, substituting chemicals that are less irritating or allergenic, establishing engineering controls to reduce exposure, using personal protective equipment such as gloves and special clothing, using barrier creams, emphasizing personal and occupational hygiene, establishing educational programs to increase awareness in the workplace, and providing health screening. A combination of several interventions, which included providing advice on personal protective equipment and educating the workforce about skin care and exposures, have proved to be beneficial for workers. Primary and secondary prevention programs that include health promotion or public awareness campaigns and education or disease awareness programs can successfully be directed toward workers in high-risk industries.[17]

> *Healthy People 2010 Objective:* Reduce Occupational Skin Diseases or Disorders Among Full-Time Workers
>
> *Target:* 47 new cases per 100,000.
>
> *Baseline:* 67 new cases per 100,000 full-time workers aged 16 years and older had occupational skin diseases or disorders in 1997.

The Cost of Occupational Diseases

The annual cost, direct and indirect, of occupational disease in the United States is calculated to be at least $6 billion.[18] Internationally, there is no completely reliable source of data on work-related injuries and deaths.

Ironically, one of the positive effects of the 1980s recession was a reduction in occupation-related mortality. With fewer people working and on the road, the 1992 accidental death toll was the lowest in sixty-nine years, with an actual work-related death toll of 9,200. The National Safety Council (NSC) estimated that 84,000 people died by accident, in and out of the workplace in 1992, 5 percent fewer than the number who died in 1991. The NSC theorized that the decline in accidents in a recession occurs because the first people to be laid off usually are the last hired and less experienced workers.

Safety Legislation

In the United States the Occupational Safety and Health Act of 1970, administered by the Occupational Safety and Health Administration (OSHA), located in the Department of Labor, was passed "to insure as far as possible every working man and woman in the nation safe and healthful working conditions." Ironically, public employees, the fourth largest group of workers in the United States, have never been covered by the federal OSHA law. The Occupational Safety and Health Act created the National Institute for Occupational Safety and Health (NIOSH), located at the CDC, whose responsibility is to conduct health hazard appraisals when requested and to conduct research regarding health and safety standards.

Three main roles of OSHA are:

1. Setting safety and health standards
2. Enforcement of the standards through federal and state inspectors
3. Public education and consultation[19]

OSHA coverage includes, but is not limited to, compliance with standards, the General Duty Clause, multi-employer responsibility, record keeping, employee rights and duties, enforcement of inspections, citation, notices of contest, abatement, degrees of violations, and penalties.[20]

A 1994 law before Congress, the Occupation Safety and Health Act reform bill, finally protects public employees. The bill required employers with at least eleven employees to organize health and safety committees run jointly by employees and employers. Employers cited by OSHA for safety violations would be required to abate the hazard immediately, regardless of whether they appeal the OSHA citation. This bill would provide whistle-blower protection, training, and accelerated standards setting process.[21]

Although protective legislation exists, success in reducing work-related illness has been difficult. Reductions in funding during the 1980s for surveillance, inspection, and compliance of OSHA regulations seem to be correlated with an actual increase in occupational injury rates even though actual numbers of deaths and injuries decreased.

In 1985, Frank Carsner, a truck painter in Portland, Oregon, incorporated the Toxic Victims Association (TVA). The TVA has been a vocal advocate for occupational health and safety in relationship to those working around toxic chemicals. In 1989 they joined forces with others to win passage of the nation's first toxic-use reduction laws.

Such activism is part of an emerging nationwide coalition to expand activism and lobbying for right-to-know laws about toxic hazards in the workplace. They aim to have community and worker representatives on investigative committees, and compel employers to develop toxic-use reduction plans. Activism around safety issues has grown out of the concerted work of labor unions that have fought for decades for a safe working environment and adequate health benefits to cover worker disability, illness, and death.

Two important regulations that help to protect the worker are the Employee Right-to-Know Law (HAZCOM) of 1983 and the Community Right-to-Know Law (Title III of SuperFund Amendment and Reauthorization Act [SARA]). Both of these laws now require that workers and communities be given timely information about the use, storage, and manufacture of toxic and hazardous chemicals. Companies must have available for all workers:

1. The chemical and common name of all substances or ingredients of all hazardous products on site
2. The characteristics of the substances
3. The physical hazards, such as combustibility of the substance
4. The health hazards associated with the substance
5. Precautions for safe handling
6. Emergency first aid procedures

This community effort targets the growing reality that workplace exposure to hazards is a serious threat to a community and that radical, vocal action is needed to assist the vulnerable worker who may be reluctant to expose his or her own risks because they fear loss of employment. It is an effort to quantify statistical evidence of work risk that until now has been less than accurate. Government data have underestimated the occurrence of occupational diseases that have long latency periods between exposure and manifestation of symptoms, and fatalities that are related to work exposure but occur off the job.[22]

Prevention

Prevention of occupational diseases requires the elimination or reduction of hazardous exposures, the detection of occupational disease in its presymptomatic stage and prevention of complications and disability of existing illness. Particular prevention can include engineering control to change design of risky machinery, use of safety gear, encouraging personal hygiene, and stress reduction on the job.

Prevention of occupational injuries and illness requires the combined efforts of community health and safety education, local and national legislation for setting standards and surveillance, more safety inspectors, protection for workers who report hazardous conditions (whistle-blower protection), changes in technology, and individual initiative in promoting health. Given the high cost of worker's compensation and health insurance benefits, the time and energy involved in safety promotion will always be cost beneficial to employers.

Education may include courses specific to the materials being used and to the overall knowledge of first aid and emergency care. Workers should have access to all information relevant to the hazards, the composition, the first aid, and the potential interactions of chemicals being used. Training on machinery should be complete and monitored for new workers. All educational materials should be written in simple language and bilingual information should be available where workers do not speak English as their first language.

Changes in OSHA standards and regulations should be made as new technology and/or chemicals are introduced in the workplace. Enforcement of legislation should be required with swift corrections demanded. There should be a renewed emphasis on inspection with an increase in hiring and training of OSHA inspectors. In 1995, there were only 2,000 OSHA inspectors for about 6 million worksites in the United States.[23]

People who report unsafe conditions should have the full protection of the law to prevent their loss of employment. Essentially, this is why the "whistle-blower" laws were enacted, to protect workers who report hazards or corruption in the workplace from retaliation. Workers should be encouraged to be involved in the safety of their workplace and should be rewarded for finding problems and making change.

Another important aspect of prevention is promotion of personal fitness of those on the job. Many businesses now have worksite health promotion programs that include weight reduction, alcohol and other drug prevention, stress management, cardiovascular fitness, and mental health programs. Keeping employees healthy, thus reducing work days lost, and improving health and energy on the job are all part of occupational health promotion.

Summary

Approximately 110 million people make up the work force in the United States, with most spending major portions of their days in their work environment. Premature death, disease, injuries, and other unhealthful conditions resulting from occupational exposure pose important national health problems.

Realization of the OSHA mandate depends upon an increase in the number of professionals trained in occupational health and safety-related professions. Progress in occupational health also requires greater emphasis on surveillance to identify high-risk groups and behaviors, as well as prevention programs.[24]

CYBERSITES RELATED TO CHAPTER 15

www.osha.gov
www.acoem.org
www.cdc.gov/niosh/homepage.html

QUESTIONS

1. Why is health and safety on the job both a boon and a bane to business and manufacturing?

2. What are the major occupational risks for people in each job category: white collar, blue collar, pink collar (traditionally women's jobs such as beauticians or maids).

3. What is the purpose of OSHA? How does it work? Why might it generate controversy in political circles?

EXERCISES

1. Select ten occupations common to your community. List the potential and real occupational risks associated with each type of employment.

2. If you work full or part time, visit the office or person in charge of safety. Review with that person the prevention programs available in your employment.

3. Describe a hypothetical occupational injury and the steps one would go through to report the injury, seek care, and compensation.

INTERNET INTERACTIVE ACTIVITY

OSHA SEARCH SITES

OSHA and its state partners have approximately 2,100 inspectors, plus complaint discrimination investigators, engineers, physicians, educators, standards writers, and other technical and support personnel spread over more than 200 offices throughout the country. This staff establishes protective standards, enforces those standards, and reaches out to employers and employees through technical assistance and consultation programs. Through its search sites one can determine where occupational health violations have occurred. The homepage for the OSHA search sites is:

www.osha.gov/

Exercise

The community health educator is interested in knowing about safety violations at airports across the country.

1. Go to home page

www.osha.gov/

2. Click on **Statistics & Inspection Data**

www.osha.gov/oshstats/

3. Click on Establishment Search

www.osha.gov/cgi_bin/est/est1

4. Enter

Airports
All States
All Offices

5. You will get something that looks like this.

Search Options							
Establishment	Date Range		RID	State	Limits	Include	Exclude
Airport	1972-07-01	2010-12-31	All	All	100/2500		

Get Detail		+	All	Reset	Found 1113—Processed 1113—Selected 1113–Displayed 100					
		Activity Nr	Open Date	Report ID	St	Type	Sc	SIC	Vio	Establishment Name
☐	1	303244024	03/31/2000	0355114	VA	UnprogRel	Part	4581		Metropolitan Washington Airports Authority
☐	2	303367262	03/28/2000	0213100	NY	OtherK	NoIn	4581		Airport Group International
☐	3	*303367288*	03/21/2000	0213100	NY	Complaint	Part	4581		Albany County Airport, Faa Airway Facilities
☐	4	303135677	03/17/2000	1054112	OR	UnprogRel	Part	4581		Airport Terminal Services
☐	5	125364687	03/08/2000	0551800	IN	Complaint	Part	4581	2	Priority Airport Parking

You now know what states had a safety violation in an airport from 1972 to 2010. You know the type of violation and the establishment's name. All definitions are given at

www.osha.gov/oshstats/est1def.html

6. If you click on the activity number you can follow the history of the reported violation.

Exercise

Using the OSHA search engine, determine what hospitals, fire departments, and laundries experienced OSHA violations during the past five years in your state.

1. What were the primary violations in each of these establishments?

2. Where were the average fines for violations of safety codes?

3. On average, how serious was the violation of the safety code?

4. Begin with the OSHA homepage, go to **Regulations & Compliance**

5. Click on **Standards**

   www.osha-slc.gov/OshStd_toc/OSHA_Std_toc.html

6. Determine three or four of the regulations regarding safe egress from a building.

REFERENCES

1. *The Nation's Health* (1994). Government health workers to be protected under OSHA reform. March, p. 5.

2. stats.bls.gov/special.requests/ocwc/oshwc/osh/os/osnr0009.txt

3. WHO (1993). Facts About WHO. Geneva.

4. stats.bls.gov/special.requests/ocwc/oshwc/osh/os/osnr0009.txt

5. Landrigan, Philip (1992). Commentary: Environmental disease, a preventable epidemic. *American Journal of Public Health*. July, Vol. 82, No. 7.

6. Goldman, Benjamin A. (1991). *The truth about where you live*. New York: Times Books, Random House.

7. Koren, Herman (1991). *Handbook of environmental health and safety*. Vol. I. 2nd Ed. Michigan: Lewis Publishers.

8. Pickett, George, & Hanlon, John J. (1990). *Public health administration and practice*. St Louis: Mosby Publishing.

9. Ibid.

10. National Institute for Occupational Safety and Health (NIOSH). *National Occupational Research Agenda*. Pub. No. 96-115. Cincinnati, OH: The Institute, 1996.

11. Ibid.

12. Koren, op. cit.

13. Miller, Dean (1982). *Safety: An introduction*. N.J.: Prentice-Hall.

14. Ibid.

15. Pickett, op. cit.

16. Miller, Dean (1992). *Dimensions of community health*. 3rd. ed. New York: Wm. C. Brown.

17. www.health.gov/healthypeople/Document/HTML/Volume2/20OccSH.htm

18. Pickett, op. cit.

19. LaDou, Joseph (1981). *Occupational health law*. New York: Marcel Dekker, Inc.

20. Rothstein, Mark A. (1983). *Occupational safety and health law*. Minnesota: West Publishing.

21. The Nation's Health, op. cit.

22. Census of Fatal Occupational Injuries Summary. (1999) stats.bls.gov/news.release/cfoi.nws.htm

23. Eldridge, Earle (1995). Study links job deaths to osha failure. *USA Today*, Sept. 5, p. D1.

24. U.S. Department of Health and Human Services (1992). *Healthy People 2000. Full report with commentary*. Boston: Jones and Bartlett Publisher.

CHAPTER 16

Mental Health, Substance Abuse, and Violence

Community Health in the 21st Century
I never would have thought of violence as a health issue until I became a
health educator. Sadly, I think the 21st Century will require more health
involvement in designing and implementing violence prevention programs,
designing the implementing programs targeting diverse populations,
programs for empowerment training, and community based substance abuse
prevention programs.

—Lori J. Stegmier, M.A., CHES, Chief Health Educator,
Kent County Health Department, Grand Rapids, Michigan

Chapter Objectives

The student will:

1. describe the impact of deinstitutional-ization on community mental health programs.

2. describe the role of community health education in terms of mental health.

3. list the most common mental illnesses in the United States.

4. explain why homelessness and mental illness are closely connected.

5. explain why minority populations, including women, are at unique risks for mental illness.

6. state their role as a community health educator in preventing violence in their lives and in the community in which they live.

7. identify acts of violence that are community health imperatives.

8. distinguish between domestic violence, emotional violence, gay bashing, child abuse, elder abuse, and hate crimes.

9. list the factors that contribute to a violent community.

10. name the ways in which alcohol and other drugs impact the mental health of communities and individuals.

Mental Health

According to the landmark Global Burden of Disease study, commissioned by the World Health Organization and the World Bank, four of the ten leading causes of disability for persons age five and older are mental disorders.[1] In any given year in the United States, 28 percent of the population have symptoms of a mental illness, everything from severe schizophrenia to mild bouts of depression. Sadly, less than a quarter of those with symptoms ever have the courage to seek help from a mental health specialist. Instead, many turn to primary care physicians who cannot always adequately treat mental illness. Of the 12 to 14 million children and adolescents with mental or addictive disorders, 80 percent never get help. Prevalence rates of adolescent mental disorders are given in Table 16.1. The role of community health education is threefold in the area of mental health:

1. Educating the public about their likelihood of being at risk for mental health stresses and helping to reduce the stigma about getting appropriate care

2. Identifying mental health practitioners in the community and helping the public seek the best care for particular symptoms

3. Creating prevention programs that anticipate high risk behaviors or stresses that may cause or aggravate mental health problems

In the 1980s, 18,571 households and 2,290 institutional residents eighteen and older were interviewed by the National Institute for Mental Health to provide prevalence rates and current population estimates for specific mental disorders and to provide incidence rates for specific time periods. Results from this study indicate that the number of persons affected sometime in their lifetime with a disabling mental disorder is 11.2 million.[2] These disorders include substance abuse (16.7 percent), schizophrenia (1.5 percent), depressive disorders (8.3 percent), anxiety disorders (14.6 percent), somatization disorder (0.1 percent), and severe cognitive impairment (1.7 percent). The total lifetime disorder rate was significantly higher for men (35.4 percent) than women (30.0 percent). Marked sex differences were found for specific disorders. Significantly higher rates of substance use disorders and anti-social personality disorders were found among men while women had higher rates of affective, anxiety, and somatization disorders.[3] Table 16.2 shows the relative severity of mental illness in terms of years lost to disability in relationship to other leading causes of disease in the United States.

History of Mental Health

The history of caring for the world's mentally ill has not been a praiseworthy part of public health. Inhumane torture, experimentation, warehousing, incarceration, lobotomies, and exorcisms were all considered the treatment of choice at various times in various locations. State mental hospitals of the nineteenth and even the twentieth century were houses of horror. Not until post-World War II, when many veterans returned from war with post-battle mental illnesses, now known as **post-traumatic stress syndrome,** did communities begin to see the need to make major changes in how the mentally ill were housed and treated. Unfortunately, many of the mentally ill have been victimized by society, government, families, and individuals. They have been warehoused in overcrowded, underfinanced institutions that have used these patients as guinea pigs in research without their ability to consent. Major changes were recommended in the 1950s in the care and treatment of institu-

Table 16.1 Children and adolescents ages 9 to 17 with mental or
addictive disorders.

	Prevalence (%)
Anxiety disorders	13.0
Mood disorders	6.2
Disruptive disorders	10.3
Substance use disorders	2.0
Any disorder	20.9

(*Source:* Mental health: A report of the Surgeon General, 1998)

Table 16.2 Disease burden by selected illness categories in established
market economies (1990).

	Percent of Total DALYs*
All cardiovascular conditions	18.6
All mental illness	15.4
All malignant diseases (cancer)	15.0
All respiratory conditions	4.8
All alcohol use	4.7<
All infectious and parasitic diseases	2.8
All drug use	1.5

*Disability-adjusted life year (DALY) is a measure that expresses years of life lost to premature
death and years lived with a disability of specified severity and duration

(*Source:* Murray & Lopez, 1996)

tionalized mentally ill people; however, as late as the 1980s private and state
hospitals were being exposed for their lack of humane, ethical care.

An important breakthrough in serving the mentally ill and recognizing the
need for training, research, and services, was the passage of the 1946 National
Mental Health Act. This act created the National Institute of Mental Health
(NIMH) and its axillary programs. At the federal level, research related to mental health is still coordinated by the National Institute of Mental Health, an
institute of the Public Health Service. In addition to the major mental illnesses,
the NIMH conducts research related to specific populations: children, minorities, criminals, and older adults.[4]

The federal government began its legislative attempts to improve mental
health care again in the 1960s. In 1963 the Community Mental Health Services
Act was passed giving funds for local community-based, as opposed to state
hospital-based, care. This plan gave patients, their families, and communities
more access and input into care and treatment and reduced the isolation and
totalitarian nature of state mental hospitals. The expectation was that community centers would provide: (1) inpatient care, (2) outpatient services, (3)
around-the-clock hospitalization, (4) emergency services, (5) consultation with
community agencies, (6) diagnostic and follow-up services, (7) alcohol and

drug rehabilitation services, and (8) research and evaluation. Since financing of such comprehensive mental health centers depended upon matching funds, all went well until the 1980s when money became tight nationwide. Most states now struggle to provide even part of the services expected by law.[5]

Deinstitutionalization

In 1971 a noble attempt was made to reduce mental hospital residency and provide more community-based mental health care among the chronically mentally ill through outpatient clinics and halfway houses. This effort was called **deinstitutionalization.** This plan was an attempt to provide appropriate working arrangements for the chronically ill in such a way that they could be medicated as needed, work as they were able, and participate in their community. Unfortunately, at the same time mentally ill people were leaving institutions, money to finance community-based programs was drying up.[6]

> *A history of mental health policy in the United States suggests that community policy was passed on the expectation that patients could be treated in non-institutional settings. Underlying this belief were several assumptions: that patients had a home; that patients had a sympathetic family or other persons willing and able to assume responsibility for their care; that the organization of the household would not impede rehabilitation; and that the patient's presence would not cause undue hardships for other family members. In 1960, however, 48 percent of the mental hospital population were unmarried, 12 percent were widowed, and 13 percent were divorced or separated. A large proportion of patients, in other words, had no families to care for them. The assumption that patients could reside in the community with their families while undergoing rehabilitation was hardly supported by such findings.[7]*

There are currently twice as many mentally ill persons on the streets and in shelters as there are in our public mental hospitals. Municipal hospitals have become the dumping ground for the mentally ill who find themselves in trouble with the law or the community at large because there are no beds available in mental facilities. However, not all the blame is in the system. Many patients refuse to take the medications prescribed them. Many also often refuse to receive treatment.[8]

The way deinstitutionalization was originally carried out, many thousands of mentally ill residents of state hospitals were discharged into inadequately prepared and programmatically deficient communities. Inadequacies include: (1) the number and range of community residential settings; (2) varying degrees of supervision and structure; (3) systems of follow-up, (4) monitoring and responsibility for ensuring that services are provided to those unable to obtain them; and (5) easy access to short- and long-term inpatient care when indicated. The consequences of these gaps in essential resources have been disastrous—one consequence was homelessness. There is a large mentally ill population among homeless persons. The American Psychiatric Association estimates a prevalence

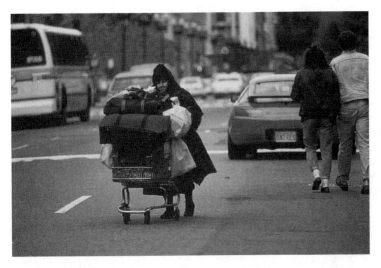

Deinstitutionalization reduced mental hospital loads but put many mentally ill people on the street without community resources or support systems.

of about 40 percent of homeless people with major mental illness. Others estimate that perhaps one-fourth of homeless persons suffer from some chronic mental illness.[9]

Homelessness

Homelessness occurs when the chronically mentally ill and others, unable to cope with the stresses of the world, become vulnerable to eviction from their residences. They may not be able to deal with ordinary landlord-tenant situations. Many drift away from their families or from care homes. Some regard leaving a controlled milieu as a necessary part of their own realization of their goals, but this process exacts a price on the ill prepared. Once the mentally ill are out on their own they will often stop taking their medications, lose touch with the Social Security Administration, and are unable to receive their Supplemental Security Income checks. Their lack of medical care on the streets and the effects of alcohol and other drug abuse are serious added complications. They may now be too disorganized to extricate themselves from living on the streets, except by exhibiting bizarre or disruptive behavior that leads to a hospital or jail.[10]

In July 1987, Congress passed the Stewart B. McKinney Homeless Assistance Act, providing funding in the initial amount of $409.2 million to include approximately twenty programs for the homeless ranging from health care to job training. Reauthorization for subsequent years has reached into the billions of dollars due to the enormous demand for government assistance for mental health.[11]

Primary health care for the homeless is less than adequate.[12] The most prevalent problems include respiratory disease, hypertensive diseases, and sexually transmitted diseases. A study of New York City homeless men found that 19.4 percent of the those tested were positive for HIV.[13] An alarming resurgence in tuberculosis among the homeless has punctuated the dire need for adequate health care as a means of preventing a community epidemic.[14]

BOX 16.1 Not in My Backyard

Even though communities acknowledge the need for outpatient care in residential homes or halfway houses to prepare some mentally ill for re-entry into a community, the prevailing attitude of most neighborhoods is "not in my backyard." This slogan has been the lobbying cry that has prevented establishing not only mental health facilities, but youth homes, penal halfway houses, waste incinerators, waste facilities, abortion clinics, and family planning clinics in communities that had the political clout (meaning economic resources), to prevent such programs. The inevitable result is that those neighborhoods with the financial resources to hire attorneys and time to attend public meetings have been successful in blocking these centers. Poorer communities, with fewer resources and even fewer allies in places of power inherit the facilities that the rich do not want in their backyard.

Classification of Mental Disorders

The mental disorders of adult life can generally be classified into three broad groups: (1) schizophrenia and allied disorders; (2) affective disorders and anxiety states; and (3) organic disorders and epilepsy. The prevalence rate of people with such disorders in 1999 is shown in Table 16.3. Some studies also include substance abuse as a classification of mental illness. Even with a clinical manual of classification, the Diagnostic and Statistical Manual (DSM) of the American Psychiatric Association, it is difficult to determine precisely and across cultures actual mental illness morbidity. What may seem to be abnormal behavior in one culture may be very healthy and appropriate in another. Further, as we learn more about the intricacies of the brain and its associated organs, conditions such as homosexuality, once thought to be a mental illness, is now more commonly understood to be part of the natural variation of the human species. Despite these diagnostic difficulties, WHO estimates that over 300 million people in the world suffer from mental or neurological disorders or from psychosocial problems such as those related to alcohol and drug abuse.[15]

The Impact of Mental Disorders It is estimated that more than 40 million citizens experience major mental illness of some kind. One-third of all families are affected by some form of mental illness which include 20 percent of adults and 12 percent of children. In 1999 there were 21 million outpatient visits to office-based psychologists and 21 million visits to psychiatrists. The cost of providing mental health care is shown in Table 16.4.

During any given month, over 15 percent of Americans will experience some mental disorder. Among the most prevalent disorders found among those seeking health care for mental illness are anxiety disorders (7.3 percent), affective disorders (5.1 percent), substance abuse (3.3 percent), and obsessive compulsive disorders (1.3 percent).

Table 16.3 Estimated 1-year prevalence rates of mental disorders ages 18 to 54 (1999).

	Best Estimate (%)		Best Estimate (%)
Any anxiety disorder	16.4	Unipolar MD	5.3
Simple phobia	8.3	Dysthymia	1.6
Social phobia	2.0	Bipolar 1	1.1
Agoraphobia	4.9	Schizophrenia	1.3
Panic disorder	1.6	Nonaffective psychosis	0.2
OCD	2.4	Somatization	0.2
PTSD	3.6	Anorexia nervosa	0.1
Any mood disorder	7.1	Severe cognitive impairment	1.2
MD episode	6.5	**Any disorder**	**21.0**

(*Source:* National Institute of Mental Health)

Table 16.4 The impact of mental illness.

Overall Cost of Mental Health Care		Types of Care and Cost	
1980	$35.3 million	Individual psychotherapy	$101
1987	$40.5 million	Psychotherapy in hospital	$120
1990	$41.4 million	Family therapy	$151
		Psychiatric diagnostic interview	$130
Coverage for Mental Health Care		Initial consultation	$131
		Group psychotherapy	$50
Insured	153 million		
Underinsured	50 million		
Uninsured	39 million		

(*Source:* National Institute of Mental Health; The Carter Center)

Stress

Stress is probably the greatest contributor to poor mental health. Community health education has found that trying to reduce stress through behavior change, in a world where the constant concern about survival is universal, is a primary preventive measure for good mental health. Many people cope with stressful life events (such as war, famine, crime, unemployment, divorce, social inequity, and poor health) through drugs, alcohol, overeating, and suicide. A 1990 U.S. study of stress found that 76 percent of those studied reported notable stress, 26 percent had anxiety disorders, 22.5 percent were diagnosed with phobias, 4.5 percent had obsessive compulsive disorders, and 2.9 percent had panic disorders.[16]

The most severe form of distress is now called **post-traumatic stress disorder syndrome (PTDS).** War has provided us with the hindsight to identify the symptoms of this mental illness that may occur with just the trauma and violence of everyday living. The symptoms include intense fatigue, nervousness, chest pains, nightmares, violence, disorientation, and emotional instability.

Community action to cope with stress when prevention does not take place includes many volunteer agencies that provide support groups and counseling to those with particular stressful conditions. Battered women's shelters, rape crisis centers, bereavement support groups, victims of violence groups, and specific health problem groups are all positive steps in providing social support.

Healthy People 2010 Objective: Increase the Proportion of Persons with Serious Mental Illnesses Who Are Employed

Target: 51 percent.

Baseline: 42 percent of persons aged 18 years and older with serious mental illnesses were employed in 1994.

It is important for those experiencing stress to regain control over situations that seem hopeless. Where stress becomes persistent or chronic and support groups are not enough, individual care may become necessary. The control of stress and violence in a community is now considered a priority of many health agencies.[17] Cutbacks in community mental health clinics have been a major concern to mental health caregivers. Without the volunteer agencies that provide group work, most communities would be overwhelmed with the problems associated with stress in society.

Suicide

A frequent result of chronic depression and the lack of mental health services by a community is suicide. The incidence of suicide is aggravated by the social pathology of our society. In a society marked by alcohol and other drug abuse, family violence, unemployment, crime, gangs and instability, the risk of depression, loss of self-esteem, and sense of worthlessness is expected. Individual illness becomes a community's malaise as these social pathologies escalate and become more overwhelming to the resources of a community. Suicide is both a symptom and a personal attempt at "treatment" for the social pathologies of the 1990s. Suicide rates for 1998 are given in Chapter 8 (See Table 8.1).

Healthy People 2010 Objective: Reduce the Suicide Rate

Target: 6.0 suicide deaths per 100,000 population.

Baseline: 10.8 suicide deaths per 100,000 population in 1998 (preliminary data; age adjusted to the year 2000 standard population).

Race and Mental Health

The association of sex, race, or gender with mental illness is explicitly found in many situations where people feel powerless. Certainly in a society that has yet to come to grips with the reality of diversity, those differently abled, people of color, women, and gay men and lesbians are often at greater risk of feelings of powerlessness. As voting activist, Fannie Lou Hammer, has said of black people, "We are sick and tired of being sick and tired."[18]

In the United States, studies have found that race and diagnosis have been strongly associated. Until the 1960s when civil rights became an important thread in our psyche, the counseling profession demonstrated little interest in or concern for the status of racial, ethnic, or other minority groups.[19] Even in the 1990s there was little evidence of changes within the mental health profession in terms of trained minority clinicians, diversity of therapeutic techniques, or community mental health outreach to minority populations. It is not unusual for a diagnosis of schizophrenia rather than affective illness to be given more frequently to African Americans than to whites.[20] Minorities tend to receive "less preferred" forms of treatment, and little or no attention has been directed to the need for developing counseling procedures that are compatible with minority cultural values.[21] Perhaps even more significant is the apparent lack of preventive and therapeutic care of mental distress among people of color who have to cope with the duel possibility of personal mental illness and the stress of surviving in a racist society.

The person of color must also live "biculturally" in a predominantly white society that may interpret anger and rage at white people and social systems as mental illness, instead of the challenge of being caught in a system that values only one set of standards. In other words, "institutional racism" exists even in the mental health profession, which basically imposes a "white" cultural standard to all behavior and expectation.[22] Add to this the lack of practitioners of different ethnic and cultural backgrounds and there is a disparity of mental health services to minority people.

There has been some debate as to whether race-specific mental health programs are appropriate in a climate of social, political, and economic reform. A study of 1,516 African Americans, 1,888 Asian Americans, and 1,306 Mexican Americans who used one of thirty-six predominantly white (mainstream) or eighteen ethnic-specific mental health centers in Los Angeles County over a six-year period compared return rate, length of treatment, and treatment outcome. Results showed that ethnic clients who attended ethnic-specific programs had a higher return rate and stayed in treatment longer than those using mainstream services.[23]

Research and clinical practice have propelled advocates and mental health professionals to press for "linguistically and culturally competent services" to improve utilization and effectiveness of treatment for different cultures. Culturally competent services incorporate respect for and understanding of, ethnic and racial groups, as well as their histories, traditions, beliefs, and value systems.

When one compares suicide rates internationally, men always have a higher rate than women. Among ten industrialized countries the male rate of suicide ranges from 12 per 100,000 to 30 per 100,000. The lowest rate among these countries is the United Kingdom with 12 per 100,000 and the highest is Denmark with 30 per 100,000. The U.S. rate is 19.9 for male suicides. The rate of suicide for women in ten industrialized countries ranges from 3.4 per 100,000 in the United Kingdom to 15.1 in Denmark. The U.S. rate for female suicides is 4.8. The question that comes to mind is, Why do Denmark and the

United Kingdom have dramatically contrasting rates given their proximity and somewhat similar cultural characteristics? It has been suggested that the long, cold, dark winters of Denmark aggravate mental illness and strict gun control in England may prevent successful suicide.

Although suicide rates are lower for women than men among all races, these rates have been increasing for women worldwide, especially among older women. This may be correlated with increasing poverty and poorer health among older women in developing countries and the greater freedom of choice afforded women in developed countries. Older people use all the usual methods of killing themselves, such as guns, hanging, and drugs, but they also use slower means that ultimately may not be classified as suicide. These "subintentional" suicide methods include not eating, not taking medicines, drinking too much, delaying treatment, and taking physical risks.

Finally, cultural differences, values, and beliefs impact the taking of one's life. Worldwide, different people define quality of life and life expectancy in such a way that suicide may be a personal choice that is accepted and assisted within the norms of any given culture. Just as one cannot easily define mental illness across cultures, one cannot place value judgments on the taking of one's own life across cultures.

> **Discussion:** Why is the suicide rate for U.S. females considerably lower than that of comparable countries?

Gender as a Mental Health Determinant

In developed countries, where diagnosis for mental illness is more openly made, women are more often found to be suffering from higher rates of mental illness than men. About 60 percent of psychiatric office visits were made by women in 1990, but women make up only 51 percent of the population.

Some attribute this difference to sex role stereotyping, where women are imposed with societal expectations of being dependent, care giving, nurturing, homebound, deferring to authority, and passive. Since the rise of feminism, the stereotypical feminine roles for all women have been studied and have proven to produce great stress and mental inconsistencies for women who have to live in a world where traditional feminine roles do not mean success.[24] Even among homemakers, women who work only in their home, the stereotypical "women's place" does not seem to produce good mental health. One study found that in terms of eleven of twelve symptoms of psychological distress, working women were found to be overwhelmingly better off than the housewives. The major reason for this difference was the status denigration that marriage brings to housewives. Further studies have confirmed that feelings of powerlessness and a sense of relative inequality of status and power may be major contributors to the greater mental distress of those women in "traditional" roles.

Social reorganization between women's and men's roles has been a goal of the women's movement worldwide. Where equity in work, wages, social, and interpersonal relationships can be found, there is the belief that mental health will improve for those who in the past have felt less equal. Equality is not the panacea for mental health problems in our community, but it is a preventive effort that can be achieved through awareness, legislation, and community action. In the general population, mental illnesses are often preventable by psychological therapy, or social change. Both women and men can be helped by changes in our society that empowers women and gives them access to the same opportunities and choices as men.

Types of Mental Illness

Schizophrenia Diagnostically, schizophrenia is considered when a person experiences thoughts that are removed, broadcast, or echoes; when one's actions or feelings are thought to be controlled by some external agency; or when one is hearing voices of people not actually present. These florid psychotic symptoms may be short lived, but typically schizophrenia impairs social interaction over long periods without medication. Schizophrenia affects one in every 100 people, or more than 2 million people in the United States.

Schizophrenia is associated with increased mortality from suicide as well as increased morbidity associated with poor nutrition, personal neglect, and increased communicable and noncommunicable infections. There is strong evidence of an inherited vulnerability to schizophrenia; however, certain "recreational" drugs and prolonged alcohol use have been shown to cause schizophrenic behaviors that are sometimes not controlled by discontinued use of the drug or alcohol.

Affective Disorders This broad group of mental disorders ranges from severe forms of illness such as manic depressive psychosis or "bipolar" illness to common forms of dysfunction such as mood disorders that include depression and anxiety.

Affective disorders, although diagnosed in all cultures, sometimes have unique manifestations that are culturally based. For example, auditory hallucinations of spirit beings are common to Native Americans, guilt and self-reproach are common in Judeo-Christian and Islamic cultures, and ideas of bewitchment are common to Yorubas.[25]

A 1989 international study among the United States, United Kingdom, Australia, Uganda, and Greece showed one month prevalence rates for anxiety states higher among females (24 percent) than males (12 percent). The percentage of bipolar incidence appeared to be the same in both sexes and vary between 0.6 percent and 0.9 percent. Depression incidences were between 4.8 percent and 7.4 percent for all countries except Uganda whose depression incidence was as high as 18.9 percent during social upheaval. Surveys in other developing countries have reported lower rates for depression.[26]

Higher depression rates are reported among those of lower socioeconomic status, the middle aged, the unemployed, those sexually and physically abused in earlier life, and among those who live in unsatisfactory housing conditions. Other aggravating variables include poverty, poor education, physical ill-health, and social isolation.

Genetic factors are important causes of severe forms of depressive illness, but environmental social adversity seems to play a greater role in less severe disorders. In developed countries, the loss of a confidant or stressful life events with the absence of an intimate relationship often contribute to depressive disorders.

In developing countries vulnerability factors may include malnutrition and parasitic infestation. Long-term social adversity is common in many developing countries, which makes accurate etiological determination difficult.

Healthy People 2010 Objective: Increase the Proportion of Adults with Mental Disorders Who Receive Treatment

Increase in Adults With Mental Disorders Receiving Treatment	1997 Baseline (%) (unless noted)	2010 Target (%)
Adults aged 18 to 54 years with serious mental illness	47 (1991)	55
Adults aged 18 years and older with recognized depression	23	50
Adults aged 18 years and older with schizophrenia	60 (1984)	75
Adults aged 18 years and older with anxiety disorders	38	50

Organic Disorders In the United States it is estimated that 1.3 percent of the adult population have severe cognitive impairment. The most common form of deterioration is senile dementia of Alzheimer type. The prevalence rate of dementia rises sharply with age, from about 2 percent in persons aged 65 to 70 years to about 20 percent in those over eighty years, and to 50 percent in those over ninety years.[27]

Huntington chorea, an hereditary disease of the brain, characterized by jerky involuntary movements and mental deterioration, affects between 4 and 7 per 100,000 and is worldwide in its distribution. In one unique population, a Scottish fishing community, the rate is 560 per 100,000 and is probably due to intermarriage since this is a genetically transferred condition. Most cases begin between ages thirty and fifty years, and its direct cause is unknown.[28]

Public health measures to reduce biological risk factors are particularly important in developing countries where there is an increased risk of organic brain syndromes or epilepsy as a result of perinatal trauma and intracranial infections. Immunization programs to reduce viral meningo-encephalitis, iodine and vitamin supplements, and good nutrition for pregnant women are important public health goals that in turn improve mental health.

Drugs and Alcohol

Substance Abuse

It may be that nothing impacts the mental health of the United States as much as the use and abuse of alcohol and other substances. It has been stated that substance abuse is the number one preventable health problem in the nation.[29] Data show that approximately 150 million people drink alcohol,[30] including 10–15 million alcoholics and another 18 million problem drinkers.[31] It is our nation's number one legal drug of choice. Tobacco use follows alcohol with

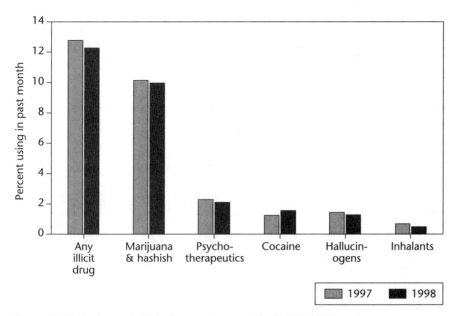

Figure 16.1 Past month illicit drug use in ages 12+ (1997–1998).

(*Source:* National Clearinghouse for Alcohol and Drug Information. National Household Survey on Drugs)

147.6 million lifetime users. Marijuana is the illicit drug of choice, followed by psychotherapeutic drugs and cocaine.

The 1999 National Household Survey on Drug Abuse found that an estimated 13.9 million Americans twelve years and older had used an illicit drug in the month prior to a national interview (Figure 16.1). Marijuana is the most commonly used illicit drug, used by 81 percent of current illicit drug users. From 1997 to 1998, drugs that increased in use among this age group were cocaine (from 0.8 percent to 1 percent) and tranquilizers (from 0.2 percent to 0.5 percent).

Table 16.5 is a list of several drugs and the percentage of their lifetime and past month use.[32] Although illicit drug use is decreasing in developed countries, heroin and cocaine use is becoming more common in developing countries. Drug injecting is also becoming common in developing countries, which means there is a concurrent increase in the risk of HIV, hepatitis, and other infections. Worldwide, between 160,000 and 210,000 deaths every year are associated with drug injecting.[33]

Alcohol as Our National Drug of Choice

Alcohol is a socially accepted drug and often is not considered a drug at all. Due to the nation's casual demeanor about alcohol, several social problems have arisen including:

- Traffic accidents
- Injuries and deaths
- Medical conditions

Table 16.5 Percent reporting lifetime and past month use of illicit substances (1997–1998).

| | TIME PERIOD | | | |
| | Lifetime | | Past Month | |
Drug	1997	1998	1997	1998
Any Illicit Drug[1]	35.6	35.8	6.4	6.2
Marijuana and Hashish	32.9	33.0	5.1	5.0
Cocaine	10.5	10.6	0.7	0.8
Crack	1.9	2.0	0.3	0.2
Inhalants	5.7	5.8	0.4	0.3
Hallucinogens	9.6	9.9	0.8	0.7
PCP	3.0	3.5	0.1	0.0
LSD	7.8	7.9	0.2	0.3
Heroin	0.9	1.1	0.2	0.1
Nonmedical use of any psychotherapeutic[2]	9.1	9.2	1.2	1.1
Stimulants	4.5	4.4	0.3	0.3
Sedatives	1.9	2.1	0.1	0.1
Tranquilizers	3.2	3.5	0.4	0.3
Analgesics	4.9	5.3	0.7	0.8
Any Illicit Drug Other than Marijuana[1]	18.9	18.9	2.6	2.5

[1]Any Illicit Drug indicates use at least once of marijuana/hashish, cocaine (including crack), inhalants, hallucinogens (including PCP and LSD), heroin , or any prescription-type psychotherapeutic used nonmedically. Any Illicit Drug Other than Marijuana indicates use at least once of any of these listed drugs, regardless of marijuana/hashish use; marijuana/hashish users who also have used any of the other listed drugs are included.

[2]Nonmedical use of any prescription-type stimulant, sedative, tranquilizer, or analgesic; does not include over-the-counter drugs.

(*Source:* SAMHSA, Office of Applied Studies, National Household Survey on Drug Abuse, 1997 and 1998)

- Birth defects (including fetal alcohol syndrome)
- Violence
- Crime
- Relationship discord
- Suicide
- Job loss
- Family destruction

Alcohol costs our nation over $90 billion yearly; about 46 percent of this amount is due to lost production, 29 percent from health and medical costs, 13 percent from motor vehicle accidents, 7 percent from violent crimes, 4 percent in community education, and 1 percent due to fire losses.[34]

In 1998, 113 million Americans age twelve and older reported current use of alcohol, meaning they used alcohol at least once during the thirty days prior to the interview (Figure 16.2). About 33 million of this group engaged in binge drinking, meaning they drank five or more drinks on one occasion during that thirty-day period. Twelve million were heavy drinkers, meaning they had five

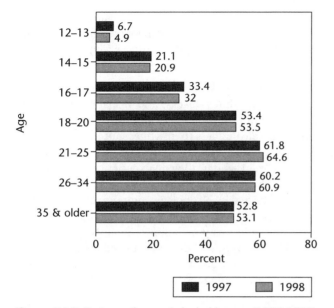

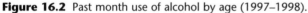

Figure 16.2 Past month use of alcohol by age (1997–1998).

(*Source:* National Clearinghouse for Alcohol and Drug Information. National Household Survey on Drug Abuse)

or more drinks on one occasion five or more days during the past thirty days.[35]

There may be a link between alcohol consumption and cancer. Researchers believe as alcohol consumption increases, so does one's risk for cancer. The National Institute on Alcohol Abuse and Alcoholism believes the strongest associations are between alcohol and cancers of the upper digestive tract: the mouth, esophagus, the pharynx, and the larynx. Alcohol may also be linked directly or indirectly to liver, breast, and colon cancers.[36]

Fetal Alcohol Syndrome and Effects

The role of alcohol on a developing fetus is a major concern of health professionals. Fetal Alcohol Syndrome (FAS) and Fetal Alcohol Effects (FAE) are major alcohol-related conditions that causes birth defects, mental retardation, other behavioral and mental abnormalities, and facial abnormalities. The National Center for Environmental Health suggests that FAS accounts for approximately 4,000 preventable birth defects in newborns each year in the United States.[37] Additionally, another 4,000 babies have FAS-related problems, but they do not meet the clinical diagnosis. Fetal Alcohol Syndrome is a particularly severe problem among minority populations, especially Native Americans. Even so, blacks and Hispanics also have a higher rate of FAS than do whites.

The best prevention of FAS is for women to abstain from alcohol when pregnant. However, since some women are at higher risk than others, prevention programs are being designed to decrease FAS in the newborn population.

By following Healthy People 2000 guidelines, community health professionals are helping by screening, counseling, and providing support services, case management and follow-up of at-risk women throughout their pregnancies.

Minority Populations and Alcohol Facts

Although statistically it appears that whites, blacks, and Hispanics use alcohol similarly as groups, there are some unique differences among these populations. For example, blacks as a group use alcohol less than whites, but they experience more medical problems associated with alcohol use. In addition, while Hispanics experience less medical problems than whites, they do experience more alcohol-related traffic accidents. Asians, on the average, use and abuse alcohol less than whites; however, they are easily affected by alcohol consumption. Among Native Americans, alcohol is a contributor in 75 percent of all accidents reported—accidents are the leading cause of death in this population.[38] Table 16.6 gives some examples of community health interventions designed to reduce alcohol and substance abuse by young Native Americans from 1988 to 1992. Figure 16.3 shows alcoholism rates by age, race, and gender for Native Americans.

Discussion: What community health programs are active in your community to reduce alcohol and substance abuse?

There may be genetic traits among some minorities that predispose them to higher risk or even protect them from the harmful effects of alcohol, although this concept is not greatly understood. Besides heredity, another possible reason for higher consumption of alcohol among some minorities may be acculturation. The longer people are in the United States, the more likely they are to approach the average consumption of alcohol (by generations). More prevention and treatment programs for minority populations must be researched and evaluated before conclusions can be reached.[39]

Women and Alcohol Use

Like other community health studies to date, most studies about alcohol have been done with male subjects. The growing consciousness about women's health has encouraged research that now includes women and their diverse characteristics. In recent studies, health care professionals are finding differences in drinking patterns between males and females. According to the Alcohol, Drug Abuse, and Mental Health Administration (ADAMHA), fewer women drink than men, and women are less likely to experience alcohol-related problems than men. However, when it comes to the heaviest drinkers, women equal or surpass men with alcohol-related problems.[40]

Consumption of alcohol also affects females and males differently. First of all, women tend to experience physiological effects of alcohol more quickly than males. According to the ADAMHA, there may be three explanations for these differences: females have a lower body water content than males, they metabolize alcohol less quickly due to the enzyme alcohol dehydrogenase, and

Table 16.6 Community interventions designed to reduce alcohol and substance abuse by young people on Native American reservations.

Program Name	Description	Program Name	Description
Children are People	Educational support for children of alcoholics.	STEP	Education program for parents of 6–12 years.
Home Education Parties	Small group discussions	SMILE	Skill building for teens
Just Say No Club	National club	Super Tots	Healthy living skills
Preparing for Drug Free Years	Education program for parents of 7–14 yrs.	Youth Leadership	1-day sessions on current issues.
School-Based Prevention	Education by request of schools	Drug Free Carnival	Annual carnival

(*Source:* Cheadle, Allen, 1995. A Community-based approach to preventing alcohol use among adolescents on an American Indian reservation. *Public Health Reports*, July–Aug, Vol. 110. No. 4)

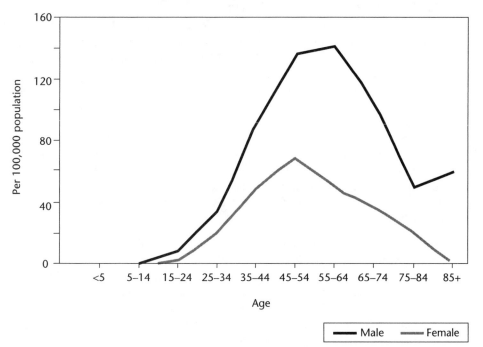

Figure 16.3 Alcoholism death rates by age and sex among Native Americans.

(*Source:* National Clearinghouse for Alcohol and Drug Information)

fluctuations in gonadal hormone levels during the menstrual cycle may affect alcohol metabolism. Chronic use also seems to affect women more dramatically and quickly than men. In fact, women have death rates 50 to 100 percent higher than those of male alcoholics.[41]

Along with the above, research has shown that white women are less likely to abstain from alcohol than their black or Hispanic counterparts. Even so, problems related to alcohol differ for women of color when compared to white women. For example, black women were shown to experience more health problems related to alcohol, while white women were shown to experience more social problems.[42]

Health risks associated with alcohol use/abuse by women range from breast cancer to reproductive problems. Preliminary data suggest a link between increased use of alcohol (one ounce of absolute alcohol daily) and breast cancer.[43] However, other studies have been inconclusive regarding this relationship, suggesting that more research is needed to make that connection. According to the National Institute on Alcohol Abuse and Alcoholism (NIAAA), reproductive dysfunctions with alcohol abuse and alcoholism include amenorrhea, anovulation, luteal phase dysfunction, and ovarian pathology.[44] These may lead to infertility, sexual dysfunction, and increased risk for spontaneous abortion. Once again, more studies about alcohol and women need to be conducted.

An Overview of Other Drugs

Although alcohol is the drug of choice for most young people and even adults, there are many other prescription, street, designer, and over-the-counter drugs that impact the health of a community. From the personal abuse of prescribed and unprescribed drugs, to the crime associated with illegal sales and distribution, the problem of drugs in our society is a major source of community health prevention programs, especially in the school. In 1993, there was a shift in teenage drug use, with an increase in marijuana use and a decrease in the belief that it is a risk to the user's health.

We have yet to adequately deal with the treatment for addiction, hoping that prevention will soon eliminate the need for treatment. Perhaps even more complex, due to lack of empirical data, is the question of whether legalizing drugs for personal or medical use, such as marijuana, would be an appropriate public health position.

> *Over the centuries our laws and social customs for regulating psychoactive drugs incorporated many fundamental scientific errors such as: (1) bad pharmacology—that marijuana is an addictive narcotic and that tobacco does not contain a drug; (2) bad psychology—that repetitive drug use can always be controlled through intentional behaviors; (3) bad sociology—that the drugs used by foreigners and minority groups are the bad drugs and that criminal laws can effectively reduce psychoactive drug use at a low cost to society; and 4) bad economics—that the increased cost of business for selling an illegal product will outweigh the increased profits to be made from selling through illegal markets.[45]*

Given these initial problems in creating health and social policy associated with drug use, it is easier to understand why new attempts to find solutions are difficult.

There are some in the profession who believe reducing penalties and decriminalizing some drug use would reduce the overall abuse problems as well as the cost of social programs associated with the criminal justice system.[46] In general, the position of the American Public Health Association is that legalization of drugs would be no panacea. "Although legalization is attractive because the adverse consequences of illicit drug use today probably stem more from the drugs' illegal status than from their chemical properties, the risks of exposing many more people to these drugs, which would occur with legalization, are large."[47]

Types of Drugs

Drugs are any substances that modify the nervous system and states of consciousness. They are currently divided into seven categories based on their chemical properties and the effects that they cause:

Depressants include alcohol, tranquilizers, and sedatives and are used as sedatives.

Stimulants stimulate physical and/or mental processes and include amphetamines, cocaine, nicotine, and caffeine.

Narcotics include opiate derivatives such as morphine, heroin, and codeine, as well as synthetic drugs like methadone. These drugs were originally designed for pain relief.

Hallucinogens distort sensory information, and include LSD, mescaline, psilocybin, and PCP.

Marijuana and its derivatives are in a separate category due to their potential multiple effects.

Inhalants are the mind-altering vapors from a variety of sources including household solvents and aerosols.

The last category includes other drugs, like designer (human-made) drugs, and anabolic steroids.

Besides these, of course, are the multiple drugs we have in our households for a variety of purposes, both prescription and over-the-counter, including caffeine. The National Institute on Drug Abuse estimates the average American household owns thirty-five drugs—an indication of our desire for the quick fix to our ailments and problems.

Historical Implications for Today's Drug Problem

As a nation, we are losing the "war on drugs." Our traditional system of punishing the dealers and users is not working. Jails are overcrowded, treatment facilities have waiting lists, and current school drug and alcohol programs like D.A.R.E. and the "Just Say No" campaign have had grim evaluations in their ability to prevent youth from using alcohol and other drugs. As a result of this overwhelming community health problem, Congress enacted stricter laws and penalties in the early 1980s. This seems to have only added to the burden of the already overtaxed judicial system, while not decreasing or preventing substance use and abuse.

Rehabilitation through punitive approaches have been "misguided, ineffective, or even counterproductive." [48] "Incarcerating drug users rarely, if ever, deters drug use. Instead, it reinforces drug careers by extending users' drug connections, makes them more familiar and comfortable with the illicit drug world, alienates them from conventional society, and hardens their attitudes against civil authorities."[49] In an era when the U.S. government is calling for more police on the streets and more jail time for users, we as a society must "just say no." Prevention of substance abuse is possible through well-designed, grassroots efforts.

Substance Abuse Prevention

From a community health perspective, prevention programs are key in reducing the use and abuse of substances in our country. In the past several years, the field of substance abuse has moved proactively from a treatment to prevention focus. Regarding substance use, there are three levels of prevention: primary prevention—efforts to preclude the onset of substance abuse; targeted prevention—efforts targeting individuals or groups which are characterized by identifiable risk factors for substance abuse; and early intervention—efforts targeting individuals or groups which are characterized by problematic use of alcohol or other drugs in order to reduce the likelihood that patterned abuse or dependence will develop.[50]

Currently, many prevention programs across the country are focusing on individual-based risk factors that place our youth and young adults at risk. Some notable risk factors for both groups are listed below:[51]

- Inadequate life skills
- Lack of self-control, assertiveness, and peer-refusal skills
- Low self-esteem and self-confidence
- Emotional and psychological problems
- Favorable attitudes toward ATOD (alcohol and other drugs) use
- Rejection of commonly held values and religion
- School failure
- Lack of school bonding
- Early antisocial behavior

Other risk factors include permissive parental attitude toward use, parental drug abuse, family history, and stress.

Promising strategies to address these risk factors are being used with relatively good success. Social and life skills training, alternative programs such as wilderness camps, individual or group therapy or counseling, tutoring and homework support activities, and mentoring programs have been implemented throughout the country and have demonstrated effectiveness in preventing substance abuse among young people.

In this complex day and age, many people are turning to different substances for a variety of reasons. If we, as community health professionals, are to change the current trends in alcohol and other drug use, we must pay close attention to those programs with proven track records, and not just those that receive the most financial and media support.

Violence as a Community Health Illness

It is a reflection of the immaturity of the public health work on violence that there is not yet unanimity on its definition.[52] However, generally, it is known as the threatened or actual use[53] of physical force against another person or against oneself, which either results in or has a high likelihood of resulting in injury or death.[54] Violence is a worldwide pandemic of devastating proportion. Violence exists in reality in every community in the form of assault, rape, gay-bashing, domestic violence, racism, anti-Semitic language and behavior, suicide, child abuse, and elder abuse. Violence exists in movies, on television, in comics, videos, music, and sports. Interpersonal violence, the use of physical force with intent to inflict injury or death, clearly represents a serious public health problem that must be addressed immediately. Considering the medical costs and productivity losses resulting from family violence, the actual financial cost of violence may be from $5–10 billion a year.[55]

The first public health research related to violence was done in the 1960s. Domestic violence became a serious health issue in the 1970s and finally, in 1985, C. Everett Koop introduced violence as a chronic disease that was targeted in the Healthy People 2000 objectives.

In 1999, violent crimes had declined significantly since 1990, with 2.2 million *reported* cases a year. Violence was perpetrated not only by criminals. In a stressful society, sometimes violent action is seen as most useful in curbing violence. In 1991, one-fifth of the population knew someone who felt they had been abused by police. The Rodney King police brutality case of 1992 was the impetus for angry, violent riots that erupted in Los Angeles when the police officers who beat him, as he lay on the ground after a police chase, were found not guilty. What the police violence and the subsequent community violence really illustrated was the frustration of a contemporary society that has been victimized by racial discrimination, massive urban unemployment, and unequal opportunities for the poor and for people of color. Violence as a public health issue requires social and economic support for prevention. Violent behavior is the result of personal, societal, familial, and environmental factors requiring long-term, intensive health promotion strategies. Such strategies demand collaborative, broad-based use of professionals and community organizations whose goals include community action intervention models based on integrated efforts which include both individual and organizational changes.[56]

Interpersonal Violence

Interpersonal violence accounts for about 350,000 hospitalizations, 1.5 million hospital days, and $638 million in health care costs annually.[57] Complete data on nonfatal injuries is difficult to collect since much violence, particularly that occuring behind closed doors, is not reported. As many as 4 million women and 2 million children a year suffer physical and sexual violence and neglect. The Child Abuse Prevention, Adoption and Family Services Act of 1988 defines child abuse and neglect as physical or mental injury, sexual abuse or exploitation, negligent treatment or maltreatment of a child by a person who is responsible for the child's welfare, under circumstances which indicate that the child's health or welfare is harmed or threatened. Neglect accounts for the greatest portion of abuse incidents (47 percent), followed by physical abuse (25 percent), sexual abuse (15 percent), and emotional abuse (5 percent).[58] Educational neglect was the most frequent category of neglect, followed by physical and then emotional neglect. There were nearly 3 million reports of suspected abuse or child neglect in 1997, a 45 percent increase since 1990 as shown in Figure 16.4.

Contributing Factors to Violence

Demographically, violent behavior is committed disproportionately by young males, particularly those in lower socioeconomic levels. Although there is an over-representation of African Americans, socioeconomic status is a greater predictor of violence than race.[59] Suicide and homicide cause about 22 percent of deaths in childhood and adolescence and 35 percent of all injury deaths.[60] Women are most

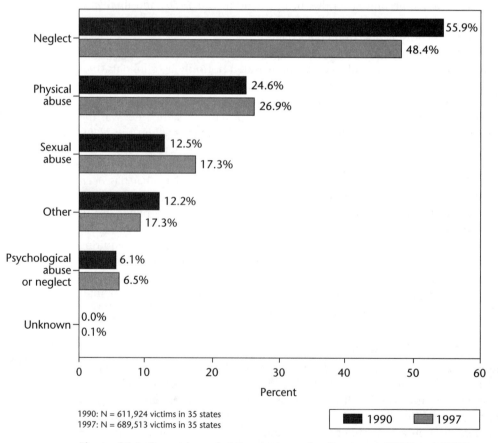

1990: N = 611,924 victims in 35 states
1997: N = 689,513 victims in 35 states

1990   1997

Figure 16.4 Comparison of victims by type of maltreatment (1990 and 1997).

(*Source:* U.S. Department of Health and Human Services. The Administration for Children and Families, "Child maltreatment victims")

often abused when they are pregnant, when they are young, and during a dating situation that appears to be a training ground for marital abuse.

Alcohol and drug use appears to increase the potential for violent behavior and victimization. The immediate access of a weapon is another critical factor. Violent children usually come from violent families; therefore violence appears to be a learned response to conflict, stress, and frustration. There is evidence that children and adolescents who use violence may mirror conflict resolution techniques they see on television since viewing aggressive acts increases aggressive behavior among children. A study of the 1991–1995 television season shows that children's programming actually featured more violence than adult prime time. The total number of violent scenes in entertainment programming increased by 74 percent in three years—from 1,002 in 1992 to 1,417 in 1994 and 1,738 in 1995—reaching an average of nearly ten incidents of violence per channel per hour during the most recent season, even after excluding commercials and all nonfiction programming. Violence involving gunplay more than tripled during the same period, rising 334 percent from 159 in 1992 to 218 in 1994 and 531 in 1995.[61] Public schools have always experienced problems with violence, but it appears that there has been an escalation of violence in the past decade. Debate continues as to whether or not media such as films, music, and TV are a cause of this increase in school violence (Figure 16.5).

Discussion: Will censoring children's TV reduce violent behavior among children?

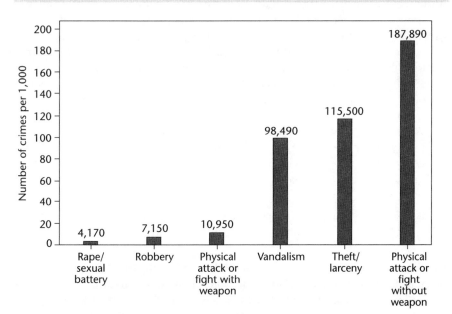

Figure 16.5 Number of various crimes occurring in public school (1997).

(*Source:* U.S. Department of Education. National Center for Education Statistics, Fast Response Survey System, "Principal/school disciplinarian survey on school violence," FRSS 63, 1997)

BOX 16.2 TV Promotes Violence and Unhealthy Lifestyles[62]

1. Number of violent acts the average American child sees on TV by age 18: 200,000
2. Number of murders witnessed by children on television by age 18: 16,000
3. Percentage of youth violence directly attributable to TV viewing: 10
4. Percentage of Hollywood executives who think there is a link between TV violence and real-life violence: 80
5. Percentage of Americans that believe TV and movies are responsible for juvenile crime: 73
6. Percentage of children polled who said they felt "upset" or "scared" by violence on television: 91
7. Percent increase in network news coverage of homicide between 1993 and 1996: 721
8. Percent reduction in the American homicide rate between 1993 and 1996: 20
9. Percent increase in number of violent scenes per hour on ten major channels from 1992 to 1994: 41
10. Number of medical studies since 1985 linking excessive television watching to increasing rates of obesity: 12
11. Percentage of American children ages six to eleven who were seriously overweight in 1963: 4.5; 1993: 14
12. Number of ads aired for "junk-food" during four hours of Saturday morning cartoons: 202

Domestic Violence

Although it has existed throughout all history in all cultures, domestic violence is a newly identified public health problem that is viewed seriously by the American Public Health Association and other private and public groups. Men of all classes and countries use violence and coercion to keep women in their place. Millions of women are beaten each year in their homes; many are killed. Some cultures encourage wife beating as a man's right; in others, the problem is hidden away as a private matter. Battered women's shelters now exist in many countries.

A ten-year study conducted by the U.S. Department of Justice found that in 1993, women age twelve or older annually sustained almost 5 million violent victimizations. In 29 percent of all violence against women, the perpetrator was an intimate (a husband, ex-husband, boyfriend, or ex-boyfriend).[63]

Discussion: Is there a women's shelter in your community? How is it funded? What does it contribute to a family's health?

Later studies have found that domestic violence is statistically consistent across racial and ethnic boundaries. Domestic violence offers within same-sex relationships the same statistical frequency as in heterosexual relationships, and battering tends to be a pattern of violence rather than a one-time occurrence.

In the time it takes to read this paragraph, a woman will have been beaten, and every eighteen seconds another woman in the United States is beaten. By the end of this year millions of women, children, and men will have been slapped, hit, shoved, thrown around, restrained, kicked, knifed, raped, choked, burned, and threatened with belt buckles, bottles, and other weapons to control or punish them.[64] This is domestic violence.

Denial, apathy, embarrassment, and guilt cause this serious public health problem to remain unreported by victims and communities. Since it is often unreported, cases often remain unsolved and future violence unpreventable. Only 5 percent of the estimated millions of violent incidents are officially identified as abuse under the current definitions of abuse, when in reality, physical, emotional, and sexual domestic abuse is an everyday occurrence in every community and in many homes. Among homeless families headed by women, 25 to 50 percent left home to escape domestic violence.[65]

Women who are battered tend to share only two characteristics: they are women and they have been abused. Demographic surveys show that battering happens in families of all racial and class backgrounds. Women are the primary victims of all forms of interpersonal violence of every type. Girls are the majority of victims of child abuse (54 percent), while white women make up the majority of abused spouses and abused elderly.[66]

In the home, women are about as violent as men. They hit, bite, and kick just as often as men, but they do not do as much damage. Men inflict more harm because of their generally greater size and strength. In addition, violence by women is often in retaliation for abuse or as self-defense. Women commit only 8 percent of all homicides in this country, but 51 percent of them are against partners with a history of wife abuse.[67]

Part of the solution is training professionals and others to recognize and report domestic violence. The *Journal of the American Medical Association (JAMA)* in 1992 reported that more than half of thirty-eight doctors in an unnamed urban HMO said they had no training in recognizing domestic violence which in this study included violence against women and children.[68]

An iconoclastic response to the public health crisis of violence is to indict a possible root cause, the family. In the United States there is a tendency to hold the family in a "see-no-evil" reverence. "Battered wives and kids who are battered or sexually abused stay silent or risk breaking the cardinal rule that says the family is above reproach. Some people would rather die than burst the myth that families are unimaginably nice places where nothing bad ever happens."[69] In fact, given the data on child and spousal abuse, elder bashing, marital rape, incest, and family murders, the family may be the most violent institution in American society.

Until all families, in all their variety, are safe places in which to grow and live, the epidemic of domestic violence cannot be abated. Although the answer is not immediately clear, it is known that changing the balance of power in relationships to one in which men are not attributed power over others by virtue of their gender, is a beginning. Laws that prohibit all violence in the home and enforcement that quickly removes violent people from the home, and punish violence in the home with the same magnitude as violence on the street, are another important step to reducing continued domestic violence. In other words, social change must be made in the home. The empowerment of women and children in our society in the last fifteen years, although seeming to make violence more common and visible, has actually been a means of confronting violence as a health issue, preventing continued violence, and treating both the victim and the abuser.

As mentioned earlier, the family is probably the most violent institution in our society. Aggression, anger, rage, hate, and hostility are usually seen as evidence of a disturbed personality, but they seem to have a normative role within families. In family settings where role stereotypes inhibit free expression of needs, particularly for women and children, aggressiveness is inevitable. Escalating violence within the family often precedes fatal injury.

Homicide

Although homicide is an important cause of death worldwide, Table 16.7 shows that the U.S. homicide rate is one of the highest in the world. Homicide was the cause of death for 19,491 Americans (7.2 per 100,000 population) in 1997.[70] Homicide is the second leading cause of death for young persons aged fifteen to twenty-four years and the leading cause of death for African Americans in this age group.[71] Homicide rates are dropping among all groups, but the decreases are not as dramatic among youth, who already exhibit the highest rates. In 1997, 6,146 young persons aged fifteen to twenty-four years were victims of homicide, amounting to almost seventeen youth homicide victims per day in the United States.[72] Of all homicide victims in 1994, 38 percent were under age twenty-four years.[73]

The homicide rate among males aged fifteen to twenty-four years in the United States is ten times higher than in Canada, fifteen times higher than in Australia, and twenty-eight times higher than in France or Germany.[74] For a U.S. citizen, the lifetime chance of becoming a homicide victim is 1 in 240 for whites and 1 in 47 for blacks and other minorities. Except for Puerto Rico, the U.S. homicide rate is many times higher than other western industrial democracies where gun ownership is legal. For example, the homicide rate in the United States is five times higher than Italy.

BOX 16.3 Lifetime Risk of Death by Homicide

U.S. total	1:133
Male	1:84
White	1:131
Black	1:21
Female	1:282
White	1:369
Black	1:104

(*Source:* U.S. Bureau of Justice, 1993)

Table 16.7 International homicide rates per 100,000.

Highest	Rate	Lowest	Rate
Philippines	38.70	Mali	.00
Lesotho	36.40	Argentina	.20
Jamaica	17.96	Ireland	.54
Lebanon	13.17	Greece	.85
Thailand	12.36	Norway	.90
Bahamas	12.20	Switzerland	.92
U.S.	7.00	Saudi Arabia	1.00

(*Source:* Adapted from *The Economist Book of Vital World Statistics,* 1990. In Almanac of World Facts, 1995: Rand McNally)

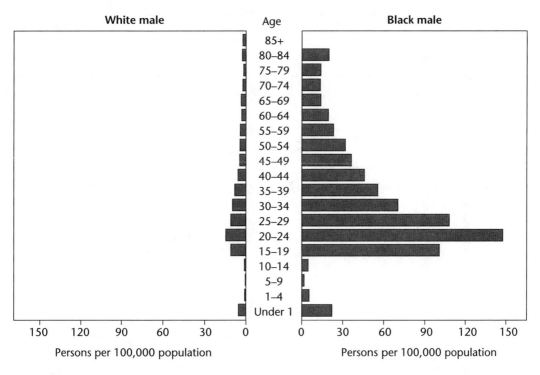

Figure 16.6 Male homicide rates by race and age (1999).

(*Source:* Chart prepared by U.S. Census Bureau)

In 1998 the homicide death rate for black males was 132.0 per 100,000, 63.5 per 100,000 for Hispanic males as compared to 16.5 for white males. Figure 16.6 shows the comparison of homicide rates between whites and blacks in the United States. In part, this reflects the added stress of being a black or Hispanic male in American society, where few minority males have role models or have access to equal economic opportunities.

Healthy People 2010 Objective: Reduce Homicides

Target: 3.2 homicides per 100,000 population.

Baseline: 6.2 homicides per 100,000 population in 1998 (preliminary data; age adjusted to the year 2000 standard population).

Figure 16.7 describes the characteristics of homicide in the United States. A small number of homicides occur during the commission of another crime (17 percent); however, the intent is usually a result of a deliberate effort to kill, maim, injure, torture, rape, or otherwise violate the physical integrity of another.[75] In about 20 percent of homicides, the victim and the assailant are members of the same family. In less than 15 percent of homicides, the assailant is a stranger to the victim. Today, more and more homicides are related to gang violence and alcohol- and drug-related violence. In fact, 60 percent of all homi-

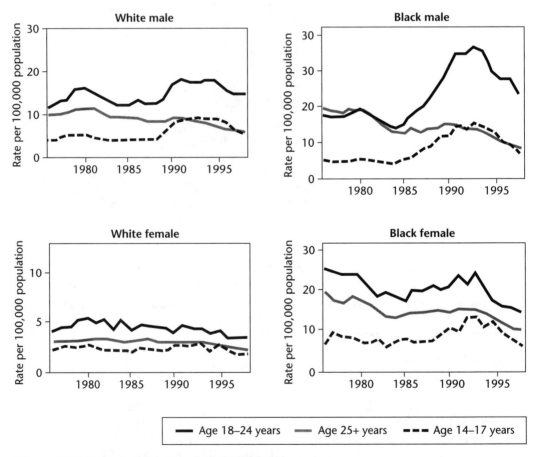

Figure 16.7 Demographics of homicide (1976–1998).

(*Source:* U.S. Department of Justice Bureau of Justice Statistics)

cides involve alcohol and drugs. Both of these factors are symptoms of family dysfunction often caused by economic and social unrest, lack of opportunity, and underlying racism that inhibits immediate and necessary social change.

Despite its enormous significance for health, responsibility for responding to homicide has been left almost entirely to the criminal justice system. There is a paucity of efforts to decrease homicide as part of a community health education program. Ironically, even with the percentage of the population incarcerated being one of the highest internationally, criminal sanctions have little preventive impact. Since this system has been less than adequate, it is time for public health providers to rise to the challenge of Healthy People 2010 and reduce violence and homicides. By stressing the sudden, unpredictable nature of homicide or its roots, such as poverty or economic despair, there is less emphasis by government to consider public health initiatives.

Reconceptualizing homicide as the by-product of interpersonal violence helps specify the targets for prevention (domestic violence or gang violence), the groups at highest risk (young adults), the major issues (gender stereotypes and male control over women and children), and the strategy (sanctions for assault and abuse, gun control, public education to reduce gender stereotypes, and protection and support for survivors of domestic violence).

In synthesizing several theoretical approaches to the issue of homicide, Stark presented the following strategy for prevention: "The saliency of homicide can be restored by emphasizing its roots in ordinary life. Homicide is a form of horrendous death that can affect anyone."[76]

Prevention

Prevention may begin by confronting the issue of unequal power that underlies interpersonal violence and homicide. Changing the sense of powerlessness among black men may be the basis for a grass roots strategy of prevention. The Centers for Disease Control and Prevention has responded by initiating a "deliberate injury" section within its "injury control branch," and the 1985 Surgeon General, C. Everett Koop, led regional conferences directed toward this health problem. Even these important health leaders have failed to impress the larger health community. A national survey called *Injury in America,* prepared in 1985, dismissed violence, homicide, and assault with a sentence or two, and completely failed to mention battering, the major source of female injury.[77]

The centerpiece of any prevention effort remains individual empowerment, recognizing that the appropriate basis for love, friendship, and parenting are autonomy and interdependence rather than dependence and domination. Attention must be focused on strengthening individuals, homes, and families. Politically affirming the right to physical integrity (having control of one's own body) is unconditional and universal.

An awareness of engineering factors is also an important aspect of injury prevention. Emphasis in prevention may be placed on preventing the creation of, use of, or the damage caused by the mechanical means of an "object of damage" (i.e., handguns). In other words, in the engineering model, public health would support gun control. This is a passive health model that requires little or no individual action for protection and contrasts with active prevention such as battered women shelters.

National governments and international bodies such as the United Nations must publicly condemn violence against women and children and work through the media and education system to decrease its cultural acceptance as an expression of male prerogative. Public health funds must be redirected to support the empowerment of women across the broad front that includes day care, schooling, access to birth control and safe, legal abortion, equal wages, meaningful job opportunities, and equal protection under the law. Prevention also means closing the gender and generational gaps that are reflections of unequal power relationships.

Prevention efforts must target the earliest signs of assaultive violence, including nonviolent behaviors designed to exercise illegitimate control over others. Education about violence should be incorporated into all professional training. Prevention programs should focus on a broader picture of health, including diet, exercise, social involvement, stress management, and education.

Racist policies that prevent equal job employment and thus put young black men on the streets earning a living in the drug industry must be eliminated. Economically viable training and job placement must be provided. Community health education interventions must include the factors of poverty, racial barriers, limited options for employment, weak ties within the family, weak ties between the family and the community, and the self-interest of powerful parties.[78]

Not all of prevention is the job of public health. It is really the combined responsibility of all those now in power at federal, state, and local levels.

Summary

Mental health is a complex, expensive, and difficult community health problem. Prevention requires major changes in how our society looks at its diverse populations and how willing communities are to be open and direct in providing treatment and support. There are many new drugs and new therapeutic techniques available that can help with serious mental illness, but access to psychological health care, the affordability of such medication, and the stigma of mental illness still prevent universal prevention, diagnosis, and treatment of mental illness.

Violence is a preventable form of death. Violence in the home and in the street begins from root causes of social, gender, and racial inequality. They grow from the frustration of powerlessness and the hopelessness of any future opportunity. Changes in social expectations of the roles of men and women, changes in economic opportunity patterns, changes in availability of guns to children, and changes in educational programs that identify risk behavior and introduce preventive coping skills may reduce the increasing rates of violence.

CYBERSITES RELATED TO CHAPTER 16

Violence
   www.famvi.com
   www.ojp.usdoj.gov/vawo

Mental Health
www.mentalhealth.org
www.behavior.net

QUESTIONS

1. What are some examples of sociopathology in our society?

2. In the past century how has the definition of mental illness changed? What conditions are no longer considered illness and what conditions are sometimes included as illness?

3. How does an individual select appropriate psychological health care? What is available in your community?

4. What educational programs might a community health educator initiate in the elementary school to reduce violence in the lives of these children?

5. Explain why domestic violence is given so little attention in our society. How can that be changed?

6. Why is the United States so violent?

7. What are the primary consequences of alcohol abuse on women, Native Americans, African Americans, and Hispanics?

EXERCISES

1. Assume you are seriously depressed. What steps are you financially, socially, and personally able to undertake? Determine the differences in methodology and care among psychiatrists, psychologists, social workers, feminist therapists, alternative healers, and health counselors. Which would you choose and why?

2. Describe a personal incidence of violence in your life. What were the factors that led to the violence? How could they have been prevented? What were the consequences of this violence? How is your experience an example of more global violence in our society?

3. Imagine that voting for the decriminalization of marijuana was on the ballot in your community. Make a list of the positive and negative health reasons, moral reasons, economic reasons, social reasons, and other reasons for and against decriminalization. Ultimately, how would you vote and why?

INTERNET INTERACTIVE ACTIVITY

MONITORING FUTURE HEALTH TRENDS

Monitoring the Future is an ongoing study of the behaviors, attitudes, and values of American secondary school students, college students, and young adults. Each year a total of some 50,000 eighth, tenth, and twelfth grade students are surveyed (twelfth graders since 1975, and eighth and tenth graders since 1991). In addition, annual follow-up questionnaires are mailed to a sample of each graduating class for a number of years after their initial participation. The homepage is:

monitoringthefuture.org/

Example

What are the trends in cigarette use among eighth, tenth, and twelth graders in 1999?

1. Go to the **Monitoring the Future** homepage.

   monitoringthefuture.org/

2. Click on **Data Tables and Figures**

   monitoringthefuture.org/data/data/html

3. Click on **New 2000 data**

   monitoringthefuture.org/data/99data.html#1999data-drugs

4. Go to **Trends on Cigarette Smoking—Tables 1–4** and click on each **Table** to determine the trends.

Table 1 suggests that lifetime use has remained rather constant since 1991, smoking in the past 30 days has increased since 1991, and the number of cigarettes smoked have increased.

Table 2 suggests that among tenth graders, females smoke more than males, whites more than blacks, more in the northcentral part of the United States, more often in nonmetropolitan areas, and the lower the parent's educational level, the greater the risk of smoking.

Exercise

What are the trends for various drug use among tenth graders, attitudes toward drug use among eighth graders, and long-term trends in availability for twelth graders?

1. Use the **Monitoring the Future** database for your trend analysis.

2. Using the figures from **Monitoring the Future,** compare marijuana, LSD, cocaine, crack, and inhalant use for all three grade levels. What do these data suggest?

3. How would your prevention program differ for eighth, tenth, and twelth graders based on the data provided?

REFERENCES

1. Message from Donna E. Shalala, Secretary of Health and Human Services. www.nimh.nih.gov/mhsgrpt/home.html

2. Bourdon, Karen H. et al (1992). Estimating the prevalence of mental disorders in U.S. adults from the epidemiologic attachment area survey. *Public Health Reports*, Nov./Dec., Vol. 107, No. 6, p. 663.

3. Ibid.

4. Johnson, Ann (1990). *Out of bedlam: The truth about deinstitutionalization.* New York: Basic Book.

5. Glob, Gerald N. (1991). *From asylum to community: Mental health policy in modern America.* New Jersey: Princeton University Press.

6. Levine, I. S. & Rog, D. J. (1990). Mental health services for homeless mentally ill persons: Federal initiatives and current service trends. *The American Psychologist, 45*(8), 963–68.

7. Glob, op. cit.

8. Isaac, Jean, (1990). *Madness in the streets: How psychiatry and the law abandoned the mentally ill.* New York: The Free Press.

9. Levine, op. cit.

10. Bender, David L. (1990). The homeless. *Opposing Viewpoints* Series. San Diego: Greenhaven Press.

11. Quigley, E. (1992). The homeless. *Congressional Quarterly Researcher, 2*(29), 676–678.

12. Doblin, B. H., Gelberg, L., & Freeman, H. E. (1992). Patient care and professional staffing patterns in McKinney Act clinics providing primary care to the homeless. *The Journal of the American Medical Association, 267*(5), 698–701.

13. Susser, E., Valencia, E., & Conover, S. (1993). Prevalence of HIV infection among psychiatric patients in a New York City men's shelter. *The American Journal of Public Health, 83*(4), 568–570.

14. Cousineau, M. R., & Lozier, J. N. (1993). Assuring access to health care for homeless people under national health care. *American Behavioral Scientist, 36*(6), 857–870.

15. WHO (1992). *Facts About WHO.* WHO. Geneva.

16. Bourdan, op. cit.

17. Green, Lawrence (1990). *Community health,* 6th ed. St. Louis: Mosby Press.

18. White, Evelyn C. (1990). *The black women's health book.* Seattle: Seal Press.

19. Belkin, Gary S. (1988). *Counseling: The art and science of helping.* Dubuque: Wm. C. Brown, Publishers.

20. Turshen, Meredeth (1989). *The politics of public health.* Rutgers University.

21. Belkin, op. cit.

22. White, op. cit.

23. Takeuchi, David, Sue, Stanley, & Yeh, May (1995). Return rates and outcomes from ethnicity-specific mental health programs in L.A. *AJPH*, Vol. 85, (5), p. 638.

24. Freeman, Jo (1989). *Women: A feminist perspective,* 4th ed. Calif.: Mayfield Publishing.

25. Goldberg, David (1991). The public health impact of mental disorders. In *Oxford textbook of public health.* Vol. III, pp. 267–280.

26. Ibid.

27. Ibid.

28. 132.183.145.103/neurowebforum/

29. Coombs, R. H., & Ziedonis, D. (1995). Preface. *A handbook on drug abuse prevention*. Boston: Allyn and Bacon.

30. SAMHSA (1997). National drug survey results released. www.dhs.state.utah.edu.

31. Hanson, G., & Venturelli, P. J. (1995). *Drugs and society*, 4th ed. Boston: Jones & Bartlett Publishers.

32. National Institute on Drug Abuse. *National household survey on drug abuse, Highlights 1993*. Rockville, Maryland.

33. Who (1992), op. cit.

34. Arkin, E. B., & J. E. Funkhouser, eds. *Communicating about alcohol and other drugs: Strategies for reaching populations at risk*. Office of Substance Abuse Prevention, U.S. Department of Health and Human Services.

35. National Household Survey on Drug Abuse.   www.samhsa.gov/OAS/NHSDA/ 98SummHtml/NHSDA98Summ.htm#TopOfPage

36. International Agency for Research on Cancer. *IARC monographs on the evaluation of carcinogenic risks to humans, 44*. United Kingdom: World Health Organization, 1988.

37. National Institute on Alcohol Abuse and Alcoholism. (1990). *Alcohol and women*. No. 10, PH 290. U.S. Department of Health and Human Services.

38. Wilsnack, R. W., Wilsnack, S. C., & Klassen, A. D., Jr. (1984). Women's drinking and drinking problems: Patterns from a 1981 national survey. *American Journal of Public Health, 74*.

39. National Institute on Alcohol Abuse and Alcoholism (1994). Alcohol Alert. No. 23, PH 347, January.

40. National Institute on Drug Abuse op. cit.

41. Ibid.

42. Ibid.

43. Ibid.

44. Mello, N. K., Mendelson, J. H., & Teoh, S. K. (1992). Alcohol and neuroendocrine function in women of reproductive age. In J.H. Mendelson & N. K. Mello (eds.). *Medical diagnosis and treatment of alcoholism*. McGraw-Hill, Inc.

45. Robins, Lee N. (1995). Editorial: The natural history of substance use as a guide to setting drug policy. *American Journal of Public Health*, 85, 1, p. 12.

46. Des Jarlais, Don C. (1995). Editorial: Harm reduction—A framework for incorporating science into drug policy. *American Journal of Public Health*, 85, 1, p. 10.

47. Ibid.

48. Coombs, op. cit.

49. Ibid.

50. National Institute on Drug Abuse, op. cit.

51. Schwenzfeier, B. (1993). *Partners in prevention*. Salt Lake City: University of Utah. Alcohol and Drug Education Center.

52. *American Journal of Public Health* (1994). Editorial: Reducing violence—How do we proceed? April *84*, (4). p. 539.

53. Ibid.

54. Let's be clear: Violence is a public health problem (1992). *JAMA*, June 10, Vol. 267, No. 22, p. 3071.

55. Stark, Evan (1991). Preventing primary homicide: A reconceptualization. In *Horrendous death, health and well-being* by Daniel Leviton. New York: Hemisphere Publishing, pp. 109–135.

56. Page, Randy M. et. al. (1992). Interpersonal violence: A priority issue for health education. *Journal of Health Education*, July/Aug., Vol. 23, No. 5, p. 286.

57. Ibid.

58. National Committee for the Prevention of Child Abuse; American Association for the Prevention of Child Abuse cited in *USA Today*.

59. Page, op. cit.

60. Editorial, Reducing violence, op. cit.

61. parentingteens.miningco.com/parenting/parentingteens/gi/dynamic/offsite.htm? site=http://www.tvfa.org/stats.htm.

62. Ibid.

63. World Health (1995). Facts, figures and estimates about substance use. July/Aug, No. 4, p. 16.

64. Whitehorse Cochran, Jo (1988). *Changing our power*, 2nd ed. Dubuque: Kendall/Hunt Publishing.

65. Stark, op. cit.

66. Whitehorse, op. cit.

67. Gable, op. cit.

68. McAvoy, Brian, & Donaldson, Liam. (1990). Health care for Asians. In *Oxford textbook of public health*. New York: Oxford Press.

69. Minkowitz, Donna (1992). Family values? No, thanks. *The Advocate*, June, p. 17.

70. NCHS. *Mortality data tapes*. Hyattsville, MD: The Center, 1994.

71. Stark, op. cit.

72. NCHS, op. cit.

73. CDC. *National summary of injury mortality data, 1987–1994*. Atlanta, GA: National Center for Injury Prevention and Control, 1996.

74. World Health Organization. *World health statistics annual, 1994*. Geneva, Switzerland: WHO, 1995.

75. Page, op. cit.

76. Ibid.

77. Stark, op. cit.

78. Page, op. cit.

CHAPTER 17

Comprehensive School Health Programs

Community Health in the 21st Century
Accessibility of community health services for all people,
young and old. Affordable disease prevention and treatment services.
Providers must be accountable and competent.

—Judith K. Luebke, M.A. Editor, *The Health Educator*

Chapter Objectives

The student will:

1. define a comprehensive school health program.

2. list the eight components of a comprehensive school health program.

3. state the difference between a comprehensive school health program and comprehensive health education.

4. state the key person/organizations involved in planning a CSHP.

5. list barriers to the implementation of a CSHP.

6. state the how-to's of successful CSHP implementation.

The School as Community

Today, children, youth, and teenagers face a number of personal and community threats that put their health at risk. Among such threats to teenagers are behaviors that include drinking, drug use, unprotected sexual intercourse, risky recreational activities, violence, tobacco use, unhealthy dietary behaviors, inadequate physical activity,[1] and the stresses associated with youth. With one million teenage pregnancies each year in the United States, and 2.5 million sexually transmitted diseases, something appears to be terribly wrong.

In 1999, 70 percent of all deaths among teens were due to vehicle crashes, other unintentional injuries, homicides, and suicides. Childhood and young adulthood are also the years that may lead to the precursors of adult heart disease and cancer, chronic diseases that can lead to an unhealthy adulthood through poor eating, exercise, and personal health habits.

Table 17.1 Leading causes of death, ages 5–14 (1998).

Unintentional injuries	3,254
Malignant neoplasms	1,013
Homicide and legal intervention	460
Congenital anomalies	371
Diseases of heart	326
Suicide	324
Bronchitis, emphysema, and asthma	152
Pneumonia and influenza	121
Benign neoplasms	84
Cerebrovascular diseases	82

(*Source:* National Center for Health Statistics)

Table 17.2 Leading causes of death, ages 15–24 (1998).

Unintentional injuries	13,349
Homicide and legal intervention	5,506
Suicide	4,135
Malignant neoplasms	1,699
Diseases of heart	1,057
Congenital anomalies	450
Bronchitis, emphysema, and asthma	239
Pneumonia and influenza	215
HIV	194
Cerebrovascular diseases	178

(*Source:* National Center for Health Statistics)

The National Center for Health Statistics Research has computed the leading causes of deaths for different age groups. Tables 17.1 and 17.2 list the leading causes of death for children ages five through fourteen, and youth/young adults ages fifteen through twenty-four.

A Need for School Health

The importance of including health instruction in education curricula has been recognized since the early 1900s. Children are influenced by the institutions to which they belong from their earliest ages. Community groups (such as religious institutions, governmental agencies, and clubs), family, and school all help (or hinder) a child's beliefs, attitudes, and values about the importance of health. Given the many demands on the average family and the vast amount of information associated with health, it is no longer realistic to think that the family can be the sole source of providing health information to children. In

For homeless children, school is often a coveted resource. Health and safety skills are an essential part of the homeless school curriculum. These children wear reflector jackets on their walk.

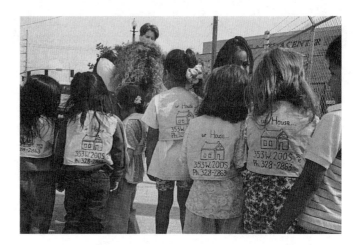

fact, the National Commission on the Role of the School and Community (1990) reported that this is the first time in our country's history where young people are less healthy and less prepared to take their place in society than their parents.[2] There are no easy solutions. Since 46 million youth attend school daily in the nation's 100,000 schools, this institution may be in the most advantageous position to help improve the health status of the nation's youth. The school is continually trying to play a leading role in providing children what they need to make informed health choices while delegating what they can to other institutions. Essentially, improving the health of youth is still a nationwide challenge. The reader might find it surprising that despite a need and a history of school health education, the American Librarians Association president has said that, the three areas that seem to be the focus of a great deal of censorship are sex education, Satanism/witchcraft, and health education. Can school health education compete with this censorship?[3]

Historical Events Leading to Comprehensive School Health Programs

One of the foremost projects to assess the health education status of the nation's youth was the **School Health Education Study (SHES).**[4] Funded by both the Samuel Bronfman Foundation and the 3M Corporation, SHES was conducted from 1961 to 1973. The project was spearheaded by community health professionals in New York as they tried to grasp what was happening with school health in the United States.

The four main tasks accomplished by SHES were:

1. The development of a book entitled "Synthesis of Research in Selected Areas of Health Instruction."

2. A nationwide study of instructional practices and a study of student health behavior, reported in "School Health Education Study: A Summary Report."

3. A book on philosophies of approaches to school health education and materials entitled "Health Education: A Conceptual Approach to Curriculum Design."

4. The development of other needed curricular materials.

Among school health education professionals, SHES is recognized as a precursor to the current comprehensive school health education movement.[5]

The **National School Health Education Coalition (NaSHEC)** is another pioneer organization involved in making comprehensive school health education a reality. Founded in 1982, this organization was designed to reach local affiliations through grassroots efforts. Made up of more than fifty national organizations, NaSHEC monitors legislation in Congress that will benefit or hinder comprehensive school health education efforts. The coalition's mission is to: (1) support the establishment of state and local coalitions; (2) develop resource materials; and (3) advocate for comprehensive school-based health education.[6]

Healthy People 2000 has been a valuable means of monitoring the health of children and youth in the United States. By means of morbidity and mortality data, as well as emotional, psychological, and learning problems information, the Healthy People 2000 objectives for the nation indicated the need for comprehensive school health programs. Healthy People 2010 builds on the previous objectives and continues its emphasis on school, community, and worksite health promotion.

In 1988, the Centers for Disease Control and Prevention established the National Center for Chronic Disease Prevention and Health Promotion. Located within this Center is the **Division of Adolescent and School Health (DASH).** DASH's mission included identifying major health risks and health problems among youth, monitoring these problems, implementing national prevention programs, and evaluation of such programs.[7] Recently, the Division has become involved with HIV education at the national level.

In 1998, Congress urged the CDC to expand its support of coordinated health education programs in the schools. Today, the CDC helps all fifty states and eighteen major cities to provide HIV and school health education for youth. Fiscal year 1999 included more than $9.6 million to enable the CDC to strengthen national efforts for coordinated school health programs and provide direct support to fifteen states as shown in Figure 17.1.[8]

Professional organizations in health education and community health have also advocated for comprehensive school health programs. In 1994, more than twenty professional and voluntary organizations worked with the CDC to develop model policies and guidelines. The American School Health Association (ASHA), the Association for the Advancement of Health Education (AAHE), and the Society for Public Health Education (SOPHE) sponsored a nationwide survey in 1989 to determine what teens know about health and how they respond to the information they have.

A major effort of the CDC's involvment in school health is the Youth Risk Behavior Surveillance System (YRBSS). This survey was developed with federal, state, and private-sector partners to survey 12,000 students in junior and senior

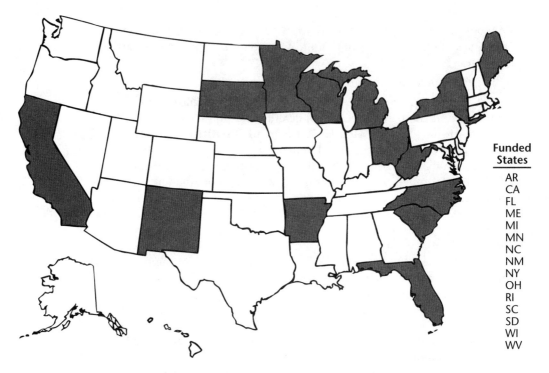

Shading denotes states funded for coordinated school health education. In addition, CDC funds all 50 states, 7 territories, the District of Columbia, and 18 major cities for HIV education for youth.

Figure 17.1 States funded for coordinated school health education (1998).

(*Source:* Centers for Disease Control)

high school.[9] The focus is on risk behaviors such as tobacco use, substance use and abuse, and sexual behavior. It is a major resource for understanding the prevalence of health risk behaviors and preparing appropriate health curriculum.

Many curriculum and teaching materials have been created and distributed by commercial businesses, private organizations, religious groups, and government agencies that are available to school districts, individual class groups, or teachers at little or no charge. Almost any organization having an affiliation with health provides factual materials and teaching materials for use in the community. Additionally, colleges and universities have increased teacher preparation courses for health instruction, as necessary for true comprehensive school health programs to be implemented.

Elements of Comprehensive School Health Programs

What is a comprehensive school health program, and how does it differ from the traditional classroom instruction on health-related issues? According to Meeks and Heit, a comprehensive school health program is an "organized set of policies, procedures, and activities designed to protect and promote the health and well being of students and staff which has traditionally included health

---

BOX 17.1 *Most Common Risk Behaviors of High School Students (Youth Risk Behavior Surveillance Study)*

Injury-Causing Behaviors
- Rarely or never using safety belts in a car
- Rarely or never wearing a helmet while riding a bicycle
- Riding with a driver who had been drinking in past month
- Carried a weapon in past month
- Involved in a physical fight in past year
- Attempted suicide in past year

Sexual Behaviors
- Had sexual intercourse during their life
- Had four or more sexual partners
- Used birth control pills at last sexual intercourse

Tobacco Use
- Smoked cigarettes in past month
- Smoked on 20 or more days in past month
- Used smokeless tobacco in past month

Alcohol, Drug Abuse
- Had a least one drink during past month
- Had five or more drinks at least once during past month
- Used marijuana in past month
- Used cocaine during past month

---

services, a healthful school environment, and health education."[10] However, in the late 1980s, it was recommended that the following also be included in such a program: guidance and counseling services, physical education, food service, social work, psychological services, and employee health promotion. Additionally, community and family involvement is also recommended. Figure 17.2 is a visual representation of a comprehensive school health program.

Discussion: Why is comprehensive school health considered a part of community health? What is the role of the community health educator in the school?

Comprehensive School Health Education

Comprehensive school health education is one of the eight components of a comprehensive school health program. Often, it is mistaken as being the bulk of the program itself. Comprehensive school health education has been defined as "one component of the comprehensive school health program which includes the development, delivery, and evaluation of a planned instructional program and other activities for students preschool through grade twelve, for parents, and for school staff. It is designed to positively influence the health knowledge, attitudes, and skills of individuals.[11] Some additional guidelines for the implementation of this particular component from the Centers for Disease Control and Prevention are:

1. Decision making and resistant skills

2. Specific amounts of instructional time for each grade

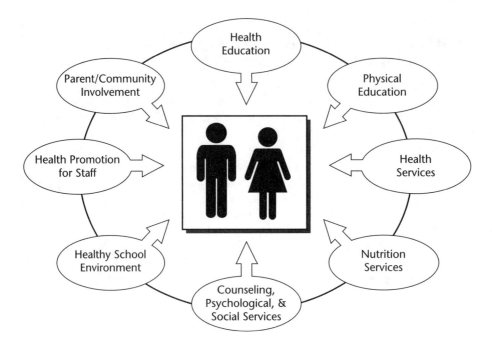

Figure 17.2 A comprehensive school health program.

(*Source:* CDC)

BOX 17.2 *National Health Education Standards*

The National Health Education Standards were adopted to help students achieve the education goals set in **America 2000: An Educational Strategy,** and **Healthy People 2000: National Health Promotion and Disease Prevention Objectives.** Health literacy is defined within the National Health Education Standards as the ability to obtain, interpret, and understand basic health information and services and the competence to use such information and services in ways which enhance health. The specific standards indicate that the student will:

1. Comprehend concepts related to health promotion and disease prevention.
2. Demonstrate the ability to access valid health information and health promoting products and services.

3. Demonstrate the ability to practice health-enhancing behaviors and reduce health risks.
4. Analyze the influence of culture, media, technology, and other factors on health.
5. Demonstrate the ability to use interpersonal communication skills to enhance health.
6. Demonstrate the ability to use goal-setting and decision-making skills to enhance health.
7. Demonstrate the ability to advocate for personal, family, and community health.

3. Trained health education coordinator for each school to manage and coordinate the program

4. Teachers providing health instruction must have appropriate training

5. Parent, health professionals, and community member involvement

6. Program evaluation, updating, and improvement.[12]

Part of the overall concept of comprehensive school health education includes the idea of comprehensive school health instruction. The CSHE Workshop (1993) states that instruction refers to the "development, delivery, and evaluation of a planned curriculum, preschool through grade twelve, with goals, objectives, content sequence, and specific classroom lessons which includes, but is not limited to, the following major content areas: community health, consumer health, environmental health, family life, mental and emotional health, injury prevention and safety, nutrition, personal health, prevention and control of disease, and substance use and abuse."[13] These areas are targeted because the Centers for Disease Control and Prevention estimates that they are the risk behaviors leading to the main causes of death later in children's lives.

The following is the CDC's Division of Adolescent and School Health's interim definition of the key elements of comprehensive health education:

- A documented, planned, and sequential program of health instruction for students in grades kindergarten through twelve

- A curriculum that addresses and integrates education about a range of categorical health problems and issues at developmentally appropriate ages

- Activities that help young people develop the skills they need to avoid tobacco use; dietary patterns that contribute to disease; sedentary lifestyle; sexual behaviors that result in HIV infection, other STDs, and unintended pregnancy; alcohol and other drug use; and behaviors that result in unintentional and intentional injuries

- Instruction provided for a prescribed amount of time at each grade level

- Management and coordination by an education professional trained to implement the program

- Instruction from teachers who are trained to teach the subject

- Involvement of parents, health professionals, and other concerned community members

- Periodic evaluation, updating, and improvement

It is estimated that over half of the nation's schools provide comprehensive school health education.[14] The CDC isn't as optimistic; they estimate the prevalence of comprehensive school health education to be as low as 5 percent.[15] The disparity in estimates may be a reflection of how schools define comprehensive school health education. Given the economic stresses of most school systems, a totally comprehensive health education program may be financially infeasible. Although the number of schools implementing comprehensive school health

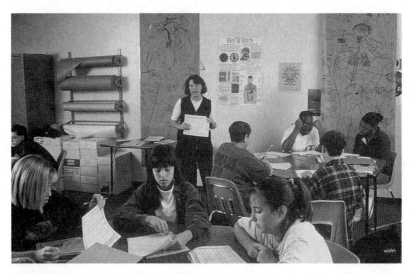

Comprehensive school health includes classroom instruction by qualified school health educators.

education appears to be less than optimal, the results of existing health education programs are encouraging. When comprehensive school health education programs work, students in schools with such programs have more knowledge and better health-related attitudes and behaviors than those with no exposure to health classes. Experts contend that to be effective, instruction must be sequential in nature from grade to grade. Research shows there is an even greater increase in health knowledge and attitudes with increase in years of exposure.[16]

Healthy People 2010 Objective: Increase School Health Education in Priority Areas

Schools Providing Comprehensive School Health Education in Priority Areas	1994 Baseline (%)	2010 Target (%)
Summary objective (all components)	28	70
Specific objectives (components to prevent health problems in the following areas):		
Unintentional injury	66	90
Violence	58	80
Suicide	58	80
Tobacco use and addiction	86	95
Alcohol and other drug use	90	95
Unintended pregnancy, HIV/AIDS, and STD infection	65	90
Unhealthy dietary patterns	84	95
Inadequate physical activity	78	90
Environmental health	60	80

Healthy People 2010 is also concerned with college age students:

Healthy People 2010 Objective: Increase College and University Education in Priority Areas

Target: 25 percent.

Baseline: 6 percent of undergraduate students received information from their college or university on all six topics in 1995: injuries (intentional and unintentional), tobacco use, alcohol and illicit drug use, sexual behaviors that cause unintended pregnancies and sexually transmitted diseases, dietary patterns that cause disease, and inadequate physical activity.

Healthy People 2010 Objective: Increase Nurse-to-Student Ratio in Elementary, Middle, and High Schools

Increase in Schools with Nurse-to-Student Ratio of at Least 1:750	1994 Baseline (%)	2010 Target (%)
All middle, junior high, and senior high schools	28	50
Senior high schools	26	50
Middle and junior high schools	32	50

Physical Education

It is estimated that one in six school children is classified as "physically under-developed" by the President's Council on Physical Fitness and Sports.[17] We have a nation of junior couch potatoes. When the Association for the Advancement of Health Education has to place advertisements in the *Journal of Health Education* for promotion of physical fitness among youth, we are in grave danger of sedentary youth turning into sedentary adults (see Figure 17.3). Certainly, we are witnessing the effects of the "Nintendo generation." It used to be that health education was considered physical education, and it was a course (or more likely part of a course) taught by the resident gym teacher. No longer is that the case. As we now know, health education is a very specific discipline from physical education that requires teacher preparation in a body of knowledge that is quite extensive and specific. Health education, like public health education, is a science, built on theory and guided through practice. Although physical education teachers still may instruct about health topics, they are increasingly receiving in-service and post-graduate education to prepare them for the health classroom.

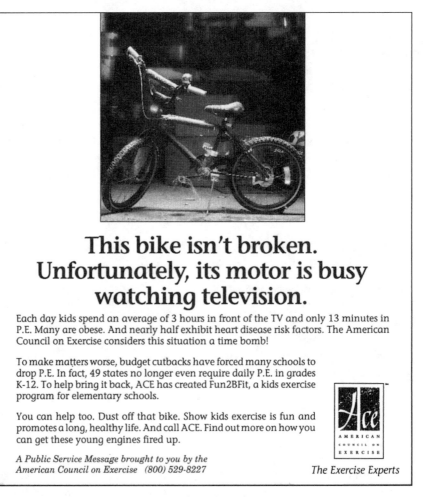

Figure 17.3 Physical activity of school aged youth.

Health Services

The objectives of the school health services include screening tests and health examinations, adjusting school programs to meet the needs of special populations, providing emergency and nursing services for those who have been injured or have become ill, counseling and advising, and coordinating efforts with participating community health agencies.

Nutrition Services

It has been well documented that children perform better in school and learn better if they are nourished. Yet, our school breakfast and lunch programs are in jeopardy by those in governmental agencies who do not see their importance or accept a role of the school environment to provide family services, such as feeding children. Breakfast and lunch programs allow children from a variety of family environments to receive one or two nutritionally adequate meals a day.

Counseling, Psychological, and Social Services

Counseling, one of the most important aspects of the school health services component, has changed dramatically over the years, from a focus on treatment to one of prevention. Ideally, a school counseling program would include the elementary grades for best chances of prevention and early intervention. Programs need to include all students, not just those with obvious signs of school, developmental, and/or social problems. School counselors would work with the personal/social development, educational development, and career development domains.[18]

Healthy School Environment

A school that is well planned and consistently maintained creates a favorable environment that enables the teaching and learning experiences to be enjoyable and free of stress. The environment of the school includes: (1) the school site and facilities, equipment, and supplies; (2) student, teacher, and staff interactions; (3) daily schedules; (4) administrative and educational policies and procedures; (5) services; (6) recreational and interscholastic activities; (7) curricula and instructional programs; and (8) student and staff development programs.[19] All of these enable students, faculty, and staff to work and learn under the best possible circumstances. Additionally, the school's policies and procedures, acceptance of diversity, conduciveness to inclusive learning, etc., are all part of a school culture that will influence those within the system.[20]

Health Promotion for School Staff

A truly comprehensive school health program involves staff who are healthy role models and active believers in healthy lifestyles. Teachers, administrators, support staff, and students should enjoy the benefits of a well structured schoolsite health promotion program. An organized health promotion program in the schools can improve productivity, decrease absenteeism, improve morale, and lower health care costs in the school system.

Implementing Comprehensive School Health Programs

School districts must not be too quick to implement comprehensive school health programs. Before such a large task is undertaken, it would be wise to take the time to formulate a well-developed plan. There are a number of steps to consider before implementing a comprehensive school health program:

1. An established need for the program
2. Heightened public awareness
3. Knowledge of the national health objectives
4. A philosophical basis for health education in the school

5. Program guidelines and models of existing programs

6. Curriculum materials

7. Prepared teachers

8. An evaluation process

9. Evidence that comprehensive school health programs work[21]

Additionally, the following steps for the implementation of a comprehensive school health program have been suggested:

1. Execute a needs assessment

2. Organize support and working groups

3. Set goals

4. Create a program status assessment

5. Do a resource analysis

6. Develop and implement a strategic plan

7. Evaluate

8. Develop a process for monitoring and managing change[22]

Local Coalition Building

The steps mentioned above are best addressed through focus groups and community awareness meetings established to get everyone involved at an early stage in the program's development. See Figure 17.4 for an ideal foundation for a comprehensive school health program.

The importance of getting key players involved, as well as the rest of the community, at the early planning stages cannot be stressed enough. Keeping community stakeholders involved and informed of developments will only help program development in the long run. It is better to know about community resistance beforehand than to rearrange things after the fact. There are many ways to achieve the goals of a comprehensive school health programs in a district, but planning is crucial. See Figure 17.5 for a flowchart of involvement of key players at different stages of the program's development.

Family and Community Values and Aspirations	Community, School, and Family Resources	Epidemiologic Data	Educational and Behavioral Research

Figure 17.4 Foundation of a school health program.

(*Source:* Kane, W. M. (1994). Planning for a comprehensive school health program. In P. Cortese & K. Middleton, *The comprehensive school health challenge: Vol. I.* Santa Cruz: ETR Associates. For information about this and other related materials, call 1-800-321-4407)

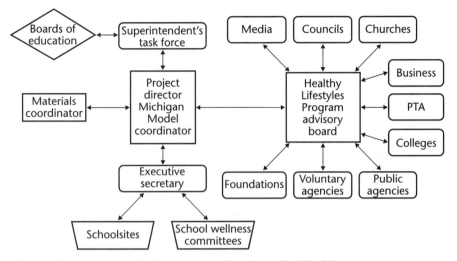

Figure 17.5 Flowchart of planning comprehensive school health.

(*Source:* Berryman, J. C. (1994). Health promotion at the school worksite. In P. Cortese &
K. Middleton, *The comprehensive school health challenge: Vol. I.* Santa Cruz: ETR Associates.
For information about this and other related materials, call 1-800-321-4407)

Discussion: At what point in planning does the community health educator participate?

Barriers to Comprehensive School Health Programs

If the above steps are taken and carefully planned programs are demonstrating
benefits in the school community, then why aren't comprehensive school health
programs a reality in many of our nation's districts? There are many barriers to
these types of programs. As you can imagine from your reading thus far, financial support is a must. For any comprehensive school health program to operate
and be evaluated successfully, there must be a financial commitment among the
agencies involved. A "top ten" list of barriers to comprehensive school health
was developed by the Harvard School Health Education Project in 1993:[23]

1. Society does not appreciate the relationship between healthy living and
   happy and successful living.

2. Schools themselves have relatively little appreciation for health instruction.

3. Teachers who teach health have not generally been trained to do so.

4. Too much instruction/texts devote disproportionate time to anatomy/phys-
   iology and disease process. This creates a permanent distaste for health
   among students.

5. There is too much focus on knowledge and not enough on skills and competencies.

6. Instruction is not well organized or standardized through grades.

7. There are no clear goals or objectives for health in schools. Hence, there is little systematic planning for results.

8. The nation's schools are under unprecedented scrutiny and pressure to improve student performance in the academic disciplines.

9. Health is too categorical and fragmented. It is not comprehensive in nature and does not fit in to larger social systems.

10. The concepts of comprehensive school health programs and comprehensive school health education are too often confused.[24]

Timing is everything, and perhaps the time is not right for some districts to change. Often, there is a lack of support from those in influential positions in the districts. School policy makers may be unaware of what comprehensive school health programs mean. Often from state to state, there are varying policy recommendations and mandates from the state education departments. Also, as mentioned above, there is a lack of teacher training. Only about half of the teachers instructing health courses have been trained in the subject matter through preparation courses or teacher in-services. Often times there is also a question of who is in charge. Since comprehensive school health programs should be interdisciplinary with other school subjects and community efforts, there needs to be a health education coordinator.[25] Table 17.3 lists barriers to schools providing comprehensive school health. All of the above reasons make the hopes for comprehensive school health programs among all our nation's schools grim. There are, however, ways to overcome these hurdles.

Moving Beyond Barriers to Healthier Schools

In order to overcome some of the major barriers to a comprehensive school health program, community health and health education professionals must join the reform efforts in their local school districts.[26] Often times, those who are happy with reform measures are the least likely to speak up in favor of programmatic changes. What happens then is that the minority who are unhappy are heard loud and clear and often have the say in the decisions being made. All community health professionals must advocate for changes to help improve the health status of our nation's young people.

Certainly, decision makers and the public need to be more informed about the need for comprehensive school health programs.[27] Community health professionals should work in conjunction with the schools to market health programs within the schools to the community. Second, government structures must coordinate their efforts for implementation of programs at the local level. State education departments and state health departments are two such agencies that should be collaborating on behalf of our children's health. Third, other nongovernmental agencies must join efforts for comprehensive school health

Table 17.3 Barriers to comprehensive school health.

Barriers

→ Lack of administrative/faculty time
→ Lack of funds
→ Lack of time for student counseling
→ Lack of community integration
→ Need lower student/counselor ratio
→ Need more time for nurses to conduct education
→ Lack of coordination between commodity food program and district menu planners
→ Insufficient amount of federal subsidy for school meal program

(*Source:* Wiley, D. et al. Comprehensive school health programs in Texas public schools. *Journal of School Health*, vol. 61, no. 10, p. 423, December, 1991. Reprinted with permission. American School Health Association, Kent, OH)

programs. The American Heart Association, Planned Parenthood, and the American Cancer Society are examples of organizations that could be advocates for program efforts, if not presently involved. Local and state universities must also take part in efforts for comprehensive school health programs. Often, health education departments within state universities can be contracted to partake in program evaluation efforts. Other resources may be found at the universities that the districts would otherwise not be able to access. Lastly, philanthropic organizations must be contacted for resource support. Many of the nation's charity organizations' mission statements include the welfare and health of our children. These particular organizations may then be approached for funding and other forms of program support. Again, the more solutions to potential obstacles thought out ahead of time, the less hardships as implementation of comprehensive school health programs take place.

Evaluation of the Comprehensive School Health Program

Much like the problems with evaluation encountered by the Michigan Model for Comprehensive School Health Education, many wonderfully designed programs are floundering due to lack of adequate evaluation. Proper and complete evaluation of such programs requires sufficient funding. If resources are tight, many districts may opt to spend more on curriculum materials or other program services. Evaluation of such programs is a must. Without proper evaluation, proof of their effectiveness does not exist. Without numbers backing the program, future funding and support for further programs are jeopardized.

There are important reasons for conducting evaluations of school health programs: (1) information needs to be gathered to prove the effectiveness of the program; (2) this information will also help to modify and improve the existing program; (3) determine how many students (the target population) the program is reaching; (4) determine if the effects of the program demonstrate a need to expand the program; (5) to be able to do a cost-benefit analysis; and (6) to be able to inform others about the program's success.[28]

Michigan Model for Comprehensive School Health Education

Although the Michigan Model is not a comprehensive school health program, it is an example of a state's effort to get quality, comprehensive school health education in every public school room. Many state agencies are involved in making the program run efficiently. There are ten health topics discussed in a sequential manner from kindergarten through twelfth grade.

The program known as the Michigan Model began in 1984, although much background work preceded its inception.[29] Curricula were developed, teacher in-servicing began, and evaluation components were developed. Implementation has been a gradual process, starting with the lower grades.

Evaluation results are promising. For example, students receiving the Michigan Model substance abuse lessons were not as likely to drink alcohol, smoke cigarettes, or try marijuana. In addition, parental surveys show that 98 percent of those responding felt school health was important and that the Michigan Model made a difference in their child.

The Michigan Model is not without its problems. Continual funding through legislation has been a problem, and the evaluation component had to be drastically scaled down. Controversy surrounding certain units and lesson plans were also a concern and public hearings were held. Examples of the challenge to community health educators and school systems are as follows: One community member complained about a unit teaching small children fire prevention. The children were supposed to draw their home and figure out how they'd exit in an emergency. This opponent stated "it is not the school's business where we sleep in our house." Should kids not be taught how to escape a fire? Another opponent stated that teaching three deep breaths for stress and anger management was teaching a new-age religion. It was removed from the curriculum. Most states would die for the Michigan Model in their state. Some in Michigan would die to see it revoked. These and other problems will be faced in almost any district due to the amount of change required.

Even so, proponents of the Model have done a good job explaining the value of a comprehensive school health curriculum. This Model is recognized as a leading program of its type in the United States.

Summary

Even if comprehensive school health programs were put into all 100,000 of America's schools today, children and young people would still be at risk for death and injury due to their behaviors. It is predicted that by the year 2000, 13 percent of all high school students will still drink regularly, 8 percent will have used other drugs, 4 percent will smoke regularly, 95 percent will still not wear bike helmets, and 62 percent will not use safety belts. There will still be a gap between knowledge and behavior. The schools are only one institution from which our young people get their information. Consistent and constant messages are needed to reinforce the information and skills learned within the comprehensive school health program. Reform is needed within society in general, along with the schools, if our nation's young people are going to have a chance at a healthier future than what they are faced with today.

Cybersites Related to Chapter 17

www.cdc.gov/nccdphp/dash/ataglanc.htm

www.ashaweb.org

Questions

1. Since funding for comprehensive school health programs is always a potential problem, who's responsibility is funding? The federal government? The state? Local school districts?

2. How is a comprehensive school health program different from comprehensive school health education? Should comprehensive school health education be implemented without the entire program?

3. Why is evaluation so critical for comprehensive school health programs? Why is it lacking?

4. Name five community agencies/organizations you would involve in a coalition to discuss comprehensive school health programs.

Exercise

Survey various schools to find out how school health is taught within the districts in your community. Is it comprehensive? Is appropriate time given to its instruction? Is it sequential from grades K through 12? How could it be improved?

Internet Interactive Activity

Youth Risk Behavior Surveillance System (YRBSS)

The YRBSS is an annual health risk behavior survey administered to school-age children across the United States. Developed by the CDC in cooperation with federal, state, and private-sector partners, this voluntary system includes a national survey of about 12,000 students and smaller surveys conducted by state and local education agencies. The YRBSS focuses on priority risk behaviors such as tobacco use and provides vital information to improve health programs. The homepage is:

www.cdc.gov/nccdphp/dash/yrbs/index.htm

Example

The community health educator can find out the status of the health of school-age children in her or his state by using the YRBSS results.

1. To get an overview of the status of health of youth in Kentucky, go to

www.cdc.gov/nccdphp/dash/yrbs/index.htm

2. Click on Leading Causes of Mortality and Morbidity and Contributing Behaviors by State, 1997 and then on **Kentucky**.

You now have a snapshot of the leading causes of mortality and disease and some high-risk alcohol, injuries, tobacco, sexual behavior, nutrition, and physical activities among youth ages ten–twenty-four in Kentucky in 1997.

Exercise
1. Using the YRBSS data found at

   www.cdc.gov/nccdphp/dash/yrbs/index.htm

   compare your state's youth with the National Data Results.
2. Show a comparison table for Unintentional Injuries, Dietary Behaviors, Physical Activity Behaviors, and School Related Violence.
3. In what areas does your state show improvement over national statistics?
4. In what areas does your state show higher risks than national statistics?
5. Compare the youth data with tables from the **Youth Risk Behavior Surveillance, 1999**
6. Look at the five-year trends in youth risk behavior. What five trends do you notice?

   www.cdc.gov/nccdphp/dash/yrbs/trend.htm
7. What is the status of the health of undergraduate students?

REFERENCES

1. USDHHS (1995). School health programs: An investment in our future. Public Health Service, CDC.
2. Hamburg, M. V. (1994). School health education: What are the possibilities? In P. Cortese & K. Middleton (eds.), *The comprehensive school health challenge: Volume one.* Santa Cruz: ETR Associates.
3. Clark, Noreen M. (1994). Health educators and the future: Lead, follow, or get out of the way. *Journal of Health Education.* May/June Vol. 25, No. 3, p. 136.
4. Nolte, A. E. (1994). School health education today: Highlights and milestones. In P. Cortese & K. Middleton (eds.), *The comprehensive school health challenge: Volume one.* Santa Cruz: ETR Associates.
5. Ibid.
6. Ibid.
7. Kolbe, L. J. (1994). An essential strategy to improve the health and education of Americans. In P. Cortese & K. Middleton (eds.), *The comprehensive school health challenge: Volume one.* Santa Cruz: ETR Associates.
8. CDC (1999). School health programs: An investment in our nation's future. USDHHS.
9. Ibid.

10. Meeks, L., & Heit, P. (1992). *Comprehensive school health education: Totally awesome strategies for teaching health.* Blacklick: Meeks Heit Publishing Company.

11. Materials from the CSHE Workshop (1993). Sponsored by the American Cancer Society, the Utah State Office of Education, and the Utah Department of Health.

12. Ibid.

13. Ibid.

14. Hamburg, op. cit.

15. Meeks, op. cit.

16. Cortese, P., & Middleton, K. (1994). Preface. In P. Cortese & K. Middleton (eds.), *The comprehensive school health challenge: Volume one.* Santa Cruz: ETR Associates.

17. Comprehensive school health: A student fact sheet. (1995). Salt Lake City: University of Utah.

18. Perry, N. S. (1994). Integrating school counseling and health education programs. In P. Cortese & K. Middleton (eds.), *The comprehensive school health challenge: Volume one.* Santa Cruz: ETR Associates.

19. Henderson, A. C. (1993). *Healthy schools, healthy futures: The case for improving school environment.* Santa Cruz: ETR Associates.

20. Ibid.

21. Hamburg, op. cit.

22. Kane, W. M. (1994). Planning for a comprehensive school health program. In P. Cortese & K. Middleton (eds.). *The comprehensive school health challenge: Volume one.* Santa Cruz: ETR Associates.

23. Lavin, A. T. (1993). Harvard School Health Education Project.

24. Ibid.

25. Hamburg, op. cit.

26. Kolbe, op. cit.

27. Iverson, D. C. (1994). Program evaluation versus research: More differences than similarities. In P. Cortese & K. Middleton (eds.), *The comprehensive school health challenge: Volume two.* Santa Cruz: ETR Associates.

28. Michigan Department of Education. Information about the Michigan Model.

29. Ibid.

Section V

The Community and Its Environmental Health Issues

Although community health educators probably spend most of their time working with individuals or groups of people on health promotion and disease prevention programs, the environment is an essential part of making a community a healthy place to live. Community health educators often become environmental health specialists, addressing the quality of a community's air and water; keeping food free from contamination, and helping a community dispose of its waste. Chapters 18 through 21 complete the introduction to community health in the twenty-first century by presenting the difficult problems our environment faces as our planet becomes more populated and our possessions become more disposable. How will we keep our air, water, and food clean and safe if we do not dispose of contaminants properly? How can we make a community a healthy place to live in the twenty-first century?

CHAPTER 18

The Air We Breathe

Community Health in the 21st Century
Pollution prevention and air quality will be a must. Better methods of mass transportation to reduce pollution. People will have to find alternatives for mobility that do not emit pollutants, perhaps electric cars will become common.

—Eleanor Divver-Shields, MPH, Environmental Health Educator

Chapter Objectives

The student will:

1. discuss the extent of the air pollution problem in the United States.

2. discuss the purpose of the Clean Air Act.

3. name and define the criterion pollutants.

4. explain the health risk associated with each of the criterion pollutants.

5. list the ways communities can reduce air pollution.

6. name five indoor air pollutants and describe how their health risks can be reduced.

7. discuss the political controversy regarding regulation of air quality.

Air Pollution

In Romania trees and grass look as if they have been soaked in ink. In northern Czechoslovakia the government pays a bonus to anyone who will work there more than ten years; euphemistically it is called burial money. In much of Eastern Europe drivers must use their headlights in the middle of the day and in industrial areas 75 percent of children have respiratory disease.[1]

In more developed countries (MDC), including the United States and Japan, pollution has its own destructive history. The bad news is that cities like Los Angeles and Tokyo have some of the worst air pollution on the planet. The good news is that some cities, such as Pittsburgh and London, have made dramatic clean-up efforts proving that pollution problems can be ameliorated through community efforts.

Pollution, any undesirable change in the characteristics of the air, water, soil, or food that can adversely affect the health, survival or activities of human

BOX 18.1 Air Pollution In Eastern Europe

No sooner had the political dust of Eastern Europe's revolution against communism settled in 1989 than the world gasped in horror at the unbelievable levels of pollution, especially air pollution, throughout the communist world. We learned that in some areas of Poland, children are regularly taken underground into deep mines to gain some respite from the buildup of gasses and pollution of all sorts in the air.[2]

or other living organisms, can have many other unwanted effects. In addition to the spread of infectious diseases, irritation and diseases of the respiratory system, genetic and reproductive harm, and cancer, pollution is an aesthetic insult that damages property, plants, and nonhuman animal life and disrupts natural life-support systems at all levels.[3]

Air pollution kills, as has been demonstrated in London, New York, and Donora, Pennsylvania. In each of these cities epidemics of respiratory distress and actual mortality among high-risk groups such as the very young, the very old, and those with chronic respiratory illness occurred during weather inversions when high pressure kept industrial pollution in the air, creating deadly air quality. A 1996 U.S. study looking at death related to air pollution estimated that 64,000 people died prematurely in 239 surveyed areas due to heart and lung ailments caused by particle air pollution.[4] Air pollution impairs health by constricting the bronchi and alveoli of the lungs, choking an individual with emphysema, bronchitis, and asthma. Air pollution also leads to lung cancer and heart attacks. It stings the throat, reduces visibility, spoils scenic areas, and deteriorates house plants and metals. The Environmental Protection Agency (EPA) estimates that air pollution costs the United States $16 billion a year in lost property and health.

A major form of air pollution is industrial pollution, which makes women, minorities, and the poor of this country its primary victims. For lack of wealth, mobility, and leisure, they are deprived of healthful living conditions, and they, disproportionately, breathe polluted air. The amount of toxic industrial pollutants released into the air in each state in 1990 is described in Figure 18.1. Again, health and economics fight for primary attention.

Discussion: Why are businesses allowed to release toxins into the air? How does one decide how much is allowable?

Sources of Air Pollution

Air pollution is the presence in the air of substances in sufficient concentrations to interfere with health, safety, comfort, or use of property. Human-created air pollutants can be divided into gases and aerosols; the latter include solid particles and liquid droplets (Table 18.1). Pollutant gases range from ozone that pro-

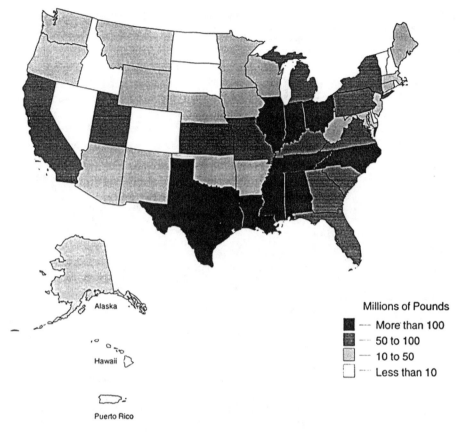

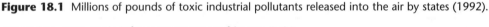

Figure 18.1 Millions of pounds of toxic industrial pollutants released into the air by states (1992).

(*Source:* EPA, 1992. Toxic Release Inventory, Washington, D.C.)

duces lung irritation, to agents such as carbon dioxide that contribute to the warming of the planet, known as the "greenhouse effect."

Natural sources of air pollution include fog, dust, airborne soil, salt spray, fissures, volcanoes, forest fires, lightning, and pollen. More than half the nation's air pollution comes from mobile sources such as cars, trucks, boats, and planes. Stationary sources include electric utilities, factories, and fuel stations.

Contributing Factors to Air Pollution

Air pollution is also aggravated by air currents, air movement, air temperature, air pressure, urban and topographic effects, and weather. When the weather is stagnant there is a sharp increase in the pollutants found in the ambient (sur-rounding) air. An inversion occurs when the temperature increases rather than decreases with altitude. When temperature near the ground is colder than the air a few hundred feet high, a surface inversion exists. This creates a lid that stops vertical mixing.

Table 18.1   Some urban air pollutants and their effects on health.

Pollutant	Effect
Smoke	Can penetrate lungs, some retained: may irritate bronchi.
Sulphur dioxide	Readily absorbed on inhalation: possibility of bronchospasm.
Sulphuric acid	Highly irritant if impacted in upper respiratory tract. Acid absorbed on other fine particles may penetrate.
Polycyclic aromatic hydrocarbons	Mainly absorbed on to smoke; can penetrate with it to lungs.
Photochemical hydrocarbons	Pollutants from traffic sources, or other hydrocarbon emissions. Non-toxic at moderate concentrations.
Nitric oxide	Capable of combining with hemoglobin in blood, but no apparent effect in human.
Nitrogen dioxide & ozone	Neither gas is very soluble. Can penetrate to lungs to cause edema. Urban concentrations show evidence of reduced resistance to infections in animals.
Aldehydes	Eye irritation, odor.
Carbon monoxide	Combines with hemoglobin in blood, reducing oxygen-carrying capacity.
Lead	Taken up in blood, distributed to soft tissues, and to bone.
Los Angeles Smog Complex:	
Nitric oxide	Primary eye irritation. Reduced athletic performance. Small changes in deaths, hospital admissions.
Nitrogen dioxide	Increased onsets of respiratory illnesses in children, increased asthma attacks in adults. No clear indication of increased bronchitis.
Carbon monoxide	Possible effects on CNS. Some evidence of effects on perception and performance of fine tasks at moderate concentrations. Enhances onset of exercise angina in patients.
Lead	Indications of neurophsycological effects on children.

(*Source:* Waller, Robert E., 1991. Field investigations of air. In *Oxford textbook of public health.* Vol. 3, p. 71. Oxford Press, London, p. 438, with permission of the Oxford University Press)

Urban areas react as heat islands or reservoirs by storing heat through absorption from the sun's rays during the day and releasing stored heat at night. As the warm air rises it carries pollutants, expands, flows toward the edges of the city, cools, and sinks. Cooler air that is loaded with pollution flows toward the center of the city dropping pollution. What the city has is a self-contained circulatory system of dust and haze. Only a strong wind can then interrupt this pattern.

Emissions and Ozone Depletion

Emissions of carbon dioxide and other gases into the atmosphere from the burning of fossil fuels and other human activities may raise the average temperature of the Earth's lower atmosphere several degrees between now and the year 2050 as a result of the greenhouse effect. A particular threat may be the manufacture of fast-food packaging that uses polystyrene foam (Styrofoam). Besides the fact

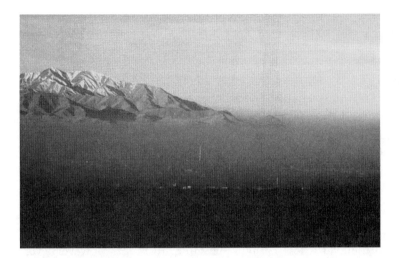

A weather inversion traps criterion pollutants in a valley where 750,000 people live. This inversion lasted 60 days.

that polystyrene is not biodegradable and presents a deadly hazard to marine and bird life, the way polystyrene is manufactured raises an even greater problem than its disposal. To create its bubble-like texture, a special chemical called chlorofluorocarbon 12 (CFC-12) is blown into the raw plastic.

Upper ozone depletion occurs as a result of the emission of CFC pollution through this manufacturing process and the CFC used in the cooling systems of refrigerators and air conditioners escaping into the atmosphere and ultimately destroying the protective upper-level ozone layer that surrounds the planet. People living in South America and Australia are already exposed to dangerous levels of ultraviolet radiation. The United States EPA announced in 1991 that the ozone layer had thinned by as much as 5 percent since 1978 over the northern hemisphere's middle latitudes, where most of the industrial world's population now lives. In October 1992, satellite measurements found that the level of ozone measured over the South Pole was the lowest ever recorded. Measured in Dobson units it was 105; the previous record low was 120 in both 1987 and 1991. The measurements found that the area of ozone depletion was 8.9 million square miles, the largest ever recorded.

BOX 18.2 *The Greenhouse Effect*

The greenhouse effect is caused when carbon dioxide, water vapor, and trace amounts of ozone, methane, nitrous oxide CFC and other gases act somewhat like panes of glass in the atmosphere. They allow light, infrared radiation (heat), and some ultraviolet radiation from the sun to pass through the troposphere. The Earth's surface then absorbs much of this solar energy and degrades it to infrared radiation, which escapes back into the atmosphere, thus warming the air.[5]

BOX 18.3 A Short History of Air Sanitation

1274 First smoke abatement law passed in England.

1473 Ulrich Ellenbog published tract on poisonous gases and fumes.

1624 Louis Savot improves the fireplace (inside air and flue).

1874 Fryer builds furnace incinerator for refuse at Nottingham.

1881 Chicago passed the first smoke regulation ordinance in the United States.

1963 Passage of the Federal Clean Air Act.

(*Source:* The Environmental History Timeline. www.runet.edu/~wkovarik/history1/timeline.text.htm)

In 1988, polystyrene manufacturers agreed to stop using CFC-12 for food packaging, switching to a less harmful substitute, HCFC-22. However, even HCFC-22 attacks the ozone, although it is only 5 percent as destructive as CFC-12. Also, when HCFC-22 is burned, it gives off chlorinated carbons, powerful and dangerous pollutants, even in tiny quantities. Some research suggests that HCFC-22 was producing benign tumors among those working with the chemical.[6]

The Dupont company, which manufactures CFCs under the trademark Freon, estimates that to restructure its methodology to produce ozone friendly alternatives (HCFCs) would cost about $1 billion in the United States alone. Even HCFCs may ultimately cause the greenhouse effect. Beginning in 1995, new cars were no longer permitted to use Freon in air conditioning. As of July 1, 1992, under the Clean Air Act, anyone servicing or disposing of refrigerators or air-conditioners had to capture the CFCs in the refrigerant chemicals.

It is believed that another source of ozone depletion is our space exploration program. Some research suggests that the space shuttle which uses ammonium perchlorate as fuel may contribute by breaking off chlorine in the upper atmosphere, affecting the ozone layer from above, and thus creating the same problem in space that humans create on earth.

The thinner ozone layer lets in more ultraviolet radiation from the sun and this has already appeared to have increased the incidence of skin cancer and eye cataracts, and to have weakened our immune system defenses against many infectious diseases. The EPA estimates that a 5 percent ozone depletion would cause an extra 170 million cases of skin cancer by the year 2075. This includes 2 million extra cases of basal and squamous cell skin cancers and an additional 30,000 cases of often-fatal melanoma skin cancer, which now kills almost 9,000 Americans each year. A 5 percent ozone depletion would also increase eye cataracts, a clouding of the lens that causes blurred vision and eventual blindness if not treated, suppression of the human immune system, and cost the United States $3.5 billion in health care.[7] Scientists predicted 1.6 million cases of cataracts a year and 300,000 new cases of skin cancer as a result of ozone depletion by the year 2000.[8]

BOX 18.4 CFC Emissions Statistics

According to preliminary EPA estimates of domestic CFC emissions, home refrigerators and freezers contribute more than 5,000 metric tons annually, while cold storage represents 8,000 metric tons, retail food refrigeration more than 12,000 tons, and industrial processes nearly 30,000 tons. In the United States, 1.3 kg of CFCs per person per year is used. The United States produces 96 percent of the world's CFCs, followed by western European countries, and Japan. Seventy-five percent of CFCs are consumed by industrial countries. Vehicle air conditioners account for about 75 percent of annual CFC emissions in the United States.

Smoke and Smog

Smoke is not a chemical entity although it is one of the most widespread components of urban air pollution. "Smoke" is applied to the black suspended particulate material in the air that is dominated by products of incomplete combustion. A dense mixture of smoke and fumes combined with fog that is formed when air pollutants are trapped at ground level by a temperature inversion is known as **smog.** An illustration of the smog/acid rain process is given in Figure 18.2.

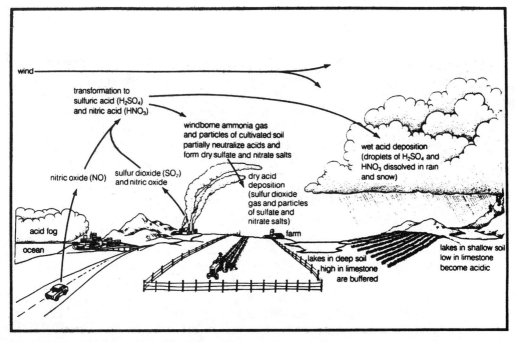

Figure 18.2 Transformation of chemicals into acid rain.

(*Source:* Miller, G. Tyler, 1992. *Living in the environment,* 7th ed. Belmont, CA: Wadsworth Publishing Company. Reprinted by permission.)

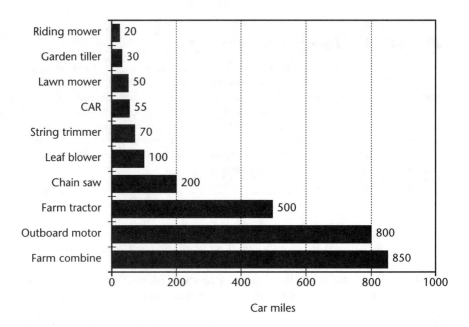

Figure 18.3 Amount of pollution created in one hour of use as compared to how far a car would travel to create the same pollution.

(*Source:* Environmental Protection Agency)

In 1992 the EPA submitted regulations to control the release of hydrocarbons that contribute to smog, from lawn mowers, weed eaters, leaf blowers, chain saws, and other off-road gas-powered machinery. For example, a lawn mower can spew as much smog-causing hydrocarbon into the air in an hour as a modern car, as shown in Figure 18.3. During the summer, lawn mowers contribute 15 percent to 20 percent of the hydrocarbons that create summer smog. A chain saw operating for two hours emits as many hydrocarbons as a new car driving 3,000 miles.

Health Impairment in Humans

The complex relationship of gas-aerosol pollutants is responsible for air pollution disasters in the world and for both acute and chronic respiratory disease. The high overall bronchitis rates in some countries with severe air pollution has been seen as an indicator of the role of pollution in the development of chronic respiratory disease (see Table 18.1). It is estimated that about 10 percent of Americans suffer from chronic bronchitis, emphysema, or asthma either caused or aggravated by air pollution. Since the mid-1980s, asthma rates in the United States have risen to the level of an epidemic. Asthma and other respiratory conditions often are triggered or worsened by substances found in the air, such as tobacco smoke, ozone, and other particles or chemicals. Based on existing data, an estimated 17.3 million people in the United States had asthma in 2000, including more than 5 million children aged eighteen years and under.

Ever since a substantial increase in lung cancer mortality was first noted in the 1930s, it has been apparent that death rates are generally higher in urban than in rural areas. While the smoking habits of lung cancer patients are probably the primary source of etiology, the outcome of most studies to date has found that once smoking has been taken into account, the differential between urban and rural dwellers in the incidence of lung cancer seems to have some relationship to the quality of the air.[9]

The Clean Air Act

The federal Clean Air Act (Box 18.5) first passed in 1963, amended in 1970, 1977, 1990, and again in 1999, was the first law established to set strict air quality standards based primarily on health rather than economic considerations in response to this country's deteriorating air quality. This law had two main purposes: (1) to limit the amount of smog by reducing concentrations of six major pollutants in the air, and (2) to regulate the emissions of hazardous toxic air pollutants, such as benzene, from chemical plants. The Act empowered the EPA to set limits on several of the 300 known air pollutants. In addition, strict emission standards for the manufacturing of new automobiles and the building of power plants and factories were established. Compliance time has been set, but pressure from industry keeps changing and delaying compliance deadlines, extending the date. Although the EPA has the power to enforce the Clean Air Act, cutbacks in federal funding and pressure from industry seems to have immobilized the EPA in terms of actual enforcement.[10]

The 1999 EPA's final air quality standards were the first update in twenty years for ozone (smog) and the first in ten years for particulate matter (soot). The updated standards, a major step forward in public health protection, will protect 125 million Americans, including 35 million children, from the health

---

BOX 18.5 The Clean Air Act

History: Enacted in 1970 and amended in 1977, 1990, and 1999.

Purpose: The overall goal is to reduce the pollutants in our air to safe concentrations. By the year 2005 the goal is to reduce pollution in our air by 56 billion pounds a year.

Goals:

1. Cut acid rain by reducing emission of sulfur dioxide and nitrogen;
2. Reduce smog or ground-level ozone; Regulate diesel-powered buses in urban areas; New emission standards for motor vehicles and adopt new clean fuel programs;
3. Reduce air toxins in chemical plants, steel mills and other businesses;
4. Protect the ozone layer by eliminating CFCs and CFC recycling.

Problems: 1995 House of Representatives voted to reduce environmental standards and cut EPA power.

Funding: Funding authorization comes through annual appropriations bills which were threatened by Congress in 1995.

(*Source*: What you can do to reduce air pollution, Salt Lake City Health Department, 1993.)

hazards of air pollution. Each year, these new, updated standards will *prevent* approximately:

15,000 premature deaths

350,000 cases of aggravated asthma

1 million cases of significantly decreased lung function in children

---

Healthy People 2010 Objective: Reduce the Proportion of Persons Exposed to Air That Does Not Meet the U.S. Environmental Protection Agency's (EPA's) Health-Based Standards for Harmful Air Pollutants

Reduction in Air Pollutants	1997 Baseline (%)	2010 Target (%)
Ozone	43	0
Particulate matter	12	0
Carbon monoxide	19	0
Nitrogen dioxide	5	0
Sulfur dioxide	2	0
Lead	<1	0

Discussion: There are some who think the Clean Air Act is too restrictive and, therefore, it is too expensive for industry to comply. What do you think?

Approximately 113 million people live in U.S. areas designated as non-attainment areas by the EPA for one or more of the six commonly found air pollutants for which the federal government has established health-based standards. The problem of air pollution is international in scope. Most of the U.S. population lives in expanding urban areas where air pollution crosses local and state lines and, in some cases, crosses U.S. borders with Canada and Mexico.[11]

The 1963 and 1970 Clean Air Act modifications set National Ambient Air Quality Standards for criterion pollutants and hazardous pollutants. **Criterion pollutants** are ozone, carbon monoxide (CO), particulate matter (PM10), sulfur dioxide (SO_2), lead, and nitrogen oxides (NO_x) (see Table 18.2). **Hazardous pollutants** are asbestos, beryllium, mercury, vinyl chloride, arsenic, radionuclides, benzene, and coke oven emissions. The 1990 Clean Air Act amendments increased the hazardous air pollutant list to 189 chemicals for which regulations were modified in 1999. The Act also established National Ambient Air Quality Standards, which required states that are not in attainment with standards to prepare federally approved State Air Quality Implementation Plans (SIP) to meet air quality standards, regulate auto emissions, and require technology based standards for new emission sources.[12]

You can determine the quality of the air in your state at this very moment by going to www.epa.gov/airnow/where and then clicking on your state.

Table 18.2 Air emissions by source (1988). (In million metric tons except lead in thousand metric tons)

Emission	Total	Vehicles	Elec.	Individual	Solid Waste
Carbon monoxide	61.2	34.1	.3	4.7	1.7
SO$_x$	20.7	.6	13.6	3.4	0
VOC	18.6	4.9	—	8.5	.6
PM	6.9	1.1	.4	2.6	.3
NO$_x$	19.8	6.1	7.1	.6	.1
Lead	7.6	2.4	.1	2.0	2.5

(*Source:* Vital Statistics, 1991)

Table 18.3 Non-attainment status.

Pollutant	Original # of Areas	1999 # of Areas	1999 Population (in 1,000s)
CO	43	20	33,230
Pb	12	8	1,116
NO$_2$	1	0	0
O$_3$	101	32	92,505
PM$_{10}$	85	77	29,880
SO$_2$	51	31	4,371

(*Source*: National Air Quality and Emissions Trends Report, 1999).

Unfortunately, the concern for the air in the 1970s and the concern for jobs in the 1980s have conflicted and limited the EPA's ability to enforce clean air standards when industry has had the ear of the administration.

Discussion: What do the cities and counties that exceeded pollutant standards have in common?

Although the 1970 law did help to reduce smog somewhat, it didn't achieve its goals. The EPA reported in 1999 that 121 urban areas had not attained permissible air levels. By 1999, thirty-two cities in the United States still had not attained the national standard for ozone (the primary ingredient in smog), twenty cities did not meet the standard for carbon monoxide, and seventy-seven did not meet the standard for particulate matter (Table 18.3). The Los Angeles basin exceeded standards for nitrogen dioxide and continues to have the nation's most unhealthful air quality. In 1998, 113 million people still lived in places with unhealthful air. Pollution indirectly contributes to their poor health by weakening the human immune system and increasing susceptibility to disease.[13]

In 1990, the Reauthorization of the Clean Air Act was passed. The legislation has three broad goals: (1) smog reduction in urban areas through regulation of the auto industry; (2) acid rain controls through regulation of the

Table 18.4 Particle size ranges for aerosols.

Type of Particle	Minimum Mean Size (Microns)	Maximum Mean Size (Microns)
Raindrops	500	5,000
Natural mist	60	500
Pollens	10	100
Plant spores	10	100
Human hair	35	200
Cement dusts	3	100
Red blood cells	7.5	
Insecticide dusts	.05	10
Oil smoke	.1	1.0
Paint pigments	.1	5
Bacteria	.3	35
Tobacco smoke	.01	1.0
Photochemical smog	.01	1.0
Normal air impurities	.01	1.0
Combustion nuclei	.01	.1
Silicosis dusts	.05	5
Metallurgical dusts	.001	100
Virus and protein	.003	.05
Gas molecules	.0001	.0006

coal-mining and utility industries; and (3) elimination of cancer-causing toxins from the air through industry implementation of clean air technology.

The Clean Air Act of 1990 placed tighter control on tailpipe exhaust starting with 1994 cars. Industries are now required to reduce by 90 percent the use of 189 chemicals known to be carcinogens and reduce CFCs and carbon tetrachloride by the year 2000, methyl chloroform by the year 2002, and hydrochlorofluorocarbons by the year 2030.

In June 1992, new regulations were enacted that allow manufacturers to increase the pollutants they emit by 245 tons a year without public hearings or judicial review. The act required states to negotiate new pollution limits by 1995.[14]

The Six Criterion Pollutants

Particulate Matter (PM10) The air we breathe contains not only the mixture of elements we are familiar with—oxygen, carbon dioxide, and nitrogen—but other chemicals and actual particles. Particles range in size from about 0.1 micron (.00004 inches) such as paint pigments, to 500 microns (.02 inches) such as raindrops (Table 18.4). Particles less than 10 microns in diameter are not respirated by the lungs and can lodge deep in the alveoli causing scarring. The larger particles, defined as aerosols, are generated as stoker fly ash, industrial dusts, and pollens. The smaller particulates (less than 0.1 micron) include smoke, fumes from combustion, and viruses.

Approximately 10 million tons of particulate matter enter the atmosphere daily from natural sources and about 700,000 tons are created by anthropogenic

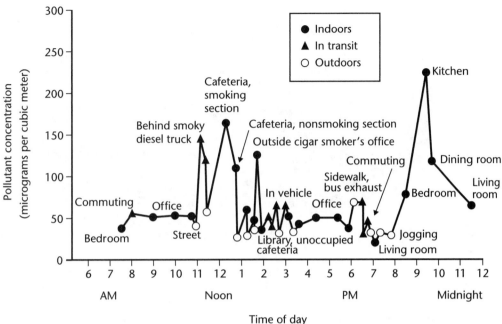

Figure 18.4 One person's potential daily exposure to respirable particles.

(*Source:* Environmental Protection Agency)

sources, including windblown dust and woodburning stoves. Look at a day in the life of one person's exposure to respiratory particles as illustrated in Figure 18.4.

Discussion: What does a day in your life look like in terms of exposure to particulate matter?

Roughly one percent of the particulates carry small amounts of lead, cadmium, chromium, arsenic, nickel, and mercury. It is known that these metals can be quite toxic when inhaled in significant quantity.

The degree of danger posed by inhalation of particulates depends not only on the composition but also on the size of particles. Particles larger than 15 microns normally are expelled by breathing. Smaller particles not only pose the risk of being retained within the lungs, destroying or damaging protective cilia, but may penetrate deep within the lung tissue and then be passed into the blood supply. Particle toxicity also depends upon such factors as chemical composition, solubility, and pH. The highest particulate concentrations by county are given in Figure 18.5.

Discussion: How does your state rank in terms of particulate matter? What is the source of this concentration in your state?

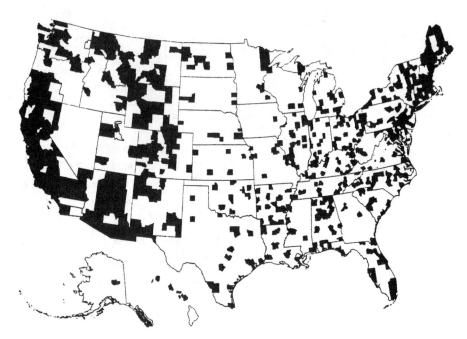

Figure 18.5 Highest maximum 24-hour PM10 by country (1996).

(*Source:* Environmental Protection Agency. National Air Quality and Emission Trends Report, 1996)

The best control for particulate matter is the use of scrubbers on smoke stacks and/or electrostatic precipitators that moisten particulates prior to releasing smoke through the chimneys. Additionally, having complete combustion of fuels, watering down dust areas such as gravel and sand pits, and avoiding "fugitive sources" (dust blown out of areas other than approved stacks), and the use of bag houses are required controls in most areas. Major sources of particulate matter are shown in Figure 18.6.[15]

Sulfur Dioxide Sulfur dioxide (SO_2) formation is associated with smoke or suspended particles since it is dependent upon the sulfur content of fuel. It is caused by the burning of coal and oil, especially high sulfur coal from the eastern United States. It is produced in the industrial processes of paper and metal products. It causes nose and throat irritation and may cause permanent damage to the lungs.

Sulfur dioxide is absorbed in the upper respiratory tract and has little direct effect on the vulnerable lower airways of the lung. It is a primary cause of respiratory ailments, coughs, asthma, and bronchitis. However, it is a precursor of more potent sulfates, including sulfuric acid, formed by oxidation of sulfur dioxide in the atmosphere. This pollutant can reach deeply into the lung by loading onto inhalable particulates. Control of sulfur dioxide can be maintained by scrubbers, fluidized bed combustion, lime slurry scrubbers, washing and crushing coal before combustion, and the use of low sulfur coal. Major sources of sulfur are shown in Figure 18.7.[16]

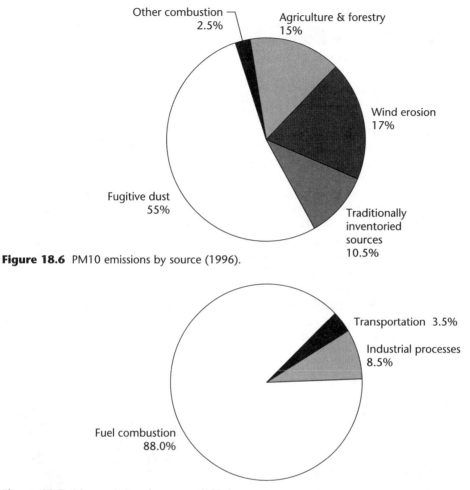

Figure 18.6 PM10 emissions by source (1996).

Figure 18.7 SO$_{10}$ emissions by source (1996).

(*Source:* Environmental Protection Agency. National Air Quality and Emission Trends Report, 1996)

When Eastern Europe became available to the rest of the world for travel and study, the tragic effects of air pollution, especially sulfur dioxide emissions, became evident and an omen of what uncontained air pollution may do to our own cities. Emigrating from Poland, East Germany, and Czechoslovakia are not only political, but environmental refugees, trying to get to the less polluted west. For example, in Krakow, Poland, 10 percent of all children have chronic bronchitis; 33 percent of the population of Leningrad has upper respiratory tract disease.[17]

The destruction of the air and soil in Poland is not an isolated problem. **Acid rain** (pH as low as 2.6 compared to normal rain pH of 6) that is produced by sulfur dioxide emission from coal factories blows into other countries from Poland, just as it blows into Canada from the northeastern part of the United

States. The highest levels of sulfate SO_2 (1,075 grams/m^3) were found in Chorzow, Poland, in 1989. The national average of SO_2 in Poland is 13(g/m^2). High levels of sulfur dioxide are reported in Sweden, Denmark, the former USSR, and Czechoslovakia. Air is a global issue, not a provincial issue.

Ozone   Ozone is a colorless gas with a pungent odor produced by an electrical discharge from virtually any electrical source. It is a powerful, toxic, oxidizing agent, and the principal component of smog. It is the most persistent of the criterion pollutants. Among the major U.S. cities, only Minneapolis, Minnesota, is in compliance with the national health-based standards for ozone. Ozone non-attainment areas for 1997 are shown in Figure 18.8.[18]

Ozone causes inflammation and congestion of the respiratory tract. Autopsies performed on over 100 Los Angeles youths who were killed in car accidents and homicides in 1988 revealed that four out of five had notable lung tissue abnormalities and nearly one-third had severe lesions in the lungs. Dr. Russell Sherwin, the pathologist, said they were simply "running out of lung." Dr. Sherwin concluded that "air pollution, in particular, high levels of ozone, was the principal culprit."[19]

Ozone is by far the most toxic component of photochemical air pollution. It is produced by a chemical reaction that occurs when hydrocarbons and nitrogen oxides are exposed to sunlight. Hydrocarbons and nitrogen oxide com-

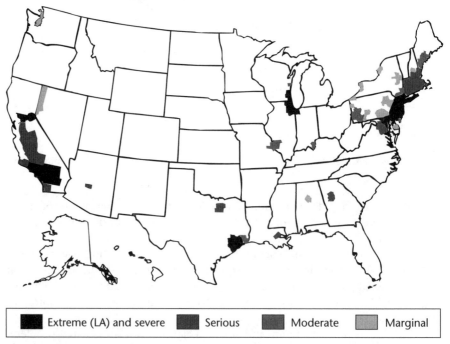

| ■ Extreme (LA) and severe | ■ Serious | ■ Moderate | ■ Marginal |

Figure 18.8 Classified ozone non-attainment areas (1997).

(*Source:* Environmental Protection Agency. National Air Quality and Emission Trends Report, 1997)

pounds are broken up, and oxygen atoms are released into the air joining other oxygen atoms already present to form ozone. Ozone appears to be affected by warm weather. The 1988 drought, which affected most of the United States, brought about ozone levels higher than those observed in 1987.

Ozone is highly irritating to the lungs, producing an inflammatory response and reacting in a manner which suggest that chronic loss in lung function may result from repetitive ozone exposure. It can cause structural and chemical changes in the lungs and some blood components. Chronic respiratory diseases are aggravated by ozone.

Since some hours are required for concentrations to build up to a peak within the daylight hours, the maxima are not necessarily at the point of emission. Ozone and nitrogen dioxide both have the ability to potentiate bacterial respiratory tract infection in mice, though the relevance to humans is unclear.[20] Ozone is prevented by controlling NO_x and hydrocarbon emissions, especially from automobile combustion or high temperature combustion manufacturing.

Volatile Organic Compounds (VOC) (smog formers such as compounds released from burning gasoline, oil, wood, or coal) are not regulated as a criterion pollutant; however, their emissions are controlled and monitored by state agencies because of their role in the formation of ozone. VOCs occur as natural biological processes in soil and vegetation or in combustion. Their photochemical reaction with NO_x are involved in the production of ozone. In addition to smog effects, many VOCs can cause serious health problems such as cancer.

Carbon Monoxide   Emissions of carbon monoxide (CO), the colorless, odorless gas formed as a by-product during the incomplete combustion of fossil fuels, are common to a wide range of sources including motor vehicles, cigarettes, and other combustion sources. Ground level concentrations in city streets are affected most by motor vehicle emissions although diesel engines produce little. The gas is relatively inert and does not play an essential part in the photochemical process, but it is readily absorbed by the blood. Because of hemoglobin's affinity for carbon monoxide, normal oxygen supply is replaced by carbon monoxide. This causes a reduction of oxygen supplied to various body cells and organs.

Exposure to carbon monoxide is a particular problem to those with preexisting cardiovascular disease. Carbon monoxide exposure produces a decrease in exercise tolerance of patients with angina at levels as low as 2 to 3 percent carboxyhemoglobin (the ability of the red blood cells to pick up oxygen).[21]

A major means of prevention of carbon monoxide is catalytic convertors in automobiles. The catalytic converter oxidizes CO to CO_2 when excess air is pumped into exhaust gas and through the converter.

Nitrogen Oxides   Nitrogen oxides (NO_x) are produced when fuel is burned at high temperatures. Automobiles burn at about 1200°F and contribute to NO_x emissions. Nitrogen oxides are required for the creation of ozone. Alone they can cause structural and chemical changes in the lungs. NO_x can be prevented by specially designed "low-NO_x" engines and catalytic convertors.

Nitrogen dioxide is a major source of indoor pollution. It is most frequently found in the exhaust of internal-combustion engines, and indoors, in the gas

Table 18.5 Percentage of African American, Hispanic, and white populations living in air-quality non-attainment areas, 1992.

Pollutant	African American	Hispanic	White
	Percent		
Particulates	16.5	34.0	14.7
Carbon monoxide	46.0	57.1	33.6
Ozone	62.2	71.2	52.5
Sulfur dioxide	12.1	5.7	7.0
Lead	9.2	18.5	6.0

(*Source:* Environmental Protection Agency)

stove. Animal studies suggest that nitrogen dioxide exposure may increase the risk of pulmonary infections and may enhance the likelihood of a fatal bacterial pneumonia.[22]

Lead   Diseases caused by lead poisoning are among the oldest identified diseases to plague humans. Egyptians suffered from lead poisoning from potters' wheels and lead leached into the aqueducts in Rome. Lead (Pb) compounds are dispersed into the atmosphere as fine particulates. The most universal source of lead has been gas-engine vehicles, through the use of lead alkyds as antiknock agents in the fuel. Concentrations are highest close to busy roads that often are the neighborhoods of poorer communities. Children in these neighborhoods have been found to have toxic levels of lead in their blood.

The EPA estimates that 1.7 million children are affected by lead from old paint, water pipes, soil, and other sources. This is 4.4% of all children and 22 percent of African American children.[23] Table 18.5 reports the percentage of people living in non-attainment areas by race in 1992.

Responding to new medical concerns about the harmful effects of exposure to even low levels of lead, in 1992 the federal government began requiring that all young children on Medicaid be screened for lead poisoning. Unfortunately, the federal directive allows states to continue using a test known to be inaccurate in measuring small amounts of lead in the blood. Poor children are at particular risk for asymptomatic lead poisoning because they live in homes that were once painted with paint that contained as much as 50 percent lead, and now this paint is chipping off walls as old buildings deteriorate. Children often ingest this loose, leaded paint. Lead poisoning is one of the most common child health problems in the United States, afflicting 3 to 4 million young children—one in six children under six years old. Exposure to lead can cause mental retardation, learning disabilities, stunted growth, hearing loss, and behavior problems in children.

Regulation allows for only 50 micrograms of lead exposure per person per day in the workplace. It can be sampled from blood, bone, urine, hair, and sweat. Other recommendations for lead reduction are shown in Table 18.6. Highest lead by county in 1996 is shown in Figure 18.9.

Table 18.6 Sources of lead and remedies.

Source of Lead	Description	Remedies
Paint	Homes build before 1950	Contain or remove lead
Water	Lead pipes, faucets, wells	Run tap for 2 minutes; use cold water for cooking
Soil	Gasoline and house paint; pesticides	Removal, cover with grass or plants
Hobbies	Artist's paint, fishing weights, bullets	Use care when handling Choose art products marked CP or AP
Glazes	Tile, pottery, ceramics, acidic drinks may leach toxins out of lead crystal	Monitor for signs of decay; don't store food in lead containers

(*Source:* Environmental Protection Agency)

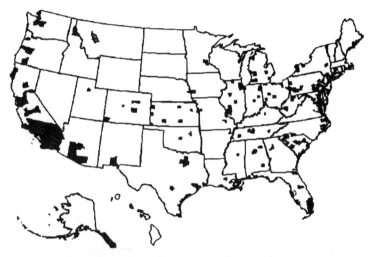

Figure 18.9 Highest Pb maximum quarterly mean by state.

(*Source:* Environmental Protection Agency. National Air Quality and Emission Trends Report, 1996)

> ***Healthy People 2010 Objective:*** Increase the Proportion of Persons Living in Pre-1950s Housing That Have Tested for the Presence of Lead-Based Paint
>
> *Target:* 50 percent.
>
> *Baseline:* 16 percent of persons living in 1998 in homes built before 1950 had tested for the presence of lead-based paint (preliminary data; age adjusted to the year 2000 standard population).

Indoor Air Pollution

By its very nature, indoor air pollution leads to maximal exposure of individuals. People spend 70 to 90 percent of their time indoors, and the infirm, elderly, and very young are indoors most of the time. Among indoor pollutants are asbestos, radon, cigarette smoke, formaldehyde, and microorganisms and allergens.

Table 18.7 Odds of dying from asbestos as compared to other risks.

Cause	# of Deaths per 100,000
Smoking	21,900
Motor vehicle	1,600
Indoor radon	400
Diagnostic x-ray	75
Lightning	3
Asbestos in building	1

(*Source:* Environmental Protection Agency)

Asbestos

Asbestos comprises a series of natural fibrous materials so small that when they get into the lungs they cannot be expelled through respiration. Ironically, the control or the attempt at elimination of asbestos has the potential of a greater public health threat than no action at all. When asbestos that may insulate pipes or fireproofing asbestos is disturbed, it becomes **friable** (flaking), making it more apt to be inhaled than if it were allowed to deteriorate naturally. Increased demand to remove asbestos, with perhaps too quick a response, has actually increased the risk of contamination. Asbestos trouble spots in the home are shown in the box below.

In the mining profession asbestos use has led to a fibrous lung disease, **mesothelioma,** a pleural or peritoneal tumor relatively specific to asbestos. The interactive effect between cigarette smoking and asbestos exposures multiplies the risk of lung cancer.

Actually the public health problem for communities is not as great for asbestos contamination in schools and public buildings as it is for the occupational hazard of asbestos removal. The asbestos removal industry is a multi-billion dollar industry whose expansion may prevent sufficient high-level sophisticated training of removal personnel. A comparison of risk of death from asbestos compared to other risks of death is given in Table 18.7.

BOX 18.6 Asbestos Trouble Spots

Ceilings:	Cottage cheese or popcorn textured paint; troweled or sprayed-on soundproofing
Walls:	Joint compound and spackle; insulation and soundproofing
Kitchens:	Linoleum and vinyl flooring and adhesives
Basement:	Furnace ducts; insulation board; door gaskets; wood and coal stoves; boilers coated with asbestos cement mix; hot water pipe insulation
Outside:	Shingles and siding
Miscellaneous:	Artificial embers for gas fireplaces; fireproof gloves

Radon

In many parts of the planet, the natural radiation levels in rock and soil give rise to an appreciable risk of lung cancer due to **radon-222** gas. This gas is the odorless, colorless, decay product of uranium–238, which itself has a relatively short half-life before forming very short-lived alpha-emitting radon daughter particles, called progeny, of high carcinogenic potential. Radon emitted outdoors rapidly dissipates. However, when emitted into the home it will tend to accumulate, particularly in the lowest floor. The isotopes of polonium, lead, and bismuth for the most part attach to tiny particles of household dust and smoke, penetrate our lungs, and become lodged there. The extent of accumulation is dependent upon a number of factors, but perhaps the most important is ventilation characteristics. Limitation schemes and values vary, but annual doses above 10–20 mSv (Sv is the symbol for **sievert,** the special name for the unit of ionizing dose equivalents among different types of radiation) are generally deemed undesirable.

Sealing cracks in basement floors and walls or installing a subslab exhaust system beneath the basement floor may be the most immediate means of controlling radon in homes with high levels. The EPA does not recommend the use of filtration systems to control radon decay in houses, but an inexpensive fan will often reduce the dose of radon to the lungs.

Although building materials such as brick and concrete do produce radon, the main source of high indoor levels is the ground. The atmospheric pressure inside homes tends to be slightly lower than outside, and radon is drawn into the home through gaps and cracks in the floor. High concentrations are more likely to occur around granite masses or on uriniferous shales. A 1993 EPA study found that in miners, about 40 percent of all lung cancer deaths may be due to radon exposure, accounting for 70 percent of lung cancer deaths among never-smokers and 39 percent among smokers.

While some scientists are not sure that we can attribute any casualties to household radon, estimates of radon-related illness now range from 2,000 to 20,000 cases of lung cancer annually in the United States. It is believed that as many as six million houses have radon concentrations at or above the dangerous levels of 4 picocuries per liter.[24]

Healthy People 2010 Objective: Increase the Proportion of Persons Who Live in Homes Tested for Radon Concentrations

Target: 20 percent.

Baseline: 17 percent of the population lived in homes in 1998 that had been tested for radon (preliminary data; age adjusted to the year 2000 standard population).

Cigarette Smoke

One factor consistently associated with a high prevalence of respiratory illness in young children is parental smoking. Clearly, cigarette smoke is a widespread problem in indoor environments, leading to odor, eye and throat irritation, and to more specific effects on respiratory illness and lung conditions, especially among young children. There is also mounting evidence indicating a small increase in lung cancer among non-smokers through prolonged exposures to environmental tobacco smoke.[25] Chemicals found in cigarette smoke and household items containing chemicals found in tobacco are given in Box 18.7.

> **Discussion:** The FDA wants to make tobacco a regulated drug. Given what you know about tobacco, should it be regulated as a drug?

Formaldehyde

A further indoor air pollutant that has gained some prominence in recent years is formaldehyde, arising in some circumstances from the urea-formaldehyde foam used for insulation in cavity walls. Formaldehyde is a colorless, pungent

---

BOX 18.7 Chemical Compounds Found in Cigarette Smoke (partial list)

Acetaldehyde	Cresol	Nickel
Acetone	Formaldehyde	Nicotine
Acrolein	Hydrogen cyanide	Nitrogen dioxide
Ammonia	Hydrogen sulfide	Nitrogen oxide
Arsenic	Methanol	Nitrosamines
Benzo pyrene	Methylchrysenes	Nornicotine
Butane	Methyl chloride	Phenol
Cadmium	Methyl ethyl ketone	Pyridine
Carbon monoxide	Methyl nitrite	Stearic acid
Chrysene	N-hetercyclic hydrocarbons	Vinyl chloride

Household Items Containing Chemicals Found in Tobacco

Stearic Acid
Elastin collagen
Cover Girl Mascara
Colgate Aftershave
Vaseline Intensive Care Lotion
Wondra Skin Lotion

Butane
Right Guard Deodorant
Brut Faberge Deodorant
Aqua Net Hair Spray
Hair Spray Glitter

Formaldehyde
Faberge Organic Wheat Germs Oil & Honey Shampoo
Revlon Nail Enamel

Ammonia
Magic Sizing Fabric Finish
Windex Window Cleaner

Acetone
Cutex Nail Polish Remover

Phenol
Carmex Lip Balm

Stearic Acid and Butane
Gillette Foam Shaving Cream

(*Source:* Physicians for a Smoke-Free Canada)

gas that is both suffocating and poisonous in high dosages and is found in binding materials and adhesives used in chipboard furniture and some other materials around the home. Eight billion pounds of formaldehyde are produced in the United States each year. It is found in cosmetics, deodorants, solvents, disinfectants, and fumigants. The most obvious effects are eye and throat irritation. There is no indication at the present time that the concentrations liable to be encountered in the home lead to any long-term effects, but the removal of chipboard furniture has solved some people's immediate respiratory problems.

More and more attention is being placed on the ill health effects of the volatile organic compounds (VOCs) arising from consumer products found in the home such as paints, polishes, and cleaning solutions. These include benzene from tobacco smoke and perchlorethylene emitted from dry-cleaned clothing. VOCs can also be emitted from drinking water. Twenty percent of drinking water has discernible amounts of VOC although only 1 percent exceed the Safe Drinking Water Act Standards for VOC.

Microorganisms and Allergens

The architectural designs of the 1970s produced buildings that were fully enclosed and windowless. The emphasis was on preventing loss of energy. Unfortunately, poor or faulty ventilation systems have aggravated a condition called sick building syndrome that includes mysterious ailments suffered by those who live or work in these buildings and the aggravation of bacterial and hypersensitivity infections to pollens, molds, hair, dust, fungi, and other contaminants that are not properly vented from such buildings. Tightly sealed buildings enhance the growth of molds and fungi and increase airborne concentrations of microorganisms in buildings.

Summary

More people die on bad air days even though the actual amount of pollutants should not kill. Air pollution "hastens the death of people who are somehow primed by disease to die." [26] Although air pollution rates for the criterion pollutants have been declining in the major cities in the past few years due to strict governmental control and consciousness by community citizens, vigilance must be maintained. Efforts by Congress in 1995 to reduce air pollution standards put the health of citizens at greater risk. Reduction of air pollutants require a concerted community effort.

Despite strict laws and attempts at enforcement, contaminants in the ambient environment still exist in concentrations that are sometimes lethal and more often hostile to living things. Cleaning the air will require the cooperation of industry, government, business, and consumers. It will be costly and require some sacrifices in the amenities we now enjoy. The result will be overwhelmingly positive, necessary, and appreciated by future generations.

Perhaps the greatest attention placed on indoor air pollution has been the state laws regarding the removal of asbestos from public buildings and the elimination of smoking in indoor public environments. Both have been controversial, but it is estimated that the long-term health benefits will outweigh the short-term financial implications by many businesses.

CYBERSITES RELATED TO CHAPTER 18

Environmental Health
    www.epa.gov
    www.cehs.siu.edu
    www.ncs.org/ehc.htm

QUESTIONS

1. How much more would you be willing to spend on an automobile to guarantee clean exhaust? What would be your limit? Should the price of gasoline be increased to curb auto use? How else might auto emissions be decreased?

2. What are the criterion pollutants that create the greatest health risk in your community?

3. What causes acid rain? What are the effects?

EXERCISE

Go through your home, place of recreation, and workplace and make a checklist of all the chemicals, appliances, and "toys" you use that potentially pollute the air. After you have made the checklist, find an alternative product or activity to eliminate the pollution risk. If the risk cannot be eliminated, what efforts can you make to reduce the air pollution?

INTERNET INTERACTIVE ACTIVITY

THE AMERICAN LUNG ASSOCIATION—DATA SOURCES

The American Lung Association has prepared trend reports (most from February 2000) depicting available prevalence, incidence, hospitalization, and mortality data for lung disease and cigarette smoking. Data are gathered from national surveys, databases, and reports and are examined by age, gender, race/ethnicity, and, in some cases, educational attainment and economic impact.

The data files are available in PDF format. To view and/or print the documents in Acrobat® PDF file format, you need a copy of *Acrobat® Reader™*. The homepage for the ALA is:

www.lungusa.org/data/index.html

Exercise

1. Click on **Data and Statistics**.

2. Click on **State Specific Lung Disease DATA**. Using the tables available, describe lung disease characteristics in your state.

3. Using the data available on **COPD (Narrative and Tables)**
    www.lungusa.org/data/copd/copd1.pdf

What is the rate of COPD by race and gender for 1998? What significant difference do you notice among these data?

4. Compare the rates of chronic bronchitis from 1982 and 1998. What do these data tell you?

5. What do you notice in the trends for emphysema for men and for women in the past ten years? Why would these trends occur?

6. Using **Asthma, Trends**

   Describe the rate of asthma in both genders.

   What do you notice about prevalence of asthma by sex, race, and age?

   How does asthma differentiate by geographical region and income? Why are there such distinctions?

7. Find your state among those reported on **Estimated Prevalence and Incidence of Chronic and Acute Lung Disease by Lung Association, State Specific Lung Disease.**

   www.lungusa.org/data/lae_00/EstPrev2.pdf

   Using the data available through the American Lung Association, peruse the documents available through the pdf files and answer the following questions:

   What is the prevalence and incidence for lung cancer, emphysema, and asthma for two urban and two rural counties in your state?

   What is the percent change for each of these diseases from 1995–1996?

   Explain the difference between prevalence and incidence for these diseases.

REFERENCES

1. Munson, Halsey (1990). "Pollution in the Soviet Union." ECON: Environmental Contractor, 5:8, 24–29.

2. Gore, Al (1992). *Earth in the balance.* New York: Houghton Mifflin.

3. Miller, G. Tyler (1992) *Living in the environment.* Belmont, CA: Wadsworth Publishing.

4. *USNWR (1996).* Our breath-taking air. May 20, p. 15.

5. Miller, op. cit.

6. Weisskopf, Michael (1992). Study finds alternatives more damaging than believed. In *Earth's eleventh hour* by William O. Dwyer. Boston: Allyn & Bacon.

7. Miller, op. cit.

8. Weisskopf, op. cit.

9. Waller, Robert E. (1991). Field investigations of air. In *Oxford textbook of public health,* Vol. II.

10. Bryner, Gary C. (1993). *Blue skies, green politics: The Clean Air Act of 1990.* Library of Congress Cataloging-in-Publication Data.

11. National Air Quality and Trends Report, EPA, Office of Air and Radiation, Washington, DC, 1997.

12. Committee on Public Works and Transportation (1993). Provisions of H.R. 3030, the Clean Air Act Amendments of 1989, that fall within the jurisdiction of the Committee on Public Works and Transportation. U.S. Government Printing Office.

13. Bryner, op. cit.

14. Goldstein, Bernard D. (1991). Environmental applications and interventions in public health. In *Oxford textbook of public health.* Vol. 1, pp. 17–28.

15. National Air Quality and Emissions Trends Report, 1997. EPA. Washington D.C.

16. Ibid.

17. Adamson, David (1990). *Defending the world.* London: Tauris and Co.

18. National Air Quality and Emissions Trends Report op. cit.

19. Goldman, Benjamin A. (1991). *The truth about where you live.* New York: Times Books, Random House.

20. Goldstein, op. cit.

21. Ibid.

22. Ibid.

23. Spake, Amanda, & Couzin, Jennifer (1999). In the air that they breathe. *U.S. News and World Report,* Dec. 20, p. 54.

24. *Environmental health perspectives* (1995). Mining the radon studies. Vol. 103, no. 10, Oct. p. 895.

25. Waller, op. cit.

26. Manning, Anita (1995). Death rates rise with air pollution. *USA Today,* March 16, p. A1.

CHAPTER 19

Water Quality

Community Health in the 21st Century
*With more and more people recreating near drinking water sources, and the
federal government placing fewer restrictions on industry that dumps its
wastes into water sources, the nation's water may be at great risk. Imagine
not being able to depend on your tap water as clean, pure, and safe. In some
cities this is happening already. It may be worse in the next century.*

—Luci Malin, M.S., Office of Mine Reclamation

Chapter Objectives

The student will:

1. account for the increasing pollution of the world's water sources.

2. explain common sources of ground-water pollution.

3. list the eight types of water pollutants.

4. identify the cause and result of acid rain.

5. describe the water treatment process for drinking water and waste water.

6. list common waterborne diseases.

The Hydrosphere

Although over 70 percent of the earth's surface is water, less than one percent is accessible as fresh water. Ninety-seven percent of the water is contained in the world's oceans with almost 2.25 percent locked up in snow and ice. The 0.8 percent that is accessible is found in the form of groundwater (0.77 percent), surface water in lakes and inland seas (0.02 percent), and finally, 0.0001 percent in rivers and streams. In other words, if the world's water supply were only 100 liters (twenty-six gallons), our usable supply of freshwater would be only about 0.003 liter or one-half teaspoon.[1] Compare that figure to the actual use of water in an average home as shown in Table 19.1. Given these figures, the protection of rivers, streams, and watersheds is absolutely necessary for the planet.

Discussion: How can you conserve water in your home?

Table 19.1 Use of water in an average home (liters/person/day).

Use	Liters
Washing machine	130–270 (load)
Flushing toilet	10–30
Dishwasher	15–20
Brush teeth	8
Shower	20–30 (minute)
Sprinkler	110–910 (hour)
Wash car	400–800 (20 min.)
Silent leak	150+ (day)
Drinking	12–15
Cooking	12–15

(*Source:* Gleick, Peter H. (1993). *Water in crisis.* Pacific Institute for Studies in Development, Environment and Security. Oxford University Press, Oxford. P. 412)

The amount of available water required to meet the needs of an industrial society has increased dramatically. During the 1930s, 99 gallons of water per person per day were used. The current value is 192 gallons per person per day. Of this amount, almost 40 gallons per capita are used each day directly in the home. Observe the comparison of U.S. water use and annual water use in other regions and countries given in Figure 19.1.[2]

Some 4.2 trillion gallons of water reach the United States in the form of rain or snow every year. However, about 92 percent of this evaporates imme-

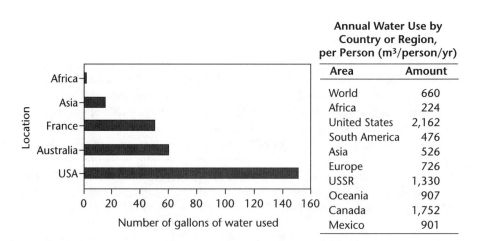

Annual Water Use by Country or Region, per Person (m³/person/yr)

Area	Amount
World	660
Africa	224
United States	2,162
South America	476
Asia	526
Europe	726
USSR	1,330
Oceania	907
Canada	1,752
Mexico	901

Figure 19.1 Average daily water use.

(*Source:* Gleick, Peter H. (1993). *Water in crisis.* Pacific Institute for Studies in Development, Environment and Security. Stockholm Environment Institute. Oxford University Press, Oxford)

diately or runs off, unused, into the oceans. We withdraw about 450 billion gallons a day (BGD) to irrigate, power, and bathe the country; 65 percent comes from freshwater sources such as lakes, rivers, marshes, reservoirs, and springs; 20 percent from underground aquifers; and 15 percent from salt water sources such as inland seas.[3] The primary uses of water are for:

- Drinking
- Industrial cooling
- Agriculture
- Recreation
- Human waste removal
- Transportation

Industry and Agriculture

The two major users and polluters of water in the United States are industry and agriculture. Industry alone is responsible for 50 percent of all freshwater use. Industry uses water in the manufacturing process to cool equipment and it also converts water to steam to provide heat and generate electricity. In New Jersey, for instance, leakage of chromium, copper, zinc, and other toxic metals and chemicals from industrial lagoons have contaminated millions of gallons of groundwater. Organic chemical and plastics industries are the largest sources of toxic chemical pollution, with metal finishing and the iron and steel industries next in line.[4] The majority of drinking water contains low levels of potentially cancer-causing volatile organics.

Agriculture is the second largest user of water in the United States. Water is consumed by livestock and for irrigation. Agriculture's use of water is also part of the pollution problem. Up to one-fourth of organic pesticides and fertilizers are lost in surface runoff before plants use them. Runoff from barnyards and feedlots contribute to pollution since livestock produce five times as much waste as humans, and twice as much organic waste as industry.[5] They are carried to streams or rivers and become part of the downstream water supply.

The U.S. Geological Survey figures show that water use has more than doubled in the past thirty years, to about 450 billion gallon per day (BGD). It is estimated that the demand for water by the United States alone will exceed 1 trillion gallons each day by the year 2010. That sum will be 50 percent more than can be provided from all the world's natural sources combined.

BOX 19.1 *Use of Water by Farming and Industry*

14,935 gallons of water to grow a bushel of wheat

62,000 gallons to produce a ton of steel

(*Source:* Environmental Protection Agency, 1999)

In parts of China, India, Africa, and North America, groundwater is withdrawn faster than it is replenished by precipitation. In the United States one-fourth of the groundwater withdrawn each year is not replenished. Yet, even if additional sources of water were somehow to be located, there is still the problem of water pollution that must be met head on. "We now recognize that a good deal of the precious drinking water supply of this country in underground aquifers has been put in jeopardy by irresponsible disposal practices ..." said then Representative Albert Gore, Jr. during a hearing before the House Science and Technology Subcommittee.

Biological Magnification

Environmental contamination moves up the food chain in a process known as **biological magnification.** For example, relatively small amounts of mercury in lake water can be magnified in concentration of biota living in the sediment, followed by even greater concentration in fish. Ultimately, fish are consumed by mammals which include humans, who store the mercury in their fat tissue.

Wetland Depletion

The United States has lost 56 percent of its wetlands (a tract is a wetland if water can be found for fourteen straight days within one foot of the surface during growing seasons). Approximately 350,000 acres of wetlands are lost each year to draining, pollution, or development. The loss of wetlands means the extinction of many migrating birds and other wetland species. Wetlands encompass a variety of wet environments—coastal and inland marshes, wet meadows, mudflats, ponds, bogs, bottom land hardwood forests, wooded swamps, and fens.

Water Pollution

The pollution of a community's water is one of the greatest concerns of public health. When drinking water becomes contaminated from discharge of toxins, pesticides, debris, human or animal waste into water sources, the ultimate result is morbidity and possibly mortality. Children and older adults are usually most at risk for the consequences of water pollution because of their frail immune systems. The ultimate betrayal of a community's preventive health efforts is the contamination of its water.

There are eight types of water pollutants:

1. Disease-causing agents
2. Oxygen-demanding wastes
3. Water-soluble inorganic chemicals
4. Inorganic plant nutrients
5. Organic chemicals
6. Sediment
7. Radioactive substances
8. Heat

The cumulative effect of these pollutants is that more than 1.7 billion people worldwide do not have an adequate supply of safe drinking water, and 1.4 billion people have no facilities for sanitary waste disposal.[6] More than 3 billion people do not have proper sanitation and are at risk of having their water contaminated. In India, for example, 114 towns and cities dump their human waste and other untreated sewage directly into the Ganges River.[7] This kind of water pollution contributes to the death of at least 5 million people, mostly children under five years, every year from waterborne diseases that could be prevented.[8]

According to the World Health Organization, 97 percent of people in developed countries have access to safe water, compared to only 53 percent of developing countries. Regionally, 74 percent of Asia has safe water, 72 percent of Latin America, and only 36 percent of Africa has safe drinking water.[9]

In 1989, the Atlantic Ocean dumped its debris on the coast of North America. From Maine to Florida, medical waste, discarded blood products, and used syringes floated from their illegal ocean garbage dumps to public and private beaches. Oil slicks from leaking oil tankers such as the *Exxon Valdez* into Prince William Sound, the oil released by Saddam Hussein into the Persian Gulf, and toxic oils spilled by various leaking oil barges have contaminated fish and shellfish, polluted estuaries, and made recreational use of our Atlantic Ocean, gulfs, and Pacific Ocean impossible. In 1990, broken sewers along the San Diego coast sent millions of gallons of raw sewage into the beach resorts of southern California.

Waterborne Disease-Causing Agents

Many diseases are known to be communicable through water. Bacteria, viruses, protozoa, and parasitic worms that enter water from domestic sewage and animal wastes (Table 19.2) are the greatest cause of sickness and death. They kill an average of 25,000 people worldwide each day, half of them children under five years.

BOX 19.2 Case Example—The San Francisco Bay

The August 1992 issue of *Smithsonian* magazine told the tragic tale of the loss of an important wetland and water system, the San Francisco Bay. More than a century ago "fishermen harvested the bay's Dungeness crabs, shrimp, salmon, sturgeon, and flatfish to feed hungry fortyniners." Today, overfishing, discharges of sewage and industrial wastes, runoff from auto emissions on urban streets, diversion of river water to agriculture, and devastating oil spills have threatened the bay into ecological death.

Only 6 percent of the original wetlands are left. San Francisco Bay has shrunk by one-third. About 7 million people live around the Bay and nearly 200 industries and municipalities have permits to discharge wastes into the Bay. Each year as much as 185 tons of toxic trace metals and 30,000 tons of hydrocarbon runoff end up in the Bay. The river diversions have changed the Bay's ratio of saltwater to fresh, reduced its ability to flush out pollution, and contributed to a 75 percent reduction in salmon and striped bass populations over the past thirty years. Can this Bay be saved?

Table 19.2 Waterborne diseases transmitted by ingestion.

Disease	Transmission/Symptoms
Cholera	Initial epidemic waterborne. Secondary cases by food and flies. Diarrhea, vomiting.
Typhoid fever	Food and water vehicles. Diarrhea, vomiting, swollen spleen, inflamed intestines.
Bacillary dysentery	Fecal/oral transmission. Milk, food, flies. Diarrhea. Rarely fatal except in children.
Paratyphoid fever	Fecal/oral transmission.
Giardiasis	Carried in over 20% of U.S. states. Diarrhea, abdominal cramps, flatulence.
Amebic dysentery	Personal contact, food, and flies. Severe diarrhea, headache, chills, fever. Can cause liver abscess, bowel perforation.
Infectious hepatitis	Water, milk, food. Fever, headache, loss of appetite, enlarged liver. Rarely fatal, but can cause permanent liver damage.

(*Source:* Environmental Protection Agency. Office of Water)

The most important measure of the quality of water is its freedom from pathogens, infectious bacteria, and viruses. There are many pathways by which viruses and bacteria from infected animals or humans may enter water supplies, but the primary source is excreta. A cattle feedlot holding 10,000 head of cattle produces as much waste as a community of 160,000 people. Runoff from these feedlots and grazing livestock are serious contributors to water pollution.

It is very difficult to measure specific pathogens in water, so a primary standard used to measure quality of water is the number of measurable **coliform** bacteria (fecal contamination) per unit volume of water. Table 19.3 describes the EPA coliform standards for water use. Since coliform bacteria are present in the fecal material of all warm-blooded animals in as much as billions of bacteria per gram of material, the tracking of coliform levels provides an indirect method of estimating the presence of other pathogens in water supplies. Current U.S. drinking water standards permit levels of coliform bacteria of 1 per 100 milliliters of water. This is not a universally accepted standard, which accounts for the pandemic of dysentery that exists around the world.

> **Discussion:** What changes in a community's environment can increase coliform in the local water?

The classic discovery of the role played by microorganisms in feces of warm-blooded animals in causing human illness was first documented in 1854 by Dr.

Table 19.3 Coliform bacteria and water use.

Coliform Level	Water Activity Permitted
1 coliform or fewer per 100 milliliters of water	Water safe for drinking
4 coliform or more per 100 milliliters of water	State must be notified and action taken
2,300 coliforms or fewer per 100 milliliters water	Swimming is allowed
10,000 coliforms or fewer per 100 milliliters water	Boating is allowed

(*Source:* Environmental Protection Agency)

Table 19.4 Favorable and unfavorable environmental factors for the
survival of human pathogens.

Favorable	Unfavorable
Moisture	Drying
Low temp	High temp
pH 5–9	pH <5 and > 9
Shade	Sunlight
Freshwater	Saline water
Clean water	Polluted water
Sterile soil	Natural soil

(*Source:* Food Safety Risk Analysis Clearinghouse)

John Snow, an English physician. Snow found that the common link in a cholera epidemic was the drinking water from which infected people drank. Snow removed the handle from the Broad Street pump and essentially ended the epidemic. This discovery was the beginning of the public health emphasis on clean water, and germ theory of disease associated with water.

Epidemiology has shown us that excretions from the nose, lungs, mouth, and our urinary and intestinal tracts all may contain eggs, larvae, and adults of the organisms that cause illness. When water sources and landfills become contaminated with these infected materials, a favorable environment for reproduction may put entire communities at risk. Table 19.4 shows the favorable and unfavorable environmental factors that impact human pathogens.[10] Essentially, pathogens live best in moist, low acidic, clean, fresh, cool water, and soil. Table 19.5 is a good example of the ability of two common water pathogens, salmonella and vibrio cholera, to live in varied environments.

> **Discussion:** What locations in your community lend themselves to the viability of pathogenic survival?

Some infections, formerly thought to affect only farm animals, have begun to emerge as diseases transmissible from livestock to humans. Water is often the pathway to this transmission. One recognized only in the past decade is *Cryptosporidium*. This is a protozoan that has probably always existed in domesticated animals, but in the 1980s, outbreaks among human populations occurred.[11]

Cryptosporidium has been identified in human stool specimens in twenty-five of forty-nine state diagnostic laboratories. Although it is being seen more frequently in municipal water supplies, testing for the parasite is not yet required by the EPA.[12] This lack of testing may have led to the epidemic that occurred in 1993. In 1993 the largest outbreak of waterborne disease ever reported in the United States occurred in Milwaukee, Wisconsin, with 400,000 cases of gastroenteritis in fourteen days. The contaminant was *Cryptosporidium*. *Cryptosporidium* is characterized by watery diarrhea, abdominal cramping, nausea, vomiting, and fever. In otherwise healthy persons, the infection is usually

Table 19.5 Survival data on two intestinal pathogenic bacteria in the open environment.

Survival Time	Salmonella typhi	Vibrio cholera
in feces	Min. 8 days General, 30 days	7–14 days unlimited if frozen
in water	tap: 4–7 days river: 1–4 days	tap: 1–2 days river: 2–3 days
on food	vegetables and fruits: 15 days +	meat: 7–14 days fish: 3–4 days milk: 1–2 days
on soil	1 day; 2 years in moist frozen	tropical: 7 days winter: 4 months
with heating	in milk @ 80°: 2 sec. in milk @ 60°: 82 sec.	water @ 100°: 0 water @ 40°: 3 days

(*Source:* U.S. Food and Drug Administration, Center for Food Safety and Applied Nutrition)

self-limited; however, in immunocompromised persons, such as those with AIDS, neoplasms, cirrhosis, or viral hepatitis, the disease can be unrelenting and fatal. Such contamination is actually quite common, with *Cryptosporidium* oocysts present in 67 percent to 97 percent of surface waters in the United States. Because the cost of testing for this protozoa is great and requires large volumes of water, testing is not a regular procedure in municipal water treatment. Nevertheless, this policy is being reconsidered to prevent future morbidity and mortality.

Oxygen-Demanding Wastes

Organic wastes, wastes decomposed by aerobic bacteria, can deplete water of dissolved oxygen and kill fish and other forms of oxygen-consuming aquatic life. The quality of oxygen-demanding wastes in water can be determined by measuring the dissolved oxygen content or the biological oxygen demand (BOD). From a prevention perspective, the first step is to repair or replace aging, leaky water supply systems in most industrial cities. Aged septic tank systems need to be replaced with modern sewage disposal systems. Industrial water use could be cut by 5 percent through good practices such as adopting innovative irrigation techniques, such as "drip irrigation" and recycling. Although drastic and expensive, increased research on removing salt from seawater and prohibiting the use of toxic chemical on farms and in factories should be considered.

Inorganic Chemicals

Acids, salts, and compounds of toxic metals such as mercury and lead are inorganic chemicals that can make water unfit to drink, harm fish and other aquatic life, depress crop yields, and accelerate corrosion of equipment that uses water. Maximum permissible levels for inorganic chemicals in drinking water are given in Table 19.6.

Table 19.6 Maximum permissible levels for inorganic chemicals in drinking water.

Element	Level	Risk
Arsenic	.05	Poison, skin cancer
Barium	1.00	Toxic on heart, vessels, and nerves
Cadmium	.01	Acute poisoning via foods; smoking a source; kidney and liver damage
Chromium	.05	Carcinogenic on inhalation
Lead	.05	Poison with food, water, air, and tobacco smoke
Mercury	.002	Poison at work; poison in food
Nitrates as nitrogen	10.00	Causes methemoglobinemia in infants on milk formulated from such water
Selenium	.01	Occupational poison; livestock poisoning
Silver	.05	Causes argyria

(*Source:* Environmental Protection Agency. National Primary Drinking Water Regulations)

Discussion: How do you feel about knowing that there are viable pathogens in your drinking water?

Mercury   An important inorganic water-soluble pollutant is mercury. Mercury enters the water supply from many industrial sources, particularly pulp and paper mills. In fishing waters, inorganic mercury is transformed into organic mercury that is then consumed by fish. Mercury found in fish off the Japanese coast are attributed to the high incidence of stomach cancer in Japan.

Lead   Lead is a serious inorganic water-soluble pollutant still found in the home and in other water sources. Lead was used to manufacture water pipes and as solder for copper water pipes and tin food cans, to enhance pigmentation in house paints, commercial paints, ceramic glazes, and as an additive in gasoline. It has no known useful function in the body. Although any use of lead that involves the risk of human consumption or ingestion is now generally prohibited in the United States, lead has leached into drinking water and food, it has been expelled from auto exhaust into soil and onto garden vegetables, it has flaked off house and school walls, and has dissolved from ceramic dishes. All these exposures cause gradual lead poisoning among exposed persons, especially children. Each year in the United States, 12,000 to 16,000 mostly poor and non-white children are treated for acute lead poisoning and about 200 die.

Recently health departments have included the added risk of lead exposure by old drinking fountains found in schools and public buildings that were part of the plumbing process and are now corroding and leaching into the drinking water. According to the EPA, nearly one in five Americans drink tap water containing excess levels of lead. Water departments can test home drinking water for lead. The problem of lead in residential water can, in many instances, be corrected by flushing the pipes for three to five minutes in the morning or after any prolonged period of non-use. If home pipes are lead, water softeners should be avoided. Harder water leaches far less lead than does softened water.

Healthy People 2010 Objective: Reduce the Number of Persons Who Have
Elevated Blood Lead Concentrations from Work Exposures

Target: 0 per 1 million.

Baseline: 93 per million persons aged 16 to 64 years (25 states) had blood
lead concentrations of 25 µg/dL or greater in 1998.

Nitrates Water-soluble inorganic plant nitrates and phosphate compounds can
cause excessive growth of algae and other aquatic plants which then die and
decay, depleting water of dissolved oxygen and killing fish. Excessive levels of
nitrates in drinking water can reduce the oxygen-carrying capacity of the blood
and kill unborn children and infants, especially those under three months.

Organic Chemicals Some of the more than 700 synthetic organic chemicals
found in trace amounts in surface and underground drinking water supplies in
the United States can cause kidney disease, birth defects, and various types of
cancer in laboratory animals. These chemicals include oil, gasoline, plastics, pesticides, cleaning solvents, detergents, and many other chemicals that threaten
life. Table 19.6 describes the permissible threshold levels of common chemicals
found in water.

   Organic materials are the largest source of water pollution. There are now
an estimated 70,000 chemicals in commerce. It is difficult to protect the public
against 70,000 chemicals and their infinite number of permutational effects.
Attempts to approach multiple chemicals in the same medium or even a single
mixture have been hampered primarily by the complexities of understanding
interactive effects. In most western nations, air, water, and land pollution are
handled by completely separate organizational units. The result is a failure to
integrate efforts. For example, it is not unusual for policy makers in water pollution to recommend removal of solvents by using the technique of air strip-
ping, which cleans the water at the cost of dirtying the air.[13]

Sediment Insoluble suspended particles of soil and other solid particles are
called **sediment.** Sediments cloud the water, reduce the ability of some organisms to find food, reduce photosynthesis by aquatic plants, disrupt aquatic food
webs, and carry pesticides, bacteria, and other harmful substances that can get
into the food chain.[14]

Groundwater The primary source of all water on the planet comes from rain,
snow, and sleet. Of the existing waters, only 3 percent is non-saline and potentially potable (suitable for drinking). Unfortunately, two-thirds of this potential
drinking water is in the form of ice caps and unavailable. **Groundwater** is that
precipitation that infiltrates the ground and fills pores and cracks in the soil and
rock in the earth's crust. Groundwater is the invisible underground sea that is
recharged by rain that percolates through the pores of soil and moves into fractures of bedrock. There is forty times as much groundwater below the earth's
surface as there is in all the world's streams and lakes.[15] In the United States,

groundwater supplies nearly 50 percent of the total drinking water, and makes up about 0.8 percent of the potential water available for drinking.

You can click on a state in the map at this web site and see what your state SuperFund sites are:
www.epa.gov/superfund/sites/npl/npl.htm

Groundwater contamination has been documented from Silicon Valley in California, to Minneapolis, Minnesota, to the rural areas of the southeast. No part of the country, urban or rural, is spared. This is partially due to the natural hydrologic cycle by which many air pollutants that are brought down with rain contaminate lakes and streams. It is also the result of abandoned dumps, military sites, municipal landfills, toxic waste pits, underground tanks and injection wells, pesticide applications, mining and oil exploration sites, transportation accidents, and even septic tanks and hazardous household wastes that leak into water supplies that tap rivers, streams, lakes, and underground water sources called aquifers.[16]

The 1999 EPA groundwater risk assessment concluded that:

1. There are about 29,000 hazardous waste sites for the EPA SuperFund cleanup program. Many of these are leaking toxins into nearby water supplies.

2. Millions of septic systems (25 percent of homes in the United States use septic systems) are potential contaminators of groundwater.

3. Over 280,000 surface impoundments (ponds, lagoons, pits) could leach into groundwater.

4. There are 500 hazardous waste land disposals and 16,000 municipal landfills that may leach into groundwater.

5. There are 6 million underground storage tanks of which hundreds of thousands are estimated to be leaking.

6. There are thousands of underground injection wells (disposing of waste into deep core waste wells).

7. Millions of tons of pesticides and fertilizers are spread on the ground and may be sources of leaching (dissolve out and pass into the water supply).

The 1990 national Healthy People 2000 objective was that there should be virtually no preventable contamination of groundwater, surface water, or the soil from industrial toxins associated with wastewater management systems after 1990. The goal was far from met. National SuperFund priority sites by region are shown in Figure 19.2.

Health People 2010 Objective: Increase the Proportion of Persons Served by Community Water Systems Who Receive a Supply of Drinking Water That Meets the Regulations of the Safe Drinking Water Act.

Target: 95 percent.

Baseline: 73 percent of persons served by community water systems received drinking water that met SDWA (Public Law 93-523) regulations in 1995.

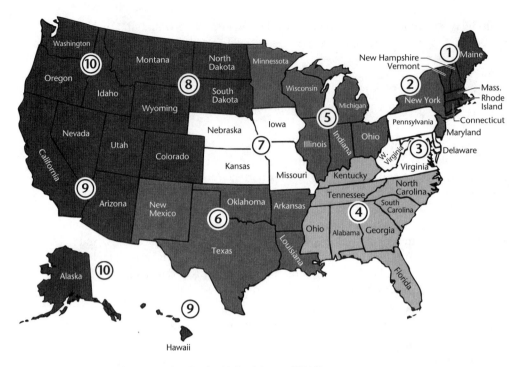

Figure 19.2 SuperFund priority sites in the United States (2000).

(Source: www.epa.gov/superfund/sites/npl/npl/htm)

The Worldwatch Institute and the World Resources Institute reports that our water resources are at great risk of destruction. The major worldwide threat from water contamination remains bacterial infection, however, there is increasing concern about the health impact of chemicals in drinking water. Only 54 of 164 countries in the world have safe drinking water. Most of these are found in North America and Europe.[17] In developing countries, 61 percent of the people living in rural areas and 26 percent of urban dwellers do not have access to safe drinking water. Each year, 5 million people die from preventable waterborne diseases. Table 19.2 describes common diseases transmitted to humans through contaminated drinking water.

In the United States, pesticides contaminate some groundwater deposits in thirty-eight states. In most other developed countries groundwater supplies are threatened by toxic waste dumps, gasoline, and municipal landfills. An example of the severity of pesticides and water is told in the Faustian pesticide story reported by Al Gore:[18]

> *The environmentalist Amory Lovins tells the troubling story of how a powerful pesticide was used in Indonesia to kill mosquitoes that were spreading malaria. The spraying also killed the tiny wasps that controlled the insect population in the thatched roofs of houses. Before long, the roofs all fell. Thousands of cats were also poisoned by the pesticide, and after they died the rat population burgeoned, which in turn brought on an epidemic of bubonic plague.*

The Clean Water Act

Laws protecting groundwater are weak in the United States and non-existent in most countries. The Federal Water Pollution Act of 1972, renamed the Clean Water Act of 1977, was designed to clean up and maintain the quality of the nation's rivers and streams; however, the challenge to cleaning up leaking waste sites that are contaminating water is massive. For example, twenty-five years ago the Cuyahoga River in Cleveland became so polluted that it caught fire. Today, while it is still polluted, it is no longer flammable. By 1990, only thirty-eight of the several hundred chemicals found in U.S. groundwater were covered by federal water quality standards and routinely tested for their presence in municipal drinking water supplies.

The Clean Water Act and the 1987 Water Quality Act require the EPA to establish national effluent standards and to set up a nationwide system for monitoring water quality. Point source dischargers, such as factories and sewage treatment plants must get a permit specifying the amount of each pollutant that a facility can discharge. In 1996 the EPA found that more than 17 million people were served by sewage treatment plants that still had water quality or public health problems, despite the efforts of water safety legislation.[19]

Although it has been over twenty-five years since the Safe Drinking Water Act became law, about 40,000 of the 170,000 water systems—serving about 58 million people—still violate testing requirements and purity standards. About 9,500 water systems serving 25 million people had "significant violations" and only 10 percent of those drew enforcement from government regulators. Most violations result from failure to do proper testing or reporting (82 percent), exceeding contamination limits (25 percent), or failure to filter or properly treat water (9 percent).[20] Current carcinogenic contamination of drinking water supplies in the United States ranges from 1 percent to 2 percent. This may expose as much as 10 percent of the population to potentially carcinogenic materials. From over 2,200 contaminants of all kinds identified in water, 765 have been identified in drinking water. Of these, twelve chemical pollutants were recognized carcinogens, thirty-one were suspected carcinogens, eighteen were carcinogenic promoters, and fifty-nine were mutagens. It is not known what the additive effects of these chemicals will be on the total incidence of cancer.[21]

The EPA found that 1 percent of the wells tested in 1997 contained water with pesticide levels that can cause health problems.[22] The most frequently detected pesticide was a breakdown product of **DCPA,** a herbicide used mostly on lawns.[23] Groundwater contamination is a major concern with pesticide use. The pesticide **Sevin** can change the behavior of large schools of fish in concentrations of one billionth.

Groundwater Treatment

All surface waters should receive complete treatment before they are used as potable water sources. The general treatment includes initial removal of large materials, chemical treatment by coagulation, sedimentation, filtration, and disinfection. Some lakes and streams are clean enough that no filtration is necessary; however, chlorination may be required.

Steps in Groundwater Treatment

Step one in treating groundwater for daily use is flash mix. Here aluminum sulfate is added to incoming water and forms a flaky hydrate, or floc. Basically, coagulation is accomplished and large particles rapidly settle. Chlorine is added here.

Step two is flocculation, whereby particles are trapped by absorption of suspended solids. Here, floc particles settle at a fast rate. Flocculation tanks are round and have large, winglike wooden paddles that move the water in even and continuous mixture which encourages the settling of floc.

Step three is sedimentation. Water is retained in sedimentation tanks for about two hours to allow the floc to settle to the bottom of the tanks, where it is scraped into troughs. Sediment is eventually hauled to landfills as solid waste. If this water has an odor, activated carbon is sometimes added.

Step four is filtration. The filtration systems used may be either diatomaceous earth, slow sand filters, or sand filters. This process filters out particles and bacteria. If sedimentation is great, preliminary settling chambers precede the filtration process. Sand filters must be cleaned by back washing with purified water every twelve to seventy-two hours using about 2 percent of water produced by a purification facility.

The final step is chlorination and sometimes fluoridation and disinfection. Ozone, a form of oxygen that has three atoms in the molecule, in a gas form, is used to remove color, taste, and odors from drinking water. It also oxidizes and

---

BOX 19.3 A Short History of Water Sanitation

Circa 4500 B.C.	Privies were used at dawn of civilization in Sumer.
Circa 3000 B.C.	Mosaic Code of Hygiene developed.
Circa 2800 B.C.	Water pipes, water closets, and flushing used in Crete.
Circa 3000 B.C.	Filtration, distillation, boiling known to Egyptians.
18 B.C.	Roman Baths opened by Vipsanius Agrippa.
1183	Paris constructed an aqueduct to supply water to the city.
1350	In France, the first sanitary police program was established.
1524	First ordinances for control of human excreta in new world issued by Cortez for Spanish colonies.
1596	Sir John Harington in *The Metamorphosis of Ajax* described the first modern valve water-closet.
Circa 1800	First use of chlorine to treat water
1871	First water filtration plant in the United States in Poughkeepsie, N.Y.
1872	The trickling filter was introduced for sewage treatment in England.
1914	Lockett discovered the activated sludge process.
1956	Federal Water Pollution Control Act.

(*Source:* Adopted from Olsztynski, Jim, 2000. *A short course in plumbing history.* PMEngineer)

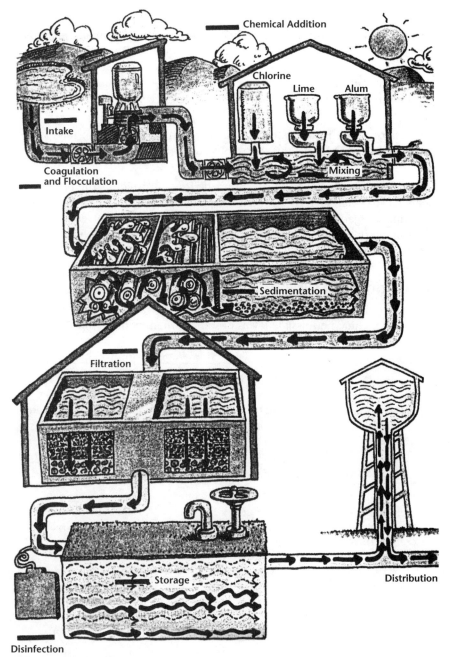

Figure 19.3 Flow chart for a water treatment plant.

(*Source:* Reprinted from *The story of drinking water,* by permission. Copyright © 1990, American Water Works Association)

allows for the removal of iron and manganese. Chloroamination (chlorine and ammonia) acts as a disinfectant. Aeration removes volatile organic materials. Chlorine or chlorine dioxide disinfects the water, leaving a residual level between 0.25 and 0.7 ppm (parts per million). Fluorides in 1 ppm are often added to water at this stage as a preventive measure for dental caries. A typical water treatment process plant is described in Figure 19.3.

Discussion: How is the water in your community treated? Is it filtered or just chlorinated? What is the source of your water?

The result is that all drinking water must be free of turbidity (the presence of suspended material such as clay, silt, or plankton), color caused by algae or aquatic microorganisms, taste affected by inorganic salts or dissolved gases, odor and foamability (due to detergents added to the water), and should have a desirable temperature.

Purification of Drinking Water

Primary drinking water standards established by the U.S. Safe Drinking Water Act of 1974 include permissible levels of some contaminants (Table 19.7)

BOX 19.4 How Often Is Your Drinking Water Tested?

Federal and state rules required different testing frequencies based on population size. Here are three examples of population size and their testing requirements.

	City Population Examples		
Contaminants	**25 to 1,000**	**25,000 to 33,000**	**97,000 to 220,000**
Bacteria	Once a month	30 times per month	120 times per month
Inorganics & metals	Once every 3 years	Once every 3 years	Once every 3 years
Lead & copper	5 times per 6 months[1] for 1st year	60 times per 6 months[2] for 1st year	100 times per 6 months[3] for 1st year
Nitrates	Once a year	Once a year	Once a year
Volatile organic compounds	Once a year for 1st year[4]	Once a year for 1st year[4]	Once a year for 1st year[4]
Sulfates	Once every 3 years	Once every 3 years	Once every 3 years
Radioactives	Once every 4 years	Once every 4 years	Once every 4 years
Pesticides & organics	4 times a year for 1st year[5]	4 times a year for 1st year[5]	4 times a year for 1st year[5]

[1]If no positives, then 5 tests are required every 3 years.
[2]If no positives, then 30 tests are required every 3 years.
[3]If no positives, then 50 tests are required every 3 years.
[4]If no positives, then every 6 years.
[5]If no positives, then 2 tests are required every 5 years.

(*Source:* Environmental Protection Agency)

Table 19.7 Permissible levels of some contaminants.

Contaminant	Amount in MCL(mg/L)
Microbiological (coliform)	1 per 100
Benzene	.005
Arsenic	.05
Barium	1.00
Mercury	.002
Lead	.05
Nitrate	10.00
Selenium	.01
Fluoride	4.00
Carbon tetrachloride	.005

(*Source:* Environmental Protection Agency)

Treatment of water for drinking by urban residents is much like wastewater treatment. Areas depending on surface water usually store it in a reservoir for several days to improve clarity and taste by allowing the dissolved oxygen content to increase and suspended matter to settle.

The water is then pumped to a purification plant, where it is given the treatment needed to meet federal drinking water standards. Usually, it is run through a sand filter, through activated charcoal, and then disinfected. This natural biodegradation process has worked well until recently. Compounds such as DDT, other pesticides, plastics, and industrial solvents have been introduced into the environment only in the past forty years. All are resistant to metabolizing or biodegrading microorganisms in the natural world. In fact, strong slugs of these compounds entering a wastewater treatment plant from an industrial discharge have disrupted the colonies of bacteria in the activated sludge process. Bacteria are often killed by the strength and toxicity of these chemicals.[24]

Sewage Water and Treatment

Sewage Water

Sewage waters include the liquid and solid wastes from households and commercial, and industrial effluents and wastes. The strength of sewage is measured by its biochemical oxygen demand (BOD). BOD is the amount of dissolved oxygen needed by aerobic decomposers to break down the organic materials (effluent) in a certain volume of water over a five-day incubation period at 68°. The higher the BOD, the greater the organic sewage. To say that BOD is reduced from 500 to 50 implies a 90 percent reduction and still needs more oxygen to dispose of the rest of the effluent present. In 1973, 27.1 million pounds of BOD were collected per day in sewers. After treatment, 8.6 million pounds were released into streams. Unfortunately, even with more sophisticated methods the rate after treatment remained the same in 1998.[25]

Sewage Treatment

The primary purpose of sewage treatment is to prevent the spread of disease among human beings by treating sewage liquids before they are recycled into rivers, irrigation, industrial use, and even household use.

Primary treatment of sewage (human and animal waste) is a large holding tank where sewage is sent through a grit chamber to remove sand, small rocks, or other nondigestible solids. In this primary step about half the solids are settled out and there is a BOD reduction of about 40 percent. Dried sludge is then used for fertilizer or landfills, or dumped.

The secondary treatment includes an activated sludge process, trickling filters, or a waste stabilization pond. Bacteria have been used to biodegrade sewage and wastewater generated by human and some industrial wastes. Sewage oxidation ponds are large, shallow, lined ponds exposed to the air that hold waste sufficiently long for microbial decomposition. The activated sludge process consists of an aerator and clarifier. In the aerator, suspended microbes are provided air or pure oxygen to metabolize the biodegradable wastes. The microbes are separated from the wastewater in a settling tank or clarifier; and a portion of them are recycled to maintain metabolics in the aerated tank. The rest are removed as sludge and incinerated or applied to land as soil amendment, or landfill. About 42 percent by weight of the sludge produced in the United States is dumped in conventional landfills where it decomposes. Another 6 percent is dumped into the ocean. The 21 percent of the sludge that is incinerated can pollute the air with traces of toxic chemicals and the resulting toxic ash is also put in landfills. Although this is the conventional method of cleaning water, there is the potential problem of contaminated sludge polluting water and air.

Trickling filters are the secondary treatment of sewage and use a biological process similar to activated sludge. The growth of microbes is encouraged to biodegrade water passed through the medium. The microbes are attached to a fixed medium such as rocks or a synthetic medium over which the wastewater is constantly recycled. The excessive microbial growth is sloughed off the media and captured in a clarifier, after which it is handled as sludge (see Figure 19.3). About 70 percent of BOD is removed from a trickling filter plant.

Stabilization ponds operate anaerobically at the lower levels and aerobically at the upper levels. They retain wastewater that is continuously digested for thirty to eighty days. When ponds fill with sludge they are cleaned and refilled.

The final stage of water treatment is basically the purification of water system, which includes the use of chemicals, particularly chlorine, in the antibacterial treatment of drinking water. A study in 1992 has, unfortunately, drawn some question about the carcinogenic potential of chlorine in drinking water. Chlorinated hydrocarbons are frequently found where municipal water sources use **chlorination,** the purification process that involves the addition of a chlorine compound to disinfect drinking water supplies or where industry contaminates with solvents such as trichlorethylene.[26] Two studies published in July 1992 in the *American Journal of Public Health* reported that chlorine used in municipal water supplies may create chemical compounds that make people more susceptible to cancers of the bladder and rectum. Precise cause and effect was not determined; however, it may be associated with the reaction of chlorine and other impurities in the water. Newer treatment plants have replaced chlorine with activated charcoal as their primary disinfectant.

Fluoride

Another chemical often added to a community's drinking water is fluoride. Fluoride has been shown to be very effective in the prevention of dental caries, particularly if taken systemically during the period of tooth formation and mineralization, and applied topically after eruption. Water fluoridation has been the most common means of distributing fluoride to the population in the recommended optimal level of 0.7 to 1.2 parts per million in a community's water supply. Today, 64 percent of people in the United States who are on community water supplies drink fluoridated water. More than 150 published fluoride studies worldwide, spanning more than forty years, have documented the efficacy, safety, and cost-effectiveness of community water fluoridation. In fact, a study from August 1992 suggested that fluoride at levels commonly found in drinking water (1 part per million) may have a deleterious effect. The study found that long-term exposure to fluoride may cause formation of bone in the hip region that is deficient in tensile strength and may lead to hip fractures among the elderly. The process of fluoridation is still controversial among those who would prefer "pure" water at the expense of tooth decay, which has stood the test of time in terms of fluoridation. Outside the United States fluoride is added to water in Sweden, the Netherlands, Germany, and Japan.

The 1990 national health objective was to decrease the proportion of nine-year-olds who have experienced dental caries in their permanent teeth to 60 percent. This objective has been achieved. The Healthy People 2010 objective is to reduce dental caries to no more than 42 percent among children aged six to eight years. The percentage is now 52 percent.

Septic Tanks

Of the 90 million U.S. citizens not served by a centralized sewage system, an on-site septic tank is used for waste disposal. Septic tanks are concrete receptacles that allow solids to settle to the bottom and undergo anaerobic digestion. After settling and decomposing, the liquid waste is discharged into an absorbent field. Remaining solids are removed every few years from the tank.

There are certain criteria that septic tank systems must meet before they can be considered safe and efficient. These criteria involve design, construction, and environmental safety.

A soil porosity test is the first step to be evaluated before installing a septic tank. This test determines how porous the soil is. The soil porosity test in Utah requires that water is absorbed one inch at a rate no faster than two minutes and no slower than sixty minutes. Another test requires that the bottom of the drain field is at least two feet above groundwater. Disposal of wastewater must occur at least four feet above a clay layer or bedrock layer.[27]

The construction process starts with a line that transports household wastewater from the house to a tank. The tank is typically constructed of concrete or plastic. At the bottom of the tank there are rocks that allow the liquid wastewater to move out into leach lines and the solid waste to stay in the tank. The leach lines are long tubular-shaped plastic pipes with holes drilled on one side. The side with the holes are turned down in a gravel bed to allow filtering to occur as the wastewater is leached into the soil.

Despite regulations and environmental acceptability, septic tank systems are a major source of groundwater pollution in the United States. In fact, the greatest pollutant to drinking water is the exudate from septic tanks, estimated to be some 800 billion gallons of effluent in U.S. soils annually.

People are often lax in updating their system. The average life of a septic tank is fifteen years.[28] Most people think, "if it isn't broken, don't fix it." Checking a septic tank system is essential because the cost of contaminated groundwater is much worse than the costs of updating. A slow leak or a broken leach line may go undetected for a long time.

It should be noted, however, that a well-maintained septic tank in soil containing 10 percent silt or clay would probably be safe at very small distances between a disposal field and freshwater supply. Soil absorbs pathogens such as viruses and bacteria. It filters waste and renovates it into nutrients used by plants. The cleaned water then moves through the soil and either empties into aquifers or rivers, is evaporated, or is digested by plants.[29]

Overcrowding of septic systems is another potential community health problem. Forty or more septic tank systems per square mile may be considered to be a high-risk contamination situation. Crowding tends to occurs in low economic communities in the northeastern and southeastern states.[30]

Another reason for septic tank systems causing groundwater pollution is the increased use of household cleaning agents. Synthetic chemicals are showing up in groundwater in alarming quantities across the United States. Household cleaning agents are highly concentrated with human-made chemicals that the soil cannot properly filter or eliminate. Also, chemicals in these products can kill the organisms that break down solid waste left in the tank causing buildup and a potential health hazard.[31]

Swimming Pools and Beaches

Although the risk from waterborne infectious diseases has diminished in developed countries, the large scale use of swimming pools for recreation carries specific risks of infections. These include skin, ear, eye, gastrointestinal, and respiratory infections. Among the diseases of these organs are athlete's foot, otitis externa caused by *Pseudomonas aeruginosa*, conjunctivitis, and chlorine inflammation.

Pool water, in effect, is diluted sewage because it is contaminated by swimmer's skin, mucus, feces, urine, dirt, and a vast variety of contaminants that may come in the water from a variety of sources. It is necessary, therefore for the swimming pool or natural bathing area to be frequently tested, properly constructed and adequately protected by means of good filtration and good disinfection techniques.[32]

The steps to water treatment in a pool include:

1. A trap to catch coarse material as water leaves the pool.

2. Addition of fresh water in a makeup tank to replace the water being expelled.

3. Pumping water continuously through the system.

4. The use of alum or filter aid material to assist infiltration.

5. Addition of soda ash to maintain proper pH between 7.2 and 7.8.

6. Filtration through sand filters or diatomaceous earth filters.

7. Back washing by reversing the flow of water through the filters and then removing the filtered material to the sewer.

8. Addition of chlorine or bromine as a disinfectant.

9. Heating of water where necessary.

10. Recirculating the water back to the pool.

Pool problems occur in six ways: (1) the operator, (2) design and construction defects, (3) water quality, (4) inadequate service and maintenance, (5) disease, and (6) lead safety hazards.

Swimmer to swimmer diseases that may be transmitted through pools include, typhoid fever, paratyphoid fever, amoebic dysentery, bacillary dysentery and giardiasis, colds, sinusitis, and septic sore throats. Eye, ear, nose, throat, and skin infections may occur because of the presence of the organisms that cause each infection or due to excessive amounts of water-treatment chemicals.

As for public beaches, in 1999 local or state officials either closed or advised against swimming at the nation's coastal beaches almost 6160 times up 50 percent from 1997. Beach closings have occurred because of fecal contamination, sewage spills, medical waste contamination and marine disease. About 35 percent of all U.S. sewage ends up in marine waters. It is estimated that 5.4 trillion gallons of sewage was discharged into marine waters by the twenty-first century.[33]

During the first half of the decade (2001–2010), the EPA plans to focus on conserving and enhancing the nation's waters and aquatic ecosystems so that 75 percent of waters will support healthy aquatic communities. Part of this effort will include developing a national beach-closing survey to monitor efforts to improve the quality of water used for recreational purposes. Small streams, private lakes, and ponds will not be addressed by the EPA beach-closing survey.

Despite the many possible pollutants and risks to human health by beach contamination, according to the National Resources Defense Council, only six states comprehensively test the water along their shores. Eight do not test at all. Despite the massive amount of pollution being washed, dumped, and rained into our oceans, states have no obligation to test the quality of beachside waters.[34]

> ### BOX 19.5 Beach, Lake, River, and Stream Debris in 1994[35]
>
> 4,400 syringes
> 7,200 condoms
> 10,266 diapers
> 16,300 tampon applicators
> 64,185 packs of cigarette butts

Summary

In 1995 the U.S. House of Representatives proposed to reduce the restrictions on industry and agriculture in terms of environmental water pollution. In essence, the House wished to reduce the criteria for water pollution with the agreement that industry and agriculture would clean up after themselves. Community health was outraged with this threat to drinking water. The incidence of waterborne pathogenic morbidity and subsequent mortality has increased in the past decade and any reduction in vigilance of water safety is reprehensible. Vocal opposition by public health and even citizens has made such reductions in water pollution laws less likely in the twenty-first century.

Cleaning groundwater or purification of wastewater has become more difficult as toxic chemicals such as lead and pesticides have been found in our water. More sophisticated techniques are becoming necessary to rid water of these toxic chemicals. The use of certain polymers on raw sewage has improved primary treatment. Another serious concern is the removal of viruses and some pathogenic bacteria. Conventional treatment, however, removes only about 90 percent.

All facilities that use water, such as pools, households, factories, agriculture, or other recreational facilities, must be aware of the potential for contamination by pathogens, chemicals, or wastes. Proper use and disposal is essential for keeping the immediate use water sanitary and preventing pollution of groundwater.

Finally, the whole issue of water conservation is a serious question for water treatment. New methods of reducing water waste and treating used water must be created.

CYBERSITES RELATED TO CHAPTER 19

Water
www.nal.usda.gov/wqic
www.epa.gov/safewater

QUESTIONS

1. Name the most common bacterial pathogens found in water and the diseases they cause.

2. Describe the risks to groundwater in your own community.

3. Describe the stages of water purification for drinking groundwater and for sewage water.

4. What are the steps in maintaining a safe pool?

EXERCISE

Visit the water purification or reclamation facility in your community. Walk through the whole process from incoming water to outgoing. Where is sludge shipped and stored in your community? What chemicals are added to your drinking water? Is fluoride added to your community's drinking water? How secure do you feel about the safety of your drinking water?

INTERNET INTERACTIVE ACTIVITY

SHOULD I DRINK THE WATER?

The Office of Water at the EPA provides information about drinking water, groundwater, and well water in selected areas. One can also find out what the U.S. water quality standards are beginning at this homepage site:

www.epa.gov/safewater/

Example

The community health educator wants to determine if the drinking water in her or his community meets national standards as compared to a less developed part of the country.

1. Go to the homepage

   www.epa.gov/safewater/

2. Click on **Local Drinking Water** icon

   www.epa.gov/safewater/dwinfo.htm

3. Select any state and click on that state on the map. For instance:

   Washington

4. If you know the name of your water system, enter it; if not, select a county

   SNOHOMISH

5. Click

   Search

   You now have a list of all the water systems in Snohomish County. If you click on a Water System ID you will have a description of any water quality violations for that system.

6. For instance, for Ceder Springs Camp you now know the water source is groundwater that serves seventy-five people. On Dec. 31, 1998 there was a **health-based violation** of coliform contamination that had three follow-up reports. There was a **monitoring and reporting violation** on August 1, 1998.

Exercise

1. Go to the EPA safewater homepage

   www.epa.gov/safewater/

2. Look up the water systems in your state by using the steps in the example above.

3. Compare three or four unique geographical locations in your state noting

   sources of water
   types of contamination
   types of violations
   the state's drinking and groundwater quality
   the number of people served by different water systems

4. Go to the current drinking water standards page and review the national regulations.

   www.epa.gov/safewater/mcl.html

5. How much arsenic, asbestos, cyanide, fluoride, lead, and PCB are allowed in the water? What are the primary means these chemicals get into the water based on the table? Were there any surprises about the national water quality standards?

References

1. Miller, G. Tyler (1993). *Environmental science: Sustaining the earth,* 4th ed. Belmont, CA: Wadsworth Publishing.

2. Corson, Walter H. (1990). *The global ecology handbook.* Boston: Beacon Press.

3. Coffin, Tristram (1985). Water in agriculture: The irrigation debate. Found in *Protecting water quality* by McCuen, 1986, pp. 14–20.

4. Corson, op. cit.

5. Ibid.

6. Ibid.

7. Gore, Al (1992). *Earth in the balance.* New York: Houghton Mifflin.

8. Miller, op. cit.

9. Corson, op. cit.

10. Neal, Homer A. (1987). Lead in drinking water: Is there a national epidemic? *ACSH News and Views.* March/April.

11. Hunter, Beatrice Trum (1993). Cyptosporidium: An emerging human health hazard. *Consumers' Research,* March, pp. 8–9.

12. Annual Report on Water Quality (2001). www.fcwa.org/water/ccr/p.7 pdf.

13. Neal, op. cit.

14. Miller, op. cit.

15. Ibid.

16. Goldstein, Bernard (1991). Environmental applications and interventions in public health. In *Oxford textbook of public health,* New York: Vol. I, pp. 17–28.

17. Miller, op. cit.

18. Gore, op. cit.

19. Copeland, Claudia (1999). Wastewater treatment. National Council for Science and the Environment. pp. 98–323 ENR.

20. Eisler, Peter (1998). Lax oversight raises tap water risk. *USA Today,* Oct. 21 p. 15A.

21. Ibid.

22. Peterson, T.L. (1997). Pesticide residues in drinking water. UCD Extexnet FAQ team.

23. Miller, G. Tyler, Jr. (1992). *Living in the environment.* Belmont, CA: Wadsworth Publishing.

24. Hynes, H. Patricia (1989). *The recurring silent spring.* New York: Pergamon Press.

25. www.epa.gov/globalwarming/publications/emissions/us2000/waste.pdf. p. 8

26. Goldstein, op. cit.

27. Kennington, John (1994), Director of Water Quality, Salt Lake County, Utah.

28. Knox, Robert C (1991). *Evaluation of septic tank systems on ground water quality,* EPA 600/s2-91-097. July.

29. Winneberger, J. (1984). *Septic-tank practices.* Butterworth Publishers.

30. Knox, op. cit.

31. Ibid.

32. Koren, op. cit.

33. Corson, op. cit.

34. Galifiankis, Nick (1995). How safe are our beaches? *USA Today,* June 30.

35. *Environment* (1995). Salvaging our seashores. Vol. 37, no. 7, Sept., p. 22.

CHAPTER 20

Food Safety

Community Health in the 21st Century
In our fast paced society, less time is devoted to meal preparation at home so
more people are relying on restaurants. Restaurant patrons who think food
safety and good sanitation practices are just common sense have not seen too
many restaurant kitchens. The food service profession is characterized by high
employee turnover, little employee job training, low wages, no health benefits
or sick leave. The food service industry has a real need for more food safety
training and foodborne illness prevention strategies.

—Amy Piddington, Environmental Health Educator, Kent
County Health Department, Grand Rapids, Michigan

Chapter Objectives

The student will:

1. name those illnesses associated with contamination of food from bacterial, viral, parasite, and chemical agents.

2. list ten potential food safety hazards found in any eating establishment.

3. list ten ways to reduce food preparation risks.

4. name three vectors that contaminate food.

5. differentiate between raw and pasteurized milk.

6. discuss the politics of milk.

7. explain the problems associated with "smell and poke" meat inspection.

Food Health and Hazards

People dining at home or away from home assume that they will eat safe, healthy, well-prepared food. Unfortunately, even among the cleanest homes or restaurants over 10 million people a year get sick from what they eat. Environmental community health is concerned primarily with controlling these outbreaks of foodborne illness among people in public eating establishments or public gatherings through a variety of educational, investigative, and legal means. Because responsibility for the safety and wholesomeness of food has moved away from the individual to the industries that process food, new potential for large scale outbreaks of foodborne diseases are ever present. Most cases of foodborne illness are not reported to authorities, leaving less than 1 percent of the over 10 million cases of acute gastroenteritis in the United States investigated and the necessary sanitary corrections made. When unreported cases are taken into account, an estimated 76 million illnesses, 325,000 hospitalizations, and 5,000 deaths each year may be associated with microorganisms in food. Three pathogens, *Salmonella, Listeria,* and *Toxoplasma,* are responsible for 1,500 deaths each year, more than 75 percent of those caused by known pathogens, while unknown agents account for the remaining 62 million illnesses, 265,000 hospitalizations, and 3,200 deaths.[1]

Epidemiological analysis indicates that 93 percent of all reported cases of food poisoning are due to water, milk, and food. Since air, water, and food are universal needs of all human beings, they become the primary concerns of community health specialists. In 2000 the CDC reported food disease outbreaks due to contaminated fruits and vegetables that most of us assume are safe: apples, cabbage, cantaloupe, onions, lettuce, watermelons, and pineapples.

> **Foodborne illness** is a disease that is carried by the vector—food—and proliferates under the proper conditions of moisture, time, and temperature. Diseases transmitted by foods are frequently classified either as poisoning or infections.
>
> **Poisonings** are caused by ingesting toxins that are found in the tissues of certain plants and animals, metabolic products formed and excreted by microorganisms, or poisonous substances that may be added to foods during the processing, transporting, or storing.
>
> **Infections** are caused by the introduction of pathogenic microorganisms into the body and the reaction of the body tissues to their presence or to the toxins they generate within the body.[2]

Common foodborne disease incidence and fatalities reported and estimated in 1999 by the CDC are given in Table 20.1.

The U.S. Public Health Service identifies potentially hazardous food as any food that consists in whole or in part of milk or milk products, eggs, meat, poultry, fish, shellfish, edible crustacea, baked or boiled potatoes, rice, tofu and other soy-protein foods, or other ingredients, including synthetic formulas, in a form capable of supporting rapid and progressive growth of infectious or toxigenic microorganisms. Since so much of social interaction takes place around food, poisoning or infection often affects large groups. Examples of such outbreaks include:

1. A nursing home had an E. coli outbreak when a food handler who was preparing meatloaf failed to wash his hands properly after mixing the meat. Proper cooking killed the E. coli in the meat, but the food handler filled drinking glasses with ice cubes that were contaminated with the E. coli from his unclean hands, killing three residents and hospitalizing seventeen.

Table 20.1 CDC reported and estimated illness, frequency of foodborne transmission, and hospitalization for foodborne pathogens, United States (1999).

Disease or Agent	Estimated Total Cases	Reported Cases by Surveillance Type		
		Active	Passive	Outbreak
Bacterial				
Bacillus cereus	27,360		720	72
Botulism, foodborne	58		29	
Brucella spp.	1,554		111	
Campylobacter spp.	2,453,926	64,577	37,496	146
Clostridium perfringens	248,520		6,540	654
Escherichia coli O157:H7)	73,480	3,674	2,725	500
E. coli, non-O157 STEC	36,740	1,837		
E. coli, enterotoxigenic	79,420		2,090	209
E. coli, other diarrheogenic	79,420		2,090	
Listeria monocytogenes	2,518	1,259	373	
Salmonella Typhi[b]	824		412	
Salmonella, non-typhoidal	1,412,498	37,171	37,842	3,640
Shigella spp.	448,240	22,412	17,324	1,476
Staphylococcus food poisoning	185,060		4,870	487
Streptococcus, foodborne	50,920		1,340	134
Vibrio cholerae, toxigenic	54		27	
V. vulnificus	94		47	
Vibrio, other	7,880	393	112	
Yersinia enterocolitica	96,368	2,536		
Subtotal	5,204,934			
Parasitic				
Cryptosporidium parvum	300,000	6,630	2,788	
Cyclospora cayetanensis	16,264	428	98	
Giardia lamblia	2,000,000	107,000	22,907	
Toxoplasma gondii	225,000		15,000	
Trichinella spiralis	52		26	
Subtotal	2,541,316			
Viral				
Norwalk-like viruses	23,000,000			
Rotavirus	3,900,000			
Astrovirus	3,900,000			
Hepatitis A	83,391		27,797	
Subtotal	30,883,391			
Grand Total	38,629,641			

[a]Numbers in italics are estimates; others are measured.

[b]>70% of cases acquired abroad.

2. A major restaurant in a big city rushed three patrons to the hospital when the chef, who was cooking omelettes, sprayed "Easy Off" (an oven cleaner), instead of "Pam" (a non-stick cooking spray) onto his skillet.

3. An inspector at the local health department received a call soon after lunch time reporting that four people had become ill after eating at a local restaurant. The only clue the inspector had was that these four people were the

Healthy People 2010 Objective: Reduce Infections Caused by Key Foodborne Pathogens

Reduction in Infections Caused by Microorganisms	1997 Baseline	2010 Target
	Cases per 100,000 Population	
Campylobacter species	24.6	12.3
Escherichia coli 0157:H7	2.1	1.0
Listeria monocytogenes	0.5	.025
Salmonella species	13.7	6.8

last people to eat in the restaurant before closing. When the inspector
arrived at the restaurant she discovered that the restaurant had run out of
rice in the kitchen and had supplemented the last four lunches with rice
from the sushi bar. The rice at the sushi bar was being stored out of the
cooler at room temperature, which was 72 degrees. Bacteria had multiplied
and infected the last four patrons.

The prevention of foodborne illness requires the avoidance of contamination or
spoilage damage through safe growing conditions, careful purchasing of safe
food, proper storage, preparation, and correct serving. Figure 20.1 is an example of a foodborne transmission route via food handlers and consumers.

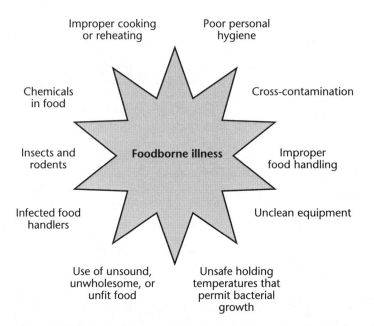

Figure 20.1 Factors that contribute to the transmission of a foodborne illness.

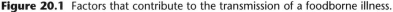

(*Source:* Reproduced, by permission of WHO, from: Jacob, M. *Safe food handling: A training
guide for managers in food service establishments.* Geneva, WHO, 1989)

BOX 20.1 Some Milestones in U.S. Food and Drug Law History

From the beginnings of civilization people have been concerned about the quality and safety of foods and medicines. In 1202, King John of England proclaimed the first English food law, the Assize of Bread, which prohibited adulteration of bread with such ingredients as ground peas or beans. Regulation of food in the United States dates from early colonial times. Federal controls over the drug supply began with inspection of imported drugs in 1848. The following chronology describes some of the milestones in the history of food and drug regulation in the United States.

1862 **President Lincoln** appoints a chemist, Charles M. Wetherill, to serve in the new Department of Agriculture. This was the beginning of the Bureau of Chemistry, the predecessor of the Food and Drug Administration.

1883 **Dr. Harvey W. Wiley** becomes chief chemist, expanding the Bureau of Chemistry's food adulteration studies. Campaigning for a federal law, Dr. Wiley is called the "Crusading Chemist" and "Father of the Pure Food and Drugs Act." He retired from government service in 1912 and died in 1930.

1906 The original **Food and Drugs Act** is passed by Congress on June 30 and signed by President Theodore Roosevelt. It prohibits interstate commerce in misbranded and adulterated foods, drinks and drugs.

The **Meat Inspection Act** is passed the same day.

1938 The **Federal Food, Drug, and Cosmetic (FDC) Act** of 1938 is passed by Congress, containing new provisions.

Delaney Committee starts congressional investigation of the safety of chemicals in foods and cosmetics, laying the foundation for the 1954 Miller Pesticide Amendment, the 1958 Food Additives Amendment, and the 1960 Color Additive Amendment.

1954 **Miller Pesticide Amendment** spells out procedures for setting safety limits for pesticide residues on raw agricultural commodities.

First large-scale **Radiological Examination of Food** carried out by FDA when it received reports that tuna suspected of being radioactive was being imported from Japan following atomic blasts in the Pacific. FDA begins monitoring around the clock to meet the emergency.

1958 **Food Additives Amendment** enacted, requiring manufacturers of new food additives to establish safety. The Delaney proviso prohibits the approval of any food additive shown to induce cancer in humans or animals.

FDA publishes in the Federal Register the first list of **Substances Generally Recognized as Safe (GRAS)**. The list contains nearly 200 substances.

1969 FDA begins administering **Sanitation Programs** for milk, shellfish, food service, and interstate travel facilities, and for preventing poisoning and accidents. These responsibilities were transferred from other units of the Public Health Service.

Low-Acid Food Processing regulations issued—after botulism outbreaks from canned foods—to ensure that low-acid packaged foods have adequate heat treatment and are not hazardous.

continues

Vitamins and Minerals Amendments ("Proxmire Amendments") stop FDA from establishing standards limiting potency of vitamins and minerals in food supplements or regulating them as drugs based solely on potency.

1988 Food and Drug Administration Act of 1988 officially establishes FDA as an agency of the Department of Health and Human Services with a Commissioner of Food and Drugs appointed by the president with the advice and consent of the senate, and broadly spells out the responsibilities of the secretary and the commissioner for research, enforcement, education, and information.

1990 Nutrition Labeling and Education Act requires all packaged foods to bear nutrition labeling and all health claims for foods to be consistent with terms defined by the Secretary of Health and Human Services. The law preempts state requirements about food standards, nutrition labeling, and health claims and, for the first time, authorizes some health claims for foods. The food ingredient panel, serving sizes, and terms such as "low fat" and "light" are standardized.

1994 Dietary Supplement Health and Education Act establishes specific labeling requirements, provides a regulatory framework, and authorizes FDA to promulgate good manufacturing practice regulations for dietary supplements. This act defines "dietary supplements" and "dietary ingredients" and classifies them as food. The act also establishes a commission to recommend how to regulate claims.

1997 Food and Drug Administration Modernization Act reauthorizes the Prescription Drug User Fee Act of 1992 and mandates the most wide-ranging reforms in agency practices since 1938. Provisions include measures to accelerate review of devices, regulate advertising of unapproved uses of approved drugs and devices, and regulate health claims for foods.

(*Source:* Food and Drug Administration, Backgrounder Information Sheet)

Of the four Healthy People 2000 food safety objectives targeted to reducing foodborne illness, only one was met in 2000: reducing the incidence of disease caused by four key pathogens (*Salmonella* species, *Campylobacter* species, *Escherichia coli* O157:H7, and *Listeria monocytogenes*).

Discussion: What food contamination outbreaks have occurred in your community? Why did they occur?

The Partnership for Food Safety Education was formed in 1997 as a part of the National Food Safety Initiative. The partnership, composed of industry, state, and consumer organizations and government liaisons, cooperatively developed the FightBAC campaign whose message is simple but most important for food safety. The message is based on four key food safety practices:

1. Clean: Wash hands and surfaces often.

2. Separate: Don't cross-contaminate.

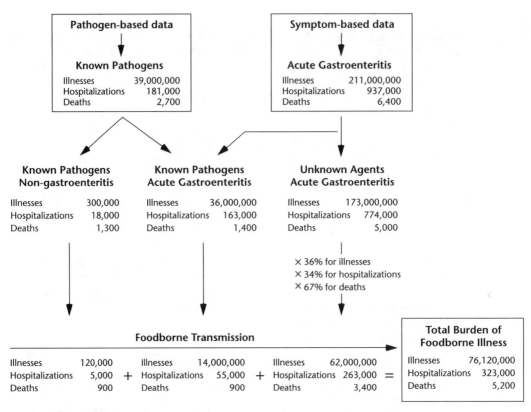

Figure 20.2 Estimated frequency of foodborne illness in the United States.

(*Source:* Mead, Paul S. et. al. Food-related illness and death in the United States, CDC, 1999)

3. Cook: Cook to proper temperatures.

4. Chill: Refrigerate promptly.

Figure 20.2 is an example of foodborne transmission estimated in 1999.

Sanitarians and food inspectors spend most of their field work trying to prevent the following most frequently cited factors involved in outbreaks of foodborne illness in public establishments: unsafe growing conditions, improper storage, improper preparation, and incorrect serving. Figure 20.3 is a sample Food Service Establishment Inspection Report form used by food inspectors to identify these high-risk situations, conditions, and behaviors to prevent illness outbreaks. As violations are found, they are marked and tallied at the end of the inspection. When an eating establishment exceeds its maximum amount of violation points, it is closed. Fewer than maximum points usually requires that the establishment make the necessary changes within a given time period.

Probably the most frequent sources of foodborne illness occur in the storage and handling of food (Table 20.2). Microorganisms are most often passed to humans because of the following food preparation errors:

ITEM NO.	DESCRIPTION	Repeat Viol.	Wt.
FOOD			
*01	☐ Source ☐ Sound condition-no spoilage ☐ Adulterated		5
02	☐ Original container ☐ Properly labeled		1
FOOD PROTECTION			
*03	Potentially hazardous foods meet temperature requirements during: ☐ Preparation ☐ Storage ☐ Display ☐ Service ☐ Transportation		5
*04	Facilities to maintain product temperature		4
05	☐ Thermometer provided ☐ Conspicuous ☐ Accurate ☐ Properly located		1
06	Potentially hazardous foods properly thawed		2
*07	Unwrapped and potentially hazardous food not re-served		4
08	Food protection during: ☐ Storage ☐ Preparation ☐ Display ☐ Service ☐ Transportation		2
09	Handling of food (ice) minimized		2
10	In use: ☐ Food and ☐ Ice dispensing utensils properly stored		1
PERSONNEL			
*11	Personnel with infections restricted		5
*12	☐ Good hygenic practices		5
13	☐ Clean clothes or apron ☐ Hair restraints ☐ Beard neat ☐ Food Handlers Permits		1
FOOD EQUIPMENT & UTENSILS			
14	Food (ice) contact surfaces: ☐ Designed ☐ Constructed ☐ Maintained ☐ Installed ☐ Located		2
15	Non food contact surfaces: ☐ Designed ☐ Constructed ☐ Maintained ☐ Service ☐ Located		1
16	Dishwashing facilities: ☐ Designed ☐ Constructed ☐ Maintained ☐ Installed ☐ Located ☐ Operated		2
17	Accurate thermometers ☐ Chemical test kits ☐ ¼ " IPS gauge cocks ☐ FINAL Rinse 15-25 psi		1
18	Utensils: ☐ Pre-flushed ☐ Scraped ☐ Soaked		1
19	Wash/Rinsewater: ☐ Clean ☐ Proper temperature		2
*20	Sanitation rinse: ☐ Clean ☐ Temperature ☐ Concentration ☐ Exposure time ☐ Equipment/utensils sanitized		4
21	Wiping cloths: ☐ Clean ☐ Stored ☐ Use restricted		1
22	Food-contact surfaces of equipment and utensils: ☐ Clean ☐ Free of abrasives ☐ Detergents		2
23	Non-food contact surfaces of equipment and utensils clean		1
24	☐ Storage ☐ Handling of clean equipment and utensils		1
25	Single-service articles: ☐ Storage ☐ Dispensing ☐ Used		1
26	No re-use of single service articles		2
WATER			
*27	Water source: ☐ Safe ☐ Hot and cold under pressure		5
WASTE WATER			
*28	☐ Sewage and wastewater disposal		4
PLUMBING			
**29	☐ Installed ☐ Maintained		1
*30	☐ Cross-connection ☐ Back siphonage ☐ Backflow		5
TOILET & HANDWASHING FACILITIES			
*31	☐ Number ☐ Convenient ☐ Accessible ☐ Designed for easy cleaning ☐ Installed		4
32	Toilet Rooms: ☐ Enclosed ☐ Self closing doors ☐ Fixtures good repair ☐ Clean ☐ Hand cleaner ☐ Sanitary towels/towels/hand drying devices provided ☐ Proper waste recps.		2
SOLID WASTE DISPOSAL			
33	Containers or Receptacles: ☐ Covered ☐ Frequency ☐ Insect/rodent/animal proof ☐ Clean		2
34	Outside storage area enclosures: ☐ Properly constructed ☐ Clean		1
INSECT—RODENT—ANIMAL CONTROL			
*35	☐ Insect/rodents ☐ Outer openings ☐ Animals		4
FLOORS, WALLS & CEILINGS			
36	Floors: ☐ Constructed ☐ Drained ☐ Clean ☐ Good repair ☐ Coved ☐ Dustless cleaning method		1
37	Walls, ceiling, attached equipment: ☐ Constructed ☐ Good repair ☐ Clean surfaces ☐ Dustless cleaning methods		1
LIGHTING			
38	☐ Lighting provided as required ☐ Fixtures shielded		1
VENTILATION			
39	☐ Rooms ☐ Equipment ☐ Clean Air Act (UICAA)		1
DRESSING ROOMS			
40	☐ Clean ☐ Provided ☐ Used		1
OTHER OPERATIONS			
*41	Toxic items properly: ☐ Labeled ☐ Used ☐ Located		5
42	Premises maintained ☐ Free of litter ☐ Unnecessary articles ☐ Cleaning, maintenance equipment properly stored ☐ Authorized personnel ☐ Safety		1

Food Service Inspection Report

Based on an inspection this day, the items marked below identify the violations in operations of facilities which must be corrected by the next routine inspection. Failure to comply with any time limits for correction specified in this notice may result in cessation of your Food Service operations.

Received by: name _____

Inspected by: name _____

Figure 20.3 Sample food service inspection form.

(*Source:* Salt Lake County Health Department)

Table 20.2 Percentage of foodborne illness due to specific risk factors, United States (1989).

Improper handling	62.4%
Inadequate cooking	17.3%
Personal hygiene	28.2%
Contaminated equipment	17.8%
Unsafe source of food	8.0%
Other	27.6%

(*Source:* Food and Drug Administration)

1. Failure to refrigerate properly at less than 40 degrees (a few states set the minimum at 45 degrees) (Figure 20.4).

2. Failure to initially cook food or reheat leftovers at 165 degrees.

3. Failure to hold cooked food at 140 degrees or higher.

4. Employees who practice poor personal hygiene or who have open wounds.

5. Foods prepared a day or more before serving.

6. Raw, contaminated ingredients incorporated into other foods.

7. Foods allowed to remain at bacteria-incubating temperatures.

8. Cross-contamination of foods through improperly cleaned equipment or improper storage (i.e., dripping meat that is stored over a tub of salad).

Discussion: Have you ever been a food handler? How were you trained about food safety? Did you always practice these principles?

During a food inspection in an eating establishment, appropriate hot and cold temperatures (the danger zone) are checked.

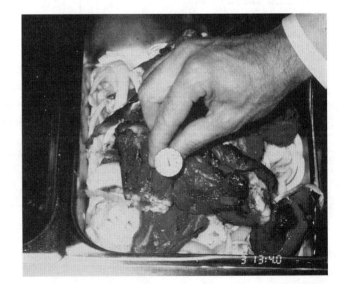

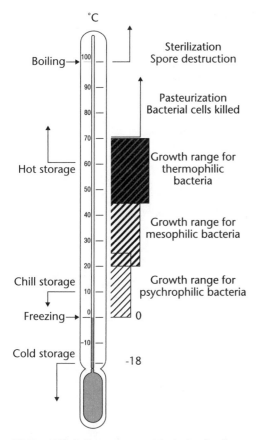

Figure 20.4 Temperature risks in food safety.

(*Source:* Reproduced, by permission of WHO, from: Jacob, M., *Safe food handling: A training guide for managers in food service establishments.* Geneva, WHO, 1989)

Microorganisms and Foodborne Illness

Food material in its natural state keeps sound and edible for only a comparatively short time. As populations have become concentrated within towns and cities, the problem of the quality of transported food products has greatly intensified. Greater handling time, from source to table, increases the waste of food through contamination, its destruction by pests, its inefficient utilization, and spoilage. All too frequently the end product is not a wholesome meal, but a potentially deadly contaminated meal. Food contamination can be from many sources, including bacteria, parasites, viruses, fungi, pests, and chemicals, as shown in Table 20.3.

Table 20.3 Foodborne and waterborne diseases and hazards.

Bacterial infections	Parasite diseases
Salmonella	Trichinosis
Shigella	Cysticerosis
Streptococcus	Plant and fungal hazards
Campylobacter jejuni	Mycetismus
Listeria	Mycotoxicosis-aflatoxins
Vibrio	Favism
Enterophathic E. coli	Plant phenolics
Clostridia perfringens	**Chemical hazards**
Bacillus cereus	Aluminum
Legionnaires' disease	Cadmium
Bacterial toxins	Lead
Staphylococcus aureus	Antibiotics
Botulism	PCB's
Viral infections	Pesticides
Infectious hepatitis	
Lymphocytic choriomeningitis	
Haemorrhagic fever	

(*Source:* Fairweather, Frank, 1991. Field investigations of biological and chemical hazards of food and water. *Oxford book of public health,* 2nd ed. Used by permission of Oxford University Press, London)

BOX 20.2 A Short History of Food Sanitation

1371 Royal order forbidding slaughtering of animals in London and suburbs.

1486 Henry VII regulates slaughterhouses.

1518 Nuremberg ordinance regulating sale of food.

1599 Vienna prohibits the sale of milk, butter, and cheese because of an epidemic.

1704 Slaughterhouse regulations passed in Massachusetts.

1730 Sale of meat from tuberculous cows forbidden in Munich.

1810 Nicholas Appert of France discovered the canning process for food preservation.

1850 Carre discovered the ammonia-absorption process for refrigeration.

1854 First milk law in Massachusetts.

1863 Louis Pasteur demonstrated the process of pasteurization.

1881 New York State enacted first effective food Control Laws in the United States.

1906 Federal food laws enacted in the United States.

1938 Enactment of the Food, Drug, and Cosmetic Act.

1959 Enactment of the Poultry Products Inspection Act.

The symptoms of all foodborne illness are similar. Five bacterial infections and their foodborne associations are shown on Table 20.4. Many symptoms of foodborne illness include diarrhea, abdominal pain, nausea, and possibly vomiting although individuals will not manifest all the symptoms all the time and in

Table 20.4 Major foodborne diseases of bacterial origin.

	Agent	Foods Involved	Prevention
Staphylococcal	*Staphylococcus aureus*	Custards, dairy, meat, poultry	Sanitation, pasteurization, proper heating, cooling
Salmonella	*Salmonella*	Meat, chicken, egg custards	Sanitation, heating, no fecal contamination
Clostridium perfringens	*Clostridium perfringens*	Meat	Isolation of raw meat, temperature control
Botulism	*Clostridium botulinum*	Canned foods, beans, corn, tuna, figs	Pressure cooking at high temperature, boiling
Shigellosis	*Shigella*	Beans, potatoes, shrimp, cider	Personal hygiene, insect and vermin control

(*Source:* Reprinted from Mariott, N. G., 1994. *Principles of food sanitation,* 3rd ed. New York: Chapman & Hall)

some cases, additional signs and symptoms may occur. The common pathogens that cause these symptoms are sometimes found in raw meat and poultry, and ubiquitously in human beings, such as staphylococcus that is found in nasal secretions. They are passed to food products vis-à-vis nasal passages and throat, on the hands and skin, and through infected cuts, abrasions, or pimples.

> **Discussion:** Why, when you report a suspected foodborne illness, may the health department want to know all the places you have eaten during the past week?

Bacteria

Microorganisms are responsible for more than 90 percent of diseases transmitted by food. Of all microorganisms, bacteria are the more commonly involved agents of disease (refer to Table 20.3). Table 20.5 reports the relative risk of consuming food that could lead to a bacterial, foodborne illness.

Table 20.5 Bacteria and their occurrence in food risk.

Staph aureus	20% of raw milk and cheese 30–50% of human population
Salmonella	15–30% of poultry and eggs 0.2% of human population
C. Perfringens	50% of red meat 80% of human population
Listeria	Fish 1–10% of human population
E. coli	Intestinal tract of animals 6.4% of food handlers

(*Source:* Center for Food Safety and Applied Nutrition)

Bacteria in food cause illness in two ways by using food as a medium for growth and as transportation to the human body, and by spores discharging toxins as they die. These toxins are poisonous to humans. It takes only twenty to thirty minutes for most bacteria to reproduce in the right food environment. There are four phases to this spoilage: the *lag* phase, which lasts about two hours; the logarithmic or *growth* phase where growth is at a maximum rate; the *stationary* or resting phase where bacteria die at the same rate as they are being produced (spores are produced in this phase); and the period of *decline,* which may occur in eighteen to twenty-four hours.

Bacteria occur in three basic shapes, spherical (cocci), rod-shaped (bacilli), and spiral (spirilla). Cocci and bacilli are the most common bacteria found in foodborne illness. Some of the rod-shaped bacteria have the ability to produce spores that can survive boiling water for an hour or more. A **spore** is a thick walled formation within the bacterial cell that is resistant to heat, cold, and chemicals.

Bacteria survive best in warm, moist environments that are neutral to slightly acidic (Table 20.6). Most bacteria will not grow well at pH levels below

---

BOX 20.3 *Examples of Multistate Foodborne Outbreaks in the United States, 1994–1997*

Year	Organism	Number of States	Food Source
1994	*Shigella flexneri*	2	Green onions, probably contaminated in Mexico.
1994	*Listeria monocytogenes*	3	Milk, contaminated after pasteurization and shipped interstate.
1995	*Salmonella* Enteriditis	41	Ice cream premix hauled in trucks that had previously carried raw eggs.
1996	*Cyclospora cayetanensis*	20	Raspberries from Guatemala, mode of contamination unclear. Cases were also reported in the District of Columbia and two Canadian provinces.
1996	*Escherichia coli* O157:H7	3	Unpasteurized apple juice, probably contaminated during harvest.
1996	Norwalk virus	5	Oysters, contaminated before harvest.
1997	*Salmonella* Infantis	2	Alfalfa sprouts, probably contaminated during sprouting.
1997	*C. cayetanensis*	18	Raspberries imported from Guatemala, mesclun lettuce, and products containing basil. Cases were also reported in the District of Columbia and two Canadian provinces.
1997	Hepatitis A	4	Strawberries from Mexico distributed through the USDA Commodity Program for use in school lunches.

(*Source:* Centers for Disease Control)

Table 20.6 pH of some foods (< 4.5 = nonhazardous).

Food	Approx. pH
Ham	6.0
Chicken	6.2–6.7
Fish	6.6–6.8
Crab	7.0
Butter	6.1–6.4
Milk	6.6–7.0
Vegetables	4.2–6.5
Fruit	2.0–6.7
Mayonnaise	3.0–4.1

(*Source:* Center for Food Safety and Applied Nutrition)

Table 20.7 Refrigerated storage temperature and shelf life.

Product	Temperature °F	Maximum Storage Time
Meats		
Bacon	28–30	15 days
Beef	30–32	7 days
Fish	5–10	15 days
Pork	30–32	15 days
Poultry	28–30	10 days
Misc.		
Butter	35	6 months
Cheese	32–34	15 months
Cream	5–10	60 days
Eggs	38–45	2 months
Milk	35–40	5 days
Oleo	34–36	90 days

(*Source: Handbook of environmental health and safety, volume I,* by Herman Koren. Copyright 1991. Chelsea, MI: Lewis Publishers. Used by permission)

a pH of 4.6 or above 9. Most **Mesophile bacteria** survive a wide range of temperature, and thrive between 60 degrees and 110 degrees. **Thermophilous bacteria** survive above 110 degrees and **psychrophiles** can multiply at refrigerator temperature.

Refrigeration retards the growth of bacteria in foods; it cannot, however, correct damage already done. Perishable and potentially hazardous items can be kept in a refrigerator only on a short-term basis. A maximum refrigerator temperature of 40 degrees F or lower should be maintained and regularly checked. Refrigerated storage temperatures and shelf life for common products are given in Table 20.7.

Bacterial growth may be stopped or hampered by sanitizers such as sodium hypochlorite (bleach), iodine, and quatanary ammonium which are used on food surfaces. There is some research being conducted on the use of ultraviolet light, high intensity sound waves, and applied pressure as other sources of bacterial death.

Types of Bacterial Foodborne Illness

Toxin-Producing Bacteria

Escherichia coli is spread primarily through a fecal-oral route. The incubation period is anywhere from twelve to seventy-two hours. The reservoir is primarily the gastrointestinal tract of cattle and people. Communicability is from person to person through water, food, or fomites (inanimate objects such as cutting boards or utensils). The incidence rate is 2.1 per 100,000.

Staphylococcus aureus is most frequently found in meat dishes, custards, cheeses, an other moist, high-protein foods. Staphylococcus incubation is one to eight hours. Its reservoir is people or animals. These organisms are readily transmitted to foods such as creams, hams, mayonnaise, chicken, poultry, custards, cream pies, and warmed-over foods. They grow best at 50 to 120 degrees F.

Clostridium perfringens has an incubation period of six to twenty-four hours. Its reservoir is soil, and the gastrointestinal tract of people and animals. Most outbreaks are associated with mass meals, such as banquets.

Clostridium botulinum is the most deadly toxin known to humans. A small amount could kill thousands of people. In the last twenty years, 399 reported cases resulted in 122 deaths. Spores are found in the soil and are resistant to heat, chemicals, and physical stress. Spores cannot really be killed, but the toxin can be destroyed by boiling food for a few minutes. Botulism symptoms include vomiting, pain, double vision, and progressive respiratory paralysis that will often cause death. Foods that may be a source of Clostridium botulinum usually include low-acid foods and smoked vacuum-packed fish.

Non-Toxin-Producing Bacteria

Salmonellosis, first described in 1885, is a gram-negative bacillus whose symptoms are slower to appear than those of a staph infection. It is found in domestic and wild animals and in domestic pets such as turtles and ducklings. It is often found in meat and poultry, eggs, unpasteurized milk, shellfish, and fish from polluted water. The incubation period is from six to seventy-two hours. Reservoirs include poultry, rodents, turtles, cats, dogs, and people. It is communicable from days to weeks. An average of 35,000 isolates are reported each year to the CDC, a figure that has been increasing in recent years. The incidence rate is 13.7 per 100,000. These increases may be due to wide distribution of contaminated foods, more immunocompromised persons, or better reporting. Even so, it is estimated that only 1 to 10 percent of the true incidence is ever reported since many cases are mild or asymptomatic.[3] Salmonella is the most frequent cause of foodborne illness.

Campylobacter jejuni enteritis has an incubation period of three to five days. Reservoirs are farm animals, cats, dogs, rodents, and birds. This disease spreads for several days to several weeks. Airborne outbreaks have been documented. The incidence rate is 24.7 per 100,000.

Healthy People 2010 Objective: Reduce Outbreaks of Infections Caused by Key Foodborne Bacteria

Reduction in Infections Caused by Foodborne Bacteria	1997 Baseline	2010 Target
Number of Outbreaks per Year		
Escherichia coli O157:H7	22	11
Salmonella serotype Enteritidis	44	22

Children under age 1 have the highest rate of *Campylobacter* species infections. Other high-risk populations include residents in nursing homes or chronic care facilities; hospitalized, cancer, and organ transplant patients; and individuals with AIDS, with cirrhosis, on antimicrobial treatment, or with reduced stomach acid such as due to antacid medications. Infections due to campylobactor in 1997 are shown in Figure 20.5.

Shigellosis is a serious bacillary dysentery infection characterized by diarrhea, cramps, chills and fever, and bloody stools. There is intense fluid loss, dehydration, and abdominal distention. Contaminated water is most often the source of infection that can contaminate other food products. The incubation period is from one to seven days. Its reservoir is people and it is communicable for four weeks. The incidence rate is 7.9 per 100,000.

Streptococcus has an incubation period of one to three days. The reservoir is people. It is communicable for ten to twenty-one days through feces, the nose, or throat.

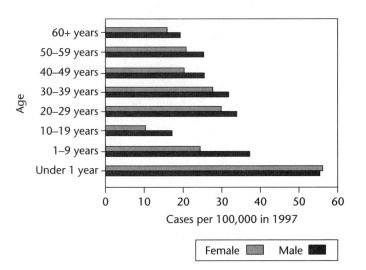

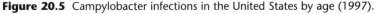

Figure 20.5 Campylobacter infections in the United States by age (1997).

(*Source:* CDC, NCHS. *Healthy People 2000 Review.* 1998–1999)

Other Foodborne Disease Transmitting Agents

Protozoa

Parasites are small or microscopic creatures that need a host to feed off, live inside, or live on. Parasites are the second most common food pathogen. They include the following protozoa and helminths:

Trichinella spiralis, found in pork, is a worm that can cause death in humans. Heating food at high temperatures or freezing food before preparation will usually kill the larvae.

Amoebic dysentery is caused by *Entamoeba histolytica* where water or food is contaminated with sewage or human feces containing amoeba. The incubation period is two to four weeks. Communicability may continue for years.

Trichinosis has an incubation period of two to twenty-eight days. The pathogen lives in larvae found in raw or poorly cooked pork.

Tapeworms have an incubation period of eight to twelve weeks for pork and beef; and three to six weeks for fish. Beef is communicable for as long as thirty years. Fish tapeworm is not communicable from person to person.

Giardiasis is a protozoan infection. The incubation period is five to twenty-five days. A person is communicable throughout the infection.

Toxoplasmosis is a protozoan spread from mother to child through the placenta, through uncooked pork or mutton, or through water or dust contaminated by cat feces. The incubation period is ten to twenty-three days.

The parasite *Toxoplasma gondii* causes toxoplasmosis and may cause miscarriage, stillbirth, or fetal abnormality. Although results of *Toxoplasma gondii* testing are not generally reported by clinicians, results from national surveys that include blood testing suggest that toxoplasmosis may be one of the most common infections associated with food. Blood tests reveal toxoplasmosis infections at a rate of 7.2 percent for children aged 6 to 10 years. Preliminary data from a European study showed that a majority of toxoplasmosis cases were foodborne.[4] Another study found that food consumption and preparation practices accounted for five of the top six practices by pregnant women that were significantly associated with congenital toxoplasmosis. The food practices were eating raw or undercooked minced meat products, eating raw or undercooked mutton, eating raw or undercooked pork or lamb, eating unwashed raw vegetables, and washing kitchen knives infrequently after preparation of raw meat and prior to handling another food item. Changing the cat litter, although often thought to be the major cause of toxoplasmosis, ranked fifth in importance of the six practices.[5]

Viruses

The relationship between viruses and foodborne disease is not clearly understood. Since viruses do reproduce in food, the food seems to serve to transport the viruses to a human host. Fish and shellfish found in tainted water may carry viral illness.

The most common foodborne virus is **Hepatitis A.** The virus is present in blood and feces during the acute phase and can be spread through poor hygiene vis à vis food preparation. Outbreaks commonly occur in day care centers where proper hand washing is not practiced after changing diapers.

Fungi

Fungi are plants or molds that may cause metabolic changes and produce toxic substances in other plants. Fungi include molds and yeasts that are naturally found in air, soil, plants, animals, water, and some food. Most molds are not harmful to humans; however, certain molds produce toxins that have been shown to cause cancer in animals. Often the potential for foodborne illness occurs before it reaches the preparer as a result of ergot poisoning from moldy grain, algae toxins in seafood from red tides, natural psoralens in celery, or even the natural carcinogens present in many foods.

Dry storage should be maintained at temperatures of sixty to seventy degrees farenheit, although fifty degrees farenheit increases the shelf life. Dry storage should keep food stuffs off floors and away from vermin, in clean, uncrowded storerooms. **Aflatoxins** are formed by molds on food at harvest time, in storage, or in conditions of water damage. It is a potent carcinogen and may be a cause of liver cancer in Africa. Aflatoxin is a product of fungi that contaminates peanuts, corn, and other human and animal foods. **Lectins** agglutinate red blood cells. They are present in seeds, leaves, bark, and roots. **Hepatoxins** contaminate wheat and corn and are poisonous to livestock and humans.

Pests as Agents of Illness

The presence of pests in urban areas is often associated with other social problems such as crowding, housing decay, poor sanitation, and a lack of vector control. There are two general categories of urban pests, those that adversely affect people's health directly through bites, or indirectly through contaminated fecal waste in food products, and those that affect aesthetic and economic value of property. Both types of pests are important to public health.

Recently, pestborne diseases have caused epidemics in Europe, Asia, and Africa. Outbreaks of up to several hundred cases of encephalitis, dengue (often brought to the United States by immigrants), yellow fever, and malaria occur almost annually in various parts of the United States. The possibility of major outbreaks of pestborne disease could occur in cities and towns where people are exposed to insects and other animals that bite, suck blood, sting or puncture the skin, deposit their feces, urine, saliva or their secretions on human food or water, or in places where such secretions are inhaled.[6]

Cockroaches Cockroaches are among the most frequent and most bothersome insect pests in relation to foodborne illness. Efforts to control them are complicated by their resistance to chemicals and population dynamics. They are known to be carriers of disease organisms such as Salmonella, the most frequent cause of food poisoning, and the viruses that cause poliomyelitis.

Roaches tend to hide and lay eggs in dark, warm, moist, hard-to-clean places. They are found between pipes and walls or where pipes pass unsealed through walls. Cockroaches leave a strong, oily odor, scurry away when lights are turned on, and leave small, black or dark brown, spherical feces practically everywhere they go.

Preventing cockroach infestation requires elimination of food and water sources through frequent cleaning, depriving roaches of shelter and hiding places, and preventing roaches from entering food preparation locations in cartons or paper goods. Exterminators spend an estimated $10 million annually on traps to kill roaches, one of the most elusive of all pests. A pair of cockroaches can generate 100,000 offspring in just one year, outproducing the ability to terminate their existence. A new approach to cockroach destruction is a new, environmentally safe trap that permits bacteria-carrying nematodes—microscopic wormlike organisms—to enter the roach's body through body openings. The nematodes release a bacteria that kills the insect but allows the nematodes to continue to reproduce inside the carcass. The newly produced nematodes then migrate to new insects to continue this bioinsecticide process.

Flies The common housefly is an even greater menace to human health than is the cockroach. A single fly is a veritable repository for a large variety of bacteria and can carry disease-causing viruses as well. Flies can transmit typhoid, dysentery, infantile diarrhea, streptococcal, and staphylococcal illnesses.[7]

Flies feed on human and animal wastes. These wastes stick on the mouth, footpads, and hairs of flies and may then be deposited in food when the fly lands. Flies defecate every four to five minutes and can infect food products with their own feces, spittle, or vomitus.

Flies are drawn to moist, warm, decaying material protected from sunlight. They enter through torn screens or screens greater than 16 mesh per inch. Garbage that is left out longer than three or four days attracts flies that breed and leave maggots.

Rodents Rats and mice are among peoples' most cunning and capable enemies. They have highly developed senses of touch, smell, and hearing. They are good swimmers and have good balance. Rats are prolific breeders, and they do enough damage to their environment to cause anywhere from $1 to 10 billion a year in economic loss to this country through consumption and contamination of food and structural damage to property.[8]

Rodents can be directly or indirectly involved in the transmission of such diseases as salmonellosis, leptospirosis, and murine typhus. One rat fecal dropping contains several million bacteria. Rats and mice defecate and urinate, with frequency, as they move around. All body wastes can be blown or carried to food.

The first step in rat-proofing an establishment is to find and eliminate all possible ways for rodents to enter. Rat nests should be destroyed by eliminating hiding places. Starve rodents by removing all garbage or stored food that can be made accessible to the hungry rat.

Chemical Contamination

There are a number of chemicals and metals that can be leached into food produce that may be harmful to humans. Eighty to 90 percent of total human exposure to most chemicals, including heavy metals, pesticides, and radionuclides come from food consumption. The Food Quality Protection Act of 1996 requires the EPA to reassess all existing standards for pesticides by the year 2006. Under this act, the EPA considers the risk from dietary exposures from all food uses of pesticides and drinking water; nonoccupational exposure, such as the use of pesticides for lawn care; and any special sensitivities for children. FDA monitors domestic and imported foods to ensure compliance with these pesticide safety standards.[9]

A good example of the use of pesticides is from "America's breadbasket":

The San Joaquin is no ordinary valley. Half of the fruit, nuts, and vegetables consumed in the United States are grown in the valley's 30,000 square miles of central California. It is one of the most intensely cultivated areas in the world ... and among the most laden with pesticides. Seven percent of all pesticides used in this country are sprayed onto crops in the San Joaquin Valley, even though the valley comprises just 1 percent of the nation's cropland. Geographical statistical maps indicate that four of the top five counties posing the greatest potential pesticide hazards are in the valley. So are a disturbing number of counties with excess deaths from acutely hazardous exposures and child cancers.[10]

Aluminum is the third most abundant earth element and is incompatible with life process. It is found in soil, air, and water and can get into the food chain to humans. Some researchers have linked high aluminum levels in the brain with Alzheimer's disease.[11] Aluminum is also present in some baking powder, processed cheese, firming agents, packaging, and antacids. However, aluminum-free baking powder is available in the United States. **Antimony** is leached from chipped gray enamelware by acidic foods. Although antimony poisoning is not common, tourists sometimes bring gray enamelware home from trips abroad and are later poisoned by the worn dishes. Other elements also pose a problem for food illness. **Arsenic** is found in ant, roach, or rodent baits and herbicides, while **cadmium** is present in plating materials of containers and trays and is leached by acidic foods. **Copper** is leached from food contact with copper tubing. **Lead** is found in paint, pesticides, and glazed pottery vessels and utensils. **Mercury** is found in fish and shellfish that have consumed mercury in contaminated waters. It is found in many industrial processes. **Zinc** is leached from galvanized containers. **PCBs** are found in wildlife in much of the world. They are found in fish and animal feed and paints that have leached into feed and cardboard cartons from recycled paper. At any given time, fully one-third of the nation's oyster, clam, and other shellfish beds are closed because of contamination. Twenty-seven marine mammals and birds in American coastal waters are now listed as threatened or endangered and the rising phenomenon of mass die-offs of dolphins and seals is blamed on toxins such as PCB.

PCB is the common abbreviation of the chemical name polychlorinated biphenyl, which applies to 209 mixtures of organic compounds produced by the reaction of chlorine with biphenyl. It is widely used as a lubricant and heating transfer fluid in electrical equipment, especially transformers. PCBs are toxic and resist decomposition. PCBs in the milk of Canadian Beluga whales, "the most polluted animal in the world," are 3,400 times the safe levels for drinking water.[12] PCBs have been detected in human adipose tissues and in the milk of cows and humans. The estimated percentage of the U.S. population with detectable levels of PCBs was nearly 100 percent in 1981.[13]

Other Mediums of Foodborne Diseases

Milk, meat, shellfish, and eggs are four common sources providing environments that are quite hospitable to pathogens that cause foodborne diseases in humans. In fact, they are probably the most common transmitters of food pathogens.

Milk

Milk is one of the most high-risk sources of foodborne illness in the United States because it produces such an amenable environment for pathogenic growth. Despite regulations the primary problems associated with safe, clean milk include cleaning of equipment and improperly operated and calibrated instruments. The everyday risks that must be carefully monitored include waste handling, flies, pesticides, improper storage, improper cleaning of pipelines, and milking equipment.

Milk is tested for color, appearance, blood, viscosity, foreign matter, sediment, and temperature through microscopic counts or breed counts, amethylene blue tests, standard plate counts, and coliform tests.

Milkborne Diseases   **Brucellosis (undulant fever or Bang's disease)** is found in raw contaminated milk products or infected animals. The incubation period is five to thirty days. The reservoir is animals and there is no human communicability. **Tuberculosis** is also transmitted in raw contaminated milk or dairy products and infected animals. The incubation is four to twelve weeks. Reservoirs are people and cattle.

Pasteurization   Pasteurization is the process of killing pathogenic organisms in milk that may be carried to the milk through unclean hands, flies, sick milkers, or sick cows. Pasteurization requires heating milk at 145 degrees for thirty minutes or 194 degrees for seventy-five seconds. Even with pasteurization, drugs, pesticides, and some chemicals that can be passed into milk through the food chain are not destroyed and are not part of the testing by government inspectors. A General Accounting Office (GAO) report prepared for a 1992 FDA subcommittee stated that the FDA tests for just four of eighty-two drugs that can be used in milk cows. According to the GAO, thirty-five of the most commonly used drugs have never been approved for use in dairy cows. New regulations were enacted in 1996.

Milk is marked Grade A if it contains less than 10,000 bacteria per milliliter. Grade B or raw milk may contain 100,000 bacteria per milliliter. Unpasteurized milk and eggs are potential sources of salmonellosis. Large outbreaks of Salmonella have contaminated shell eggs, especially in New England and the Mid-Atlantic areas of the United States.[14]

The Politics of Milk Milk is one of the most political of all food products. Its production has been protected by milk subsidies and its safety has been demanded by many strict regulations. There are enormous surpluses of milk, butter, cheese, and nonfat milk in U.S. storage facilities, but the cost of disseminating these surpluses to the hungry appears to be too costly according to those who legislate this action. Instead, under a 1985 farm bill, the U.S. Department of Agriculture paid dairy farmers to remain out of dairying for five years. The government buyouts are intended to reduce the amount of dairy products by 8 percent. At the same time that dairy cows are being slaughtered for meat and exported because too much milk is being produced, a bovine growth hormone is about to be approved for commercial use in the United States.[15]

Scientists at major chemical companies have isolated the genes in a cow's cells that control the synthesis of bovine growth hormone (BGH). Through biotechnology the BGH has been transplanted into microbes that manufacture commercial quantities of the hormone. The synthesized hormone is injected on a daily basis into dairy cattle. The increased growth hormones boost the cow's appetite, increase her milk production 10 to 25 percent, and ultimately burn her out so rapidly that within a few years she is exhausted from the speeding up of her biological process. Cows with BGH enhancement have more infections, particularly mastitis, an infection of the mammary glands. Cows become more at risk for heat stress, and their fertility is reduced.[16]

This biotech approach to agriculture should remind the reader of previous hormonal attempts to increase meat production with hormones such as DES, a synthetic estrogen, and the ultimate effect on human beings. There is evidence that estrogen-like hormones in cattle and chicken (i.e., DES), may cause precocious sexual development in children who eat these products. Cattle that have been treated with antibiotics cause hypersensitivity to antibiotics in some who eat this meat. In 1992 the GAO urged the FDA to withhold commercial approval of synthetic BGH because of increased residues of antibiotics in meat and milk. There is no requirement that hormones in meat and milk be labeled when sold to the consumer.

The continued research in bovine milk biotechnology at a time when milk is in surplus causes one to wonder about the commercial reasons, versus the animal and human health outcomes, of biotech agriculture, dairy farming, and fast food production. Further, greater inspection and testing of milk should be considered. Again, at present, only four of eighty-two drugs used to treat dairy cows are routinely tested in milk.

Meat

Virtually all meat and poultry in the United States has been inspected by the U.S. Department of Agriculture. Testing occurs at many stages of the meat processing. Tests include total plate counts, tests for yeasts and molds, and microscopic examinations of pH, salt, and nitrite levels. This does not, however, guarantee freedom from pathogens. Attempts to prevent contamination has been less than adequate. Problems related to safe meat include removal of solid waste, intense fly populations, presence of rodents, unclean equipment, walls, floors, and appurtenances and unsanitary handlers.

Annually, 7 million meat animals are inspected at several stages of production. Before slaughter, each animal is inspected by a veterinarian or one of the 7,800 Food Safety and Inspection Service (FSIS) meat inspectors in some 6,500 plants.[17] The inspectors look for sickly cows, fresh injection marks, open wounds or other potentially contaminating sources.[18] This inspection system is not considered very sophisticated, having changed very little since its establishment under President Theodore Roosevelt in 1906. It has been called, euphemistically, the "sniff and poke" method of meat testing. The CDC estimates that 5 million illnesses and 4000 deaths occur annually as a result of eating meat and poultry contaminated with microbial pathogens, and 90 percent of these could be eliminated through improved inspection of raw meats at the processing plants.[19]

In 1998 the science-based meat inspection system called HACCP was enacted at the nation's 300 largest meat plants, requiring them to identify critical points along their production lines and ensure that practices at those points minimize bacterial contamination and growth. Very small plants, those with fewer than ten employees, implemented HACCP in January 2000.[20] Even with HACCP, only 1 in 300 beef carcasses, 1 in 3,000 turkeys, and 1 in 20,000 chickens will be tested. No microbial testing is required in meat and poultry processing plants.

However, to the credit of the FSIS inspectors, during the routine nationwide statistical monitor for residues of 133 animal drugs and pesticides, only .3 percent of the 40,252 samples showed illegal residue limits. It was found that these residue levels fell well within the margins of safety established by the FDA. Also, noticeably the residues were mainly found in the kidney, livers, and other organs; rarely in the muscle of the meat.[21]

If a carcass is suspect it is sent to the laboratory for additional inspection. A lab tests for all residues and bacteria the meat may have. The FSIS may then prevent all related meat products or cattle from entering the human consumption market. A controversy exists surrounding these tests because of the length of time it takes a colony of bacteria to grow (from three to seven days) and the fact that other suspect meat affected by the same sources may have already gone to market.[22]

A company called Leatherhead Food RA has developed a sensor that can detect the quality and freshness of raw meat in one hour.[23] A sensor of this type could potentially be used at all sites of raw meat inspection and may eliminate all bacterial infections. Beyond inspection, meat handling must include proper sanitation, refrigeration, and cooking of meat to ensure safety.

In 1994 the Clinton administration released a long-range plan to modernize the nation's huge meat and poultry inspection system. The plan was called the "Pathogen Reduction Act" and would require that all meat and poultry passing through federal inspection sites be tested for invisible bacteria or pathogens. The plan would give the government new power to recall tainted meat or hold it at the processing plant, allowing the Agriculture Department to track infected animals back to the farm. On the other hand, new congressional plans would given more power to slaughterhouses to do their own inspections and thus reduce government inspectors. Most in public health find this a very risky plan.

Meatborne Illnesses   An indirect illness associated with meat is **tularemia.** Tularemia is spread by wild rabbits, squirrels, and animals through the bites of infected ticks and deer flies that live on these mammals. Incubation is two to ten days. The reservoir is wild animals and hard ticks. There is no transmission from person to person.

Poultry

The primary problems associated with poultry production of 7 billion birds a year are cleanliness of walls, floors, drains, equipment, conveyor belts, and surroundings. Examples of problems include: (1) excessive solid waste, causing overloaded sewage systems which flush back into production areas; and (2) rats frequently invading chicken slaughter plants. Chickens are a major source of *Salmonella* bacteria and *Campylobacter jejuni* bacteria, and today, over 25 percent of all chicken purchased contains *Salmonella* bacteria, and 70 percent to 90 percent have been tainted with Campylobacter despite regulations that attempt to keep poultry safe. Testing is done by holding a clean bird for four days at 32 degrees F and checking bacterial count in developed slime.

Prevention of Salmonellosis and Campylobacter involves careful handling of foods and good personal hygiene. Consumers should assume that poultry, eggs, and meats are contaminated and should cook these foods thoroughly. In addition, care should be taken to avoid contamination of other foods. Most cases occur in the home setting, and if a single case is reported in a household, one-third of other household members are likely to get ill as well.

Egg Processing   Americans consume an average of 234 eggs per person per year. Cracked eggshells are at risk for penetration of the eggshell by organisms, pesticides, and other contaminants. Pasteurization of eggs is usually performed in a high temperature-short time pasteurizer similar to milk pasteurization. This process of getting eggs from hen to consumer is illustrated as an example in Figure 20.6.

In 1999 the Clinton administration announced a new egg safety program to reduce *Salmonella* illnesses (S.E.). Under the new plan, egg producers and processors will implement one of two strategies to improve egg safety. Strategy I requires rigorous on-farm agricultural and sanitation practices, extensive testing for SE, and diversion of eggs to pasteurization or cooked product based on positive SE testing. Strategy II requires implementation of new technologies to kill the potentially dangerous organism, such as "in-shell pasteurization," at the packer stage of production.

WHOLE SHELL EGGS

HEN →   SHELL EGGS →

CANDLE →   CLEAN →   SHELL TREATMENT →
Classify; eliminate spoiled   Spray wash with water   Immerse eggs at 75°F in oil.
eggs, blood spots; separate   at same temperature   Rotate for 10 min.
cracked eggs   as eggs

STORE →   SUPERMARKET
40°F well-ventilated area;
clean area; relative
humidity 85–90%

FLOW CHART FOR LIQUID OR FROZEN EGGS

HEN →   SHELL EGGS →   CANDLE →

CLEAN →   SANITIZE SHELLS →   BREAK SHELLS →
                              Spray   Separate white from yoke
                              Rinse off excess sanitizer

MIX THOROUGHLY →   CLARIFY OR FILTER →   COOL →
                                                               40°F

FERMENT →   PASTEURIZE →   ADD ADDITIVES →
To remove sugar   140°F for 1.75 min. for whole   Salt, sugar, adjust pH
                              eggs; 134°F at pH9 for 1.75 min.
                              for liquid egg whites; 142°F for
                              1.75 min. for liquid yolk

PACKAGE →   FREEZE →
                              Rapidly to 0°F; defrost when
                              needed in refrigerator at 45°F

FLOW CHART FOR DRIED EGGS

HEN →   SHELL EGGS →   CANDLE →

CLEAN →   STORE →   SANITIZE →
                              40°F for 72 hours before
                              sanitizing

BREAK SHELLS →   MIX →   CLARIFY →

HOLDING VAT →   PASTEURIZE →   SPRAY DRY →
40°F for maximum of   Under high pressure; drying
48 hours   temperature 340°F

COOK →   STORE →
Final cooling to 50°F   In sterile barrels or cartons

Figure 20.6 Egg processing diagram.

(*Source:* Koren, Herman, 1991. *Handbook of environmental health and safety, volume I.* Copyright 1991. Chelsea, MI: Lewis Publishers. Used with permission)

Shellfish

Shellfish receive their food by pumping water from their environment through their bodies. Along with food, sand, and dirt, a variety of bacteria and viruses are found. Two recent epidemics directly related to contaminated shellfish have been hepatitis A and 14,000 cases of cholera originating in Peru and spreading north. Additionally, shellfish absorb pesticides, metals, radionuclides, and other hazardous waste. Consumed shellfish should be certifiably from a non-polluted growing area to prevent shellfish poisoning. Typical processing of shellfish is shown in Figure 20.7.

Cholera vibrio is associated almost exclusively with seafood and found in nearly all seafood products. Cases in Japan range from 10,000 to 14,000 annually. Incubation is twelve to fourteen hours. Reservoirs are marine areas during the cold season in water, and in fish and shellfish in the warm season. It is not spread by people.

GROWING AREA →
Sanitary survey by Public Health Service; evaluate sources of actual or potential pollution, bacteriological study of water and shellfish; chemical analysis of water and shellfish; graded as approved, conditional approval, restricted, or prohibited

HARVEST →
From approved area only; from conditionally approved area only under supervision of health authorities, to ensure that shellfish are purified; from restricted areas only under controlled purification and supervision of health authorities; never from prohibited areas; human body waste must not be discharged from the harvest boat into the water

TRANSPORT →
Boats and truck; shellfish stored in thoroughly cleaned bins and away from bilge water; bins must be sanitized

WASH SHELLFISH →
Wash away mud; use potable water under pressure

SHUCK →
Separate from packing operation; not subject to flooding; fly tight screening

PACK →
Clean room; surfaces washed, sanitized; impervious floors and walls; fly control measures; adequate safe sanitary water supply; approved plumbing—avoid cross connections and submerged inlets; strict hand-washing procedures; use clean sanitized single-service containers; label with packer's name, address, number, state, and date

REFRIGERATE →
Refrigerate quickly below 40°F; freeze quickly

CLEAN EQUIPMENT AND SANITIZE
Washing sinks, made of impervious, non-toxic materials; storage, shucking, and packing rooms cleaned within two hours after completing operations; sanitize with 100 ppm available chlorine

Figure 20.7 Shellfish processing diagram.

(*Source:* Koren, Herman, 1991. *Handbook of environmental health and safety, volume I.* Copyright 1991. Chelsea, MI: Lewis Publishers. Used with permission)

Summary

The monitoring of food safety has become a common and well-established process. The result is one of the safest food supplies in the world. From the FDA and USDA inspection of meat, poultry, dairy products, and processed foods, to state and local public health regulations of restaurants and retail food sales, an unprecedented level of safety and assurance has been achieved for consumers. The greatest risk to food safety now lies with the personal hygiene of food handlers due to high turnover and lack of education. Good education of food handlers and consumers will reduce any foodborne illness significantly.

Although the United States works hard to keep food safe, in 1999, 70 percent of all fruits and vegetables came from Mexico. It is very difficult for U.S. food inspectors to regulate what comes from out of the country. Further, new pathogens, not routinely cultured, are being introduced through foreign import. Today, due to cost, lack of laboratory capability, and lack of government commitment, we are not looking for all the possible agents that may cause foodborne disease. While not discussed in this chapter, the community health educator should consider irradiation to be an important means of food safety in the twenty-first century.

CYBERSITES RELATED TO CHAPTER 20

Food Safety
> vm.cfsan.fda.gov/list.html
> www.fsis.usda.gov

QUESTIONS

1. What are common ways milk might be contaminated from the cow to the table?

2. What are ten things you can do in your home to prevent foodborne disease?

3. From an epidemiological viewpoint, why should you call your local health department if you suspect you are ill from a foodborne disease?

EXERCISE

Take the food inspection form (Figure 20.3) from this chapter and inspect a food service operation on your campus or in your neighborhood. (With their permission, of course!)

INTERNET INTERACTIVE ACTIVITY

FOODBORNE DISEASES ACTIVE SURVEILLANCE NETWORK: CDC'S EMERGING INFECTIONS PROGRAM

The Foodborne Diseases Active Surveillance Network (FoodNet) is the principal foodborne disease component of CDC's Emerging Infections Program (EIP). FoodNet is a collaborative project of the CDC, nine EIP sites (California, Colorado, Connecticut, Georgia, New York, Maryland, Minnesota, Oregon, and Tennessee), the U.S. Department of Agriculture (USDA), and the Food and Drug Administration (FDA). The project consists of active surveillance for foodborne diseases and related epidemiologic studies designed to help public health officials better understand the epidemiology of foodborne diseases in the United States. The Homepage is

> www.cdc.gov/ncidod/dbmd/foodnet/what_is.htm

Example

Given the survey data, the community health educator wants to know what meats, fruits and vegetables, dairy or eggs, or other exposures were reported for a foodborne illness outbreak during the survey period.

1. Under **Reports and Studies,** click on **Food Data Sources**.
2. Start at the bottom on the pyramid and click on E**xposures in General Population.**
3. Under the 1998–1999 population survey, click on **View the Atlas of Exposures.**
4. Start with **Table 1** and click through the **Tables** to get an idea of foods associated with exposure.

From the tables we now know that most were exposed to lettuce, oven-roasted chicken, hamburger and bacon, runny eggs, and some international travel.

Exercise

Select two states from the seven that were surveyed and compare their exposure variables for foodborne illness outbreaks.

1. Use the most recent **FoodNet Population Survey.**
2. Compare all the variables associated with **Exposure Frequency by Site.**
3. For your two states, compare all the variables associated with **two fruits and vegetables, two meat products, and either eggs or milk, international travel in the past 14 days, contact with a cat, and one of the consumer knowledge questions from Stratified Exposure Frequency.**
4. Based on your search of this database, what are the primary sources of foodborne illness in the states surveyed? How would the community health educator prevent other foodborne outbreaks based on your survey information?

REFERENCES

1. Paul S. Mead, Laurence Slutsker, Vance Dietz, Linda F. McCaig, Joseph S. Bresee, Craig Shapiro, Patricia M. Griffin, and Robert V. Tauxe (1999). *Food related illness and death in the United States.* Atlanta: Centers for Disease Control and Prevention.

2. Bryan, Frank (1982). *Diseases transmitted by foods.* Atlanta: U.S. Department of Health and Human Services.

3. *Epidemiology Newsletter* (1994). Salmonellosis in Utah. Utah Department of Health, May, p. 1.

4. Kapperud, G., Jenum, P. A., Stray-Pederson, B., Melby, K. K., Eskild, A., and Eng, J. Risk factors for *Toxoplasma gondii* infection in pregnancy. Results of a prospective case-control study in Norway. *American Journal of Epidemiology* 144(4):405–412, 1996.

5. Ibid.

6. Committee on Urban Pest Management (1980). Urban Pest Management. Washington, DC: National Academy Press.

7. *Foodservice sanitation,* 3rd ed. John Wiley, with National Institutes for Food Service Industries.

8. Ibid.

9. FDA. *Pesticide program residue monitoring, 1997.* Washington, DC: Food and Drug Administration, 1998.

10. Goldman, Benjamin A. (1991). *The truth about where you live.* New York: Times Books, Random House.

11. Fairweather, Frank A. (1991). Field investigations of biological and chemical hazards of food and water. In *Oxford textbook of public health,* Vol. II, p. 451.

12. Stix, Gary (1993). Red banner burger. *Scientific American.* June.

13. Some federal action that protects our foods (1993). *Consumer's Research,* 76(1), January.

14. Salmonellosis in Utah, op. cit.

15. Hynes, H. Patricia (1989). *The recurring silent spring.* New York: Pergamon Press.

16. MacKenzie, Debora. (1988). Science milked for all it's worth. *New Scientist,* 22 March, 28–29.

17. Some Federal Action, op. cit.

18. *Consumers' Research* (1992). Residues in meat and poultry. 77(1), January.

19. Welch, William (1995). Meat inspection plan faces delay. *USA Today,* July 11, p. 6A.

20. www.fsis.usda.gov/OA/news/salmrel.htm

21. Some Federal Action, op. cit.

22. Campylobacter enteritis outbreaks associated with drinking raw milk during youth activities (1992). *Journal of the American Medical Association.* 268(22), Dec 9.

23. Kress-Rogers, Erika (1993). Making sure your food is good to eat. *Chemtech,* May.

CHAPTER 21

The Throwaway Society

Community Health in the 21st Century
The key element underlying recycling, reusing, and reducing is awareness.
Awareness takes us out of our habitual or reactive patterns, so that we can be
more proactive and situationally specific. The more informed, conscious, and
vigilant we are, the better are our decisions and courses of action, which in
turn helps to establish a better relationship with our environment.

—Eric P. Trunnell, Ph.D., University of Utah

Chapter Objectives

The student will:

1. list the types of solid wastes and discuss their potential risks to human health.

2. list the pros and cons of landfills, incineration, ocean dumping, and recycling.

3. draw a diagram of a landfill with its proper requirements.

4. list those items that can be recycled in her or his community.

5. define what constitutes a hazardous waste.

6. explain the role of SuperFund and discuss barriers to its implementation.

7. define "ecological racism."

Trashing the Planet

No place on earth is too remote for garbage. If you walk through a typical village in east Greenland today or the scientific community of McMurdo Sound in Antarctica you will find the evidence of human existence. In Greenland, there are hills of beer cans, rubber boots, and tires. In Antarctica the refuse may seem more sophisticated, yet just as ugly—gas tanks, crates, metal scraps, and soda machines. In many developing countries thrown away trash and refuse is recycled as human abode, food, and clothing. As sad, unsanitary, and deprecating as this reuse of "unusable" trash by the world's poor obviously appears, at least foodstuff, fabric, newspaper, cardboard, and tin are in some sense recycled at this primitive level.

In 1955 *Life* magazine reported on a new American habit—the "throwaway society." Products could be produced so cheaply that it became more economical to throw away a razor, a cigarette lighter, even a VCR or telephone than to

---

BOX 21.1 *America's Garbage: Packaging Materials*

In just one day, Americans toss out 50,000 tons of packaging material. This mound would fill about 10,000 tractor trailers. If all the trucks were lined up end to end, they would stretch for 120 miles.[1]

---

repair or adjust it. There are approximately 2,000 new products created each year. Each new product sharply increases the level and amount of solid waste. In 1998 the United States disposed of 238 million tons of municipal solid waste (MSW) that averaged 1.272 tons per person, according to *Biocycle* magazine. Chicago alone created more than 7,500 tons of garbage each day; New York City produced more than 25,000 tons a day; and Los Angeles County more than 50,000 tons a day. South Dakota won first place as the nation's "Best" at managing their municipal waste for 1997, and Nevada won the "Worst" place position. New York was the leading exporter of waste at 4.0 million tons; Pennsylvania imported the most waste, at 6.3 million tons; and California was the leading generator of waste, at 45.0 million tons. Washington recycled the most waste, at 48% of their municipal waste stream[2] (Table 21.1). A comparison of MSW by selected countries is shown in Figure 21.1.

A History of Waste

The first municipal dump was in Athens in 500 BC. Ancient dumps contained simple components that were more easily decomposed. Nevertheless, these dumping sites were still odorous, unsightly, and unhealthy. Vermin that visited the dumps often moved on to nearby households, transmitting disease and

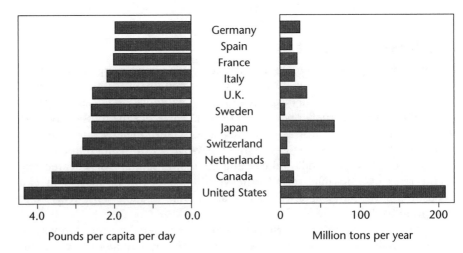

Figure 21.1 International waste production.

(*Source:* Statistical Abstracts of the United States)

Table 21.1 Best and worst of waste management in the United States (1998).

Rank	Best Management tons/person/yr	Worst Management tons/person/yr	Generates Most tons/yr	Recycles Most (% of generation)	Imports Most (tons/yr)	Exports Most (tons/yr)
1.	South Dakota 0.400	Nevada 2.132	California 45,000,000	Washington 48%	Pennsylvania 6,300,000	New York 4,000,000
2.	Wisconsin 0.580	Kansas 1.879	New York 28,800,000	New Jersey 45%	Indiana 2,674,000	New Jersey 2,300,000
3.	North Dakota 0.628	South Carolina 1.588	Florida 23,617,000	Minn/S. Dakota 42%	Michigan 1,838,000	Missouri 1,756,000
4.	Colorado 0.649	Delaware 1.491	Texas 21,738,000	Maine 41%	Illinois 1,300,000	Maryland 1,200,000
5.	Oklahoma 0.663	Utah 1.484	Georgia 14,645,000	Florida/Tenn. 40%	Oregon 1,067,000	Washington 989,000
6.	Minnesota 0.679	New Hampshire 1.471	Michigan 13,500,000	New York 39%	Kansas 1,000,000	Ohio 600,000
7.	Idaho 0.732	Indiana 1.432	Illinois 13,386,000	Arkansas 36%	Mississippi 800,000	Massachusetts 549,000
8.	Missouri 0.761	Hawaii 1.342	Ohio 12,339,000	Virginia 35%	New Hampshire 700,000	Minnesota 412,000
9.	Lousiana 0.769	Georgia 1.333	North Carolina 9,843,000	South Carolina 34%	Ohio 668,000	California 408,000
10.	Maine 0.784	Missouri 1.316	Tennessee 9,496,000	Georgia/Missouri/ Massachusetts 33%	Wisconsin 656,000	North Carolina 330,000

(*Source:* Zerowasteamerica.org)

plagues over large areas. Garbage archaeologists estimate that the street level of the ancient city of Troy rose almost five feet per century as a result of debris accumulation. Present street levels on the island of Manhattan are typically six to fifteen feet higher than they were in the seventeenth century; it wasn't until 1895 that the city undertook systematic garbage removal.[3]

During the Industrial Revolution, from 1700 to the mid 1800s, garbage disposal took on an added dimension. Rapid urban development led to widespread pollution of the soil, air, and streams in most industrial areas because of the inadequacy of existing systems for collection and disposal of massive amounts of garbage and trash, as well as human and industrial wastes. Landfills became a common and necessary means of preventing such obvious hazards.

A twenty-first century problem is the continued discovery of landfills that were filled in the twentieth century in primitive ways and in absorbent marshes, old quarries, gravel pits and desert lands. In the mid-twentieth century, many subdivisions were built on landfills that over the decades have leaked and sunk, ruining property and the health of residents.

Since 1973 a group of anthropologists at the University of Arizona has been conducting a series of systematic archaeological digs, excavating more than fourteen tons of garbage. The garbage project discovered a phenomenon they called the Lean Cuisine Syndrome—to appear more socially correct, people consistently underreport the quantities of junk food they eat, and overreport the amount of fruit and diet soda they consume. Most people also underreport their consumption of alcohol by 40–60 percent.[4]

Another finding of the garbage archeologists is that we are often misdirected by our incorrect beliefs. Most people believe that expanded polystyrene foam, which is used in fast-food packaging, coffee cups, packing "peanuts," and the molded forms that are used as packing around equipment—constitutes a major proportion of our garbage. The garbage project discovered that polystyrene foam accounted for less than one percent of the volume of garbage dumped in landfills between 1980 and 1989. Similarly, disposable diapers average no more than 1.4 percent, by volume, of the average landfill's total solid waste contents from 1980 to 1989. These are not major contributors to the U.S. solid waste problem.

Solid Waste

Solid waste is defined by the Resource Conservation and Recovery Act (RCRA) as garbage, refuse, sludge, and other discarded material. Exceptions include domestic sewage (untreated sanitary wastes), industrial wastewater discharges, irrigation return flows, nuclear material or byproducts, and mining materials not removed from the ground during the extraction process.

With only 4.5 percent of the world's population, the United States produces 33 percent of the world's **solid waste**—any unwanted or discarded material that is not a liquid or gas. The United States generates about 10 billion metric tons of solid waste per year, about 1,280 pounds per person per year, and now

---

BOX 21.2 America's Garbage

Daily Trash

Every day each American throws out an average of about four pounds of garbage. If everyone's daily trash were piled in a giant heap it would weigh 438,000 tons.[5]

Disposable Diapers

People in the United States get rid of 48 million disposable diapers everyday. Eighteen billion are thrown out every year and take up about 2 percent of the volume of solid waste dumped into landfills. They take more than 200 years to degrade.

Tires

Americans throw out 280 million tires each year. Laid out in a single line, these tires would stretch for about 140,000 miles . . . nearly four and half times around the world at the equator.

Table 21.2 Discards of municipal waste by weight (1996).

	Thousand Tons	Percent of Total	Cumulative Percent		Thousand Tons	Percent of Total	Cumulative Percent
Food wastes	21,380	14.0%	14.0%	Plastic wraps	1,820	1.2%	87.5%
Yard trimmings	17,200	11.3%	25.3%	Paper bags & sacks	1,710	1.1%	88.6%
Miscellaneous durables	11,270	7.4%	32.7%	Magazines	1,490	1.0%	89.6%
Corrugated boxes	9,690	6.4%	39.1%	Glass wine & liquor bottles	1,470	1.0%	90.6%
Furniture and furnishings	7,320	4.8%	43.9%	Other paper packaging	1,340	0.9%	91.5%
Wood packaging	5,990	3.9%	47.8%	Major appliances	1,320	0.9%	92.3%
Other commercial printing	5,750	3.8%	51.6%	Plastic bags & sacks	1,300	0.9%	93.2%
Newspapers	5,640	3.7%	55.3%	Steel cans & other packaging	1,300	0.9%	94.0%
Clothing and footwear	4,640	3.0%	58.3%	Plastic other containers	1,090	0.7%	94.7%
Paper folding cartons	4,410	2.9%	61.2%	Paper plates & cups	950	0.6%	95.4%
Other non-packaging paper	4,070	2.7%	63.9%	Aluminum cans & other packaging	940	0.6%	96.0%
Third class mail	3,840	2.5%	66.4%	Trash bags	860	0.6%	96.6%
Glass beer & soft drink bottles	3,530	2.3%	68.8%	Plastic plates & cups	800	0.5%	97.1%
Office-type papers	3,470	2.3%	71.0%	Books	770	0.5%	97.6%
Miscellaneous non-durables	3,450	2.3%	73.3%	Small appliances	760	0.5%	98.1%
Miscellaneous inorganic wastes	3,200	2.1%	75.4%	Towels, sheets & pillowcases	620	0.4%	98.5%
Rubber tires	3,180	2.1%	77.5%	Paper milk cartons	460	0.3%	98.8%
Disposable diapers	3,050	2.0%	79.5%	Plastic milk & other bottles	460	0.3%	99.1%
Tissue paper and towels	2,980	2.0%	81.4%	Plastic soft drink bottles	430	0.3%	99.4%
Glass food & other bottles	2,870	1.9%	83.3%	Telephone directories	410	0.3%	99.6%
Carpets and rugs	2,290	1.5%	84.8%	Other paperboard packaging	230	0.2%	99.8%
Other plastic packaging	2,270	1.5%	86.3%	Other miscellaneous packaging	150	0.1%	99.9%
				Lead-acid batteries	110	0.1%	100.0%
				Paper wraps	50	<0.1%	100.0%
Total MSW Discards	152,330	100.0%					

(*Source:* Statistical Abstracts of the United States)

faces an enormous garbage problem. Types of municipal solid waste are reported in Table 21.2.

Landfills are full or quickly running out of room for more garbage. States refuse to dump the trash of other states, countries, or major waste producers. Today, barges filled with garbage that cannot be dumped in one state sail around the hemisphere looking for a willing landfill such as the most famous example, the so-called garbage barge. This barge left Islip, Long Island, in early 1987 and wandered for six months in search of a port that would accept its

This "trash heap" is actually
a metal recycling plant.
While the idea of recycling
is a plus, having such an
eyesore in one's neighborhood is less than desirable.

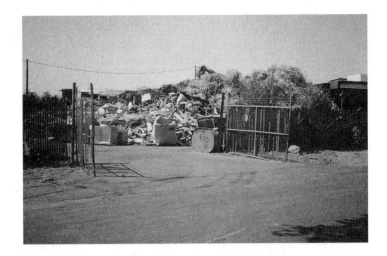

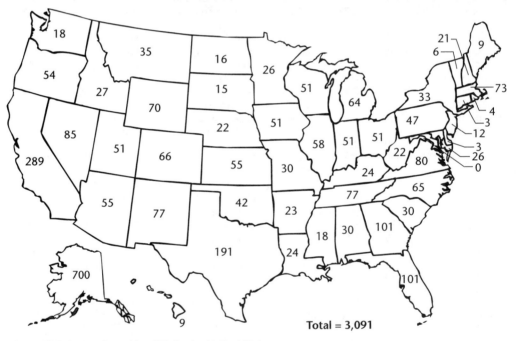

Figure 21.2 Number of landfills in the United States.

(*Source:* Environmental Protection Agency, Office of Solid Waste)

3,186 tons of commercial garbage. For many, this mock-epic garbage journey
became a symbol of the crisis.

By 2010 over three-quarters of all the landfills in the United States will shut
down. In 1979, the United States had 18,500 landfills. In 1998 the EPA estimated
that there were only 2,400 still in operation. Three states report having less than

Table 21.3 Landfill facilities in 1996.

Region	Number of Landfills*	Number of States with Years Capacity Remaining		
		>10 yr	5 to 10 yr	<5 yr
Northeast	208	5	1	3
Southeast	857	11	5	0
Midwest	490	8	4	0
West	827	11	0	0
*U.S. Total**	2,382	35	10	3

*Excludes landfills reported in Alaska (700) and Hawaii (9).

(*Sources: Biocycle,* April 1997 and *Waste Age,* May, 1996)

Table 21.4 Rates of recycling, incineration, and landfilling.

State of Garbage Survey Year	Total Tons Generated	Recycled (%)*	Incinerated (%)	Landfilled (%)
1989	250,000,000	n/a	n/a	n/a
1990	260,000,000	8	8	84
1991	293,613,000	11.5	11.5	77
1992	280,675,000	14	10	76
1993	291,742,000	17	11	72
1994	306,866,000	19	10	71
1995	322,879,000	23	10	67
1996	326,709,000	27	10	63
1997	327,460,000	28	10	62
1998	340,466,000	30	9	61

*Incudes yard trimmings composting

(*Source: Biocycle,* State of Garbage in America)

five years' capacity left (Figure 21.2) (Table 21.3). Waste-management expert, Iraj Zandi believes that this overstates the problem. He says that the landfills that have closed were relatively small and the remaining sites are quite large. The trend is toward operating fewer but larger landfills.[6] The percent of waste, using alternate systems of disposal to dumping, are reported in Table 21.4.

> **Discussion:** Where is the landfill in your community? Does it meet the standards set for the model landfill?

The most common solid wastes as a percentage of total discards is given in Figure 21.3. Paper takes up over 40 percent of the contents of landfills by volume. The two runners-up are construction debris and yard waste, which consists of grass clippings and leaves. Newspapers alone constitute about one-third of the

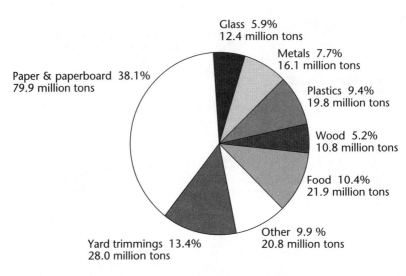

Figure 21.3 Materials generated in landfills by weight.

(*Source:* Environmental Protection Agency, Solid Waste Handbook)

volume of discarded papers; a year's worth of the *New York Times* takes up about 1.5 cubic yards; as much space as 18,660 crushed aluminum cans or 14,969 crushed Big Mac clamshells.[7]

The Healthy People 2000 Objective was to reduce human exposure to solid waste-related water, air, and soil contamination, as measured by a reduction in average pounds of municipal solid waste produced per person each day to no more than 3.6 pounds compared to 4.4 pounds in 1996.

Types of Solid Waste

Most people can identify solid waste when they empty their trash cans. There is much more than household waste that is considered to be solid waste:

1. **Residential**—garbage, trash, food, tires, refrigerators, yard stuff (81.5 million in 1996)

2. **Commercial**—garbage, refuse, wastes, scraps

3. **Municipal**—street litter, auto bodies, sludge, dead animals, fly ash

4. **Institutional and research laboratory**—dressings, blood products, refuse, chemicals

5. **Industrial**—369 tons a year increasing by 3 percent annually. Industrial waste (wood, asphalt, brick, dirt, drywall) should be removed daily to central stations where industrial incinerators' burial sites are located.

6. **Food**—12.5 million tons; decreased from 14.9 in 1960 to 14 million tons in 1996.

7. **Yard**—grass clippings, prunings, 29.8 million tons.

8. **Food processing**—growing, harvesting, processing, and packaging food.

9. **Metal**—scrap metal, 20 million tons a year.

10. **Paper**—41 percent of all waste.

11. **Glass**—2.2 percent of all waste.

12. **Chemical**—145 million pounds include organic and inorganic chemicals.

13. **Rubber**—tires.

14. **Radioactive waste**—low level and high level. Low level are packaged and then shipped for storage to sites licensed by the Energy and Research Development Authority of the United States. By the year 2000, 7.8 million cubic meters of low-level waste will be stockpiled in the United States. High-level waste used to be packaged and shipped. Today it is isolated. No one knows exactly how much radioactive waste exists.

15. **Mining**—2 billion tons of solid waste.

16. **Agricultural waste**—1.5 billion tons of fecal material; 600 million tons of liquid waste. An additional 900 million tons of other agricultural waste.

17. **Recreational waste**—campgrounds = one pound per visitor a day.

18. **Abandoned vehicles**—14.6 million vehicles discarded. A typical vehicle weighs 3,574 pounds. There are 1,309 lbs of light steel, 1,222 lbs of heavy steel, 511 lbs of cast iron, 31 lbs copper, 54 lbs of zinc, 50 lbs of aluminum, 20 lbs lead, 145 lbs rubber, 87 lbs glass, 127 lbs other combustibles, 15 lbs non-combustibles.

19. **Packaging materials**—only 10 percent recycled. In 1990 the average per capita consumption was 680 lbs. 79 million tons produced a year. 66.5 million tons become solid waste—paper, glass, metals, wood, plastics and textiles.

Solid Waste Disposal

The United States produces more garbage and trash than any other nation on earth. On the average, an individual generates nearly 1,300 pounds of solid waste a year. Of the waste produced, 67 percent is disposed in landfills or ocean dumping, 27 percent is recycled, and 6 percent is incinerated.[8] The result of uncontrolled waste disposal is human contamination by toxic residues. Breast milk in nursing women has been found to contain DDT and other pesticides and industrial hydrocarbons that go directly into the fetus, not to mention the accumulation in women's bodies.

Landfills, incineration, and deep well injection are all serious risks to the health of the environment. The United States presently spends about $90 billion per year on pollution control. Despite this attempt to contain pollution, thousands of locales are dangerously polluted by municipal garbage and industrial wastes that contaminate land and air.

Landfill Construction   The modern, state-of-the art, sanitary landfill is designed to eliminate or minimize environmental problems that plagued older landfills. Location is restricted to geologically suitable and stable areas. Many landfills do not meet the current federal and state standards for safe design and operation; only 25 percent monitor groundwater for pollution, and less than 16 percent have natural or artificial liners. Only 5 percent collect the polluted leachate, the gases and fluids that are created by decaying waste. Of those that collect leachate, only 50 percent treat it. Over 50 percent lack controls for water pollution that results from runoff of rainwater from their sites. Less than 50 percent impose restrictions on receipt of bulk liquid waste. Today, 22 percent of sites on the SuperFund list are municipal waste landfills.[9]

Healthy People 2010 Objective: Minimize the Risks to Human Health and the Environment Posed by Hazardous Sites

Target: 98 percent of sites on the following lists:
   National Priority List sites
   Resource Conservation and Recovery Act facilities
   Leaking underground storage facilities
   Brownfield properties

Baseline: 1,200 National Priority List sites; 2,475 Resource Conservation Recovery Act facilities; 370,000 leaking underground storage facilities; 1,500 brownfield properties in 1998.

Landfills are enormous holes situated downwind from major living areas where a community's trash is dumped. The bottom of such a hole is usually covered with a stratified lining of clay or plastic between layers of sand, which in theory prevents the leakage of contaminated fluids known as leachate to be absorbed into the soil and then into the water supply. Overflows of the leachate from the landfills are prevented by drainpipes that are installed at the bottom of the landfill where leachate is pumped out, only to be dumped into another landfill.[11]

Landfills are safeguarded by wells and probes outside the landfill that detect leachate or methane leaks. Methane, nitrogen, and hydrogen sulfide are the by-products of the digestion process of bacteria and fungi that live on rotting food and organic scraps. The average methane molecule can remain in the atmosphere for 12.5 years. While the biodegradation by bacteria and fungi is probably preferable to eternally buried refuse, the combination of methane and carbon dioxide under pressure can explode and be flammable when combined with air in a 5–15 percent concentration. In 1999 there were about 190 methane recovery plants operating in the United States. Pipes that collect explosive methane gas are often pumped from the landfill into a furnace, which heats up a steam generator and produces electricity that can be used in nearby communities. A single large landfill can meet the energy needs of 10,000 families.

Landfills are covered with a six-inch layer of soil daily. When the landfill is full, layers of sand and clay seal in the trash for the next centuries. This land is

---

BOX 21.3 America's Garbage: Shoreline

There are 84,000 miles of shoreline in the United States. Along these shorelines in 1991, 667 pounds of garbage were collected per mile of beach. The most common item left behind was cigarette butts. Smokers seem to think that the world is their ashtray.

In 1990 there were 3,738 syringes found along U.S. shorelines. Although new regulations were made to prevent illegal ocean dumping, there were 8,280 syringes collected from U.S. beaches in 1991.[10]

---

sometimes reclaimed as golf courses, parks, or even housing developments. While covering the landfill may prevent the problem of smelly environments, bacteria need more than just a good supply of biodegradable material to digest garbage. Bacteria need plenty of oxygen from air or water to do their job. Deeply covered landfills may not have enough oxygen to encourage the biodegradation process.[12]

In September 1993, the EPA announced long-awaited requirements for municipal sold waste landfills under Subtitle D of the Resource Conservation Recovery Act. These new rules set stricter requirements for location of landfill, facility design and operation, groundwater monitoring, corrective action, and conditions for closing a landfill.[13] Among the specific requirements:

- Landfills may not be located near wetlands, flood plains, fault areas, seismic zones, or unstable terrain. They may not be located near an airport if birds will present a hazard to airplanes.

- Landfills must keep out regulated hazardous waste, control disease vector populations, monitor methane gas, restrict public access, and keep appropriate records.

- Landfills must have a synthetic liner covering a two-foot clay liner and leachate collection system.

- Landfills must have monitoring wells to detect groundwater contaminations for forty-five organic chemicals and fifteen metals.

- Landfill owners or operators must show they have the financial means to close, care, and clean up landfills.

On-Site Volume Reduction Alternatives[14]   There are a few suggestions for reducing the need for landfills that include disposing of solid waste on site. These include:

1. **Composting**—reduces solid waste to one-quarter of its original volume. It also may be used as a soil conditioner. The first municipal composting took place in India in 1925. They are popular in Europe but not very successful in the United States.

2. **Pulping**—paper wastes are ground in water and squeezed semi-dry.

3. **Compacting**—creates a reduction of waste by 75 percent.

4. **Incineration**—reduces volume up to 90 percent. Remainder must be disposed as solid waste. Approximately 2 to 15 percent of municipal waste in the United States is incinerated in combustion facilities.

Incineration   Burning trash has universally been a method of garbage disposal for centuries. This practice, utilized in the 1950s, led to fires that burned for weeks. Today, approximately 150 facilities burn between 50 and 1,000 tons of trash a day at about 1,500 degrees in the primary chamber.

Unfortunately, the product of burning has been air pollution and many cities ultimately chose to use landfills instead of burning, especially as trash became far more toxic and hazardous to human health. However, as landfills became filled to overflowing, the idea of burning waste and trash seemed to become a viable option. Approximately 70 to 80 percent of residential and commercial solid waste is combustible. If all the solid waste in the United States were converted into energy, and pollution were prevented, it would equal more than 206 million barrels of oil per year. See Figure 21.4, an illustration of a typical, modern incinerator.

> **Discussion:** Is there an incinerator in your community? What does it burn? If you do not have an incinerator, would you promote and encourage a community incinerator?

Modern incineration involves controlled burning at very high temperatures (over 1,000 degrees) in special facilities called resource recovery plants. These facilities create essentially no visible emissions or odors and produce ash that must be disposed. Figure 21.5 on page 586 is a schematic of a modern resource recovery plant.

There are presently 150 incinerators now operating and about 200 under construction in the United States. Battles by communities against medical waste incinerators are being waged nationwide. In the South Bronx, New York, community leaders have called a new $20 million, 48 tons a day, medical waste incinerator "a classic form of environmental racism. You have a community that is already saturated with toxic wastes and industrial facilities and this is just another health hazard."[15] Location for such facilities is not an easy decision.

Medical tests and studies show links between toxic pollution and birth defects, heart problems, and other illnesses, but rarely have the federal health agencies drawn the same conclusions. This may be a result of sampling errors, biased researchers, and studying wrong symptoms the Campaign Fund reports by agency studies.

In addition to the environmental and personal health effects of hazardous waste, class and race issues need public attention as well, as mentioned earlier. Few communities want to serve as a dumping ground for toxic waste; studies have noted the disproportionate number of landfills and hazardous waste facilities in poor and minority areas. A study, *Toxic Wastes and Race in the United States*, came to the following conclusion:

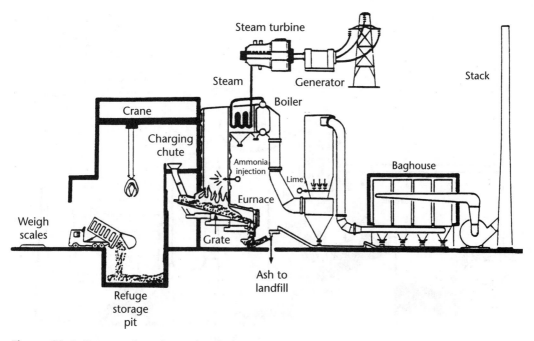

Figure 21.4 Cutaway view of a modern incinerator.

(*Source:* U.S. EPA, Guidelines for local governments on solid waste management, Washington, DC, 1971, p. 84)

> *Race proved to be the most significant factor among variables tested in associa-*
> *tion with the location of commercial hazardous waste facilities. This represents*
> *a consistent national pattern. In communities with two or more facilities or one*
> *of the nation's five largest landfills, the average minority percentage of the pop-*
> *ulation was more than 3 times that of communities without facilities (38 per-*
> *cent vs. 12 percent). (p. 149).*[16]

Nearly one in six Americans lives within four miles of a hazardous waste site. Those living so close to hazardous sites are often people of color and/or low income. They are often those who do not have the political clout to prevent the intrusion of this risk into their neighborhood. Often, these communities, like small Native American reservations, encourage toxic waste dumping near their neighborhoods to assist in economic survival of dying communities. These sites often provide much needed employment and an improved economic base.

Burning gets rid of a huge volume of garbage—at least three-quarters of it goes up in smoke. One-third is dumped as ash in a landfill. In theory, inciner-ators should be able to create enough heat to create steam which then can be used as a resource for heating buildings or driving turbines that generate elec-tricity. Although this may sound like a great idea, incinerators still pose the

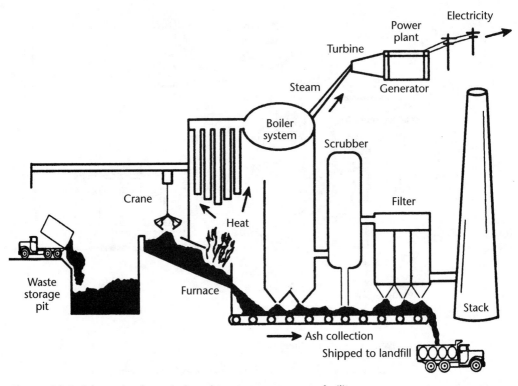

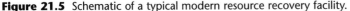

Figure 21.5 Schematic of a typical modern resource recovery facility.

(*Source:* Environmental Protection Agency)

problems of potentially smelly, sooty neighborhoods, and potentially deadly air pollution. Medical waste, biological waste, chemical waste, and many human-made products, such as plastics, that are burned emit dangerous and deadly chemical by-products. High standard incinerators of the types used in Europe or Japan may make incineration a viable option, however, until incineration proponents can convince communities of their safety, it will be a slowly emerging technology in the United States.

The controversial Bronx incinerator is said to remove "99 percent of *most* pollutant particles. Critics of incineration believe that emissions that may be acceptable elsewhere are not necessarily acceptable in a community that already has the highest rate of tuberculosis and asthma in the country."[19] Further, because 85–95 percent of all medical waste is not truly contaminated, opponents say incineration is unnecessary. Proponents believe new high-tech scrubbers and filters make incineration the safest way to get rid of medical waste at a time when overflowing landfills are being forced to close.

The principal consequence of incineration is the transporting of the communities' garbage, in gaseous form, through the air to neighboring communities, across state lines, and indeed to the atmosphere of the entire globe, where it will linger for many years. A second consequence is the 10 percent of remaining ash that is highly toxic, and actually more hazardous than the larger volume of waste before incineration.[20]

Off-Site Alternative to Landfills[21]

Disposal at sea has been cited as an alternative to landfills. To date, inadequate data exist concerning the amount of solid waste dumped into the oceans each year. Industrial waste accounted for 5.3 million tons, sewage sludge for 6.5 million tons, construction and demolition waste for 2.3 million tons, and harbor dredging for 52 million tons. In addition, at least twenty coastal cities have utilized the ocean for dumping. These include Seattle, Portland, San Francisco, Los Angeles, San Diego, Houston, New York, Philadelphia, Baltimore, Boston, and Mobile.

Ocean dumping has included sediments from dredging of canals, industrial waste refuse from canneries, low-level radioactive material placed in weighted fifty-five gallon drums, construction and demolition waste, and contaminated products. Before 1972 ocean dumping was unregulated. A 1988 Marine Protection Act was amended to set up a framework for ending ocean disposal of sewage sludge and industrial waste by December 31, 1991.

In 1970 Jacques Cousteau, the underwater explorer, said: "In thirty years of diving I have seen this slow death everywhere under the water. In the last twenty years, life in our oceans has diminished by 40 percent. If it continues, I predict that humans have only fifty more years on the planet."[22] Some calculate the cycle time of the oceans (evaporation, clouds, rain, percolation down into groundwater, and eventual return to the rivers and back to the ocean) to

---

BOX 21.4 *Ecological Racism—Case Study*

In October 1991, 500 protesters poured into Kettleman City, California, a truck-stop community on Interstate 5 between Los Angeles and San Francisco. Led by the Rev. Jesse Jackson, the local residents of the predominantly Hispanic community joined to rally against a plan to build the state's first toxic-waste incinerator about four miles outside of town. Nobody has the right to engage in chemical warfare upon the people, Jackson thundered. This is toxic racism. Two months later a California judge temporarily blocked the plan, citing the civil rights of Hispanics as one of the reasons.[17]

The buzzword to describe these areas is LULUs or "locally undesirable land uses"

such as landfills, incinerators, petrochemical plants, and sewage treatment facilities. The controversy between environmental activists and the EPA is whether or not LULUs are the result of racism or poverty, low property values, and lack of political power since the EPA says whites are also widely victimized. The United Church of Christ, however, reported that three in five Blacks and three in five Hispanics live in neighborhoods near abandoned toxic waste sites. Data show that the minority population is 60 percent higher and population value is 38percent lower than the national average in areas where incinerators exist.[18]

be about 2,000 years. Cousteau was reporting only the first visible consequences of ocean pollution. It will take 2,000 years to learn the total impact.[23]

In 1986, a barge, the "Khian Sea," loaded 28 million pounds of toxic incinerator ash from Philadelphia. The ship attempted unsuccessfully to discharge all
over the Caribbean. After dumping 4 million of the 28 million pounds of ash in
Haiti, it continued its voyage. In September 1988, the Khian Sea was sighted in
the Suez Canal. In October 1988, the captain sent a message saying the ash had
been discharged. Since no country admits to having accepted the load of toxic
ash, it appears clear that it was dumped illegally at sea.

Sludge dumping in the ocean is more controversial because some believe it
is relatively benign. Municipal sludge is an essential part of municipal sewage disposal and much of coastal city sludge ends up in our oceans. Municipalities generate about 7 million dry tons of wastewater sludge a year. Sludge production was
expected to double to about 13 million dry tons a year by the year 2000.[24]

Unfortunately, the synergistic effect of many synthetic chemicals, pesticides,
metals, and medical wastes do, in fact, affect the health of the ocean. Sludge contains over 200 different substances including toxic metals, organic chemicals,
and pathogenic organisms. Dumped sludge has caused diseased lobsters and
crabs and a general drop in the Rhode Island fishing industry deepwater catches.

Although sludge dumping is now illegal in the U.S., it still continues
throughout the world.

Recycling

Developed countries use about 80 percent of the world's mineral and energy
resources, and generate most of the world's pollution and waste. At present,
Americans recycle, or burn to generate heat or electricity, only 28 percent of all
solid waste we collect. This leaves 89 percent for disposal. In 1999 there were
9,000 curbside recycle programs and 102 combustion-to-energy programs
(incineration) in the United States.[25]

As is often the case, when developed countries feel at risk by something, it
is shipped to poorer countries to maintain U.S. business interests. Garbage is no
exception. In February 1988, more Philadelphia incinerator ash was shipped to
Guinea on the west coast of Africa than was dumped in Philadelphia. Chemicals dumped by Italian ships contaminated large areas of farmland in Nigeria.
Spreading poisonous waste from richer nations to poorer ones makes no sense
in the global picture. Since 1989, forty-five countries have banned the import-
ing of garbage from other countries. Despite treaties, illegal dumping in developing countries continues without much reduction.

On the homefront, the United States is a throwaway society that must be
converted to a matter-recycling society. Unfortunately, recycling matter
requires high-quality energy that cannot be recycled.

Discussion: What are your state's laws regarding recycling? Are they
enforced? Are they adequate?

Some nonrenewable resources such as copper, aluminum, iron, and glass can be recycled by communities interested in reducing waste and pollution. About 70 percent of all metal is used just once and then discarded. Only 30 percent is recycled making "our refuse richer than some of our natural ores."[26] Presently one in every fifteen bottles is recycled.

> *Healthy People 2010 Objective:* Increase Recycling of Municipal Solid Waste
>
> *Target:* 38 percent of municipal solid waste generated.
>
> *Baseline:* 27 percent of total municipal solid waste generated was recycled in 1996 (includes composting).

Products That Can Be Recycled

Plastic Plastic is not a natural material. It is synthesized from petro-chemicals to create a long, complicated chain of atoms called polymers. The weight of plastics used in packaging in the United States more than doubled between 1974 and 1990 and was expected to triple by 1995. In 1990, about 25 million barrels of oil were used to produce plastic packaging in the United States. Plastics account for 8 percent of the weight and approximately 20 percent of the volume of municipal landfills. Plastic also accounts for 60 percent of debris found on U.S. beaches.

Bacteria and fungi that would usually live on the decaying waste of natural food, fauna, and flora cannot digest these polymers. Instead, toxic cadmium and lead compounds used as binders can leach out of plastics and ooze into groundwater and surface water in unlined or failed landfills. Unfortunately, plastic is one of the most common non-biodegradable wastes deposited in landfills.

There are a number of plastic items that create great decomposition problems; among them are diapers, grocery bags, balloons, and soda can rings. Today only 5 percent of all plastic containers are recycled. Typical products made from plastic are given in Table 21.5. Additionally, there are five different types of raw plastic material called resins. Each resin has different strengths or flexibility, making general recycling of plastics difficult.

As far as diapers go, the plastic lining and adhesive in a disposable diaper will survive for centuries. Public health is also concerned about the fecal material that is disposed in the diaper. The possible transmission of viral and bacte-

Table 21.5 Typical plastic scrap-molding products.

Shoe soles	Bicycle pedals
Luggage handles	Lawnmower wheels
Suction pump	Doorstops
Seals	Dog toys
Toy animals	Cable housing
Bicycle saddles	Auto parts

rial pathogens in body waste pose a health risk to sanitation workers. Although viruses will probably not survive burial in anaerobic landfills, many bacteria will thrive in such an environment and may leak into groundwater.

A washable cotton diaper can be reused up to 200 times and then be recycled. Fecal waste can be disposed of properly in the sewage system. Laundering cotton diapers, however, produces nine times as much air pollution and ten times as much water pollution as disposable diapers do in their lifetime. Over a lifetime, cloth diapers also consume six times more water and three times more energy than disposables. From an environmental standpoint, neither product has a clear edge, but economically, a diaper service is less expensive than disposable diapers.

Plastic threatens the lives of millions of marine animals who get entangled in plastic netting and soda can six-pack rings. Autopsied marine animals have revealed intestines full of non-biodegradable plastic. In one dead sea turtle was found a golf tee, shreds of bags, pieces of fishing line, a plastic flower, part of a bottle cap, and dozens of small chips of Styrofoam and hard plastic. As the turtle's stomach filled with indigestible trash, the turtle starved to death. Other marine mammals and birds have suffocated, strangled, and been poisoned by the plastic waste (such as six-pack can rings or balloons) that has been expelled into the oceans and into the air. Those who fish currently dump around 175,000 tons of plastic into the oceans each year. It is thought that as many as a million sea birds and 100,000 marine mammals in just the northern Pacific Ocean die each year from eating or becoming entangled in plastic waste. Many more marine life are poisoned in the Atlantic Ocean and Baltic Sea by raw sewage, chemical waste, and pesticide waste flowing from rivers into these water bodies.

Tires There are about 800 million old tire sitting in piles around the U.S. Ohio ranks number one in piles with 100 million. Discarded tires pose two particular vector health threats to a community: rats and mosquitoes. Tires create an excellent breeding place for rats and mosquitoes, which in turn carry diseases to humans.

An automobile tire contains about 2.5 gallons of oil, which has the potential to produce, en masse, enough electricity to serve a small town. Unfortunately, when tires burn in an uncontrolled environment, they are extremely difficult to contain or extinguish. There are actually some tire graveyards that have been burning for years. Although 15 million old tires are recycled each year, the number of recycled tires is actually going down each year as new blends of rubber and steel-belted tires cannot use recycled tires. Even some great ideas have drawbacks, however. In one community, a company is recycling tires into paving material. Unfortunately the recycling company is literally in someone's neighborhood backyard and poses a possible health risk to adjacent neighbors. Further, some paving tires have caught fire and caused smoking, toxic pavements.

Paper Paper is the single most frequently seen item in most landfills, taking up more land space than even diapers. It accounts for more than 40 percent of a

---

BOX 21.5 America's Garbage: Paper Junkmail

In 1987, 10 billion mail-order catalogs alone were stuffed into mailboxes. Most end up as trash. Add these catalogs to the enormous amount of paper junkmail that is delivered and disposed of daily in the United States.

---

landfill's contents. Newspapers alone may take up as much as 13 to 30 percent of the space in landfills. It is not enough to just change from paper grocery bags to recyclable cloth bags. Garbage archeologists from the University of Arizona have discovered that most materials buried deep in a landfill change very little. Newspapers from the 1950s could still be read in 2001. Paper in landfills does not biodegrade; it mummifies.

Paper may be one of the most recyclable waste products. Typical products made from recycled paper are shown in Figure 21.6. If the *New York Times* printed just one Sunday edition on recycled instead of new paper, 75,000 trees would be saved.[28] It is not surprising to environmentalists who seek this kind of recycling to discover that the *Times* is part owner of three paper mills that manufacture only new paper. Business interests and government regulations often

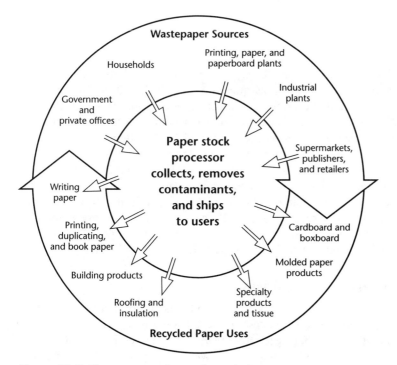

Figure 21.6 The sources and uses of recycled paper.

(*Source:* Lipták, B. (1991). *Municipal waste disposal in the 1990s.* Radnor, PA: Chilton, p. 334)

Table 21.6 Generation and recovery of municipal wastes (1996).

	Weight Generated	Weight Recovered	Recovery as a Percent of Generation
Paper & paperboard	79.9	32.6	40.8%
Glass	12.4	3.2	25.7%
Metals			
Ferrous metals	11.8	4.5	38.0%
Aluminum	3.0	1.0	34.3%
Other nonferrous metals	1.3	0.8	66.8%
Total metals	16.1	6.4	39.6%
Plastics	19.8	1.1	5.3%
Rubber & leather	6.2	0.6	9.5%
Textiles	7.7	1.0	12.3%
Wood	10.8	0.5	4.5%
Other materials	3.7	0.8	21.2%
Total Materials in Products	156.6	46.0	29.4%
Other wastes			
Food wastes	21.9	0.5	2.4%
Yard trimmings	28.0	10.8	38.6%
Miscellaneous inorganic wastes	3.2	Neg.	Neg.
Total Other Wastes	53.1	11.3	21.3%
TOTAL MUNICIPAL SOLID WASTE	209.7	57.3	27.3%

(*Source:* Natural Resources Defense Council)

make it easier for manufacturers to rely on new materials than to recycle used ones. President Ronald Reagan was quoted as saying that "trees pollute." His administration felt that the protection of the logging industry was in the best interest of America, despite its impact on the environment. Admittedly, the issue is a difficult one, especially during the 1980s and 1990s when jobs were scarce and the economies of lumber states like Oregon and Washington were in crisis.

A concurrent problem is the cost of recycling paper. To establish a newsprint recycling mill it takes three to five years and costs from $300 to $500 million to build. Can the capital investment be recouped if there is no community plan to market the recycled paper? If economic incentives were given to creative entrepreneurs, more products could easily be developed. The amount of waste recovered and recycled from most sources is given in Table 21.6.

Infectious and Medical Waste

In the summer of 1988, syringes, IV tubing, and prescription bottles washed up on the shores of five east coast states. The result was that beaches were closed and the population was outraged. Investigation of this pollution found that infectious wastes from medical institutions were largely unregulated and that the ocean was one of the most common waste dumps for infectious waste.[28]

Many wondered if the deaths of many marine mammals such as whales, dolphins, and seals was not directly related to now infectious waters. A result of this incident was the Medical Waste Tracking Act of 1988. This act requires the EPA to reduce the threat posed by medical wastes to human health and the environment. New regulations now impose certain packaging requirements as well as require the tracking of medical waste from point of generation to point of disposal. Few states have issued their own regulations. It is estimated that 3.2 million tons of infectious and medical waste are generated every year. Classification of regulated medical wastes is given in Table 21.7.

Medical waste can be divided into two main categories, regular medical waste and infectious waste. Regular medical wastes are generally everything non-medical used in the facility. This might include administrative waste, paper, or cafeteria discard.[29]

Infectious waste (10–15 percent of waste) includes human blood and blood products, cultures and stocks of infectious agents, pathological wastes, contaminated sharps (hypodermic needles, scalpel blades, capillary tubes), contaminated laboratory wastes, contaminated wastes from patient care, discarded biologicals, contaminated animal carcasses and body parts infected with human pathogens such as in research and training, contaminated equipment, and miscellaneous infectious waste.[30]

Regular waste goes through normal trash collection and ends up in a landfill. Infectious waste can be treated and then incinerated. Treatment includes steam sterilization, microwave heating, and chemical treatments, all followed by land filling.[31] Most hospitals have incinerators on site and have skilled individuals who run them.

The need for infectious and medical waste management now reaches beyond hospitals and medical centers to smaller waste generators such as clinics, colleges and universities, diagnostic laboratories, funeral homes, doctor's offices, and other health facilities (500,000 tons a year). Infectious and medical waste produce occupational risks such as direct exposure to blood products, needle sticks, and infectious dressings by patients, visitors, and workers. Environmental risks include the possibility of waste to groundwater, surface water, or air. Even small amounts of laboratory solvents can leach into drinking water. Incinerated medical waste may not destroy infectious agents, releasing them into the air, in the ash, or via scrubber effluent.[32]

Prevention of contamination by infectious waste requires:

1. Proper packaging of sharps, solids, and liquids.

2. Proper waste handling practices of collection and transportation.

3. Safe waste storage in sealed containers with limited access and proper labeling.

4. Proper waste treatment. Proper waste treatment may include incineration, steam, or gas sterilization.

Table 21.7 Classes of regulated medical waste.

Class	Description
Cultures and stocks	Cultures and stocks of infectious agents. Includes: ■ Cultures from medical and pathological laboratories ■ Cultures and stocks of infectious agents from research and industrial laboratories ■ Wastes from the production of biologicals ■ Discarded live and attenuated vaccines ■ Culture dishes and devices used to transfer, inoculate, and mix cultures
Pathological wastes	Human pathological wastes. Includes: ■ Tissues, organs, and body parts and body fluids that are removed during autopsy or surgery or other medical procedures ■ Specimens of body fluids and their containers
Human blood and blood products	■ Liquid waste human blood ■ Products of blood ■ Items saturated and/or dripping with human blood ■ Items that were saturated and/or dripping with human blood that are now caked with dried human blood Includes: ■ Serum, plasma, and other blood components, and their containers, which were used or intended for use in either patient care, testing, and laboratory analysis or the development of pharmaceuticals ■ Intravenous bags
Sharps	Sharps that have been used in animal or human patient care or treatment or in medical, research, or industrial laboratories. Includes: ■ Hypodermic needles ■ Syringes (with or without the attached needle) ■ Pasteur pipettes ■ Scalpel blades ■ Blood vials ■ Needles with attached tubing ■ Culture dishes (regardless of presence of infectious agents) ■ Other types of broken or unbroken glassware that were in contact with infectious agents, such as used slides and cover slips
Animal waste	Contaminated animal carcasses, body parts, and bedding of animals that were known to have been exposed to infectious agents during research (including research in veterinary hospitals), production of biologicals, or testing of pharmaceuticals
Isolation wastes	■ Biological waste and discarded materials contaminated with blood, excretion, exudates, or secretions from humans who are isolated to protect others from certain highly communicable diseases ■ Such materials from isolated animals known to be infected with highly communicable diseases
Unused sharps	The following unused, discarded sharps ■ Hypodermic needles ■ Suture needles ■ Syringes ■ Scalpel blades

(*Source:* Reinhart, Peter A., & Gordon, Judith G., 1991. *Infectious and medical waste management.* Copyright 1991. Chelsea, MI: Lewis Publishers. Used with permission)

Other Hazardous Waste

Hazardous waste is defined by the Resource Conservation Recovery Act as a solid waste or combination of solid wastes that because of their quantity, concentration, physical, chemical, or infectious characteristics may:

1. Cause or contribute to an increase in mortality or serious irreversible or incapacitating reversible illness.

2. Pose a substantial present or potential hazard to human health or the environment when improperly treated, stored, transported, or disposed.

The EPA has four characteristics of hazardous waste:

1. **Ignitability**—a flash point less than 140 degrees F, a non-liquid capable under normal conditions of spontaneous combustion, an ignitable compressed gas.

2. **Corrosivity**—a solid waste that is an igneous material with pH less than or equal to 2 or greater than or equal to 12.5, or a liquid that corrodes steel at a rate greater than one-fourth inch per year at a temperature of 130 degrees.

3. **Reactivity**—reacts violently without detonating, reacts violently with water, forms an explosive mixture with water, contains cyanide or sulfide at a pH between 2 and 12.5, capable of detonation at standard temperature and pressure.

4. **Extraction procedure (EP) toxicity**—leaching hazardous concentrations of a particular toxic into the groundwater. Many people may be surprised at how many toxic and hazardous materials are found in the home.

Discussion: How does your community assist in the collection and disposal of toxins found in the home?

In the United States, there are an estimated 650,000 commercial and industrial sources of hazardous waste. The EPA believes that 99 percent of this waste comes from only 2 percent of the sources. According to the United Nations Environmental Programme, more than 7 million chemicals have now been discovered or created by humankind. Most troubling is that many of the new chemical waste compounds are never tested for their potential toxicity.[33] According to Helen Caldicott, internationally known peace advocate, complete health studies have been done on only 1,600 of 70,000 industrial chemicals now being used by U.S. companies. Everyday, industries produce the equivalent of nearly thirty pounds of toxic waste for every man, woman, and child in the country.[34] There are an average of nineteen toxic chemical accidents a day in the United States. Seventy-five percent of these accidents are at industrial facilities and 25 percent occur in transport. The chance a person will receive an immediate injury from a chemical spill is one in sixteen.[35]

About 70 percent of our hazardous waste comes from the mid-Atlantic, Great Lakes, and Gulf Coast areas of the United States. Biological waste includes pathological hospital waste (170,000 tons annually) and biological warfare agents (anthrax, mustard gas) and pesticides.[36]

Improper disposal and discharge into surface waters is one of the greatest risks. The National Toxic Campaign Fund has concluded that the health implications of toxic waste sites have not been properly studied or considered in toxic cleanup. "There are big gaps in scientific data on what the link is between exposure and specific health effects."[37]

This is little comfort for citizens of Alsen, Louisiana, who have had breathing problems, burning eyes, nosebleeds, asthma, and cancers since a chemical dump opened in 1980 and another in 1994. The Campaign Fund reports that the Agency for Toxic Substances and Disease Registry did a general health assessment of this predominantly black, low-income community in 1991. However, it never did a cancer study, although one citizen claims to have four of nine families on her street with cancers.

Medical tests and studies show links between toxic pollution and birth defects, heart problems, and other illnesses, but rarely have the federal health agencies drawn the same conclusions. This may be a result of sampling errors, biased researchers, and studying wrong symptoms the Campaign Fund reports by agency studies.

Nuclear Waste

Nuclear energy has become our greatest source of power to generate electricity. Power from atomic fission is produced in a silent machine called a nuclear reactor, atomic reactor, or atomic pile. In this machine, splitting atoms of uranium serves as a source of heat to boil water and produce steam. Atomic reactors are like special furnaces. The primary advantage of atomic energy for power is that a small amount of fuel can produce a great deal of power.[38] The greatest drawbacks of atomic energy are the potential for human exposure and the disposal of the waste products that are produced. Since 1945 atomic energy has become not only a blessing to medicine, agriculture, and industry, but a potential community health risk.

The consumption of nuclear energy has grown rapidly, worldwide, partly due to the population increases, use of energy for industry, agriculture, and medicine. Now that we have nuclear energy, even given the potential risks and difficulties associated with waste, it is hard to imagine giving up this "clean" source energy.[39] Nuclear energy has two key advantages: nuclear power does not involve chemical combustion, and the process encloses rather than scatters wastes that are produced. When compared to coal mining, the environmental impact of uranium may be less severe because less uranium is needed for the production of energy as compared with coal. Again, the by-product of this production is "cleaner" than coal.[40]

While much good has come from radiation, especially in treating cancers, the lack of responsible environmental sensitivity to the long-term effects of radium has resulted in one of the major environmental conundrums of our time—how to dispose of radioactive waste, one of many hazardous waste products of the twentieth century.

There is no shortage of ideas on how to dispose of radioactive waste. Scientists have proposed burying it under Antarctic ice sheets, injecting it into the seabed, and shooting it into outer space. Scientists have increasingly fallen back on the idea of burying radioactive waste hundreds of meters deep in the earth's crust, arguing that geological burial is the "best, safest long-term option." Although the Nuclear Energy Commission (NEC) sees geological burial as safe, it is nothing more than a calculated risk. Future changes in geology, land use, settlement patterns, and climate will affect the ability to isolate nuclear safety. Even the NEC admits that the process is "more complicated than had been thought."[41]

The health effects of radiation exposure are known and the evidence of increases in morbidity and mortality rates in countries that now use nuclear energy, although controversial, should be considered in looking at the potential risk of the hazardous waste that clean nuclear energy produces. Nikolai Dubinian, head of the Soviet Institute of General Genetics noted that the percentage of children in industrialized countries born with congenital defects more than doubled between 1956 and 1977. In 1998 to 1999 the WHO estimated that the global human mutation rate, sometimes called the **genetic load,** averaged 6 percent of offspring, with the highest rates in developing countries. The United Nations Council for Radiation reported that the global genetic load had reached 10.8 percent by 1977, close to a doubling of the mutation rate experienced over centuries, in just ten years.[42] This genetic mutation is not isolated to humans. The increase in mistakes of reproduction also occurs in plants and animals. Half the fish in areas polluted by toxic chemicals fail to spawn and suffer from weakened immune systems.

Hazardous Waste Cleanup—SuperFund

Hazardous waste is a unique problem of the last four decades. The rate of hazardous waste generation is growing at about 10 percent annually (12 million tons a year). These waste products cannot be disposed of in traditional ways such as in municipal landfills. In 1980, the federal government passed Super-Fund legislation budgeted at 1.6 billion dollars that was aimed at cleaning up many decades of irresponsible mining and disposal of radioactive waste, hazardous ore, chemical and oil spills, dumping and refuge. Of the 35,000 identified and possibly 2 million actual chemical hazardous waste sites, only 1,300 are even eligible for review by the EPA. By 1997, only thirty of the nation's 1,252 most dangerous waste sites were cleaned up. The EPA reports construction and cleanup of 750 sites.

Most would consider the SuperFund a failure since the money spent seems to lack results. The eventual cost was estimated, in 1993, at over $400 billion. It has become a gold mine for lawyers and consultants who have been hired to represent these sites to determine who should pay for cleanup. Since many sites were created as long as forty years ago, finding records to prove who has owned and operated a waste site, who sent what waste and how much, and where this waste is has become expensive and time-consuming. There were a total of 1,227 National Priority SuperFund sites in November, 2001.

Discussion: Are there any hazardous waste sites in your community? Why have they been classified as a hazardous waste site?

Click on the map as shown at this web site and see where the SuperFund sites are in your state:

www.epa.gov/superfund/sites/npl/npl.htm

Since the cleanup costs an average of $26 million per site and some sites cost hundreds of millions, cleaning up has more often become capping a chemical dump site, storing waste elsewhere, or replacing wells with alternate water supply systems. Ergo, most hazardous sites have not been cleaned up. An administrator of the U.S. Environmental Protection Agency commented, "One of the sad truths about the program is that so much money has gone to people in three-piece suits and not moon suits."[43] In other words, there has been much talk, little action.

BOX 21.6 States with Majority SuperFund of Sites

New Jersey	100	Florida	51	Illinois	39
Pennsylvania	97	Washington	43	Indiana	37
California	88	Minnesota	40	Ohio	36
Michigan	81	Wisconsin	39	Texas	28
New York	76				

(*Source:* Environmental Protection Agency)

Summary

The two most frequently used methods of solid waste disposal in the United States are landfills and incineration. While ocean dumping still occurs, it is illegal. Unfortunately, landfills are almost full and convenient space for new landfills is scarce. The fear from many communities about incineration, as well as the cost of incineration construction, makes this method controversial and problematic. In the future, recycling may be the most correct, efficient, and safe means of solid waste disposal. It will also be a primary means of reducing air, water, and soil contamination.

Recycling, when compared to energy use and containment production of original manufacture, results in lower energy consumption, reduced water use, and less air and water contamination. Concerted efforts by private citizens; local, state and federal governments; public health departments; and community associations would facilitate achievement of the Healthy People 2010 objectives and preempt an enormous and overwhelming problem.

Technology has given the planet the gift of efficient, creative means of harnessing and using energy, especially nuclear and radioactive energy. Unfortunately, the demand for this energy and the desire to use it now appears to exceed our ability to cope with the environmental and health implications of waste disposal. Early processes left soil, water, and buildings contaminated in ways that may never be restored or cleaned up completely.

The government's primary means of correcting past problems is the Super-Fund program which in 2000 has completed the cleanup of 206 priority hazardous locations. The cost of this cleanup has escalated far beyond initial estimates and the probability of ever cleaning up the many hazardous waste sites, in the United States alone, seems slim.

The best hope for the future is to anticipate and prevent the excesses and errors of the past. Until proper, safe waste disposal is available, nuclear energy and the use of toxic, hazardous wastes must be implemented with all stakeholders, both human and non-human, considered.

CYBERSITES RELATED TO CHAPTER 21

Pollution
> www.epa.gov/tri
> www.worldbank.org/nipr

Hazardous Substances
> www.atsdr.cdc.gov/toxfaq/html (Tox FAQs)
> www.atsdr.cdc.gov/hazdat.html (HazDat Database)

QUESTIONS

1. What are the primary risks to human health associated with solid waste dumping?

2. If you could design a recycling program for your community, what would be the primary components?

3. What would be the personal, political, and social factors associated with changing behavior of others in terms of waste disposal?

4. What are the setbacks or regressions citizens make if they terminate the use of nuclear energy today and convert to other forms of energy? Do costs exceed benefits?

5. What are the pros and cons of communities allowing hazardous waster to be stored in their "backyard"?

EXERCISES

1. Recycle, reuse, and reduce solid waste for a week. Keep a diary of what you do, how you do it, and the pros and cons of each of your efforts. How are recycling, reuse, and reduction done in your community? What is the community response? What other initiatives would you suggest to your community?

2. Go to the library and look at the literature about the history of the Trojan Nuclear Power Plant in Oregon. What were the debates for building the plant? What was the economic effect of the plant on Oregon? What was the plant's history during its use? Were there accidents? What were the health implications of the Trojan plant? What happened to the plant? Would you like a nuclear power plant in your state? Why or why not?

3. Obtain from your state environmental health agency a list of toxic waste sites in your community. Compare these locations with census data on average income, racial, and ethnic demographic figures. What conclusions can you draw about your own community?

INTERNET INTERACTIVE ACTIVITY

ATSDR, THE HAZDAT DATABASE

HazDat Database

ATSDR: Hazardous Substance Release and Health Effects Database

HazDat, the **Agency for Toxic Substances and Disease Registry's** Hazardous Substance Release/Health Effects Database, is the scientific and administrative database developed to provide access to information on the release of hazardous substances from SuperFund sites or from emergency events and on the effects of hazardous substances on the health of human populations. The following information is included in HazDat: site characteristics, activities and site events, contaminants found, contaminant media and maximum concentration levels, impact on population, community health concerns, ATSDR public health threat categorization, ATSDR recommendations, environmental fate of hazardous substances, exposure routes, and physical hazards at the site/event. In addition, HazDat contains substance-specific information such as the ATSDR Priority List of Hazardous Substances, health effects by route and duration of exposure, metabolites, interactions of substances, susceptible populations, and biomarkers of exposure and effects. HazDat also contains data from the U.S. Environmental Protection Agency (EPA) Comprehensive Environmental Response, Compensation, and Liability Information System (CERCLIS) database, including site CERCLIS number, site description, latitude/longitude, operable units, and additional site information

The address for HazDat is

www.atsdr.cdc.gov/gsql/siteact.script

Example

For this exercise the community health educator wants to know what waste storage treatment sites are on the Priority list of Hazardous Substances for Louisiana.

1. Go to www.atsdr.cdc.gov/gsql/siteact.script

2. Select

   Louisiana
   All Sites
   Final, Proposed, Non Priority
   All Facility Types

3. Click **Submit**

You should get a response that looks something like this:

Query Results: 41 Records Found

site_id	site_name	to_docs	to_chems
LAD981056997	AGRICULTURE STREET LANDFILL	—» 9	—» 204
LAD000239814	AMERICAN CREOSOTE WORKS, INC (WINNFIELD)	—» 1	—» 20
LAD985172022	ASCENSION PARISH OLD HIGHWAY 429 LANDFIL		
LAD980745632	BAYOU BONFOUCA	—» 2	—» 226
LAD981916570	BAYOU D'INDE		—» 2
LA0001187491	BROUSSARD CHEMICAL CO.		
LA0002368173	CALCASIEU ESTUARY	—» 5	—» 22
LAD985169978	CAMPBELL WELLS CORPORATION		

You now know that there are forty-one hazardous waste sites in Louisiana and you know the name of the cite, its location, and how to access the documentation regarding the danger of this site.

Exercise

Using ADSTR look up the priority hazardous waste sites and non-priority waste sites for your state by

   mining
   government
   waste storage

What makes the sites on the Hazardous List in your state dangerous?

What is your city doing to clean up these sites?

What is the estimated cost to clean up the sites in your state?

Are any of the sites in your State Priority sites? Why?

Use the Data Dictionary at the end of the home page to understand the abbreviations on your printout.

REFERENCES

1. Hadingham, Evan & Janet (1990). *Garbage! Where it comes from, Where it goes.* New York: Simon & Schuster.

2. ZWA's 1998 State of the Nation's Waste. www.zerowasteamerica.org/1998StateOfNation.htm

3. Rybczynski, Witold (1992). *We are what we throw away.* *New York Times* Book Review, 5 July, pp. 5–6.

4. Rathje, William (1992). *Rubbish! The archeology of garbage.* New York: Harper Collins.

5. Hadingham, op. cit.

6. Rathje, op. cit.

7. Rybczynski, op. cit.

8. www.epa.gov/epaoswer/non-hw/muncpl/mswrpt97/msw97re.pdf

9. The whiff of discrimination (1992). *U.S. News and World Report,* May 4, p. 35.

10. *U.S. News and World Report,* June 15, 1992. Database.

11. Bonaparte, Rudolph (1990). *Waste containment systems: Construction, regulation, and performance.* New York: American Society of Civil Engineers.

12. Rathje, op. cit.

13. Guerra, Sarith (1992). EPA issues comprehensive landfill rules. *Public Management,* Vol. 74(2), pp. 13–15.

14. Koren, Herman (1991). *Handbook of environmental health and safety,* Vol. 1. Mich.: Lewis Publishing.

15. *USA Today,* August 12, 1992.

16. Gore, Al (1992). *Earth in the balance.* New York: Houghton Mifflin.

17. The whiff of discrimination, op. cit.

18. Bryant, Bunyan (1992). Race, poverty and environment. *EPA Journal.* March/April p. 9.

19. *USA Today,* op. cit.

20. Gore, op. cit.

21. Koren, op. cit.

22. Lund, M. (1971). The great sea sickness. *Signature,* Sept., pp. 36–40.

23. Liptak, Bela (1991). *Municipal waste disposal in the 1990s.* Pennsylvania: Chilton Book Co.

24. Koren, op. cit.

25. www.epa.gov/epaoswer/non-hw/muncpl/mswrpt99/msw99re.pdf

26. White, P. T. (1983). The fascinating world of trash. *National Geographic,* 193(4):424–457.

27. Hadingham, op. cit.

28. Reinhardt, Peter, & Gordon, Judith (1991). *Infectious and medical waste management.* Michigan: Lewis Publishers.

29. Hynes, H. Patricia (1989). *The recurring silent spring.* New York: Pergamon Press.

30. Reinhardt, op. cit.

31. Green, Alex E. S. (1992). *Medical waste incineration and pollution prevention.* New York: Van Nostrand and Reinhold.

32. Reinhardt, op. cit.

33. Gore, op. cit.

34. Caldicott, Helen (1992). *If you love this planet.* New York: W.W. Norton.

35. *U.S. News and World Report* (1994). Database.

36. Koren, Herman (1991). *Handbook of environmental health and safety.* Vol 1. 2nd ed. Michigan: Lewis Publishers.

37. Haynes, op. cit.

38. Gladstone, Samuel & Sesonske, Alexander (1991). "Radiation protection and environmental effects." *Nuclear reactor engineering,* 3rd ed. p. 560.

39. Bosconti, Anne S. (1993). "Two faces of nuclear energy." *Vital Speeches,* No. 10, Vol. 59, March p. 317.

40. Caldicott, op. cit.

41. Brown, Lester R. (1992). *State of the world 1992.* New York: W.W. Norton.

42. Bertell, Rosalie (1989). *No immediate danger: Prognosis for a radioactive world.* London: The Women's Press.

43. Green, Alex E. S. (1992). *Medical waste incineration and pollution prevention.* New York: Van Nostrand and Reinhold.

INDEX

Page references followed by *fig* indicate a figure; followed by *t* indicate a table; followed by *b* indicate a box.